Advances in Neurosurgery **3**

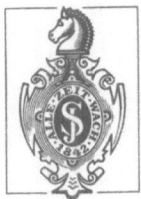

Brain Hypoxia

Pain

Edited by
H. Penzholz   M. Brock   J. Hamer
M. Klinger   O. Spoerri

With 160 Figures and 110 Tables

Springer-Verlag
Berlin Heidelberg GmbH 1975

Proceedings of the 26th Annual Meeting
of the Deutsche Gesellschaft für Neurochirurgie
Heidelberg, May 1–3, 1975

ISBN 978-3-540-07466-3   ISBN 978-3-642-66239-3 (eBook)
DOI 10.1007/978-3-642-66239-3

Library of Congress Cataloging in Publication Data. Deutsche Gesellschaft für Neurochirurgie,
Brain hypoxia, pain. (Advances in neurosurgery; 3) "Proceedings of the 26th annual meeting
of the Deutsche Gesellschaft für Neurochirurgie, Heidelberg, May 1–3, 1975."
Bibliography: p. Includes index. 1. Cerebral anoxia-Congresses. 2. Pain-Congresses.
3. Nervous system-Surgery-Congresses. I. Penzholz, Helmut. II. Title. III. Series. [DNLM:
1. Cerebral anoxia-Congresses pain. 2. Surgery-Congresses. 3. Spinal cord injuries-Congresses.
WI AD684N v. 3; WL355 D488b 1975] RC388.5.D49 1975 616.8 75–26877.

© by Springer-Verlag Berlin Heidelberg 1975
Ursprünglich erschienen bei Springer-Verlag Berlin • Heidelberg 1975

Preface

This volume contains the papers presented at the 26th Annual Meeting of the Deutsche Gesellschaft für Neurochirurgie, held in Heidelberg, Western Germany, on May 1—3, 1975.

Since at recent meetings of the German Neurosurgical Society central pathophysiological problems such as "central dysregulation" and "brain edema" had been discussed extensively, it seemed appropriate to choose another major area of cerebral pathophysiology for the meeting in Heidelberg. CEREBRAL HYPOXIA is, as LANGFITT once emphasized, "the final common denominator" of various cerebral lesions with which the neurosurgeon is confronted every day. Raised intracranial pressure, respiratory disorders and disturbances in systemic arterial blood pressure, etc. may lead, if not treated, to a focal or global lack of oxygen in the brain tissue. Anoxia finally results in cell death and thus in irreversible cerebral damage or even death. Main interest has therefore been focussed on disturbances in cerebral perfusion pressure ("ischemic hypoxia") and in arterial oxygenation ("hypoxic hypoxia"). The importance of cerebral autoregulatory mechanisms protecting the brain against tissue hypoxia, of pathomorphological alterations of the cerebral vessels (e.g. the "no-reflow-phenomenon") in the course of severe hypoxia, and of changes in brain metabolism have been discussed on a large scale. The organizing committee was particularly happy to have obtained internationally well-known scientists who presented their work in the field of cerebral hypoxia. We feel that the papers published on this important topic will have some influence on our daily pathophysiological considerations in the clinic, the operating theatre, and the intensive care unit as well.

The second main topic of the meeting was the NEUROSURGICAL TREATMENT OF PAIN. The efforts to eliminate pain by operating on the nervous system are as old as modern neurosurgery. The first successful extirpation of the Gasserian ganglion (KRAUSE 1896), the first dorsal rhizotomy to eliminate gastric crises and other intolerable states of pain (FOERSTER 1909), and the first cordotomy of the spinothalamic tract (SPILLER and MARTIN 1912, FOERSTER 1912) were important steps. The treatment of trigeminal neuralgia by alcohol injection (HÄRTL 1912) and the improvement of this method by means of partial electrocoagulation of the Gasserian ganglion by the Heidelberg surgeon KIRSCHNER (1933) are further milestones. Important methods, which have been significant for a further development, are stereotactic operations in the region of the basal ganglia, chemical rhizotomy with phenol, percutaneous cordotomy and the recent attempt to dispense with the destruction of painconducting tracts and, instead, to influence only pathological states of irritation. Methods for a successful neural blockade have been known for a long time. New, however, is the application of electric stimulation. We were very glad to see so many experts from all over the world and to enjoy their collaboration as speakers and discussants in this very important field of modern neurosurgery.

The last chapter contains miscellaneous contributions on various topics such as traumatic lesions of the spinal cord and the modern aspects of computer tomography in neurosurgery.

Finally, we want to express our thanks to all contributors who enabled us to publish this volume so quickly. We are also greatly indebted to the Springer Verlag for technical aid in the preparation of this third volume of the **Advances of Neurosurgery** and to Sharp & Dohme GmbH, Munich, for their generous financial support.

Heidelberg, June 1975   HELMUT PENZHOLZ

Contents

Brain Hypoxia

Pain

Free Communications

List of Contributors

ALBERTI, E., Neurologische Universitätsklinik, D-6900 Heidelberg, Voßstraße (Federal Republic of Germany)

ALBUS, G., Abteilung für Anaesthesiologie, Städtische Krankenanstalten, D-5000 Köln-Merheim (Federal Republic of Germany)

ASSMUS, H., Neurochirurgische Abteilung des Chirurgischen Zentrums der Universität Heidelberg, D-6900 Heidelberg (Federal Republic of Germany)

BÄR, TH., Max-Planck-Institut für Biophysikalische Chemie, Abteilung Neurobiologie-Neuroanatomie, D-3400 Göttingen-Nikolausberg (Federal Republic of Germany)

BAETHMANN, A., Abteilung für Experimentelle Chirurgie der Universität, D-8000 München 2, Nußbaumstraße 20 (Federal Republic of Germany)

BALDY-MOULINIER, M., Service de Physiopathologie des Maladies Nerveuses, Centre Gui de Chauliac, Hôpital Saint-Eloi, Montpellier (France)

BECKER, P., Neurochirurgische Universitätsklinik, D-7800 Freiburg i. Br., Hugstetter-straße 55 (Federal Republic of Germany)

BENEZECH, J., 61. Avenue de Lodève, F-34000 Montpellier (France)

BERLET, H., Institut für Pathochemie und Allgemeine Neurochemie der Universität, D-6900 Heidelberg, Im Neuenheimer Feld 220 (Federal Republic of Germany)

BETTAG, W., Neurochirurgische Klinik der Gesamthochschule, D-4300 Essen, Hufe-landstraße 55 (Federal Republic of Germany)

BETZ, E., Physiologisches Institut der Universität, D-7400 Tübingen (Federal Republic of Germany)

BOUCHARD, G., Neurochirurgische Klinik der FU, Klinikum Steglitz, D-1000 Berlin 45, Hindenburgdamm 30 (Federal Republic of Germany)

BROCK, M., Neurochirurgische Klinik der Medizinischen Hochschule, D-3000 Hannover-Kleefeld, Karl-Wiechert-Allee 9 (Federal Republic of Germany)

BROGGI, G., Division of Neurosurgery, Instituto Neurologica "C. Besta", Milano (Italy)

BUSCH, G., Neurochirurgische Universitätsklinik, D-6500 Mainz, Langenbeckstraße 1 (Federal Republic of Germany)

CALLIS, A., Laboratoire de Physique et des Gaz du Sang, Centre Gui de Chauliac, Hôpital Saint-Eloi, Montpellier (France)

CAROLI, A., Neurochirurgische Klinik der Universität, D-5300 Bonn, Venusberg (Federal Republic of Germany)

CERVOS-NAVARRO, J., Abteilung für Neuropathologie, Klinikum Steglitz der Freien Universität, D-1000 Berlin 45, Hindenburgdamm 30 (Federal Republic of Germany)

CHODKIEWICZ, A. J. P., Service de Neurochirurgie, Hôpital Saint Anne, F-75674 Paris Cedex 14 (France)

CIOLOCA, C., Service de Neurochirurgie, Hôpital Saint Anne, F-75674 Paris Cedex 14 (France)

CORREIA, A., Service de Neurochirurgie, Hôpital Saint Anne, F-75674 Paris Cedex 14 (France)

DIECKMANN, G., Abteilung für Stereotaktische Neurochirurgie, Neurochirurgische Klinik der Universität des Saarlandes, D-6650 Homburg/Saar (Federal Republic of Germany)

DIETZ, H., Neurochirurgische Klinik der Medizinischen Hochschule, D-3000 Hannover-Kleefeld, Karl-Wiechert-Allee 9 (Federal Republic of Germany)

DISTELMAIER, P., Neurochirurgische Universitätsklinik, D-5300 Bonn, Venusberg (Federal Republic of Germany)

DRAXLER, V., Institut für Anaesthesiologie der Universität, A-1090 Wien (Austria)

ENGELHARDT, P., Neurologische Klinik der Medizinischen Hochschule, D-3000 Hannover-Kleefeld, Karl-Wiechert-Allee 9 (Federal Republic of Germany)

ENTZIAN, W., Neurochirurgische Universitätsklinik, D-5300 Bonn, Venusberg (Federal Republic of Germany)

ESCURET E., Département d'Anaesthésie-Réanimation, Centre Gui de Chauliac, Hôpital Saint-Eloi, Montpellier (France)

FENSKE, A., Neurologische Abteilung des Universitätskrankenhauses, D-6500 Mainz, Langenbeckstraße 1 (Federal Republic of Germany)

FISCHER, F., Abteilung für Anaesthesiologie des Universitätskrankenhauses, D-6500 Mainz, Langenbeckstraße 1 (Federal Republic of Germany)

FRASER, R. A. R., New York Hospital, Cornell University Medical Center, 525 East 68th Street, NEW YORK, NY 10012 (USA)

FREREBEAU, PH., Service de Neurochirurgie, Centre Gui de Chauliac, Hôpital Saint-Eloi, Montpellier (France)

FUKUSHIMA, T., Department of Neurologic Surgery, Mayo Clinic, Rochester, MN 55901 (USA)

FURUSE, M., Neurosurgical Department, Nagoya-University, Nagoya (Japan)

GLEIM, F., Neurologische Abteilung des Akademischen Krankenhauses Nordwest der Universität, D-6000 Frankfurt/Main (Federal Republic of Germany)

GOBIET, W., Neurochirurgische Universitätsklinik, D-4300 Essen, Hufelandstraße 55 (Federal Republic of Germany)

GRATZL, O., Neurochirurgische Klinik der Universität München im Klinikum Großhadern, D-8000 München 70, Marchioninistraße 15 (Federal Republic of Germany)

GROS, CL., Service de Neurochirurgie, Centre Gui de Chauliac, Hôpital Saint-Eloi, Montpellier (France)

GROTE, J., Abteilung für Physiologie des Universitätskrankenhauses, D-6500 Mainz, Langenbeckstraße 1 (Federal Republic of Germany)

GUGGEMOS, L., Abteilung für Chirurgie und Neurochirurgie der Universität, D-8000 München 2, Nußbaumstraße 20 (Federal Republic of Germany)

GRUMME, TH., Neurochirurgische Klinik, Klinikum Westend, Freie Universität, D-1000 Berlin 19, Spandauer Damm (Federal Republic of Germany)

HADJIDIMOS, A., Abteilung für Neurochirurgie des Universitätskrankenhauses, D-6500 Mainz, Langenbeckstraße 1 (Federal Republic of Germany)

HAGENLOCHER, H.-U., Neurochirurgische Abteilung des Chirurgischen Zentrums der Universität Heidelberg, D-6900 Heidelberg, Kirschnerstraße (Federal Republic of Germany)

HAMER, J., Neurochirurgische Abteilung des Chirurgischen Zentrums der Universität Heidelberg, D-6900 Heidelberg, Kirschnerstraße (Federal Republic of Germany)

HARTMANN, A., Neurologische Klinik der Universität, D-6900 Heidelberg, Voßstraße (Federal Republic of Germany)

HASSLER, R., Neurobiologische Abteilung des Max-Planck-Institutes für Hirnforschung, D-6000 Frankfurt/Main, Deutschlandstraße 46 (Federal Republic of Germany)

HASUO, M., Neurochirurgische Klinik der Medizinischen Hochschule, D-3000 Hannover-Kleefeld, Karl-Wiechert-Allee 9 (Federal Republic of Germany)

HERRMANN, H.-D., Max-Planck-Institut für Hirnforschung, D-5000 Köln-Merheim (Federal Republic of Germany)

HERRSCHAFT, H., Abteilung für Neurologie und Max-Planck-Institut für Gehirnforschung, D-5000 Köln-Merheim (Federal Republic of Germany)

HOLBACH, K. H., Neurochirurgische Klinik der Universität, D-5300 Bonn, Venusberg (Federal Republic of Germany)

HOYER, S., Institut für Pathochemie und Neurochemie der Universität, D-6900 Heidelberg, Im Neuenheimer Feld 220 (Federal Republic of Germany)

HÜBNER, B., BG-Unfallklinik, Neurochirurgische Abteilung, D-6000 Frankfurt/Main, Friedbergerlandstraße 430 (Federal Republic of Germany)

HUNZIKER, O., Sandoz AG, Abteilung Medizinische Grundlagenforschung, CH-4002 Basel (Switzerland)

KAZNER, E., Neurochirurgische Klinik im Klinikum Großhadern der Universität, D-8000 München 70, Marchioninistraße 15 (Federal Republic of Germany)

KRAINICK, J.-U., Neurochirurgische Universitätsklinik, D-7800 Freiburg i. Brsg., Hugstetterstraße 55 (Federal Republic of Germany)

KOSTADINOW, G., Neurochirurgische Abteilung im Städt. Krankenhaus Berlin-Neukölln, D-1000 Berlin 47, Rudower Straße 56 (Federal Republic of Germany)

KRENN, J., Institut für Anaesthesiologie der Universität, A-1090 Wien, Spitalgasse 23 (Austria)

KÜHNER, A., Neurochirurgische Abteilung des Chirurgischen Zentrums der Universität, D-6900 Heidelberg, Kirschnerstraße (Federal Republic of Germany)

LANGE D., Universitäts-Strahlenklinik, D-6900 Heidelberg, Voßstraße (Federal Republic of Germany)

LANGFITT, TH. W., Division of Neurosurgery, Hospital of the University of Pennsylvania, 3400 Spruce Street, Philadelphia, PA 19104 (USA)

LANKSCH, W., Neurochirurgische Klinik im Klinikum Großhadern der Universität, D-8000 München, Marchioninistraße 15 (Federal Republic of Germany)

LEDENSKI, G., Institut für Tumorforschung, 4100 Zagreb, Jandriceva 17 (Yugoslavia)

LINKE, D., Neurochirurgische Universitätsklinik, D-5300 Bonn, Venusberg (Federal Republic of Germany)

LINS, E., Neurochirurgische Universitätsklinik, D-5300 Bonn, Venusberg (Federal Republic of Germany)

LORENZ, E., Neurochirurgische Universitätsklinik, D-6300 Gießen, Klinikstraße 37 (Federal Republic of Germany)

LÜCKING, C. H., Neurologische Klinik der Technischen Universität, D-8000 München 80, Möhlstraße 28 (Federal Republic of Germany)

MARGUTH, F., Neurochirurgische Klinik im Klinikum Großhadern der Universität, D-8000 München 70, Marchioninistraße 15 (Federal Republic of Germany)

MARTINS, L. F., Clinica Neurológica, Goiás (Brasilia)

MARX, P., Neurologische Klinik, Klinikum Mannheim, D-6800 Mannheim 1, Theodor-Kutzer-Ufer (Federal Republic of Germany)

MATHEW, N. T., Baylor College of Medicine, Houston, Texas (USA)

MAZARS, G., Service de Neuro-chirurgie A, Hôpital Saint Anne, Paris (France)

MENZEL, J., Neurochirurgische Abteilung des Chirurgischen Zentrums der Universität, D-6900 Heidelberg, Kirschnerstraße (Federal Republic of Germany)

MERIENNE, L., Service de Neuro-chirurgie A, Hôpital Saint Anne, Paris (France)

MÜKE, R., Neurochirurgische Abteilung der Neurologischen Universitätsklinik Hamburg-Eppendorf, D-2000 Hamburg 20, Martinistraße 52 (Federal Republic of Germany)

MUNDINGER, F., Neurochirurgische Universitätsklinik, D-7800 Freiburg i. Brsg., Hugstetterstraße 55 (Federal Republic of Germany)

OETTINGER, W., Abteilung für Experimentelle Chirurgie der Universität, D-8000 München 2, Nußbaumstraße 20 (Federal Republic of Germany)

PALLESKE, H., Neurochirurgische Universitätsklinik, D-6660 Homburg/Saar (Federal Republic of Germany)

PANITZ, C., Abteilung für Neurochirurgie der Städt. Krankenanstalten, D-6800 Mannheim, Theodor-Kutzer-Ufer (Federal Republic of Germany)

PATTERSON, R. H., New York Hospital, Cornell University, Medical Center, New York, NY (USA)

PENDL, G., Neurochirurgische Universitätsklinik, D-2300 Kiel, Weimarer Straße 8 (Federal Republic of Germany)

PENZHOLZ, H., Neurochirurgische Abteilung des Chirurgischen Zentrums der Universität, D-6900 Heidelberg, Kirschnerstraße (Federal Republic of Germany)

PERNECZKY, A., Abteilung für Neurochirurgie der Universität, A-1090 Wien, Alserstraße 4 (Austria)

PIASZEK, L., Nuklearmedizinische Abteilung des Universitätsklinikums, D-4500 Essen 1, Hufelandstraße 55 (Federal Republic of Germany)

PIOTROWSKI, W., Abteilung für Neurochirurgie der Städtischen Krankenanstalten, D-6800 Mannheim, Theodor-Kutzer-Ufer (Federal Republic of Germany)

PISCOL, K., Neurochirurgische Klinik, Krankenhaus St. Jürgenstraße, D-2800 Bremen (Federal Republic of Germany)

PRIVAT, J. M., Service de Neurochirurgie, Centre Gui de Chauliac, Hôpital Saint-Eloi, Montpellier (France)

RAY, C. D., 3055 Old Highway Eight, Box 1453 Minneapolis, MN 55400 (USA)

REDONDO, A., Service de Neurochirurgie, Hôpital Saint Anne, F-75674 Paris Cedex 14 (France)

REULEN, H.-J., Neurochirurgische Universitätsklinik, D-6500 Mainz, Langenbeckstr. 1 (Federal Republic of Germany)

ROOSEN, K., Neurochirurgische Klinik der Gesamthochschule, D-4300 Essen, Hufelandstraße 55 (Federal Republic of Germany)

ROQUEFEUIL, B., Departement d'Anesthésie-Réanimation, Centre Gui de Chauliac, Hôpital Saint-Eloi, Montpellier (France)

SALAH, S., Abteilung für Neurochirurgie der Universität, A-1090 Wien, Alserstraße 4 (Austria)

SAMII, M., Neurochirurgische Universitätsklinik, D-6500 Mainz, Langenbeckstraße 1 (Federal Republic of Germany)

SCHIRMER, M., Neurochirurgische Abteilung, Städtisches Krankenhaus Neukölln, D-1000 Berlin 47, Rudower Straße 56 (Federal Republic of Germany)

SCHMIDT, H., Abteilung für Anaesthesiologie, Akademisches Krankenhaus Nordwest der Universität, D-6000 Frankfurt/Main (Federal Republic of Germany)

SCHMIEDEK, P., Abteilung für Experimentelle Chirurgie der Universität, D-8000 München 2, Nußbaumstraße 20 (Federal Republic of Germany)

SCHMITZ, P., Neurochirurgische Universitätsklinik, D-6500 Mainz, Langenbeckstraße 1 (Federal Republic of Germany)

SCHNEIDER, R., Department of Neurosurgery, University of Michigan, C 5135 Out-. patient Bldg., Ann Arbor, MI 48104 (USA)

SCHÖTER, I., Neurochirurgische Universitätsklinik, D-5300 Bonn, Venusberg (Federal Republic of Germany)

SCHÜRMANN, E., Neurochirurgische Universitäts-Klinik, D-6500 Mainz, Langenbeckstraße 1 (Federal Republic of Germany)

SCHÜRMANN, K., Neurochirurgische Universitäts-Klinik, D-6500 Mainz, Langenbeckstraße 1 (Federal Republic of Germany)

SCHUBERT, R., Neurochirurgische Universitäts-Klinik, D-6500 Mainz, Langenbeckstraße 1 (Federal Republic of Germany)

SIEGFRIED, J., Neurochirurgische Universitäts-Klinik, CH-8091 Zürich, Rämistraße (Switzerland)

SIESJÖ, B. K., Institute for Brain Research, E-blocket, University of Lund, S-221 85 Lund (Sweden)

SOHLER, K., Institut für experimentelle Chirurgie, D-8000 München 2, Nußbaumstraße 20 (Federal Republic of Germany)

SPORN, P., Institut für Anaesthesiologie der Universität, A-1090 Wien (Austria)

STEINBEREITHNER, K., Institut für Anaesthesiologie der Universität, A-1090 Wien (Austria)

STOLKE, D., Neurochirurgische Klinik der Medizinischen Hochschule, D-3000 Hannover-Kleefeld, Karl-Wiechert-Allee 9 (Federal Republic of Germany)

STRUPPLER, A., Neurologische Klinik der Technischen Universität, D-8000 München 80, Möhlstraße 28 (Federal Republic of Germany)

SUNDER-PLASSMANN, M., Neurochirurgische Universitätsklinik, A-1090 Wien, Alserstraße 4 (Austria)

SWEET, W. H., Massachusetts General Hospital, Boston, MA 02114 (USA)

TERRAZAS, F., Service de Neurochirurgie, Hôpital Saint Anne, F-75674 Paris Cedex 14 (France)

THODEN, U., Neurologische Universitätsklinik, D-7800 Freiburg i. Brsg. (Federal Republic of Germany)

TSCHABITSCHER, M., Abteilung für Neurochirurgie der Universität, A-1090 Wien, Alserstraße 4 (Austria)

VIGUE, E., Département d'Anaesthésie-Réanimation, Centre Gui de Chauliac, Hôpital Saint-Eloi, Montpellier (France)

VLAJIC, I., Neurochirurgische Universitätsklinik, D-5300 Bonn, Venusberg (Federal Republic of Germany)

WANDT, H., Neurochirurgische Klinik der Gesamthochschule, D-4300 Essen, Hufe-landstraße 55 (Federal Republic of Germany)

WAPPENSCHMIDT, J., Neurochirurgische Universitätsklinik, D-5300 Bonn, Venusberg (Federal Republic of Germany)

WATZEK, CH., Institut für Anaesthesiologie der Universität, A-1090 Wien (Austria)

WEIDNER, A., Neurochirurgische Klinik 'der Medizinischen Hochschule, D-3000 Han-nover-Kleefeld, Karl-Wiechert-Allee 9 (Federal Republic of Germany)

WEINHARDT, F., Institut für Pathochemie und Neurochemie der Universität, D-6900 Heidelberg, Im Neuenheimer Feld 220 (Federal Republic of Germany)

WENKER, H., Neurochirurgische Abteilung des Städtischen Krankenhauses Neukölln, D-1000 Berlin 47, Rudower Straße 56 (Federal Republic of Germany)

WIEGAND, H., Neurochirurgische Klinik der Medizinischen Hochschule, D-3000 Han-nover-Kleefeld, Karl-Wiechert-Allee 9 (Federal Republic of Germany)

WHITCOMB, B. B., 85 Jefferson Street, Hartford, (T) 06106 (USA)

WINKELMÜLLER, W., Neurochirurgische Klinik der Medizinischen Hochschule, D-3000 Hannover-Kleefeld, Karl-Wiechert-Allee 9 (Federal Republic of Germany)

WOLFF, J. R., Max-Planck-Institut für biophysikalische Chemie, Abteilung Neurobio-logie-Neuroanatomie, D-3400 Göttingen (Federal Republic of Germany)

WÜLLENWEBER, R., Neurochirurgische Klinik der Freien Universität, Klinikum Char-lottenburg, D-1000 Berlin 19, Spandauer Damm (Federal Republic of Germany)

ZIERSKI, J., Neurochirurgische Universitätsklinik, D-6300 Gießen, Klinikstraße 37 (Federal Republic of Germany)

ZIMMERMANN, M., Abteilung Physiologie des Zentralnervensystems, II. Physiologisches Institut der Universität, D-6900 Heidelberg (Federal Republic of Germany)

ZSCHOCKE, ST., Neurologische Universitätsklinik, D-2000 Hamburg 20, Martinistr. 52 (Federal Republic of Germany)

Brain Hypoxia

Neuropathology of Cerebral Hypoxia

J. CERVÓS-NAVARRO and F. MATAKAS

The clinical result of cerebral hypoxia is caused by a complex interaction of different lesions which we shall try to describe separately.
The variety of effects cerebral hypoxia may produce is due to the fact
that it provokes specific reactions in all different cell types of
the brain (Table).

Astrocytes react most easily on an oxygen deficit by swelling (Fig.1).
This swelling first develops in the perivascular astrocytic processes,
but soon spreads on to the periphery. The reports (13) that severe
swelling of perivascular astrocytic processes may compress capillaries and, thus, lead to a collapse of the capillary lumen, could
not be verified by own observations. This hypothesis can be rejected
also from a mere theoretical point of view. The pressure within capillaries is always greater than that of the surrounding tissue, except
for the extreme situation in which intracranial pressure equals mean
arterial blood pressure (10). Swelling of astrocytes does not necessarily lead to brain edema. After moderate hypoxia swelling of astrocytes is associated with shrinkage of nerve cells. We, thus, have a
shift of fluid from neurons to astrocytes which does not increase
brain volumen. In severe cases, however, swelling of astrocytes may
result in brain edema.

In the border zone of necrotic lesions astrocytes multiply and mi-
grate. We, therefore, find astrocytes in areas where they originally
have been destroyed. The fact that we sometimes find areas, where
solely nerve cells have been destroyed, does not mean that nerve
cells have a greater vulnerability. They may also be the result of a
total necrosis which has been repaired by a replacement of glial cells.

The reaction of oligodendrocytes has not been examined as detailed
as that of the macroglia. There are certain indications that their
resistance towards hypoxia is rather great. In severe cases they may
participate in swelling.

The first morphological effects of hypoxia in nerve cells are swelling and destruction of mitochondria and shrinkage of the nucleus.
The nerve cells, as a whole, do not swell, but tend to reduce their
volume. An exact catalogue of lesions which hypoxia may produce in
nerve cells is important since we still lack exact knowledge about
those criteria which indicate the irreversible death of a nerve cell.
There is experimental evidence that the resistance of the nerve cell
to an oxygen deficit is rather great (5). The changes of nerve cells
which we find some hours after cerebral hypoxia may, thus, still be
reversible. This is important with respect to the therapy of ischemic
insults which, in most cases, can be started only hours after the
onset of the ischemic attack. The necrosis within the center of an
infarct is possibly not influenced by any form of therapy. However,

1

Table. Effect of hypoxia, anoxia and ischemia on different cell types of the brain

	brain parenchyma			vessel wall		vascular lumen
	neurons	astrocytes	oligodendroc.	muscle	endothelium	blood
hypoxia anoxia	functional disorder	swelling	(swelling)	vasoparalysis	swelling, blebs damage of BBB	
	death	death	death			
additional effect of ischemia	increased resistance to anoxia ?					sludging
early consequences	neurological defects	brain edema		brain swelling	obstruction brain edema	no-reflow
late conse-quences	intracranial hypertension reduction of CBF hypoxia, anoxia, ischemia				local ischemia	

within the neighbourhood of an infarct nerve cells are subjected to hypoxia which leads to cell death only after a prolonged period of time. Moreover, in these regions, we find completely undamaged nerve cells just beside nerve cells which show severe lesions (Fig. 2). There are possibly factors other than mere hypoxia which determine the extent of a necrosis and which make nerve cell destruction a process which is much slower than we thought originally. However, we still do not know exactly in what time an oxygen deficit causes irreversible changes in nerve cells.

The effect of hypoxia on the cerebral vascular system has been evaluated only within the last few years. Hypoxia affects the vascular muscle cells, the endothelium and it probably also affects the vascular nerve fibre terminals. LANGFITT et al. in 1965 (8) first stressed the clinical implications of the fact that cerebral hypoxia may lead to vasoparalysis. As a consequence of vasoparalysis extreme dilatation of intracranial vessels may increase the brain volume and, thus, lead to intracranial hypertension. LANGFITT called this mechanism brain swelling. However, he only considered the arterial branches of the vascular tree, which he thought to dilate in the absence of autoregulation. In our experiments we could verify that venous vessels, too, may contribute to brain swelling. In the case of venous hypertension the brain shows enormous and rapid swelling which is exclusively due to vessel dilatation (Fig. 3). Brain swelling develops within a few minutes after hypoxic damage while brain edema wants some hours to develop. Many acute conditions of intracranial hypertension are more due to brain swelling than to brain edema.

Another effect which, however, is observed only after ischemia is the no-reflow phenomenon. It means that after ischemia large areas of the brain are not perfused again. The no-reflow phenomenon was first described by AMES and coworkers (1968)(1). From experiments of WALTZ, SUNDT (1967)(12) and HEKMATPANAH (1973)(4) we know that the no-reflow phenomenon is caused by stasis and sludging of erythrocytes during ischemia. Aggregations of red blood cells have a greater resistance to the driving blood pressure. Because of this mechanism the no-

2

reflow phenomenon is enhanced if the postischemic recirculation is impaired, for instance by cardiac insufficiency or by intracranial hypertension. The no-reflow phenomenon is counteracted by postischemic hyperemia.

Ischemia has also an effect on the vascular endothelium. Some hours after the stop of cerebral circulation we find swelling of the endothelium and formation of blebs which may obstruct the capillary lumen (Fig. 4). Investigations of NELSON and coworkers (1974)(11) indicate that the formation of blebs may also occur in large vessels. Since they originate from protruding endothelial cytoplasm, they always result in a damage of the endothelial lining of the vessel. In brain death nearly all small vessels of the brain are obstructed by blebs.

Brain swelling, brain edema, and in the case of ischemia the no-reflow phenomenon are the effects of cerebral hypoxia. If severe, they may again cause reduction of cerebral blood flow and, thus, lead to a vicious circle (Fig. 5). They are all effects which develop rapidly and which need acute therapy. The late consequences of oxygen deficit are always cell death. However, the destruction of cells may be confined to nerve cells or include all cell elements; it may be local or general. Thus, the result of cerebral hypoxia varies enormously.

In the center of a necrotic area we find destruction of all cell elements. The marginal zone of a necrosis is built by reactive astrocytes and microglia. These cells divide and infiltrate the infarct in centripetal direction.

The second type of tissue lesion is that nerve cells undergo destruction while all other cell elements remain intact. In most cases those areas where nerve cells have vanished are small, but they may also comprise the whole cerebral cortex (Fig. 6). The pathomechanism of these conditions seems to be the following: CBF is first disturbed by a short lasting cardiac arrest, asphyxia or any similar condition. Following moderate brain swelling or brain edema CBF is reduced because intracranial perfusion pressure is lowered. The no-reflow phenomenon seems to be involved, too. As a result most of the gray substance of the cerebrum is destroyed while the medulla and brain stem are more or less intact. The patients show the symptom of an apallic syndrome. The investigations of INGVAR et al. (1972)(6) and HEISS et al. (1972)(3) have revealed that CBF in the apallic syndrome is reduced significantly and does not reach a normal level even after a prolonged period of time. This result is in accordance with our observation that many of the blood vessels in the cortical areas are obstructed. However, the same hypoxia in the child causes different lesions. Cortical destruction as described above are not found in children. Instead, we find small circumscribed necrotic areas in the brain stem. This last example demonstrates that we still lack important details which would explain the exact pathomechanism of a lesion as simple as a hypoxic necrosis.

Summary

Severe hypoxia, anoxia or ischemia affects all cell elements of the brain. The nerve cells may undergo destruction. The glial cells, predominantly astrocytes, usually swell and contribute to brain edema. The vascular muscle cells may become paralytic so that extreme vessel dilatation may produce brain swelling. If the oxygen deficit is caused by ischemia the endothelium of capillaries may swell and obstruct the lumen. Ischemia produces sludging of erythrocytes which may impair or even stop the circulation in wide areas of the brain in the postischemic period. The different reactions of different cell elements of the brain determine the development of the patient after the primary anoxic or ischemic injury. Swelling of glial cells and water efflux out of capillaries produces brain edema which may be the cause of intracranial hypertension. Vasoparalysis may lead to brain swelling which has the same effect as brain edema. All these consequences usually occur in combination. The final outcome after an hypoxic or ischemic injury depends on the degree to which all these primary lesions develop. There is a wide variety of morphological changes of the brain. The circumscribed loss of nerve cells will be the result if the hypoxic period is not too long and the postischemic circulation optimal. Local necroses may be caused by local factors, e.g. vessel stenosis or arteriosclerosis, or by the no-reflow phenomenon. Moderate brain edema may result in an apallic syndrome while severe brain edema usually results in brain death.

REFERENCES

1. AMES, A., WRIGHT, R.L., KOWADA, M., THURSTON, J.M., MAJNO, G.: Cerebral ischemia II. The no-reflow phenomenon. Amer. J. Path. 52, 437-453 (1968).

2. GARCIA, J.: Personal communication.

3. HEISS, W.D., GERSTENBRAND, F., PROSENZ, T., KREIN, J.: The prognostic value of cerebral blood flow measurement in patients with the apallic syndrome. J. Neurol. Sci. 16, 279-382 (1972).

4. HEKMATPANAH, J.: Cerebral blood flow dynamics in hypertension and cardiac arrest. Neurology 23, 174-180 (1973).

5. HOSSMANN, K.A. and ZIMMERMANN, V.: Factors influencing the recovery of the monkey brain after prolonged cerebral ischemia. In: Pathology of cerebral microcirculation (ed. J. Cervós-Navarro), p. 354. Berlin-New York: Walter de Gruyter 1974.

6. INGVAR, D.H., BRUN, A.: Das komplette apallische Syndrom. Arch. Psychiat. Nervenkr. 215, 219-239 (1972).

7. JOHNSTON, I.H., ROWAN, I.O., HARPER, A.M., JENNETT, W.B.: Raised intracranial pressure and cerebral blood flow. I. Cisterna magna infusion in primates. J. Neurol. Neurosurg. Psychiat. 35, 285-296 (1972).

8. LANGFITT, T.W., WEINSTEIN, J.D., KASSELL, N.F.: Cerebral vasomotor paralysis produced by intracranial hypertension. Neurology (Minneap.) 15, 622-641 (1965).

9. MATAKAS, F., CERVÓS-NAVARRO, J., SCHNEIDER, H.: Experimental brain death. I. Morphology and fine structure of the brain. J. Neurol. Neurosurg. Psychiat. 36, 497-508 (1973).

10. MATAKAS, F., VON WAECHTER, R., KNÜPLING, R., POTOLICCHIO, J.S.: Increase in cerebral perfusion pressure by arterial hypertension in brain swelling. J. Neurosurg. 42, 282-289 (1975).

11. NELSON, E., KAWAMURA, J., SUNAGA, T., RENNELS, M.L., GERTZ, S.D.: Scanning- and transmission electron microscopic study of endothelial lesion following ischemia with special attention to ischemic and "normal" branch points. In: Pathology of Cerebral Microcirculation (ed. J. Cervós-Navarro), pp. 267-273. Berlin-New York: Walter de Gruyter 1974.

12. WALTZ, H.G., SUNDT, T.M.: The microvasculature and microcirculation of the cerebral cortex after arterial occlusion. Brain 90, 681-696 (1967).

13. WOLFF, J.: Über die Möglichkeit der Kapillarverengung im zentralen Nervensystem. Eine elektronenmikroskopische Studie an der Großhirnrinde des Kaninchens. Z. Zellforsch. 63, 593-611 (1964).

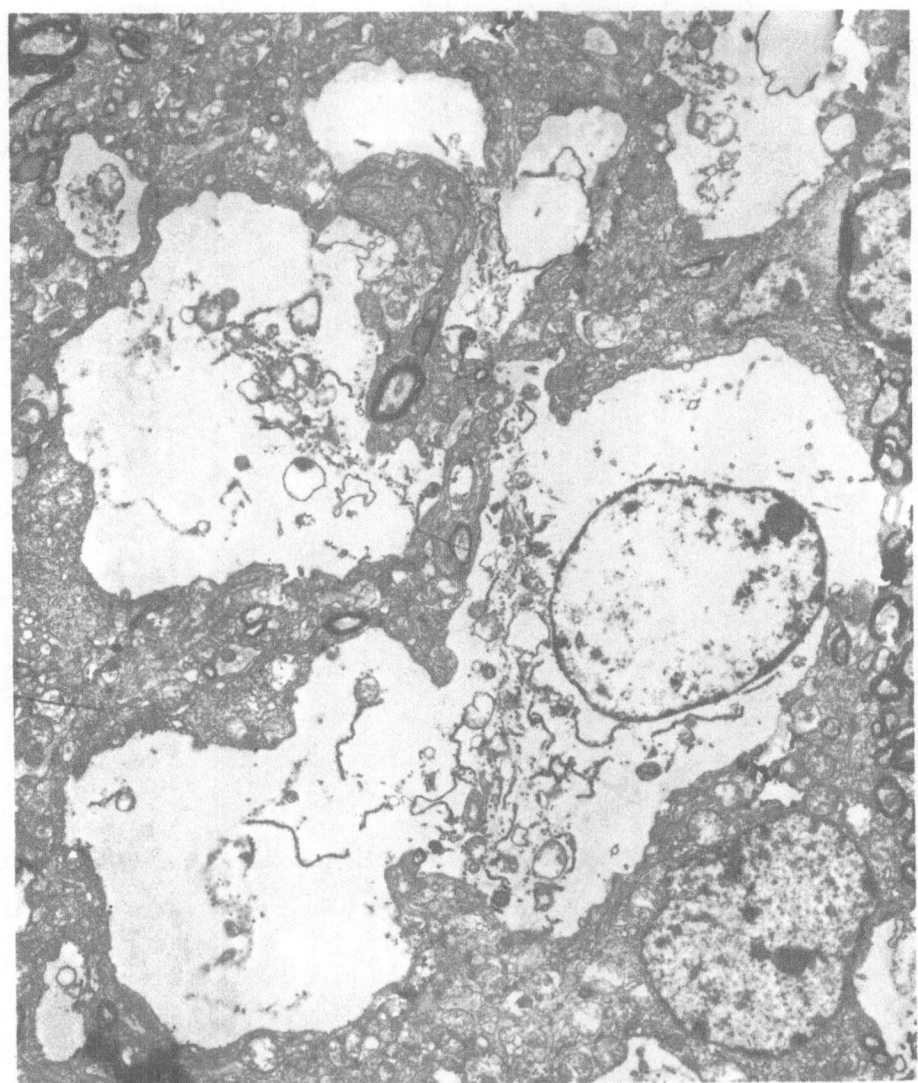

Fig. 1. Cat. Swelling of astrocytes after ischemia of 20 mins (X 5.500)

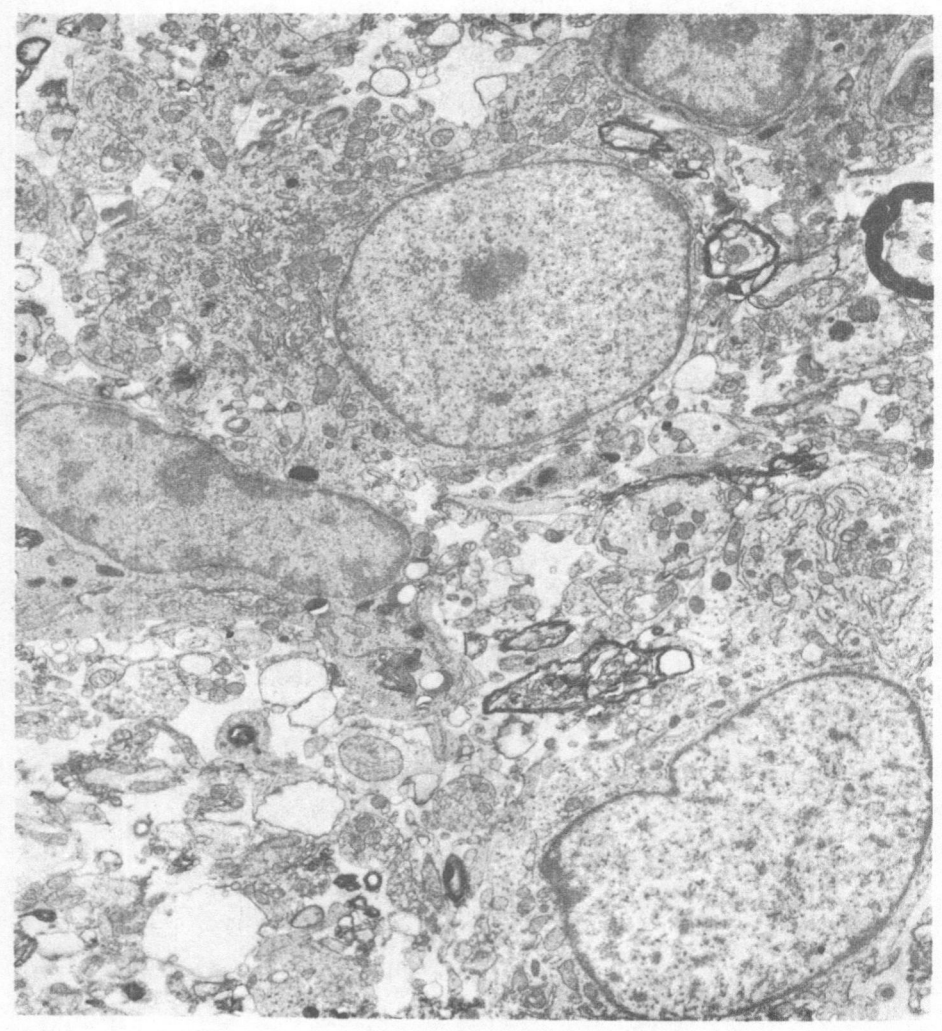

Fig. 2. Rat. Spinal cord after 20 mins ischemia and 7 days survival. Completely looseness of the neuroglia. Nerve cells and axons are concerned and show only slight changes. Two microglia cells in the neuropil (X 5.500)

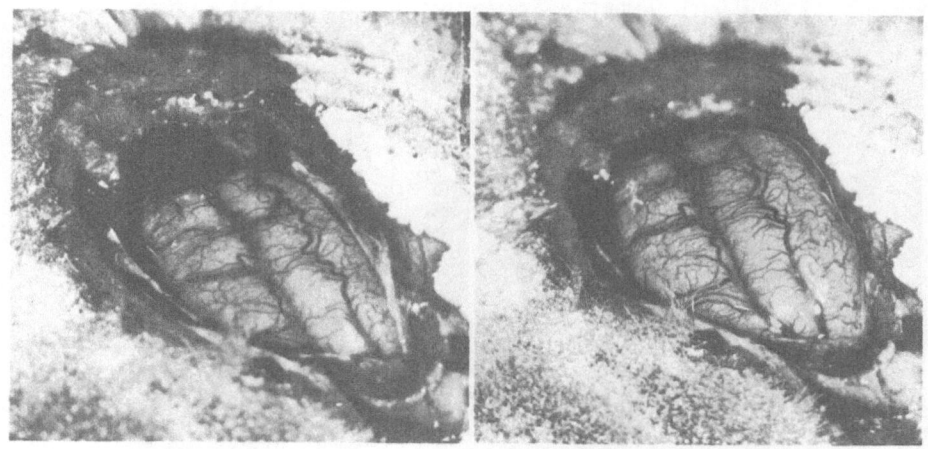

Fig. 3. Cat left: Normal surface of the brain. Right: Brain swelling during venous hypertension (central venous pressure 30 mm Hg)

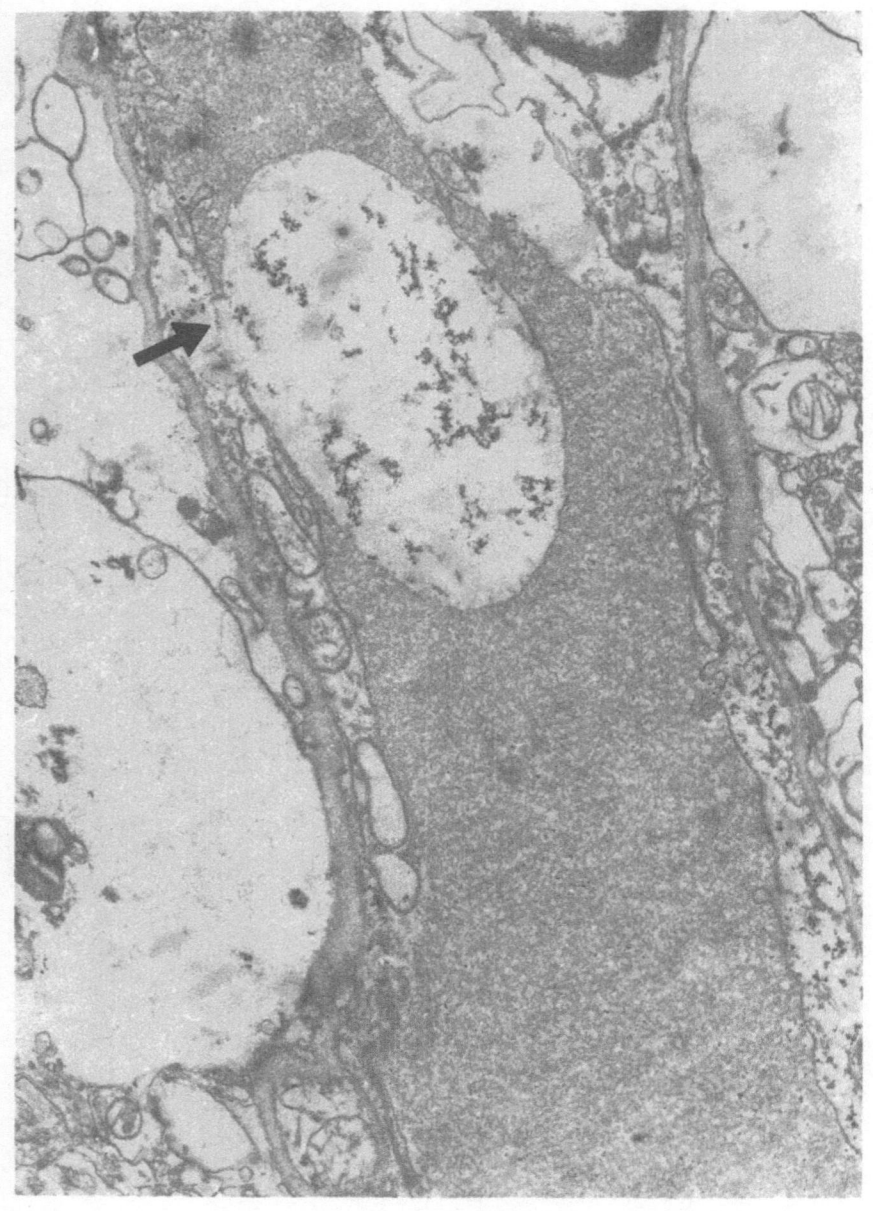

Fig. 4. Cat. One hour after cerebral ischemia for 20 mins. Endothelial bleb of capillary (X 15.000)

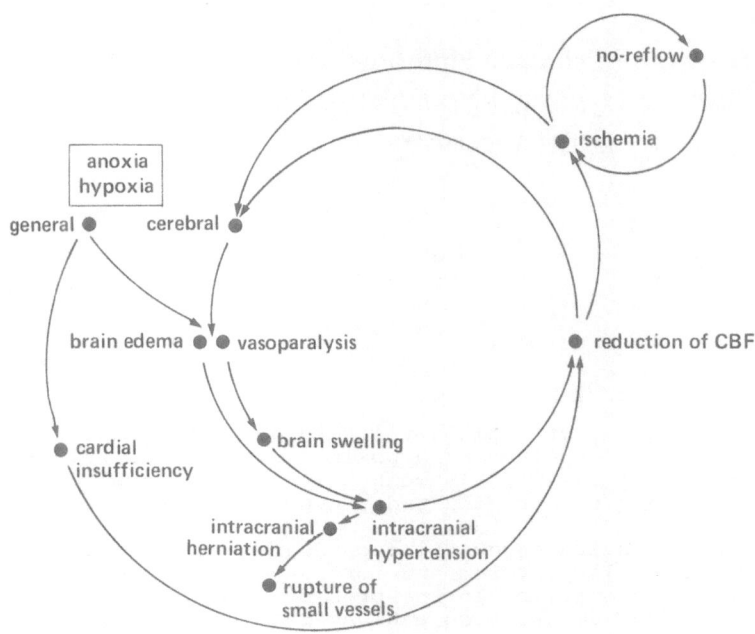

Fig. 5. Effect of hypoxia on the brain

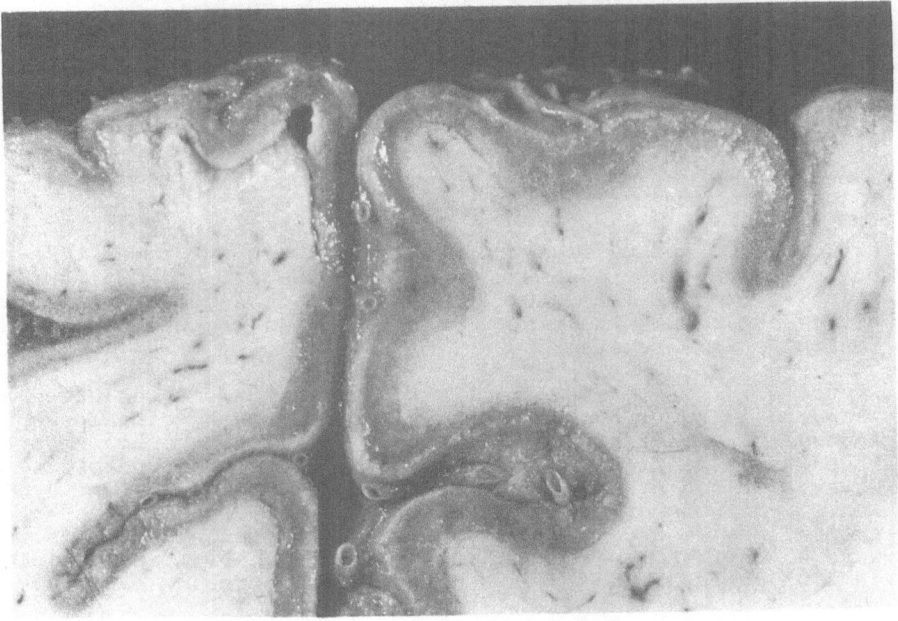

Fig. 6. Destruction of cerebral cortex. Man. Cardiac arrest. Resuscitation after about 5 mins. Survival 22 days

Effects of Different Hemodynamic Conditions on Brain Capillaries: Alveolar Hypoxia, Hypovolemic Hypotension, and Ouabain Edema

Th. Bär and J. R. Wolff

Introduction

An increase of capillary length has been described in studies on the influence of alveolar hypoxia (15, 8, 6) as well as of hypovolemic hypotension (12), although the capillaries become dilated under hypoxic and constricted under hypovolemic conditions.

These results suggest independent mechanisms for the elongation of the capillary system and for changes in the size distribution of vessel diameters. In the present study, the intracortical microvascular system has been evaluated quantitatively under various hemodynamic conditions.

Alveolar hypoxia induces a dilation of the precapillary arterial vessels (1) and consequently an increase of intracapillary pressure. In contrast, the capillary blood pressure is reduced by a *hypovolemic* decrease in the mean arterial pressure to about 40% of the normal value (12). In a third set of experiments, *ouabain* was locally applied to certain cortical regions causing a tissue swelling without a significant change in the arterial blood pressure (22), i.e. the balance between intra- and extracapillary pressure was disturbed by changing the tissue pressure.

Material and Methods

Hypoxia: Three groups of Sprague Dawley Albino rats (A, B and C, aged 14, 30, and 80 days, respectively) were subjected to a normobaric low oxygen atmosphere (10% O_2; 90% N_2; 0,05% CO_2; 40 - 60% relative humidity) for 40 days. Standard food and tap water were given ad libitum. The visual cortices of 11 chronic hypoxic and 9 control rats were examined.

Hypovolemic hypotension: 8 male cats were randomly selected and distributed in two groups of 4 cats. Hypovolemic hypotension was obtained in 4 animals by withdrawing a sufficient volume of arterial blood from the right arteria femoralis (12), to reduce systemic arterial blood pressure from 120 mmHg to 44-50 mmHg. The hypotension was maintained for 90 min. The arterial blood pressure of control animals was kept constant at 120 mmHg. The following brain regions were investigated: Area striata, frontal (A 19.5) and occipital (A 3.0) parts of the gyrus suprasylvianus anterior (20).

Ouabain: 300 mcg of the drug in a volume of 1,0 ml saline were infused over 3-6 min into a parietal branch of the middle cerebral artery of 3 anesthetized beagle dogs. The survival time was 20 - 40 minutes. The systemic arterial blood pressure was continuously recorded and did not show significant variations in the experiments under consideration. The affected areas were identified by an injection of 2% Evans blue which stains the brain tissue where the blood brain barrier has broken down. Control dogs received an infusion of 0,9% NaCl solution under the same conditions.

Preparations: After pentobarbital anesthesia all animals were killed by cardiac perfusion with either 2,5% glutaraldehyde in phosphate buffer (SOERENSEN) - ouabain experiments - or with a mixture of 3% glutaraldehyde + 3% p-formaldehyde in cacodylate buffer. Specimens were postfixed in buffered 1% OsO_4 solution, dehydrated, and embedded in Epon 812.

Measurements: In conventionally stained, semithin (1-2 μm) sections of cortical tissue the lumina of the perfused vessels were quantitatively analysed (internal diameters, number of sections per square unit) by automatic TV image analysis (Quantimet 720 'Imanco' Ltd., G.B.).[1]

The collective vascular length per mm^3 brain tissue, as calculated by stereological means (SALTIKOV, cited by 21) and the size distribution of the vessel diameters were compared in normal and experimental animals.

Results

After *chronic hypoxia* we found an increase of the mean diameter of the cortical microvessels (Fig. 1a, b). The frequency distribution of vascular diameters has shifted to greater values, i.e. a dilation of all vessels has taken place (Fig. 2a). The mean internal diameter of the capillaries (this fraction includes more than 90% of all vascular profiles) has increased from 5,31 to 6,62 μm in adult rats. In young animals (group A: 14 days after birth + 40 days hypoxia), the volume of the visual cortex was smaller after hypoxia indicating a retardation of growth. The vascular length per unit of brain volume had increased (Table 1).

In group B (30 + 40 days) the capillary length was increased, while the cortical growth seems to be not impaired (Table 1). In adult animals we neither found significant changes in the capillary length nor a reduction in cortical tissue volume after chronic (10% O_2) hypoxia (Table 1). If the O_2 concentration in the inspired air was further reduced to 7 - 8% (it occurred accidentally in one case), multiple small tissue lesions became visible (Fig. 1c). This can be taken as a first sign of brain atrophy under the hypoxic stress. Thus, the effect of hypoxia on the cortical tissue and the vascular system not only depends on the degree of O_2 deprivation, but also on the developmental stage of the tissue.

Hypotension: After hypovolemic hypotension no histological lesions were detected in the visual cortex of the cats. The frequency distribution of vascular diameters demonstrates that the terminal vascular bed is evenly constricted in the area striata (Fig. 2b). Electron microscopical observations show that the vessel wall was locally folded, and the mean thickness of the capillary wall was increased

[1] The authors like to thank the Deutsche Forschungsgemeinschaft, SFB 33, Proj. C.3 for financial support.

Table 1. Effects of hypoxia on cortical microvessels (rat)

postnatal age (days)	54		70		120	
	control	hypoxia day 14 – 54	control	hypoxia day 30 – 70	control	hypoxia day 80 – 120
thickness of visual cortex (mm)	1,28(±0,1)	1,05(±0,03)*	1,38(±0,09)	1,33(±0,12)	1,21(±0,09)	1,19(±0,08)
length of microvessels $\frac{mm}{mm^3}$	714(±48)	1008(±58)*	758(±66)	946(±108)*	832(±34)	876(±114)
'capillary' length+ $\frac{mm}{mm^3}$	652(±50)	888(±60)*	678(±58)	820(±78)*	748(±26)	780(±88)
internal diameter of 'capillaries' (µm)	5,61(±0,08)	6,48(±1,0)	5,31(±0,46)	6,46(±0,86)	5,31(±0,2)	6,62(±0,16)*
total number of intercepts	1782	1924	2110	5990	1700	1972

Values represent means ($\pm$ S.D.); * significantly different from control ($p < 0,05$); + The 'capillary' fraction includes all vessels within the range of two size classes (= 3,5 µm) on both sides of the median of the frequency distribution of diameters, i.e. about 90% of all vascular intercepts.

(Fig. 3a). The vascular alterations vary between different cortical laminae and areae. In the samples studied the hypovolemic effects were minimal in Lamina 1 in comparison to the deeper layers.

Irrespective of regional variations, the total vascular length per unit of cortical tissue remained nearly constant after hypovolemic hypotension, although the length of vessels with diameters smaller than 8 μm varied, i.e. the fraction of vessels classified as 'capillaries' increased or decreased with changes in the diameter of pre- and post-capillary vessels (Fig. 2b).

Ouabain: The drug causes the well-known swelling of astrocytes and certain presynaptic elements in the cortical grey matter (for ref. see 22). The size distribution of microvessels shows a characteristic pattern in edematous regions (Fig. 2c): Constricted capillaries (internal diameter ≤8 μm) are accompanied by dilated terminal vessels. In spite of the decrease of capillary diameters, these dilated large vessels, however, cause the total vascular cross sectional area ($\Sigma n \cdot \bar{d}^2 \cdot \mu/4$; $\bar{d}$ = mean diameter; n = number of vessel profiles) to increase by about 10%. The narrowing of the capillary lumen is interpreted as a result of compression, because endothelial swelling has never been observed, and the surfaces of the vessel wall were sometimes folded (Fig. 3b).

Discussion

Depending upon the duration and magnitude of alveolar O_2 deprivation, the resulting hypoxia causes variable changes in blood volume, hematocrit, and Hb concentration of erythrocytes (14, 1, 13). On the other hand, chronic hypoxia has been demonstrated to dilate pre- and postcapillary vessels more than capillaries (1). The latter change is responsible for the drop of precapillary resistance. Consequently, the dilation of capillaries under hypoxic conditions (15, 3) seems to result from an elevated intracapillary pressure.

To check whether a relationship between the intracapillary pressure and the capillary diameter can also be demonstrated under conditions of low blood pressure, hypovolemic hypotension was produced in cats. It is well known that the cerebral circulation is decreased after a critical arterial hypotension is reached (19). In the cat the cortical blood flow is significantly reduced at 50 mm Hg mean arterial blood pressure (10). Therefore, the reduction in the mean diameter of intracortical microvessels demonstrated by HUNZIKER et al. (12) and in the present paper seems to be one of the factors which correspond to the reduced CBF in vivo. The fact that most brain capillaries are not surrounded by perivascular extracellular spaces suggests that increase in pressure and volume of brain tissue should be able to compress brain capillaries without preceding changes in the intravasal pressure.

Changes in the capillary length per unit of brain volume can occur under different conditions (chronic hypoxia: 8, 6, 3; hypovolemia: 12; exercise training: 17; ontogenesis: 7, 5, 9, 2).

During ontogenetic development capillary growth is produced by endothelial mitosis, telescope-like separation of post-mitotic cells along the vessel axis and elongation of endothelial cells (4). Hypoxia can obviously increase the endothelial proliferation rate, when applied during the early postnatal period, when the rapid vascular proliferation normally takes place. If hypoxia is applied to adults, there is no evidence for additional endothelial proliferation (3). In animals receiving alveolar hypoxia between days 30 - 70 postnatally, a real increase of capillary length takes place which is mainly due to elongation and flattening of the existing endothelial and pericytal cells.

In adult animals a low oxygen atmosphere does not induce significant changes in the vascular length per unit of brain volume. If the lowered partial pressure of oxygen in the inspired air, however, causes brain lesions resulting in an atrophic reduction of tissue volume, a relative increase of capillary length per unit of volume can be shown. This is likely to be one of the factors in earlier studies demonstrating an increased capillary length under the above mentioned circumstances (8, 6). An elongation of the vascular system is also simulated by a retarded cortical growth, when hypoxia is applied during the early postnatal period.

Special attention must be paid to the definition of capillaries in relation to the other terminal vessels in brain tissue. If capillaries are defined as terminal vessels with a diameter less than 8 μm (16, 11, 18), the capillary length may vary with the change of the vessel diameters.

Thus, dilation of terminal vessels seems to reduce the 'capillary' fraction of the vascular bed, while constriction may cause an apparent elongation of capillaries.

It is concluded that the dynamic changes in the capillary system of the adult brain seem to be restricted mainly to variations of the vessel diameter. Dilation and constriction are accompanied by changes of the shape of endothelial cells. As far as we know, a real increase in the vascular length has not been proved in the adult brain.

Summary

Morphometric parameters of intracortical microvessels have been evaluated by quantitative image analysis after perfusion fixation of the brain in stained semithin sections.

Alveolar hypoxia (10% O_2, 90% N_2, lasting for 40 days) dilates all vessels. The influence of O_2 deprivation on the vascular length depends upon its magnitude and upon the time of onset during postnatal development. In adults, vascular length was not changed, as long as changes of cortical volume were absent. After hypovolemic hypotension, the terminal vessels are constricted in certain cortical regions, whereas the total vascular length remains nearly constant.

Brain swelling induced by application of ouabain causes simultaneously constriction of capillaries and dilation of certain other terminal (shunt-)vessels.

Average capillary diameter thus seems to depend upon the equilibrium between tissue- and intravascular pressure.

REFERENCES

1. ANTHONY, A., KREIDER, J.: Blood volume changes in rodents exposed to simulated high altitude. Amer. J. Physiol. 200, 523-526 (1961).

2. BÄR, Th., WOLFF, J.R.: Quantitative Beziehungen zwischen der Verzweigungsdichte und Länge von Capillaren im Neocortex der Ratte während der postnatalen Entwicklung. Z. Anat. Entwickl.-Gesch. 141, 207-221 (1973).

3. BÄR, Th., EINS, S., NICKSCH, E.: Morphometrische Untersuchungen an Hirnkapillaren von Ratten nach chronischem Sauerstoffmangel. Verh. Anat. Ges. 69, (in press 1975).

4. BÄR, Th., WOLFF, J.R.: Development and adult variations of the wall of brain capillaries in the neocortex of rat and cat. Erwin Riesch-Symposium on Cerebral Vessel Wall, Berlin 1975 (in press).

5. BLINKOV, S.M., GLEZER, J.: Das Zentralnervensystem in Zahlen und Tabellen. Jena: VEB Gustav Fischer 1968.

6. BURIAN, W.G.: Der Einfluß chronischen Sauerstoffmangels auf die Kapillardichte in der Großhirnrinde erwachsener Ratten. Inaugural-Diss. Med. Fak. München. Zürich: Juris Druck und Verlag 1970.

7. CRAIGIE, E.: Postnatal changes in vascularity in the cerebral cortex of the male albino rat. J. comp. Neurol. 39, 301-324 (1925).

8. DIEMER, K., HENN, R.: Kapillarvermehrung in der Hirnrinde der Ratte unter chronischem Sauerstoffmangel. Naturwissenschaften 62, 135-136 (1965).

9. DIEMER, K.: Capillarisation and oxygen supply of the brain. In: Oxygen transport in blood and tissue (eds. D.W. Lübbers, U.C. Luft, G. Thews, E. Witzleb), p. 118. Stuttgart: Georg Thieme 1968.

10. GYGAX, P., EMMENEGGER, H., DIXON, R., PEIER, A.: The effect of hypovolemic oligemia on the cerebral microcirculation and EEG in the cat (Wigger's model). In: Pathology of cerebral microcirculation (ed. J. Cervós-Navarro), p. 386. Berlin: Walter de Gruyter 1974.

11. HUNZIKER, O., FREY, H., SCHULZ, U.: Morphometric investigations of capillaries in the brain cortex of the cat. Brain Res. 65, 1-11 (1974).

12. HUNZIKER, O., EMMENEGGER, H., FREY, H., SCHULZ, U., MEIER-RUGE, W.: Morphometric characterization of the capillary network in the cat's brain cortex: A comparison of the physiological state and hypovolemic conditions. Acta Neuropathol. 29, 57-63 (1974).

13. KIRCHHOFF, H.W., MEYER-ERKELENZ, J.D.: Kreislauf und Atmung unter Hypoxiestreß. Med. Klin. 65, 2051-2059 (1970).

14. KORNER, P.J.: Circulatory adaptations in hypoxia. Physiol. Rev. 39, 687-730 (1959).

15. MERCKER, H., SCHNEIDER, M.: Über Capillarveränderungen des Gehirns bei Höhenanpassung. Pflügers Arch. 251, 49-55 (1949).

16. MÉREI, F.T., TRIXLER, M., GALLYAS, F., GOSZTONYI, G.: Brain capillaries in the rat. In: Recent development of neurobiology in Hungary, Vol. II (ed. K. Lissak), p. 153. Budapest: Akademiai Kiadó 1969.

17. PETRÉN, T.: Untersuchungen über die relative Kapillarlänge der motorischen Hirnrinde in normalem Zustande und nach Muskeltraining. Anat. Anz. 85 (Erg.H.), 169-172 (1938).

18. RHODIN, J.A.G.: Ultrastructure of the microvascular bed. In: The microcirculation in clinical medicine (ed. R. Wells), p. 13. New York: Academic Press 1973.

19. SIESJÖ, B.K., ZWETNOW, H.N.: The effect of hypovolemic hypotension on extra- and intracellular acid-base parameters and energy metabolites in rat brain. Acta physiol. scand. _79_, 114-124 (1970).

20. SNIDER, R.S., NIEMER, W.T.: A stereotaxic atlas of the cat brain. 2nd impression. Chicago-London: The University of Chicago Press 1964.

21. UNDERWOOD, E.E.: Quantitative stereology. Reading, Mass.: Addison-Wesley 1970.

22. WOLFF, J.R., SCHIEWECK, Ch., EMMENEGGER, H., MEIER-RUGE, W.: Cerebrovascular ultrastructural alterations after intra-arterial infusions of ouabain, scillaglycosides, Heparin and histamine. Acta neuropath. (Berl.) _31_, 45-58 (1975).

▷

Fig. 1. Equivalent regions of the visual cortex of a control rat (a) and of a chronic hypoxic rat (b) of the same age. After hypoxia the dilation of the perfused microvessels (white lumen) is clearly visible. Endothelial cell nuclei (arrows). (Stained semithin Epon sections; magn. 400:1). c) If the O_2 concentration falls below 10 Vol %, small fields of degenerating neuronal processes occur in perivascular positions (large arrows). Myelinated axons (small arrows) (Magn. 640:1)

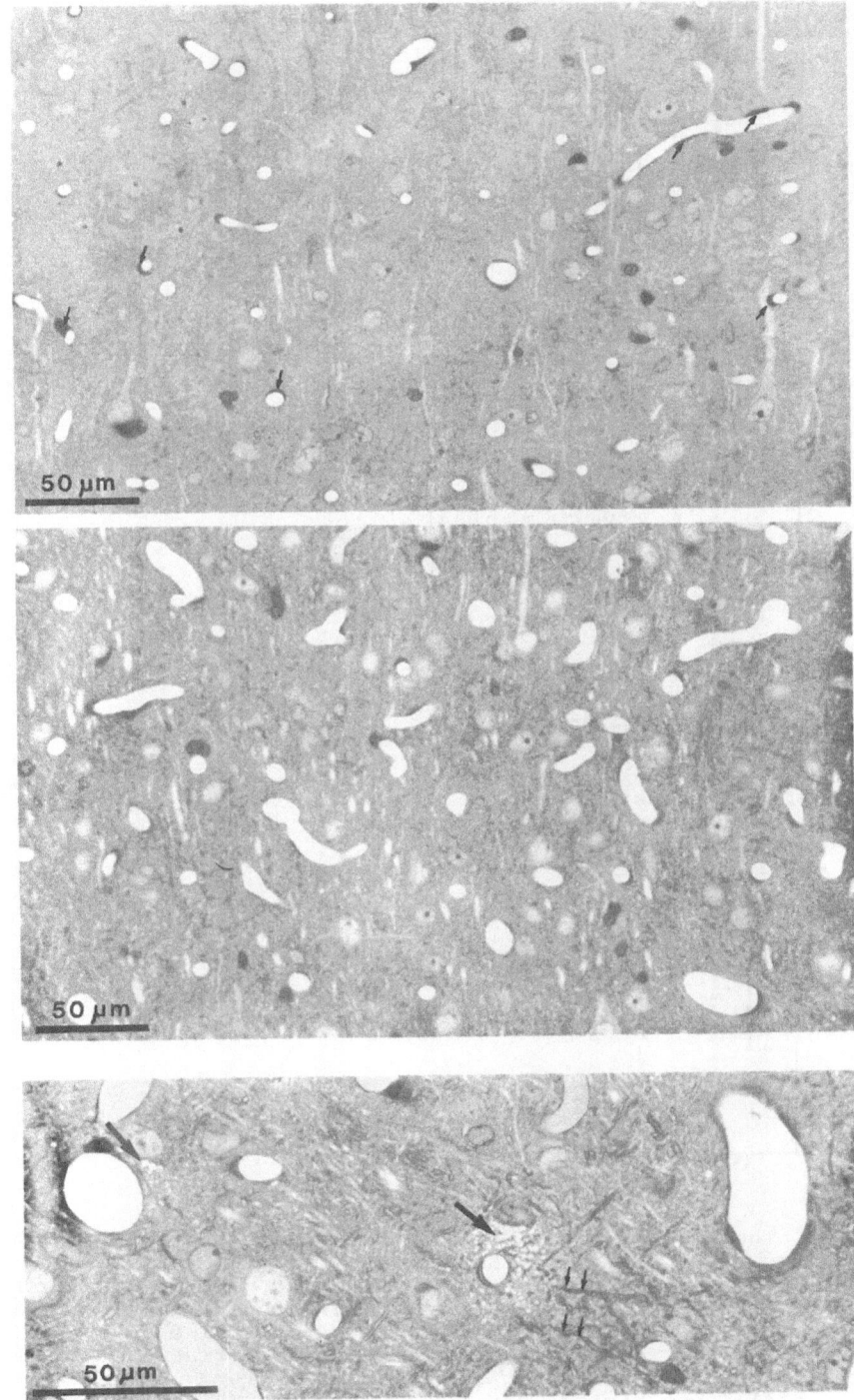

50 μm

50 μm

50 μm

17

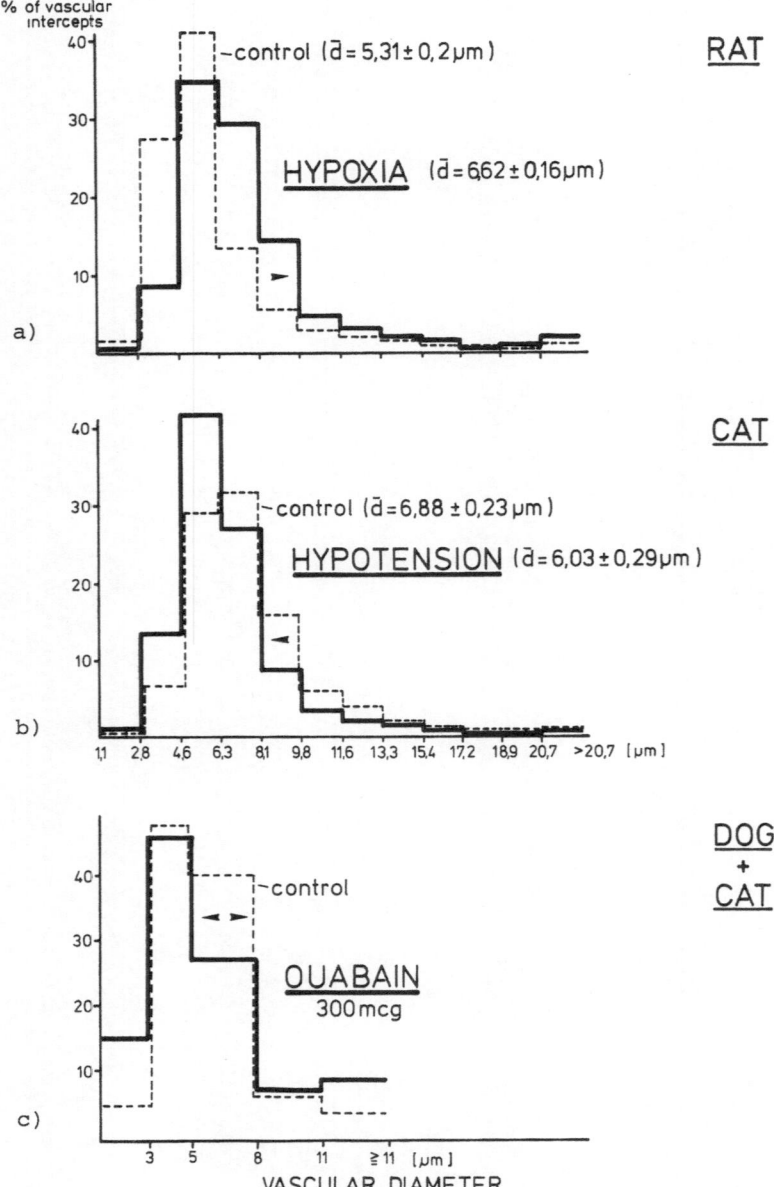

Fig. 2. The effects of different hemodynamic conditions on the size distribution of internal diameters of cortical microvessels. a) After chronic hypoxia there is a general shift to greater diameters compared with the control (adult rats). b) Hypovolemic hypotension causes the opposite effect in adult cats: the size distribution shows a uniform trend to smaller diameters. c) Histograms for normal and ouabain treated dogs do not show a uniform trend. An increase of very small (constricted) capillaries is accompanied by a decrease of larger ones (5 - 8 μm). However, about 7% of the capillaries are dilated after ouabain treatment and show diameters of more than 8 μm

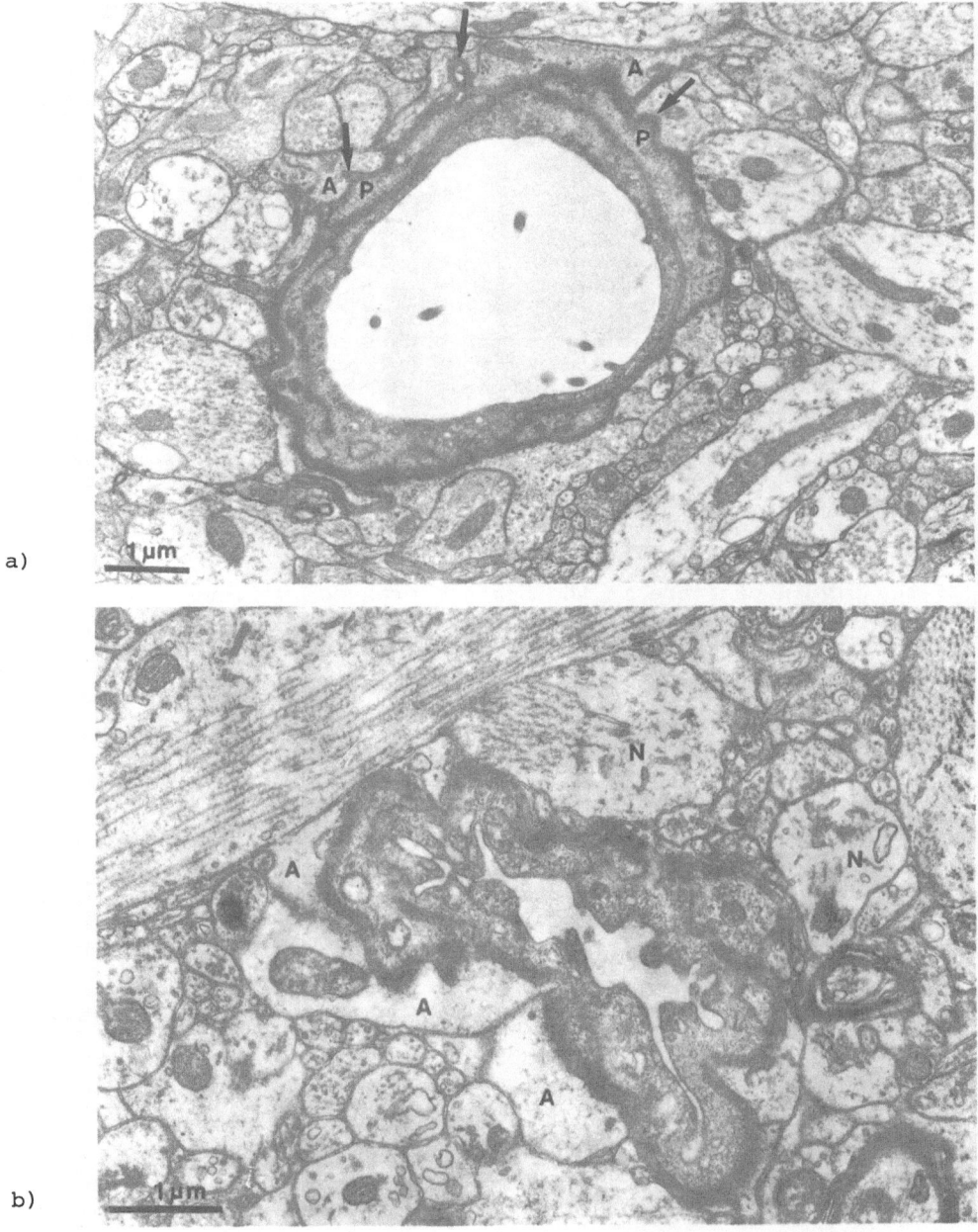

Fig. 3. a) Hypovolemic hypotension: Electron micrograph of a cross section of an intracortical microvessel showing folds (arrows) of pericytal (P) and perivascular astroglial (A) processes. Astroglia are not swollen. 15000:1. b) Infusion of ouabain into a parietal branch of the middle cerebral artery: in the affected areas astroglial (A) and neuronal elements (N) are swollen and the capillary profiles are compressed. Note the folded endothelial surface and the absence of endothelial swelling (20000:1)

Pathophysiological Aspects of Cerebral Hypoxia

E. Betz

There exists a great variety of the causes of tissue hypoxia. An attempt has therefore been made to work out principles of classifications of the various forms of hypoxia (9, 19, 28, 12).

Table 1 A-D represents a classification of hypoxic causes with clinically important examples. For neurosurgery mainly the forms of hypoxia listed under A - C are significant. The type of hypoxia listed under C can be widely reduced during neurosurgical treatment by a careful monitoring of the various parameters for the control of oxygen supply of the patient.

If the oxygen pressure in the brain decreases, various regulatory mechanisms come into play which all show a tendency to compensate for the low oxygen supply of the tissue:

1. Cerebral blood flow increases.

2. The arterial systemic blood pressure and the cardiac output increase.

3. If the P_{O_2} is low in the peripheral chemoreceptors of the carotid artery and of the aorta, ventilation is enhanced.

With these changes hypoxic cerebral tissue disturbances are prevented if the hypoxia is only of a moderate degree. During long extended exposure of animals or men to low oxygen concentrations of 10% or 8% in the air the initially increased CBF returns gradually towards normal values despite continuing exposure to the low oxygen. This gradual decrease is a sign of adaptation to hypoxic conditions. Fig. 1 shows the course of CBF adaptation in cats during chronic hypoxia produced by a decrease of O_2 in the ambient air to a concentration of 10% (in 10 cats) resp. 8% (in 10 cats) during daily repeated hypoxic periods. The animals were exposed to low oxygen concentrations every day for 4 - 6 h during 14 days. During the first period of hypoxia CBF remained high throughout the whole time (Fig. 2). It has been found that after 10 days of daily repeated hypoxic periods CBF does remain nearly normal even in the beginning of the inhalation of the low oxygen (4).

It has been found by many investigators that the adaptation to hypoxia is a complex process in which - besides the increase in ventilation (20, 22) with a change of the O_2 tension (15, 8), a decrease of the alkali-reserves (20, 31) with a fall in the total CO_2 in the blood (20), a shift in the oxygen dissociation curve (11) and an increase in Hb and the number of the erythrocytes (20, 30, 17, 1, 16, 21) - enzymatic processes (3) cause more favourable conditions for a better oxygen supply of the brain (see also 6, 7, 2). These adaptive

Table 1. A. Hypoxic hypoxidosis caused by decreases of the oxygen uptake into the blood

Types	Causes	Mechanisms	Clinical Examples
Hypoxia in the inspired air	Selective reduction of O_2 in the respired gas Decrease of atmospheric pressure	P_{O_2} is decreased in the inspired air	Anaesthesia accidents Mountain sickness
Respiratory hypoxidosis	Ventilatory insufficiency	P_{O_2} is decreased in the inspired air	Obstructive disturbances of the ventilation Restrictive disturbances of the ventilation Paralysis of respiratory muscles, tetanus, intoxication with strychnine
	Disturbance of alveolo-capillary diffusion	Impaired alveolo-capillary diffusion Blood passage through non-ventilated segments of the lung	Fibrosis or edema of alveolar walls, pneumonia, left ventricular failure, pneumoconiosis Obstruction of bronchi
	Intrapulmonary shunts	Arterio-venous shunts of unoxygenated blood in the lungs	Pulmonary. hemangioma a.-v. shunts

Table 1. B. Hypoxic hypoxidosis caused by circulatory disturbances

Types	Causes	Mechanisms	Clinical Examples
Asphyxia	Circulatory arrest, lung collapse	Complete stop of oxygen transport into the arterial blood	Adam-Stokes seizures, cardiac arrest during narcosis
Congenital heart failure with arterial hypoxia	Anomalous inflow or outflow of the heart	Venous blood routes into the left atrium or into the aorta	Transposition of great vessels, persistent ductus Botalli
	Absence of one or more cardiac chambers	Mixing of arterial and venous blood in one chamber	Cor biloculare, Cor triloculare biatriatum
	Abnormal central communications between lesser and greater circulation	Venous blood is ejected into the left heart or in the aorta	Rt-lt-shunt (ventricular septal defect) Rt-lt-shunt (atrial septal defect)
Non congenital heart diseases with arterial hypoxia	Myocardial insufficiency	Low cardiac output because of decrease in myocardial force	Myocarditis, myocardial infarction, decrease of blood pressure below critical value
	Constrictive lesion of the heart	Low cardiac output because of poor diastolic filling	Cardiac tamponade, constrictive pericarditis, deformations of the thorax
	Obstructive lesion of the heart	Low cardiac output because of increased resistance to flow	Heart valve lesions increased intrapulmonary or peripheral resistance

Table 1. B. (Continued)

Types	Causes	Mechanisms	Clinical Examples
	Obstruction of arteries	Ischemic hypoxidosis	Arteriosclerosis, arterial thrombosis, emboli, arteriitis, rupture of vessels, extrinsic pressure on arteries, peripheral disturbance of blood distribution
Vascular damage	Venous stasis	Venous hypoxia	Cardiac insufficiency, venous thrombosis, insufficiency of venous valves
	Lymph stasis	Reduced capillary blood flow as result of high tissue pressure	Idiopatic and acquired lymphatic edema
	Vasospastic states	Distal ischemia resulting from abnormal degree of angiospasm	Raynaud's disease, arterial or venous obstruction, spasms after cold injury
	Low blood volume	Low circulating blood volume	Hemorrhagic shock, burns, infections, trauma
	Inadequate distribution of blood volume	Low regional circulatory blood volume	Peripheral vascular collapse
Circulatory insufficiency	Increase of demand for oxygen	Hormonal disturbances	Thyreotoxikosis
	Abnormal peripheral	Shunting of arterial blood into peripheral veins	Arterio-venous fistula

23

Table 1. C. Hypoxic hypoxidosis caused by changes of the blood

Types	Causes	Mechanisms	Clinical Examples
Anemia	Reduction of the total circulating Hb_{O2}	Oxygen deficiency in the blood	Anemia after blood loss, bone marrow depression, hemolysis
Toxic hypoxidosis	Reduction in functional circulating Hb_{O2}	Conversion of Hb into CO-Hb, Met-Hb or Sulf-Hb	Toxicity of CO, chlorate, various derivates of tar, nitrates

Table 1. D. Histotoxic hypoxidosis

Types	Causes	Mechanisms	Clinical Examples
Encymatic	Poisoning of specific enzymes	Failure of oxygen utilizing enzymes	Cyanide poisoning

mechanisms are more economic than the above mentioned rapid responses of CBF, ventilation and systemic circulation. They replace in
the course of the adaptation so much of the nutrition-functions of
CBF that an increase of CBF becomes useless.

The example was chosen in order to demonstrate that compensatory reactions can be so effective during a chronic state of hypoxia that
existing deficits of oxygen in the inspired air are sometimes ob-
scured.

For the pathophysiology of cerebral energetics the consequences of
hypoxia become important if the compensatory mechanisms are insufficient for a normal oxygen supply of the brain. If, as a consequence
of hypoxia, disturbances of cerebral functions appear, these can
reach various degrees.

Disturbances of association or coordination pass over rapidly into a
paralysis if the hypoxia is augmented. The paralysis can be brought
back to a normal state if the brain receives sufficient oxygen within a few minutes after the beginning of the paralysis. However, if
the anoxia continues for more than 10 min, the brain functions are
damaged irreparably if no artificial aid is used for brain perfusion
and oxygenation. Meanwhile the nomenclature introduced by SUGAR and
GERARD (29) and GERARD (10) characterizing the various states of anoxic brain disturbances have become widely accepted definitions. The
sequence of events during aggravating cerebral hypoxidosis are:
Disturbance ⟶ paralysis ⟶ irreparable damage ⟶ necrosis of
the cells. The latter is the sign of cellular death. The following
terms belong also to this nomenclature: The "survival time" which is
defined as the period of time from the beginning of the anoxia until
the investigated function reappears. The "recovery latency" which is
defined as the period of time from the end of the stop of a complete
anoxia to the onset of a function, and the "recovery time" which is
the period of time beginning at the end of the anoxia and lasting
until the tested function is completely re-established.

Starting from this rough outline the following problems will be
discussed:

1. Which functional parameters characterize best the hypoxic conditions of the brain tissue?

2. How do such parameters change in the course of hypoxia or ischemia of the tissue?

In a film (blood flow measurements in the hypothalamus of a conscious
cat) it is demonstrated how spontaneous behaviour and hypothalamic
blood flow of the animal change if the O_2 concentration in the ambient air is decreased by a rate of 1%/min. At about 17 - 16% O_2, blood
flow starts to increase and it reaches its maximum at about 8% O_2 in
the inspired air. At about 7% disturbances of the behaviour can be
seen: The movements of the animal become atactic, the cat pants, it
salivates, the pupils dilate. Further decrease of the ambient O_2
leads to a collapse of the animal combined with a decrease in systemic arterial blood pressure and CBF. If at this state sufficient
oxygen is delivered, blood pressure increases, a posthypoxic hyperemia with a strong increase of CBF is seen and the animal recovers.
Finally CBF returns to its initial value.

If in such experiments the local oxygen pressure field (18, 5) is
measured in the cerebral cortex with oxygen-sensitive platinum micro-

electrodes one finds soon after the onset of the hypoxia a decrease of the oxygen pressure reaching the zero-value at many spots of the tissue despite the fact, that the P_{O2} in the arterial blood is still considerably higher than zero. The tissue consumes the oxygen which is transported into the tissue via the arterial blood, so that the resulting O_2 pressure gradient between blood and tissue is explained. It therefore is not possible to deduce directly from the arterial P_{O2} nor from local tissue P_{O2} values on the degree of tissue hypoxia, for one has to consider the demand for oxygen of the tissue. The latter differs considerably in anesthetized and non-anesthetized animals.

Which other functional parameter could be used in order to characterize the degree of brain hypoxia? In experiments of SCHMAHL et al. (25, 27) simultaneous measurements of the local cortical oxygen pressure field, the EEG, the cortical energy-rich substrates and the lactate and pyruvate of the tissue were carried out in anesthetized cats when the oxygen content in the inspired air was decreased to 5%. The EEG showed considerable disturbances despite unchanged ATP and Cr~P of the cortical tissue. As a symptom of anaerobic glycolysis of the tissue the lactate-concentration increases. If the hypoxia is intensified, Cr~P starts to decrease. When its cortical tissue level reaches about 1.5 μmol/g tissue (fresh weight) the EEG becomes iso-electric. However one may not draw the conclusion that a decrease of the energy-rich substrates would be the only condition for obtaining an isoelectric EEG. Isoelectricity can also be elicited by very high CO_2 concentration in the tissue without hypoxia. In this case lactate is lowered instead of increased. As a rule one finds during severe respiratory acidosis a reduction of Cr~P. However, there are exceptions with nearly normal tissue Cr~P and these exceptions are sufficient for the hypothesis that a certain level of Cr~P is a necessary but not a sufficient condition for the explanation of the functional disturbance. ATP is in these cases normal or even higher than normal (23).

In the analytical experiments in animals it is necessary to use as a functional cerebral control electrical parameters and it seemed useful to us to take the EEG for this purpose.

All results mentioned have been obtained under the conditions of unrestricted affluent and effluent blood. In ischemic areas the tissue energetics show very similar reactions (26). The time course of the decrease of the energy rich phosphates and the speed of the increase in tissue lactate during a sudden and complete stop of blood flow in cortical tissue is demonstrated in Fig. 3. HOSSMANN and KLEIHUES (14) reported recently on experiments in which in cats affluent vessels to the brain were ligated at their origin directly at the aorta. The ligatures were combined with an artificial decrease of arterial blood pressure below 80 mm Hg in order to prevent small cerebral inflow through spinal arteries. In these experiments flow stops in the pial vessels and the blood stream in the pial arteries is seen to be interrupted.

After re-opening of the ligatures and increasing the blood pressure by means of sympathicomimetic drugs a reappearance of an EEG could be seen after some hours in numerous cases. In our laboratory we did some similar investigations (13). K^+ and H^+ in the subarachnoideal space, the arterial blood pressure, the brain volume and the endexpiratory CO_2 were recorded. Fig. 4 shows a single experiment of a ligature which lasted 1/2 h. The EEG disappeared shortly after the ligature. It appeared again, however, about 2 h after re-opening of the ligatures.

Compared with the initial state the mean frequency of the EEG was slower than normal. In a relatively large number of experiments the EEG did not reappear, despite a normalization of K^+ and H^+.

The wide variability of the results made it possible to solve the problem of whether the reappearance of the EEG can be traced back to one single parameter. If K^+ in the extracellular space of the brain remained high or if the extracellular pH in the CSF remained very low the EEG did not appear. However, it could be seen that in some cases the EEG remained disappeared despite a normalization of sub-arachnoideal K^+ and H^+. As a rule the EEG was not present when the brain tissue volume remained high - as a sign of a severe brain edema - , but it could happen that there was no EEG when the brain volume, the K^+ and the H^+ were normalized.

SCHINDLER et al. (24) analysed the cortical energy-rich substrates, the Red/Ox-state and some amino acids before, during and 4 h after ligature-periods of 1/2 h. The brain tissue was excised by the aid of a steel punch (25). The obtained results permitted an arrangement of the results in groups. One group of results was characterized by a persisting hypoxia with reduction of tissue-ATP and tissue-Cr~P and a considerable increase of lactate because of a nonsufficient re-perfusion of the tissue with blood.

In a second group the energy-rich substrates and the energy charge potential normalized again and the EEG reappeared again. Lactate in the tissue was increased in these brains.

Finally, there were cats in which the energy-rich substrates of the cerebral tissue normalized after restoring brain circulation, the lactate was somewhat higher as in group 2, but the EEG did not reappear.

The different developments of the reactions in the same experimental procedure suggest that an EEG can develop only if numerous conditions are fulfilled. It is worth considering that in the experiments of SCHINDLER et al. (24) in which despite of normalized energy-rich substrates no EEG appeared, the tissue-glutamate was below normal. From this finding one may conclude, that an additional condition for the re-appearance of the EEG is a tissue glutamate concentration above a certain threshold.

Whether these findings will lead to a correction of the conception of the survival time can not yet be decided. Until now the proof for the conception that the reappearance of the EEG can be equated with the restoration of normal cerebral functions is not sufficient. Only if the animals survive with normal postoperative behaviour after such a long term stop of the total cerebral circulation, can it be stated whether the EEG can be used as a sign of restored complex and inte-grative cerebral functions.

Summary

After a classification of causes for cerebral hypoxia the reactions of the organisms for maintaining a sufficient cerebral oxygen supply are discussed.

The role of cerebral circulation, oxygen supply, energy rich sub-strates and extracellular ion concentration as parameters for the de-gree of tissue hypoxia are demonstrated in numerous examples. It is shown how these parameters change in the course of adaptation to hypoxic conditions and during ischemia of the brain.

REFERENCES

1. ADOLPH, E.F.: General and specific characteristics of physiological adaptation. Amer. J. Physiol. 184, 18-28 (1956).

2. ALBAUM, H.G., CHINN, H.: Brain metabolism during acclimatization to high altitude. Amer. J. Physiol. 174, 141-145 (1953).

3. BARBASHOVA, Z.I.: Cellular level of adaptation. Handbook of Physiology Sect. 4, 37-54 (1964).

4. BETZ, E.: Adaptation of regional cerebral blood flow in animals exposed to chronic alterations of P_{O2} and P_{CO2}. Acta. neurol. scand. 14, 121-128 (1965).

5. BICHER, H.I., BRULEY, D.F.: Oxygen transport to tissue. New York-London: Plenum Press 1973.

6. DAHL, N.A., BALFOUR, W.M.: Prolonged anoxia survival due to anoxia pre-exposure: brain adenosine triphosphate lactate, and pyruvate. Amer. J. Physiol. 207, 452-456 (1964).

7. DETAR, R., BOHR, D.F.: Adaptation to hypoxia in vascular smooth muscle. Fed. Proc. 27, 1416-1419 (1968).

8. DILL, D.B., CHRISTIANSEN, E.H., EDWARDS, H.T.: Gas equilibria in the lungs at high altitudes. Amer. J. Physiol. 115, 530-538 (1936).

9. DITTMAR, D.S., GREBE, R.M. (Eds.): In: Handbook of respiration, p. 272.

10. GERARD, R.W.: Anoxia and neural metabolism. Arch. Neurol. Psychiat. (Chic.) 40, 985-996 (1938).

11. HALL, F.G., DILL, D.B., GUZMANN-BARRON, E.S.: Comparative physiology in high altitudes. J. cell. comp. Physiol. 8, 301-313, (1936).

12. HIRSCH, H., SCHNEIDER, M.: Durchblutung und Sauerstoffaufnahme des Gehirns. In: Handbuch der Neurochirurgie, Bd. 1, 2. Teil (eds. H. Olivecrona, W. Tönnis), Berlin-Heidelberg-New York: Springer 1968.

13. HEUSER, D., HOSSMANN, K.-A., SCHINDLER, U., BETZ, E.: Changes of cerebral extracellular ion activities and brain volume during prolonged cerebral ischemia and recovery. Pflügers Archiv, 335, (Suppl. R 99) (1975).

14. HOSSMANN, K.-A., KLEIHUES, P.: Reversibility of ischemic brain damage. Arch. Neurol. 29, 375-384 (1973).

15. HOUSTON, C.S., RILEY, R.L.: Respiratory and circulatory changes during acclimatization to high altitude. Amer. J. Physiol. 149, 565-588 (1947).

16. HURTADO, A., CLARK, R.T.: Parameters of human adaptation to altitude. In: Physics and medicine of the atmosphere and space (eds. Benson, Strughold), pp. 352-369. New York: J. Wiley & Sons 1960.

17. HURTADO, A., MERINO, C., DELGADO, E.: Influence of anoxaemia on the hemopoetic activity. Arch. Intern. Med. 75, 284-292 (1945).

18. KESSLER, M., BRULEY, D.F., CLARK, Jr., L.D., LÜBBERS, D.W., SILVER, I.A., STRAUSS, J.: Oxygen Supply (Theoretical and practical aspects of oxygen supply and microcirculation of tissue). München-Berlin-Wien: Urban & Schwarzenberg 1973.

19. VAN LIERE, E.J., STICKNEY, J.C.: Hypoxia. Chicago-London: Univ. of Chicago Press 1963.

20. LUFT, U.C.: Die Höhenanpassung. Ergebn. Physiol. $\underline{44}$, 256-314 (1941).

21. MÜRTZ, R.: Zur Pathophysiologie des chronischen Sauerstoffmangels. Untersuchung über Anpassungsvorgänge von Kreislauf und Atmung bei Morbus caeruleus. Arch. Kreisl.-Forsch. $\underline{40}$, 167-235 (1963).

22. RAHN, H., OTIS, A.B.: Man's respiratory response during and after acclimatization to high altitude. Amer. J. Physiol. $\underline{157}$, 445-462 (1949).

23. SCHINDLER, U., GÄRTNER, E., BETZ, E.: Energy-rich metabolites and EEG in Hypoxia. In: Oxygen Transport to Tissue (eds. H.I. Bicher, D.F. Bruley), pp. 233-238. New York: Plenum Publ. Corporation 1973.

24. SCHINDLER, U., HEUSER, D., HOSSMANN, K.-A., BETZ, E.: Cat brain metabolism and EEG after recovery from long-term complete ischemia. Pflügers Archiv $\underline{335}$, (Suppl. R 99) (1975).

25. SCHMAHL, F.W., BETZ, E., DETTINGER, E., HOHORST, H.J.: Energiestoffwechsel der Großhirnrinde und Elektroencephalogramm bei Sauerstoffmangel. Pflügers Arch $\underline{292}$, 46-59 (1966).

26. SCHMAHL, F.W., BETZ, E., TALKE, H.: Effects of transient carotid occlusion on the extramitochondrial redox system in the disturbed hemisphere. In: Cerebral Blood Flow and Intracranial Pressure, Proc. 5th int. Symp. Roma-Siena 1971, part I. Europ. Neurol. $\underline{6}$, 323-328 (1971/72).

27. SCHMAHL, F.W., BETZ, E., TALKE, H., HOHORST, H.J.: Energiereiche Phosphate und Metabolite des Energiestoffwechsels in der Großhirnrinde der Katze. Biochem. Zt. $\underline{342}$, 518-531 (1965).

28. SCHNEIDER, M.: Einführung in die Physiologie des Menschen, s.210-213. Berlin-Göttingen-Heidelberg: Springer 1964.

29. SUGAR, O., GERARD, R.W.: Anoxia and brain potentials. J. Neurophysiol. $\underline{1}$, 558-572 (1938).

30. THORN, G.W., JONES, B.F., LEWIS, R.A., MITCHELL, E.R., KOEPP, G.E.: The role of the adrenal cortex in anoxia, the effect of repeated daily exposures to reduced oxygen pressure. Amer. J. Physiol. $\underline{137}$, 606-619 (1942).

31. WANG, S.I., WIRZ, H., VERZAR, F.: Die O_2-Sättigung des arteriellen Blutes bei Mensch und Kaninchen auf 1800 m ü.M. und ihr Zusammenhang mit der Erythrozytenzunahme. Schweiz. med. Wschr. $\underline{81}$, 82-95 (1951).

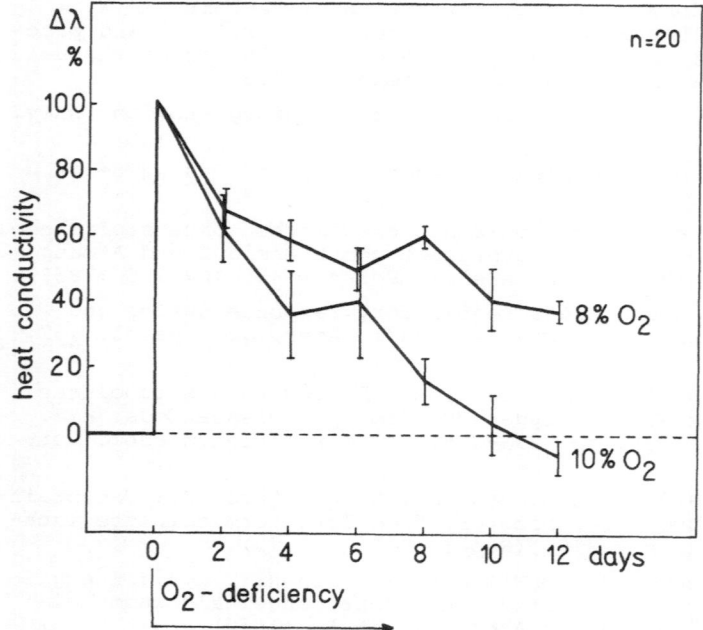

Fig. 1. Mean values of regional cerebral blood flow in 20 cats during hypoxia. Measuring site: Thalamus or hypothalamus, blood flow was measured by heatclearance probes. The initial values in normal atmosphere are indicated as $\Delta\lambda = 0$ per cent; the mean increase in cerebral blood flow during the first exposure to 8 per cent O_2 or 10 per cent O_2 as $\Delta\lambda = 100$ per cent. In the course of adaptation the mean values of CBF in the cats which were exposed to 10 per cent O_2 decreased to normal values within 10 days, whereas cerebral blood flow in those cats which were exposed to 8 per cent O_2 remained elevated

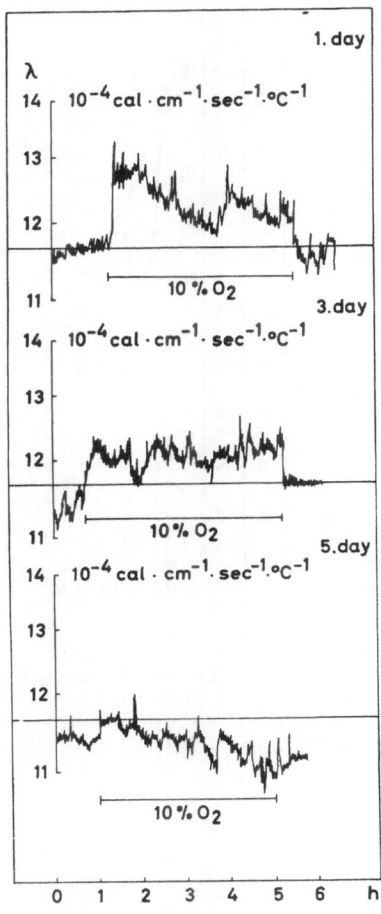

Fig. 2. Hypothalamic blood flow in a conscious cat during daily repeated exposure to 10% O_2 in the ambient air. Local blood flow was continuously recorded with a chronically implanted heart clearance probe. The exposure to low oxygen in the atmosphere lasted four hours daily (heat clearance is a relative measure of blood flow and is recorded as the apparent heat conductivity. Increased heat conductivity means increased flow)

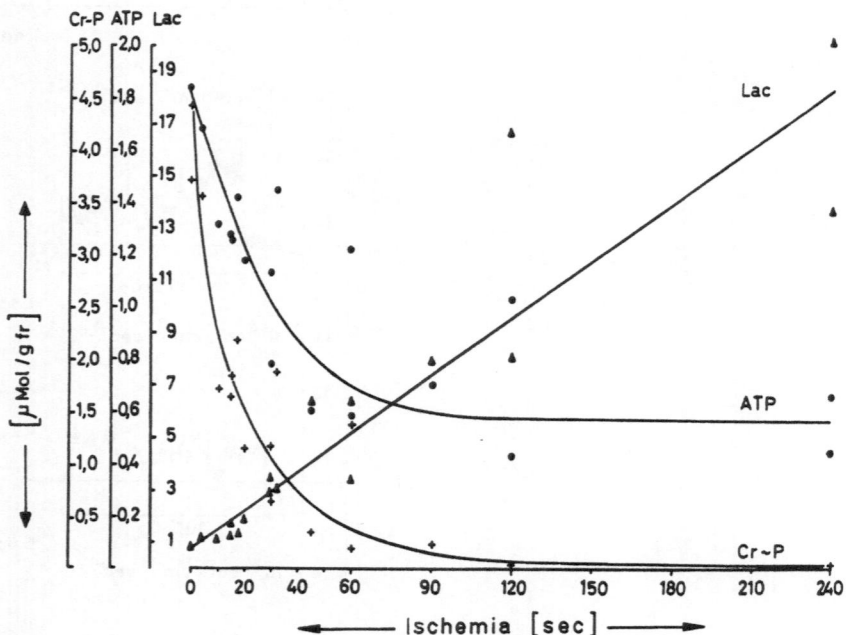

Fig. 3. Effect of complete ischemia on cerebral cortical tissue
Cr~P, ATP and lactate. The values are given in µmol/g tissue (fresh
weight). Values were obtained from 28 cats anesthetized with 25 mg/kg
pentobarbital (from SCHMAHL et al., 1965)

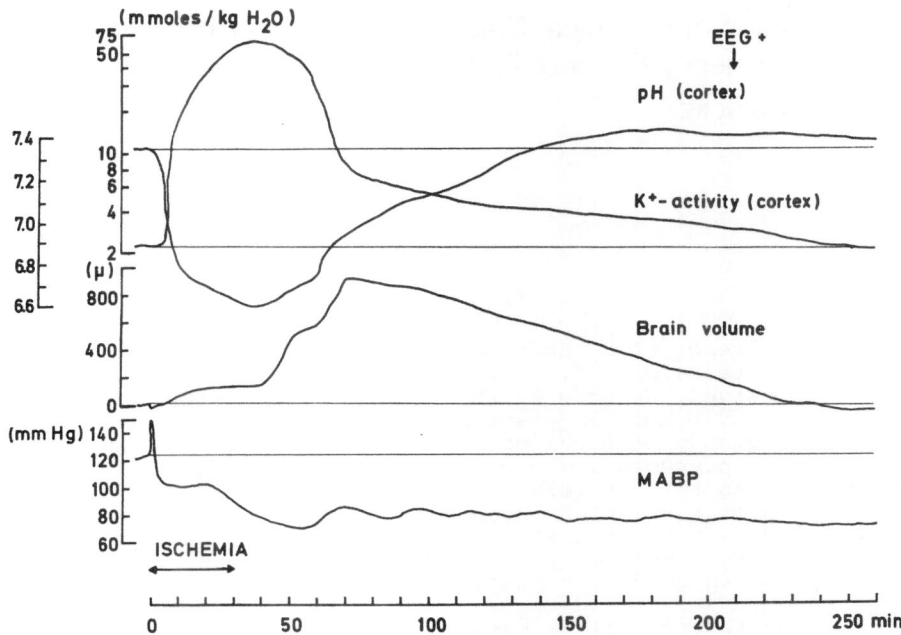

Fig. 4. Single experiment in an anesthetized cat: Cortical subarachnoideal pH and K$^+$ activity, continuously recorded brain volume and
mean blood pressure in the aorta before, during and after ligature
of the brain vessels at their origin at the aorta. Ligature lasted
30 min. EEG returned 170 min after reopening of the ligatures
(HEUSER et al., unpublished)

33

Activation of a Cortical Seizure Focus Under Hypoxia: O_2-Deficiency Effect or Result of Tissue Acidosis?

ST. ZSCHOCKE

The influence of O_2 deficiency on cerebral convulsions was examined many times before (4, 5, 6). A suppression of the convulsion activity was observed. We studied the effects of hypoxia on a cortical seizure focus. Under moderate hypoxia different results were obtained: the frequency of focal cortical seizure discharges even increased. At first we presumed a direct hypoxic stimulation of the focus. In further tests animals were exposed to hypercapnic conditions. The comparison of results of these various test series led to the conclusion that focus activation recorded under hypoxia is not an effect pertaining immediately to O_2 deficiency but the consequence of tissue acidosis induced by hypoxia.

This statement will be based on an analysis of bioelectrical data recorded epicortically. Particularly the recording of the cortical DC potential serves for a qualitative assessment of hypoxia and acidosis effects (see 1), controlled in some tests by measuring the cortical tissue pO_2.

Methods

The experiments were carried out on albino rats anesthetized with phenobarbital (80 mg/kg i.p.), relaxed by d-tubocurarin, and ventilated artificially, the body temperature being kept constant at 37ºC. The cortical seizure focus was elicited by topical application of penicillin G (-Na-K). On the top of the focus (always fronto-parietal) and from other cortical points (ipsi- and contralateral for studying the propagation of the focal discharge) the ECoG and the DC potential were recorded, with reference points in the anterior portion of the nasal bone. The seizure discharges were counted electronically (13). Special bioelectrical data such as the presentation of variations in spike sequence (interval histogram) or variations in form and rise time of seizure potentials were evaluated by processing tape recordings, partly with the aid of a digital computer. In each test the rats were exposed to gas mixtures with reduced O_2 content (12 - 6% O_2 in N_2; 49 measurements) or increased CO_2 content (5 - 30% CO_2 in air; 29 measurements). Arterial blood pressure (via a. femoralis) and heart rate were recorded for circulation control.

Results

Under phenobarbital anesthesia the cortical penicillin focus exhibits only so-called interictal discharges. Typical reactions of such a focus to hypoxia and to hypercapnia are shown in Figs. 1 and 2.

Hypoxia regularly reduces the discharge frequency, and simultaneously it enhances the irregularity in spike interval distribution (H in Fig. 1). The amplitude of the seizure potentials often slightly increases. Concomitantly there is an increase in potential rise time (Fig. 2A). The cortical DC potential shows a surface-negative shift which is typical for a direct hypoxia effect. Propagation of the focal discharges will be accelerated (Fig. 3).

An (hypercapnic) *acidosis* (10% CO_2 in Fig. 1 B and 2 B) at first leads to marked increase in spike frequency[1]. The spike interval reduction naturally reflects the frequency increase. But according to the interval histogram (H in Fig. 1) acidosis furthermore leads to marked regularisation of the interval duration: the random focus activity turns into a marked rhythmical one. The propagation of the focal discharge, however, will be delayed, paralleled by a reduction of the propagated discharge itself (Fig. 3). The spike amplitude will be decreased, and there is also a significant decrease of the potential rise time (Fig. 2 B). During the increase of the pCO_2 the cortical DC potential clearly shifts to the positive direction.

In summary, both hypoxia and hypercapnia cause clearly distinguishable changes which permit to discriminate contrary hypoxia-induced reactions of the cortical seizure focus mentioned above.

Fig. 4 shows an example, divergent from the regular hypoxic reaction: the focus responds to hypoxia by an increase in discharge frequency. In this case the negative shift of the DC potential at the beginning of the exposition to 8% O_2 (paralleled by a short increase in potential rise time) initially reveals a transient immediate O_2-deficiency effect. After two minutes, however, this negative shift will be stopped and superimposed by a tendency to a positive-going shift indicating an increasing acidosis effect. Simultaneously other data of this representative experiment also resemble an augmenting CO_2 (acidosis) effect: decrease in spike amplitudes, decrease in potential rise time, decrease in variability of interval duration (increasing regularisation or rhythmization, respectively). If such changes appear under a hypoxic state they usually outlast the hypoxia period. Moreover in the posthypoxic period they could additionally be intensified to some extent. This is remarkably evident in the course of the DC potential (see Fig. 4).

Discussion

A cortical seizure focus can be influenced by hypoxia in a twofold manner. The obvious primary effect of the O_2 deficiency is manifested by a diminuition in spike frequency. But under hypoxia the cortical seizure focus can also be activated. This activation, however, does not seem to be a direct effect of the O_2 deficiency. Comparing several bioelectrical data as shown above the results support the assumption that the activation of the focus observed under hypoxia is caused by hypoxically induced tissue acidosis.

As shown in earlier and recent studies by others (8, 10, 12) tissue acidosis can be an early and marked metabolic reaction to tissue hy-

---

[1]The focal cortical discharges will only be suppressed by more severe increase of the pCO_2 (above 30% CO_2 inspiratory) which causes a general depression of the central nervous activity (CO_2 narcosis).

poxydosis. It superimposes the hypoxia effects. Increasing cerebral blood flow partly compensates the O_2 lack. This acidosis regularly outlasts the hypoxia period. According to this the focus activation also outlasts the O_2 deficiency; the activation may even be further intensified. In some cases it will occur only in the posthypoxic period, obviously depending on outlasting acidosis.

Activation of a cortical seizure focus by increase in pCO_2 has also been recorded by others (3, 4, 7). It seems incompatible with the general view according to which acidosis inhibits seizure activity. Inhibitory effects, however, of raised pCO_2 (or acidosis) are derived from experiments with generalized seizure activity as induced by pentetrazol (2, 4, 5, 9, 14). The activating effect of acidosis is seen only in a cortical seizure focus, probably in consequence of pH-dependent inhibition of inhibitory neurons (so-called disinhibition). Propagation and generalization of the focus activity will be reduced, which is in agreement with generally accepted effects of acidosis.

In conclusion, the cortical seizure focus may be activated by the hypoxically induced (secondary) tissue acidosis even in general cerebral hypoxia as well as in general (primary) acidosis (e.g. hypercapnic acidosis), but the generalization of the epileptic process is prevented. In *circumscribed* metabolic disorders causing tissue acidosis, however, the enhanced focus activity can spread into adjacent unaffected neuronal structures. A generalization of the focal event may then occur. This hypothetical concept could be of clinical relevance in case of focal epileptic reactions due to localized circulatory disturbances, or to tissue acidosis in the vicinity of brain tumors.

Summary

The influence of O_2 deficiency on a cortical penicillin-induced seizure focus was examined in rats. Hypoxia regularly reduces the focus activity. Particularly under moderate hypoxia an increase in frequency of focal discharges could also be observed. This activation apparently does not pertain to hypoxia itself but seems to be the consequence of hypoxically induced tissue acidosis as revealed by a comparison of several bioelectrical data recorded in rats under hypoxia and hypercapnia. Possible clinical relevance of the results is discussed.

REFERENCES

1. CASPERS, H. (Ed.): DC potentials recorded directly from the cortex. In: Handbook of electroencephalography and clinical neurophysiology (ed. A. Rémond), Vol. 10, Part A (ed. C. Ajmone Marsan). Amsterdam: Elsevier 1974.

2. CASPERS, H., SPECKMANN, E.-J.: DC potential shifts in paroxysmal states. In: Basic mechanisms of the epilepsies (eds. H. Jasper, A.A. Ward, A. Pope). Boston: Little, Brown & Co. 1969.

3. GELLHORN, E., FRENCH, L.A.: Carbon dioxide and cortical spike frequency. Arch. Int. Pharmacodyn. 93, 427 - 433 (1953).

4. GELLHORN, E., HEYMANS, C.: Differential action of anoxia, asphyxia and CO_2 on normal and convulsive potentials. J. Neurophysiol. 11, 261 - 273 (1948).

5. GELLHORN, E., YESINICK, L.: The effect of oxygen-lack and inhalation of carbon dioxide on chemically induced convulsions. Amer. J. Physiol. <u>133</u>, 290 (1941).

6. JASPER, H.H., ERICKSON, T.C.: Cerebral blood flow and pH in excessive cortical discharge induced by metrazol and electrical stimulation. J. Neurophysiol. <u>4</u>, 333 - 347 (1941).

7. KORNMÜLLER, A.E., NOELLE, W.: Über den Einfluß der Kohlensäurespannung auf bioelektrische Hirnrindenphänomene. Pflügers Arch. ges. Physiol. <u>247</u>, 660 - 685 (1944).

8. LOESCHCKE, H.H., LOESCHCKE, G.: Über den Milchsäureaustausch zwischen arteriellem Blut und Gehirngewebe und seine Veränderungen im Sauerstoffmangel. Pflügers Arch. ges. Physiol. <u>249</u>, 521 - 538 (1947).

9. POLLOCK, G.G.: Central inhibitory effects of carbon dioxide. I. Felis domesticus. J. Neurophysiol. <u>12</u>, 315 - 324 (1949).

10. SIESJÖ, B.K., NILSSON, L.: The influence of arterial hypoxemia upon labile phosphates and upon extracellular and intracellular lactate and pyruvate concentrations in the rat brain. Scand. J. Clin. Lab. Invest. <u>27</u>, 83 - 96 (1971).

11. SPECKMANN, E.-J., CASPERS, H., SOKOLOV, W.: Aktivitätsänderungen spinaler Neurone während und nach einer Asphyxie. Pflügers Arch. ges. Physiol. <u>319</u>, 122 - 138 (1970).

12. THORN, W., HEITMANN, R.: pH der Gehirnrinde vom Kaninchen in situ während perakuter, totaler Ischämie, reiner Anoxie und in der Erholung. Pflügers Arch. ges. Physiol. <u>258</u>, 501 - 510 (1954).

13. ZSCHOCKE, St.: An electronic device for continuous counting of chemically induced epileptic discharges. Electroenceph. clin. Neurophysiol. <u>37</u>, 191 - 193 (1974).

14. ZSCHOCKE, St., HEYN, D.: Influence of the pCO_2 on macropotentials and single cell discharges in cortical seizure activity. Electroenceph. clin. Neurophysiol. <u>30</u>, 265 (1971).

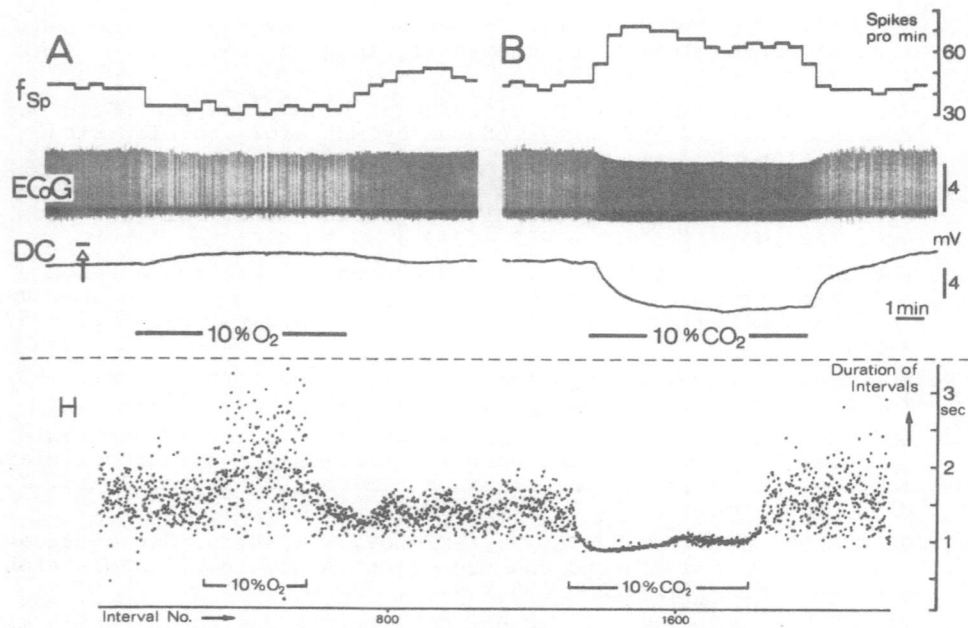

Fig. 1. Primary effect of hypoxia (ventilation with 10% O_2) and the effect of hypercapnic acidosis (ventilation with 10% CO_2) on a cortical penicillin-induced seizure focus. ECoG (Electrocorticogram) showing focal discharges from interictal type. ECoG and DC (cortical steady potential; negativity is up) recorded from the focus area at slow speed (1 cm/min). f_{Sp}: frequency histogram of the focal discharges. H: Sequential interval histogram including the consecutive intervals (each plotted as a point) of both the original recordings in the upper trace

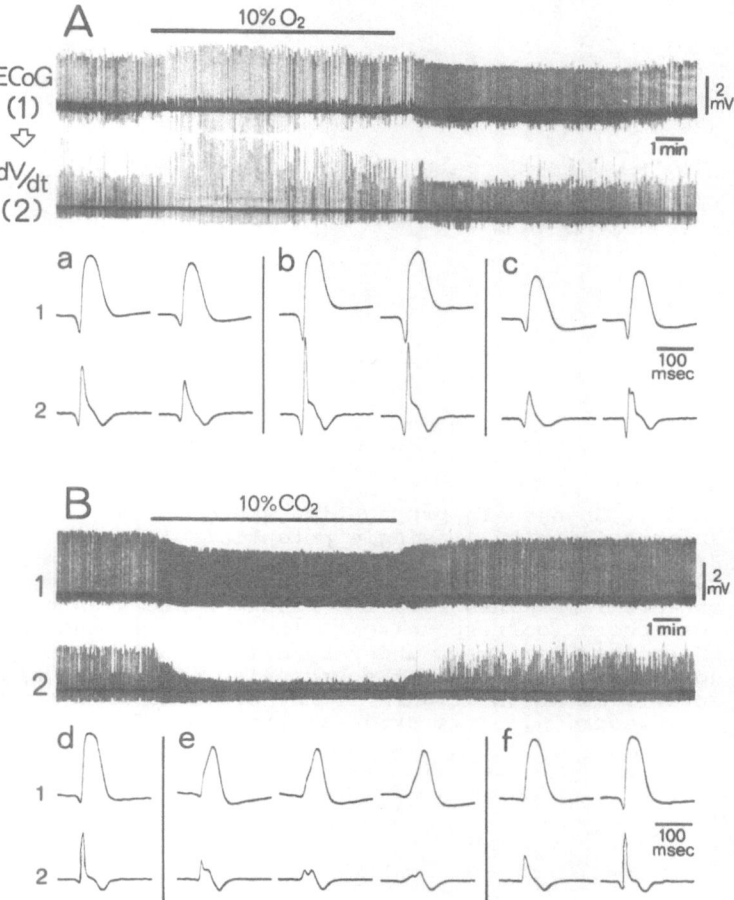

Fig. 2. Changes in potential rise time disclosed by electronical differentiation dV/dt (2) of the seizure potentials (1) as shown in upper parts of *A* and *B* in original recordings (1 cm/min): Increase in rise time as a typical primary hypoxia effect (*A*) and marked decrease in rise time during hypercapnic acidosis (*B*). Lower parts in *A* and *B*: single seizure potentials (1) and their derivates (2) of the same experiment in high-speed recordings; *a* prior to, *b* during, and *c* after ventilation with 10% O_2, *d* prior to, *e* during, and *f* after application of 10% CO_2

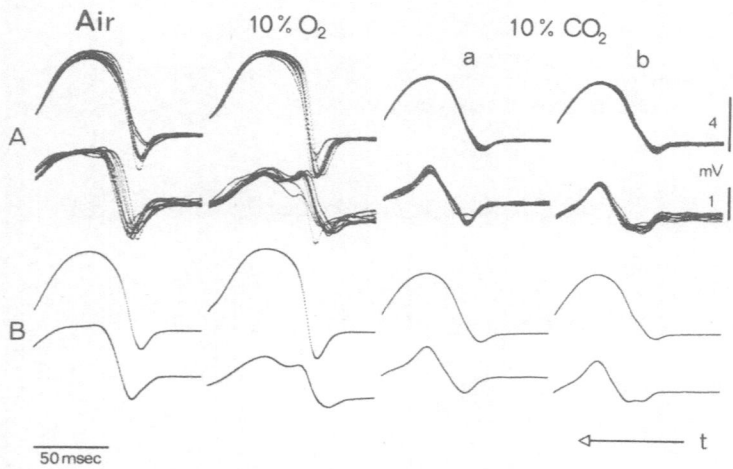

Fig. 3. Changes in propagation speed of the focal discharge. A: superposition of 10 single potentials (plot of random selections). B: computed average of 50 random selected potentials. In A and B, the focal discharge is shown in the upper trace, and the projected potential obtained from the fronto-parietal area of the contralateral hemisphere (corresponding to the focus) in the lower trace: Increase of propagation speed under hypoxia, decrease under hypercapnic acidosis (a: 2 min after the beginning of the CO_2 application, b: 6 min later). *Note*: the figure is the original of a reverse analysis of tape recording. Time axis (t) therefore from right to the left

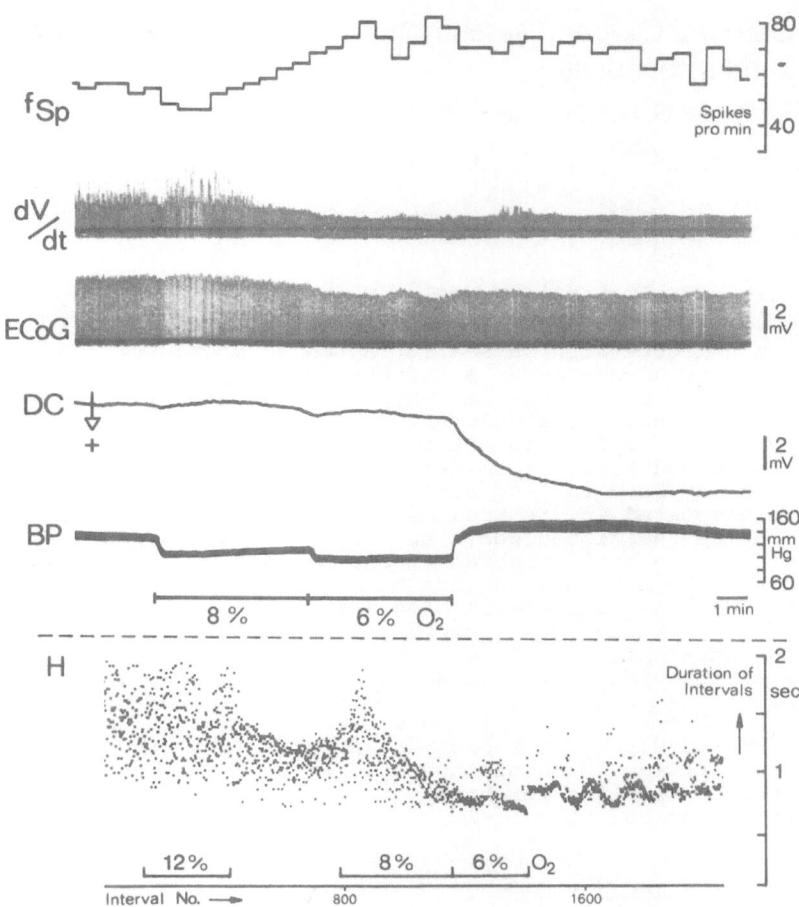

Fig. 4. Activation of a cortical seizure focus under hypoxia which, in comparison with the CO_2 effects illustrated in Figs. *1* and *2*, seems to be the consequence of the hypoxically induced tissue acidosis. ECoG and DC potential recorded in the focus area, together with the simultaneous plotted derivative dV/dt. The sequential interval histogram *H* of this test shows a hypoxia period (12% O_2) previous to the upper original recording. Note that the abscissa of the histogram is not a time scale. BP: arterial blood pressure. Further explanations see text

Cerebral Oxygen Consumption in Profound Arterial Hypoxemia and Hypocapnia

J. HAMER, S. HOYER, and E. ALBERTI

For patients with raised intracranial pressure, respiratory insufficiency always means a threatening complication because of the danger of cerebral hypoxia. Whereas a decrease of arterial PO_2 may
directly cause insufficient oxygenation of the brain tissue ("hypoxic
hypoxia"), a fall in arterial PCO_2 acts through a decrease of cerebral blood flow due to vasoconstriction of the cerebral vessels and
thus may lead to "ischemic hypoxia". As artificial hyperventilation
is advocated in the treatment of raised intracranial pressure, it
must be questioned where to set the limit beyond which hypocap-
nically induced cerebral tissue hypoxia may occur. In clinical practice, the neurosurgeon has mainly to face the resultant of different
pathogenetic factors such as intracranial hypertension, disturbances
of respiration and of blood pressure etc. To get better insight into
the intrinsic effects of markedly lowered aPO_2 and $aPCO_2$ on the brain,
investigations based on an experimental model are required. The
present experimental study contributes to the question to which degree of pure normocapnic normotensive arterial hypoxemia and normoxic normotensive hypocapnia a sufficient oxygen supply to the
brain tissue is maintained and which regulatory mechanisms are elicited to keep the cerebral metabolic rate of oxygen ($CMRO_2$) in the
physiological range.

Material and Methods

The investigations were carried out on 21 artificially ventilated
healthy mongrel dogs anesthetized with pentobarbital and 0,4vol%
halothane. In group A (n=10), aPO_2 was lowered to about 30 Torr
while keeping a PCO_2 normocapnic (38 Torr) and mean arterial blood
pressure (MABP 110 mm Hg) normotensive. In group B (n=11), $aPCO_2$
was decreased to about 18 Torr, leaving aPO_2 and MABP normoxic and
normotensive respectively. The hypoxemic phase was maintained for
about 20 minutes, the hypocapnic phase for 30 minutes. Under steady
state conditions the following measurements were carried out: Total
cerebral blood flow (CBF) was determined by the nitrous oxide method
as modified by BERNSMEIER and SIEMONS (1), the concentrations of
oxygen in the arterial and the cerebral venous blood were measured
by means of gaschromatography. Blood sampling was performed with
motor syringes extracting 1 ml of blood per minute from the aorta
and the frontal part of the superior sagittal sinus after draining
diploic veins had been occluded in order to prevent extracerebral
contamination. Blood gases and acid base parameters were checked in
short intervals throughout the whole experimental run. The investigations were performed in normothermia of the experimental animals.

Results

In profound arterial hypoxemia (aPO_2 about 30 Torr), global CBF increased for about 88%, whereas $avDO_2$ fell for about 46% as compared to the resting state. The mean cerebral metabolic rate of oxygen changed only insignificantly (see Table 1 with corresponding mean values). In profound arterial hypocapnia ($aPCO_2$ 18 Torr), CBF fell for about 55%. In a compensatory fashion, $avDO_2$ significantly increased for about 67%, and due to this increased oxygen extraction, $CMRO_2$ remained constant (see Table 2 with corresponding mean values).

Table 1.

n = 10	aPO_2 116 mm Hg	aPO_2 32 mm Hg
CBF ml/100 g min	58,8	110,9[a]
(A - V)O_2 vol%	7,97	3,76[b]
$CMRO_2$ ml/100 g min	4,70	4,22
CPP mm Hg	112	104

[a] $P < 0,001$.
[b] $P < 0,01$.

Table 2.

n = 11	$aPCO_2$ 36 mm Hg	$aPCO_2$ 18 mm Hg
CBF ml/100 g min	61,0	33,9[a]
(A - V)O_2 vol%	5,6	9,4[a]
$CMRO_2$ ml/100 g min	3,4	3,2
CPP mm Hg	103	106

[a] $P < 0,001$.

Comments

The present data clearly demonstrate that in arterial hypoxemia and hypocapnia two basically different cerebral regulatory mechanisms are elicited which keep cerebral oxygen consumption constant over a surprisingly wide range of decreasing aPO_2 and $aPCO_2$ respectively: Insufficient oxygen saturation of the arterial blood induces cerebral hyperemia, whereas the hypocapnic decrease of CBF is counteracted by an increased oxygen utilisation of the brain tissue. Hypoxemic cerebral hyperemia was observed in spontaneously breathing conscious men first by KETY and SCHMIDT (6) and studied in animal preparations by NOELL and SCHNEIDER (9). However, the hypoxic threshold for eliciting a marked increase in CBF differs with the experimental conditions. This is mainly due to the fact that even moderate arterial hypoxemia provokes spontaneous hyperventilation and that concomitant hypocapnia attenuates the hypoxic vasodilatatory effect. In agreement with recently published results of KOGURE and coworkers (7), we observed in a more extensive experimental study that even a moderate decrease of aPO_2 to 60-50 Torr is accompanied by a considerably increased blood flow of the brain provided that $aPCO_2$ was controlled and kept normocapnic. In profound arterial hypoxemia, that means at aPO_2 values about or below 30 Torr, the increase in cerebral blood flow is particularly high whereby the cerebral metabolic rate of oxygen can be kept constant. Unchanged global cerebral oxygen consumption in marked arterial hypoxemia has also been found in awake men by COHEN and associates (3) who lowered aPO_2 to 35 Torr. The same clinical investigators (2, 12) have demonstrated raised oxygen utilisation in man during respiratory alcalosis with $aPCO_2$ values between 20 and 25 Torr. The present study shows that even a decrease of $aPCO_2$ below 20 Torr must not necessarily be associated with a significant fall in total cerebral oxygen consumption. Thus it may be assumed that a moderate decrease of $aPCO_2$ to values of about 25-28 Torr as currently achieved in therapeutic artificial hyperventilation does not induce cerebral tissue hypoxia. It has been shown by other investigators (13) that the hypocapnic vasoconstriction of the cerebral vessels is a self-limiting process in so far as finally in "ischemic hypoxia" hypoxic cerebral vasodilatation will prevail. It should be emphasized, however, that the regulatory mechanisms mentioned above are closely linked to an unchanged cerebral tissue perfusion pressure. Moreover, a methodological problem must be briefly discussed: The cerebral metabolic rate of oxygen gives only a *global* value. Regional differences in tissue oxygenation are not recognized. However, local changes may be of considerable importance considering the physiological difference of blood flow and oxygen demand of various brain areas. Nevertheless, the present global values for cerebral oxygen consumption fit well with experimental investigations which were devoted to the energy metabolism of the brain in hypoxic hypoxia and profound hypocapnia. It has been shown that in the presence of an aPO_2 of 25 and an $aPCO_2$ of 20 Torr respectively the production of energy rich phosphate bounds such as ATP and CrP is not or only slightly disturbed (4, 10, 11). Whereas controlled moderate hypocapnia may be a help in combating intracranial hypertension, hypoxemic reactive cerebral hyperemia should be regarded with caution, because due to raised intracranial blood volume it may be a considerable pressure rising factor (5), in particular in the presence of space occupying lesions, which have not yet led to decompensated intracranial pressure. It is well known that in marked brain edema hypoxic cerebral vasodilatation with cerebral hyperemia as an emergency reaction is no longer elicited. One may assume that one important factor for producing intracranial plateau waves as discussed by LUNDBERG and associates (8) is hypoxic cerebral vasodilatation in those areas of the brain which are still susceptible to the hypoxic vascular stimulus. This, again, would support the daily clinical experience that adaptive mechanisms which virtually serve for a physiological homeostasis may readily be converted into the opposite effect when other interfering pathogenetic factors are present.

REFERENCES

1. BERNSMEIER, A., SIEMONS, K.: Die Messung der Hirndurchblutung mit der Stickoxydulmethode. Pflügers Arch. ges. Physiol. 258, 149-162 (1953).

2. COHEN, P.J., WOLLMAN, H., ALEXANDER, S.C.: Cerebral carbohydrate metabolism in man during halothane anesthesia. Effects of $PaCO_2$ on some aspects of carbohydrate utilization. Anesthesiol. 25, 185-191 (1964).

3. COHEN, P.J., ALEXANDER, S.C., SMITH, T.S.: Effects of hypoxia and normocarbia on cerebral blood flow and metabolism in conscious man. J. appl. Physiol. 23, 183-189 (1967).

4. GRANHOLM, L., SIESJÖ, B.K.: The effects of hypercapnia and hypocapnia upon the cerebrospinal fluid lactate and pyruvate concentrations and upon the lactate, pyruvate, ATP, ADP, phosphocreatine and creatine concentrations of cat brain tissue. Acta physiol. scand. 75, 257-266 (1969).

5. HAMER, J., ALBERTI, E., HOYER, S.: Effects of arterial hypoxemia, hypercapnia and changes in cerebral perfusion pressure on mean CSF and sagittal sinus pressure. Acta neurochir. 30, 167-179 (1974).

6. KETY, S.S., SCHMIDT, C.F.: The effects of altered arterial tensions of carbon dioxide and oxygen on cerebral blood flow and cerebral oxygen consumption of normal young men. J. of Clin. Invest. 27, 484-492 (1948).

7. KOGURE, K., SCHEINBERG, P., REINMUTH, O.M.: Mechanisms of cerebral vasodilatation in hypoxia. J. appl. Physiol. 29, 223-229 (1970).

8. LUNDBERG, N., CRONQUIST, S., KJÄLLQUIST, A.: Clinical investigations on interrelations between intracranial pressure and intracranial hemodynamics. Brain Res. 30, 69-75 (1968).

9. NOELL, W., SCHNEIDER, M.: Über die Durchblutung und die Sauerstoffversorgung des Gehirns im akuten Sauerstoffmangel. I. Die Gehirndurchblutung. Pflügers Arch. ges. Physiol. 246, 181-249 (1942).

10. NORBERG, K., SIESJÖ, B.K.: Cerebral metabolism in hypoxic hypoxia. I. Pattern of activation of glycolysis, a re-evaluation. Brain Res. 86, 31-44 (1975).

11. SIESJÖ, B.K., NILSSON, L.: The influence of arterial hypoxemia upon labile phosphates and upon extracellular and intracellular lactate and pyruvate concentrations in the rat brain. Scand. J. Clin. Lab. Investig. 27, 83-96 (1971).

12. WOLLMAN, H., ALEXANDER, S.C., COHEN, P.J.: Cerebral circulation of man during halothane anesthesia. Effects of hypocarbia and of d-tubocurarine. Anesthesiol. 25, 180-184 (1964).

13. WOLLMAN, H., SMITH, T.C., STEPHEN, G.W.: Effects of extremes of respiratory and metabolic alkalosis on cerebral blood flow in man. J. appl. Physiol. 24, 60-65 (1968).

Development and Time Course of Blood Brain Barrier Disturbances Caused by Hypoxia

W. GOBIET, L. PIASZEK, and W. SCHUMACHER

Recent investigations have shown that various pathological factors can cause break down of the blood-brain barrier (BBB). This is followed by the appearance of protein-rich, high molecular exudate in the extravascular space (2, 7, 8). Ischaemia (5), osmotic changes (12), arterial hypertension (6), toxic substances (4, 10) and arterial hypoxia (11, 3) have been named as precipitating factors.

The aim of our investigation was to examine the development and time course of hypoxic disturbances of the BBB by continuous registration.

Labelled 125-jodine albumin was used as an indicator for disturbed BBB.

Method

Experiments were carried out on 30 rabbits under general anaesthesia. All animals were passively ventilated.

Following values were recorded:

(1) Cerebral blood flow (CBF) on the arteria carotis interna by an electromagnetic flowmeter.

(2) Impulse rate of intravenous given 125-jodine-albumin through a fronto-temporal burr hole over the right hemisphere.

(3) Arterial and venous blood pressure.

(4) EEG.

(5) Rectal temperature.

Blood gases and arterial 125-jodine-albumin concentration were checked every 30 minutes and at the beginning and at the end of the hypoxia phases. Hypoxia was induced through breathing in a closed system.

The impulse rate of the radioactive tracer depends on the blood concentration, blood pressure, cerebral blood flow and cerebral 125-jodine-albumin uptake.

Knowing BP, CBF and blood concentration of the tracer, impulse rate changes over the hemisphere without altering the other factors reflect cerebral 125-jodine-albumin uptake, which indicates disturbed BBB.

In this way, continuous registration is possible

Results

The following investigations were carried out:

(1) Hypoxia for 1, 2, 3, and 6 minutes.

(2) Increased intracranial pressure (ICP) between 50 and 60 mm Hg together with a local lesion produced by an epidural balloon blown up for 45 minutes to an ICP between 40-50 mm Hg.

(3) Local lesion for 45 minutes followed immediately by hypoxia for 6 minutes.

For control the same parameters were registered in 4 animals as blind trials. Here impulse rate and the blood concentration of the radioactive tracer remained constant while CBF and BP showed a slight tendency to fall.

Hypoxia up to 3 minutes also had no significant effect on cerebral 125-jodine-albumin uptake. Here the blood gases showed a clear fall of O_2 and PH after about 2 minutes.

Hypoxia for 6 minutes produced still more pronounced changes in the blood gases. (PO_2 from 93,9 to 14,2, PCO_2 from 38,5 to 46,9 mm Hg and PH from 7,45 to 7,27 on the average).

The impulse rate attained a maximum directly after the end of hypoxia (Fig. 1). It fell slightly after about 1/2 hour. About 1 1/2 hours later 125-jodine-albumin uptake still increased. Mean values of counter rate were now higher than the initial levels. The blood concentration of 125-jodine-albumin remained constant. CBF and BP fell slightly. We found a similar course after local trauma by the epidural balloon. Here, however, the 1/2 hour and 1 1/2 hour values for the cerebral uptake of 125-jodine-albumin were equal (Fig. 2). Also here the 1 1/2 hours mean values were higher than initial levels of counter rate. Blood concentration, CBF and BP were similar to those of the hypoxia trial.

The most marked increase in cerebral uptake of 125-jodine-albumin was found after combined local trauma and hypoxia. Here the rise in impulse rate was distinctly higher than of the previous trials Fig. 3. Blood concentration and CBF remained equal, BP fell slightly.

Discussion

By continuous registration of the cerebral uptake of 125-jodine-albumin it could be shown that both hypoxia for more than 6 minutes and also raised ICP combined with a local lesion to lead to disturbance of the blood-brain barrier with an extravascular leakage of serum proteins. An increased cerebral 125-jodine-albumin uptake was already found during the impairment and was still demonstrable 1 1/2 hours later with no tendency to normalize. Since the other parameters measured did not alter significantly, the increase in impulse rate corresponds to the cerebral uptake of 125-jodine-albumin. It is consequently a measure for the degree of BBB disturbance.

The combined action of hypoxia and local trauma, according to our observations adds the effects of the individual factors on the BBB. It is also remarkable that in all trials, break down of the BBB were already observed in a very early phase, i.e. still during the hypoxia phases or the local trauma.

As has been emphasised by different authors (9, 1), the opening of
the BBB with the appearance of protein-rich extravasate is to be
considered as one of the precipitating factors for the development
of vasogenic cerebral edema. According to our observations, in clinical condition the development of cerebral edema could be promoted by
the break down of BBB either by arterial hypoxia or a local trauma.
This might be given i.e. in the shock phase of severe head injury.
The unfavorable initial position might, however, consist in the coincidence of arterial hypoxia, local damage and raised ICP, because
here the BBB disturbances have been shown to be still more pronounced.

Summary

By continuous registration of the impulse rate of intravenously given
125-jodine-albumin could be shown, that hypoxia over 6 minutes, as
well as local trauma leads to a disturbance of BBB.

Combined hypoxia and local trauma adds the effect of the individual
factors.

REFERENCES

1. BRIGHTMAN, M.W., REESE, T.S.: Junctions between intimately ap-
   posed cell membranes in the vertebrate brain. J. Cell Biol. 40,
   648-677 (1969).

2. CLASEN, R.A., SKY-PECK, H.H., PANDOLFI, S., LAING, I., HASS,
   G.M.: The chemistry of isolated edema fluid in experimental cerebral injury. In: Brain edema (eds. I.KLATZKO, F.SEITELBERGER)
   pp. 536-553. Wien-New York: Springer 1972.

3. CUTLER, R.W.P., BARLOW, C.F.: The effect of hypercapnia on brain
   permeability to protein. Arch. Neurol. 14, 54-63 (1966).

4. FLODMARK, S., STEINWALL, O.: Differentiated effects on certain
   blood-brain barrier phenomena and on the EEG produced by means of
   intracarotidally applied mercuric dichloride. Acta physiol.
   scand. 57, 446-453 (1963).

5. HOSSMAN, K.A., OLSON, Y.: Influence of ischemia on the passage of
   protein tracers across capillaries in certain blood-barrier injuries. Acta neuropath. 18, 113-122 (1971).

6. JOHANSSON, B., LI, C.L., OLSSON, Y., KLATZKO, I.: The effect of
   acute arterial hypertension on the blood-brain barrier to protein
   tracers. Acta neuropath. 16, 117-124 (1970).

7. KARCHER, D., LOWENTHAL, A.: Hydrosoluble proteins of edematous
   human nervous tissue. In: Brain edema (eds. I.KLATZKO, F.SEITEL-
   BERGER), pp. 195-201. Wien-New York: Springer 1967.

8. KIYOTA, K.: Electrophoretic protein factions and the hydro-
   property of brain tissue. II.J.Neurochem. 4, 209-216 (1959).

9. KLATZKO, I.: Pathophysiological Aspects of Brain Edema. In:
   Steroids and brain edema (eds. H.J.REULEN, K.SCHÜRMANN) p.1.
   Berlin-Heidelberg-New York 1972.

10. MAJNO, G., PALADE, G.E.: Studies on inflammation. I. The effect
    of histamine and serotonin on vascular permeability: An electron
    microscopic study. J.biophys.bioche.Cytol. 11, 571-605 (1961).

11. MOSSAKOWSKI, M.J., LONG, D.M., MYERS, R.E., RODRIGUEZ, H., KLATZKO, I.: Early histochemical changes in perinatal asphyxia. J.Neuropath.exp.Neurol. <u>27</u>, 500-516 (1968).

12. RAPOPORT, S.I., HORI, M., KLATZKO, I.: Reversible osmotic opening of the blood-brain barrier. Science <u>173</u>, 1026-1028 (1971).

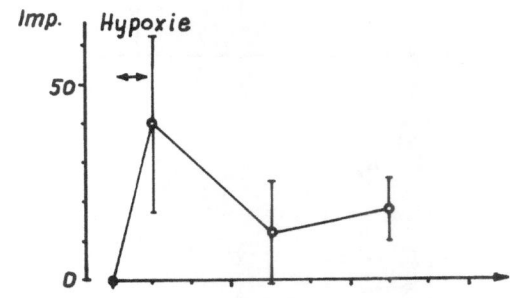

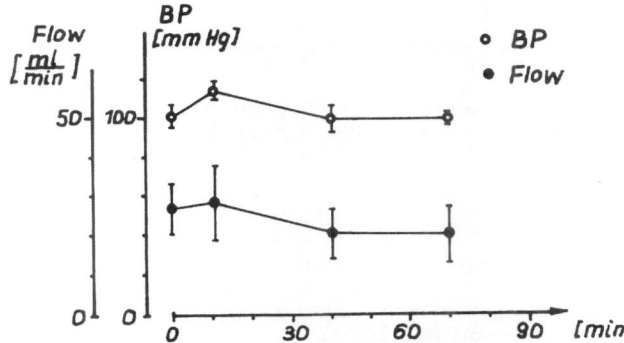

Fig. 1. Increasing Impulse Rate over the Hemisphere reflects the progressive brain 125-Jod-Albumin uptake and therefore BBB disturbance caused by hypoxia over 6 min. There are two tops, one at the end of the hypoxia phase, the second after 90 minutes.
Abbreviations: Imp = Impulse Rate difference of intravenous given 125-Jod-Albumin recorded at 24 sec intervalls. Starting values were taken as zero. BP = Mean blood pressure, Flow = cerebral blood flow

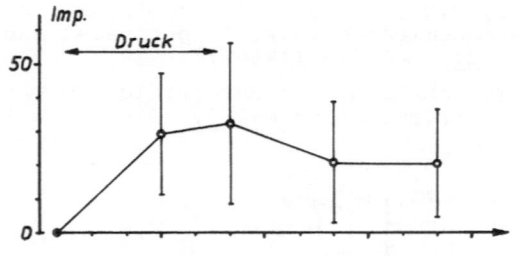

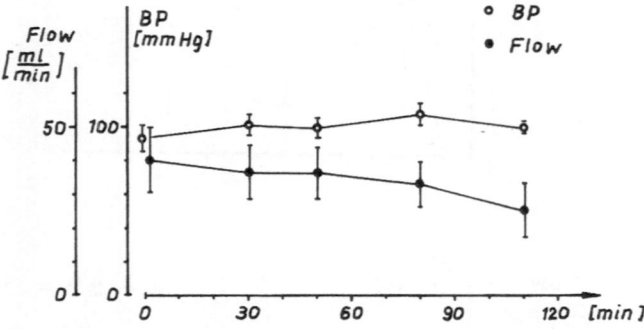

Fig. 2. Local trauma by an epidural balloon inflated for 45 minutes
leads also to an BBB disturbance, shown by an increase of cerebral
125-Jod-Albumin uptake   (Abbreviations see Fig.1)

Fig. 3. Highest values
of cerebral 125-Jod-Al-
bumin uptake were found
after combined local
trauma and hypoxia. Here
BBB disturbances was
more marked than after
hypoxia or local trauma
alone

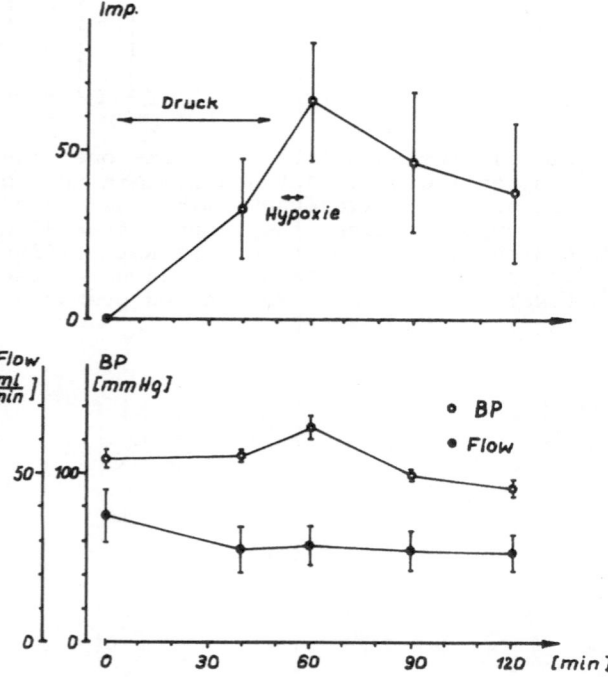

The Influence of Ventricular Perfusion on Normal Brain

R. SCHUBERT, A. FENSKE, J. GROTE, and H. J. REULEN

The prognosis and final outcome in patients with severe head injuries is closely related, among other factors, to the level of increased intracranial pressure (ICP) caused by cerebral edema as well
as to the severity of CSF lactacidosis. There exists evidence that
a clearance of substances which accumulate in edematous tissue, i.e.
proteins and lactate, without rising the ICP exerts a beneficial
effect in such cases. Previous studies by other groups (4, 5) using
a similar experimental technique but with small amounts of perfusion-
volume were concerned with the influence of various concentrations
of bicarbonate of the perfusion medium on the regulation mechanisms
of cerebral blood flow (CBF). The present study was carried out to
investigate the effect of a ventriculo-cisternal perfusion with a
flow volume leading to a ten to twelve timefold exchange of the
intraventricular cerebro-spinal fluid (CSF) volume on the normal
cerebral blood flow.

Methods

In 18 cats anaesthetized and artificially ventialted catheters were
placed in the femoral artery and vein for continously recording of
the arterial blood pressure (MABP) and drug injection respectively.
The right lateral ventricle and the cisterna magna were punctured
for ventriculo-cisternal perfusion and measuring of ICP. A small
catheter was inserted into the superior sagittal sinus for pressure
recording and withdrawing venous blood samples. The artificial CSF
had an ionic composition and osmolarity similar to the cats CSF except the absence of proteins (2) and was equilibrated with 4% and
8% CO_2 respectively. The perfusion rate was set to 1.2-1.5 ml/min.
pH, pCO_2, pO_2 were estimated in the arterial and cerebral venous
blood as well as in the CSF, and in the perfusion medium before and
after ventricular passage. Regional cerebral blood flow (rCBF) was
measured using the ^{85}Kr clearance technique in 8 animals, and in 10
aniamls by means of the ^{133}Xe method on the parieto-occipital region
of the perfused hemisphere in intervals of 30 minutes. Autoregulation was tested before and after the duration of the perfusion. At
the end of the experiments tissue samples from grey and white matter
were taken from the brain to measure the water content. Lactate and
pyruvate were estimated in arterial and venous samples as well as in
the perfusion outflow.

Results

The main results of our experimental studies are shown in form of a
diagram (Fig. 1). Artificial CSF was equilibrated with 4% CO_2 at the
beginning of the perfusion period and with 8% CO_2 after 90 minutes.

The two upper scales show CO_2 and pH. The PCO_2 of the artificial CSF is about 30 mmHg during the first perfusion period and rises to more than 50 mmHg throughout the second perfusion period. $PaCO_2$ remains constant at 28 - 30 mmHg in the course of the whole experiment. However, in the venous blood of the sinus sagittalis superior an increase of PCO_2, starting from 41 mmHg to finally 47 mmHg, was observed. In accordance with a rise of PCO_2 in the artificial CSF, pH decreases under equilibration with 8% CO_2 in the influent and effluent perfusion medium by approx. 0.3, whereas arterial pH remains unchanged. MABP is not affected either. The broken line shows rCBF measurements with the ^{133}Xe clearance technique, reflecting a combination of grey and white matter flow. rCBF was also repeatedly measured by means of the ^{85}Kr clearance method, i.e. cortical flow, on an area over the right suprasylvian gyrus under a perfusion period of 90 minutes while the perfusion medium was eqilibrated with 4% CO_2. It is interesting to notice that even in the phase of increased PCO_2, respectively decreased pH, changes of the rCBF did not occur, neither in the grey nor in the white matter.

The resulting $CMRO_2$ was 8.34 $\pm$ 0.93 for the grey matter, 2.33 $\pm$ 0.04 for the white matter and remained unaffected during the whole experimental procedure. The second autoregulation test after a perfusion period of 3 hours demonstrates the undamaged reactivity of the cerebral vessels after a mean perfusion volume of 420 ml. Water content of the grey and white matter was unchanged in the perfused as well as in the unperfused hemisphere. The intraventricular pressure was 4.7 mmHg $\pm$ 0.25 and 2.4 mmHg $\pm$ 0.2 in the superior sagittal sinus. Lactate concentration in CSF was 1.937 mmol/l H_2O at the beginning and subsided to 0.643 mmol/l H_2O at the end of the experiment (t=3.4103^{++}). Pyruvate was 0.216 mmol/l H_2O in the native CSF and 0.038 mmol/l H_2O in the effluent perfusion medium (t=8.28334^{+++}). However, lactate and pyruvate concentration did not decrease, neither in the arterial nor in the cerebral venous blood.

Comments and Summary

A ventricular-cisternal perfusion of 3 hours maintaining a high perfusion rate has no harmful effect on the normal undamaged brain. Moreover no changes are observed during an increased PCO_2 to 50 mmHg in the artificial CSF. Intracranial pressure remains unchanged, too. On the other hand lactate and pyruvate concentrations are significantly diminished.

METZEL et al. (3) showed that the intrathecal administration of sodium bicarbonate is a possible direct method of normalizing a CSF acidosis in patients. Clearance of edema proteins of the edematous tissue using a supracortical perfusion has been demonstrated by MATSEN et al. in experimental studies. (1) Ventriculo-cisternal perfusion might provide another possibility in the treatment of severely progressing brain edema which resists against conventional therapy.

REFERENCES

1. MATSEN III, F.A., C.R. WEST: Supracortical fluid: a monitor of albumin exchange in normal and injured brain. Amer. J. Physiol. 222, 532-539 (1972)

2. MERLIS, J.K.: The effect of changes in the calcium content of the cerebrospinal fluid on spinal reflex activity in the dog. Amer. J. Physiol. 131, 67-72 (1940).

3. METZEL, E., H. SCHRADER, D. SEITZ, M. HIRSCHAUER, H. ZIMMERMANN, W.E. ZIMMERMANN, F. MUNDINGER: Treatment of cerebral acidosis in post-traumatic and postoperative cerebral edema. Influence on CBF, EEG, and clinical status. In: Brain edema (eds. K. SCHÜRMANN, M. BROCK, H.J. REULEN, D. VOTH), p. 146. Berlin-Heidelberg New York: Springer 1973

4. PANNIER, J.L., WEYNE, J., DEMESTER, G., LEUSEN, I.: Influence of changes in the acid-base composition of the ventricular symptoms on cerebral blood flow in cats. Pflügers Arch. 333, 337-351 (1972)

5. SIESJÖ, B.K., KJÄLLQUIST, A., PONTEN, U., ZWETNOW, N.: Extracellular pH in the brain and cerebral blood flow. In: Brain res. 30 (ed. W. LUYENDIJK), p. 93. Amsterdam-London-New York: Elsevier 1968.

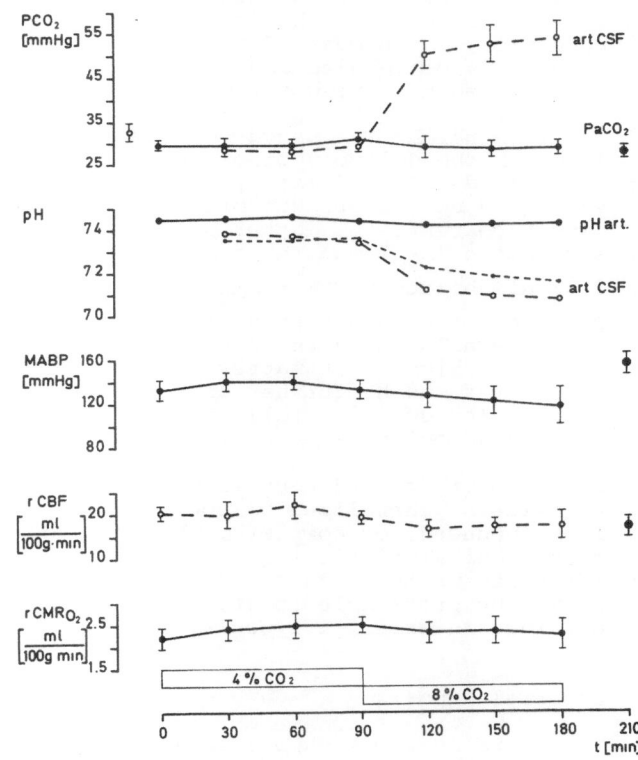

Fig. 1. Changes of PCO_2, pH, MABP, rCBF and $CMRO_2$ during perfusion. 1. period: equilibration of the artificial CSF with 4% CO_2, second period with 8% CO_2. PCO_2 scale: The isolated open circle: average of PCO_2 in the native CSF. pH scale: upper broken line for the effluent, lower broken line for the influent perfusion medium. Isolated spots: Values of $PaCO_2$, MABP and rCBF of the final autoregulation test

Biochemical Aspects of Cerebral Hypoxia

B. K. Siesjö

Introduction

In the following, an outline is given of cerebral energy metabolism
in hypoxia. Since this subject is a large one, and since the outline
must be brief, only the main biochemical aspects will be covered. By
necessity, the number of references will be small. Readers interested
in details of results and in original references are recommended to
consult recent review articles (20, 5, 29, 30, 31, 21).

The term *cerebral hypoxia* is commonly used to denote all situations
in which the delivery of oxygen to brain cells is insufficient for
their needs. This delivery ("oxygen availability") is convenniently
expressed as the product of cerebral blood flow (CBF) and arterial
oxygen content, the latter being determined by the percentage oxygen
saturation (S_{O_2}) and the hemoglobin (Hb) concentration

$$O_2 \text{ availability} = CBF \cdot S_{O_2} \cdot [Hb].$$

There are two main causes of cerebral hypoxia: (1) *ischemia*, in which
oxygen availability is reduced due to fall in CBF, and (2) *arterial
hypoxia*, which is characterized by a fall in arterial oxygen content.
The latter can be further divided into *hypoxic hypoxia* (the saturation is low due to a fall in Pa_{O_2}) and *anemic hypoxia* (there is a
reduced hemoglobin content).

In neurosurgery and neurology, the most common cause of cerebral
hypoxia is generalized or focal ischemia. However, when the ischemia
is pronounced, or complete, there is not only oxygen lack in the
tissue but also deficiency of substrates, and incomplete removal of
metabolic waste products (CO_2, ammonia, lactic acid). For that reason,
it may be profitable to start the discussion by considering results
obtained in arterial hypoxia.

Arterial Hypoxia

There are numerous experimantal results and clinical observations to
show that even a relatively moderate hypoxic hypoxia leads to symptoms of cerebral oxygen lack. Concomitantly, there are biochemical
changes that can be attributed to cellular hypoxia. Thus, when the
Pa_{O_2} is reduced below about 50 mm Hg there is stimulation of glycolytic rate with accumulation of lactate and pyruvate, and cellular
redox systems change towards a more reduced state. Secondary to the
elevated pyruvate concentration, and the redox change, there occur
a gradual increase in the citric acid cycle pool, and amino acid
changes dominated by increases in alanine and GABA, and by a reduction in aspartate (8, 22, 23). These changes, and the reduced rates
of synthesis of catechol and indole amine neurotransmitters (6, 7)
may contribute to the symptomatology of hypoxic hypoxia.

Although biochemical changes affecting carbohydrate intermediates and amino acids occur at moderate degrees of hypoxic hypoxia, even pronounced hypoxia can be tolerated without causing a detectable change in the concentrations of ATP, ADP and AMP ("energy state"). In all probability, this energy homeostasis is entirely due to the increase in CBF which occurs within seconds after the induction of hypoxia, and which may amount to 400 - 600% of normal at pronounced degrees of hypoxia (13, 1). Contrary to previous beliefs, recent results suggest that the increase in CBF is *not* caused by cellular production of lactic acid but that a neurogenic mechanism may be involved (24, 32). From a clinical point of view it is of interest that, during hypoxia, CBF varies passively with perfusion pressure. Thus, if there is a fall in blood pressure, or obstruction of a major cerebral vessel, energy balance is upset and neuronal damage can result (28, 25, 26).

Like uncomplicated hypoxic hypoxia, anemic hypoxia is characterized by a pronounced energy homeostasis which is due to an increase in CBF. In the rat, reduction in the Hb content to $3 \ g \cdot (100 \ ml)^{-1}$ gives a fivefold increase in CBF but no changes in cerebral oxygen consumption and there are few, if any, changes in cerebral metabolites (2, 14). In all probability, the low viscosity contributes to the increase in CBF, and it appears that even a drastic reduction in arterial oxygen content can be tolerated by the brain provided that an adequate perfusion pressure can be upheld (*c. f.* hypoxic hypoxia).

Ischemia

There are three main types of biochemical changes in the tissue during *complete ischemia*: anoxia, substrate deficiency and accumulation of metabolic waste products. Since the oxygen stores of the tissue only suffice for a few seconds of uninterrupted oxidative metabolism, aerobic energy production quickly ceases. When this occurs, the tissue can only obtain energy by utilizing its stores of ATP and phosphocreatine (PCr), and by metabolizing glucose and glycogen anaerobically to lactic acid. The total amount of energy ($\Delta \sim P$) that can be made available is given by the approximate equation (18).

$$\Delta \sim P = 2 \cdot \Delta ATP + \Delta PCr + 2\Delta glucose + 3\Delta glycogen.$$

In the rat cerebral cortex, the normal rate of $\sim P$ utilization is about $30 \ \mu mol \cdot g^{-1} \cdot min^{-1}$ and the stores of ATP, PCr, glucose and glycogen only suffice for about 1 min of uninterrupted utilization. However, since the rate of utilization falls during ischemia, complete energy depletion does not occur until after about 5 min (15). In the human brain the normal rate of energy utilization is lower but, since also the energy stores are smaller, the end point may be reached in a comparable period of time. The rate of energy use is decreased by anaesthesia and hypothermia. As an example: surgical anaesthesia with barbiturates and a lowering of body temperature by $10^{o}C$ both reduce $\sim P$ utilization to 50% of normal.

Energy depletion in the tissue is not synonymous with cell death. Certain brain functions may return even if the ischemia is prolonged for 30 - 60 min, at least during barbiturate anaesthesia (11, 12, 10). In rats, studied under nitrous oxide anaesthesia, the energy state of the cerebral cortex returns to near-normal values after 15 min of complete ischemia (16) and few neurons show ischemic cell changes (3). Futhermore, *in vitro* studies of mitochondria isolated from ischemic brains show that oxidative phosphorylation is not impaired until after about 30 min of circulatory interruption (27). These results demonstrate that brain cells may survive extensive periods of oxygen (and glucose) lack provided that there are optimal conditions for restitution. Usually, functional restitution is much slower than recovery of energy metabolism. It is conceivable that this may, at least partly, be due to "transmission failure" since there is a lingering perturbation in the metabolism of amino acids (9) and of indole- and catecholamines (4).

From a clinical point of view the most important condition is represented by *incomplete ischemia*. In this condition, though, the tissue changes are usually inhomogeneous hence the type and extent of metabolic abnormalities are not easy to define. Incomplete ischemia varies in severity from a degree of underperfusion that just barely affects cerebral function and metabolism to almost complete cessation of flow. It is usually recognized that extreme hyperventilation (Pa_{CO_2} < 15 mm Hg) is accompanied by mild tissue hypoxia, mainly manifested as increase in tissue lactate content (see (19)). In this condition, CBF is reduced to about 50% of normal, implying that this reduction in CBF can be tolerated without manifest energy failure, or damage to neurons. However, since the fall in CBF due to hypocapnia is probably homogeneous, it cannot be stated without further proof that tissue damage does not result if CBF is reduced to 50% of normal in other forms of incomplete ischemia. This is due to the fact that if CBF is 50% of normal in a given tissue region, there may be inhomogeneous flow at the capillary level with a larger degree of underperfusion in microflow areas.

Present evidence suggests that with moderate degrees of ischemia the metabolic changes in the tissue resemble those observed in arterial hypoxia (increased rate of glycolysis with elevation of tissue lactate, increased reduction of cellular redox couples, decrease in PCr, and minor changes in adenine nucleotides). With more pronounced degrees of ischemia, however, the supply of substrate becomes insufficient and tissue glucose levels fall. In general, incomplete ischemia may be associated with a more pronounced degree of lactic acidosis than is complete ischemia since glucose is continously carried to the tissue via the blood. Thus, it is not uncommon to find lactate levels of 40 μmol $\cdot$ g^{-1} in the tissue in cases of *e.g.* hemorrhagic hypotension. During complete ischemia, it has been possible to vary the degree of lactic acidosis by means of previous hypo- or hyperglycemia, and these experiments suggest that the lactic acidosis does not influence recovery of energy metabolism (17). The influence of even more massive acidosis is not known.

Present evidence suggests that any incomplete ischemia leads to an inhomogeneous decrease in CBF and that the tendency towards inhomogeneity is exaggerated by tissue acidosis, *e. g.* due to hypercapnia. In such situations there may be derangement of tissue energy metabolism in spite of a normal, or higher than normal, cerebral venous P_{O_2}. The results emphasize the difficulty of studying CBF and cerebral metabolism in incomplete ischemia, and of evaluating the oxygenation of the brain by any other method than direct tissue analyses.

Acknowledgements

This study was supported by grants from the Swedish Medical Research Council (Projects No. 14X - 263 and 14X - 2179), from the Swedish Tercentenary Fund, and from U.S. PHS Grant No. RO1 NSO 7838 - O6 from NIH.

REFERENCES

1. BORGSTRÖM, L., JOHANNSSON, H., SIESJÖ, B.K.: The relationship between arterial P_{O_2} and cerebral blood flow in hypoxic hypoxia. Acta physiol. scand. (in press).

2. BORGSTRÖM, L., JOHANNSSON, H., SIESJÖ, B.K.: The influence of acute normovolemic anemia on cerebral blood flow and oxygen consumption of anaesthetized rats. Acta physiol. scand. (in press).

3. BRIERLEY, J.B., LJUNGGREN, B., SIESJÖ, B.K.: Neuropathological alterations in rat brain after complete ischemia due to raised intracranial pressure. Proc. 2nd Int. Symp. on Intracranial Pressure, Lund/Sweden 1974 (in press).

4. BROWN, R.M., CARLSSON, A., LJUNGGREN, B., SIESJÖ, B.K., SNIDE, S.R.: Effect of ischemia on monoamine metabolism in the brain. Acta physiol. scand. 90, 789 - 791 (1974).

5. COHEN, P.J.: The metabolic function of oxygen and biochemical lesions of hypoxia. Anesthesiol. 37, 148 - 177 (1972).

6. DAVIS, J.N., CARLSSON, A.: Effect of hypoxia on tyrosine and trypthophan hydroxylation in unanaesthetized rat brain. J. Neurochem. 20, 913 - 915 (1973).

7. DAVIS, J.N., CARLSSON, A., MACMILLAN, V., SIESJÖ, B.K.: Brain tryptophan hydroxylation: Dependence on arterial oxygen tension. Science. 182, 72 - 74 (1973).

8. DUFFY, T.E., NELSON, S.R., LOWRY, O.H.: Cerebral carbohydrate metabolism during acute hypoxia and recovery. J. Neurochem. 19, 959 - 977 (1972).

9. FOLBERGROVÁ, J., LJUNGGREN, B., NORBERG, K., SIESJÖ, B.K.: Influence of complete ischemia on glycolytic metabolites, citric acid cycle intermediates, and associated amino acids in the rat cerebral cortex. Brain Res. 80, 265 - 279 (1974).

10. HINZEN, D.H., MÜLLER, U., SOBOTKA, P., GEBERT, E., LANG, R., HIRSCH, H.: Metabolism and function of dogs brain recovering from longtime ischemia. Amer. J. Physiol. 223, 1158 - 1164 (1972).

11. HOSSMAN, K.-A., SATO, K.: Recovery of neuronal function after prolonged cerebral ischemia. Science. 168, 375 - 376 (1970).

12. HOSSMAN, K.-A., SATO, K.: The effect of ischemia on sensorimotor cortex of the cat: Electrophysiological biochemical and electron-microscopical observations. Z. Neurol. 198, 33 - 45 (1970).

13. JÓHANNSSON, H., SIESJÖ, B.K.: Cerebral blood flow and oxygen consumption in the rat in hypoxic hypoxia. Acta physiol. scand. (in press).

14. JÓHANNSSON, H., SIESJÖ, B.K.: Brain energy metabolism in anaesthetized rats in acute anemia. Acta physiol. scand. (in press).

15. LJUNGGREN, B., SCHUTZ, H., SIESJÖ, B.K.: Changes in energy state and acid-base parameters of the rat brain during complete compression ischemia. Brain Res. 73, 277 - 289 (1974).

16. LJUNGGREN, B., RATCHESON, R.A., SIESJÖ, B.K.: Cerebral metabolic state following complete compression ischemia. Brain Res. 73, 291 - 307 (1974).

17. LJUNGGREN, B., NORBERG, K., SIESJÖ, B.K.: Influence of tissue acidosis upon restitution of brain energy metabolism following total ischemia. Brain Res. 77, 173 - 186 (1974).

18. LOWRY, O.H., PASSONEAU, S.V., HASSELBERGER, F.X., SCHUTZ, D.W.:
    Effect of ischemia on known substrates and cofactors of the
    glycolytic pathway in brain. J. Biol. Chem. _239_, 18 - 30 (1964).

19. MACMILLAN, V., SIESJö, B.K.: The influence of hypocapnia upon
    intracellular pH and upon some carbohydrate substrates, amino
    acids and organic phosphates in the brain. J. Neurochem. _21_,
    1283 - 1299 (1973).

20. MAKER, H.S., LEHRER, G.M.: Effect of ischemia. In: Handbook of
    Neurochemistry, Vol. VI. (ed. A. Lajtha). New York: Plenum Press
    1971.

21. NILSSON, B., NORBERG, K., SIESJö, B.K.: Biochemical events in
    cerebral ischemia. Br. J. Anaesthesia. (in press).

22. NORBERG, K., SIESJö, B.K.: Cerebral metabolism in hypoxic hypoxia.
    I. Pattern of activation of glycolysis; a re-evaluation. Brain
    Res. _86_, 31 - 44 (1975).

23. NORBERG, K., SIESJö, B.K.: Cerebral metabolism in hypoxic hy-
    poxia.II. Citric acid cycle intermediates and associated amino
    acids. Brain Res. _86_, 45 - 55 (1975).

24. PONTE, J., PURVE, M.J.: The role of the carotid body chemorecep-
    tors and carotid sinus baroreceptors in the control of cerebral
    blood vessels. J. Physiol. (Lond.) _237_, 315 - 340 (1974).

25. SALFORD, L.G., PLUM, F., SIESJö, B.K.: Graded hypoxia-oligemia in
    rat brain. I. Biochemical alterations and their implications.
    Arch. Neurol. _29_, 227 - 233 (1973).

26. SALFORD, L.G., PLUM, F., BRIERLEY, J.B.: Graded hypoxia-oligemia
    in rat brain. II. Neuropathological alterations and their impli-
    cations. Arch. Neurol. _29_, 234 - 238 (1973).

27. SCHUTZ, H., SILVERSTEIN, P.R., VAPALAHTI, M., BRUCE, D.A., MELA,
    L., LANGFITT, T.W.: The function of brain mitochondria after in-
    creased intracranial pressure. In: Intracranial Pressure (eds.
    M. BROCK, H. DIETZ), pp. 90 - 95. New York: Springer 1972.

28. SIESJö, B.K., NILSSON, L.: The influence of arterial hypoxemia
    upon labile phosphates and upon extracellular and intracellular
    lactate and pyruvate concentration in the rat brain. Scand. J.
    Clin. Lab. Invest. _27_, 83 - 96 (1971).

29. SIESJö, B.K., PLUM, F.: Pathophysiology of anoxic brain damage.
    In: Biology of Cerebral Dysfunction Vol. 1 (ed. G.E. GAULL),
    pp. 319 - 372. New York: Plenum Press 1972.

30. SIESJö, B.K., JÓHANNSSON, H., LJUNGGREN, B., NORBERG, K.: Brain
    dysfunction in cerebral hypoxia and ischemia. In: Brain Dysfunc-
    tion in Metabolic Disorders (ed. F. PLUM) 7, Vol. 53, pp. 75-112,
    New York: Raven Press 1974.

31. SIESJö, B.K., NORBERG, K., LJUNGGREN, B., SALFORD, L.G.: Hypoxia
    and cerebral metabolism. In: A Basis and Practice of Neuroanaes-
    thesia (ed. E. GORDON), pp. 47 - 82. Exc. Med. Amsterdam 1975.

32. SIESJö, B.K., JÓHANNSSON, H., NORBERG, K., SALFORD, L.G.: Brain
    function, metabolism and blood flow in moderate and severe arte-
    rial hypoxia. Alfred Benzon Symposium VIII. Copenhagen: Munks-
    gaard 1974 (in press).

Cerebral Metabolic Rates as Determinants of Hypoxic Survival of Adult Mice*,**

H. H. BERLET

Survival times of adult mice exposed to moderate though eventually lethal hypoxic hypoxia were recently observed to differ distinctly in relation to the maturational stage of the animals (BERLET, in preparation). Furthermore, a striking increase in hypoxic survival times was exhibited by animals pretreated with 6-aminonicotinamide (5). This compound appears to stimulate the glycolytic flux of neural tissue as judged by a steep rise of lactate levels during ischemic anoxia (13).

The following study was therefore undertaken to find out whether hypoxic survival times of young adult (17) and adult mice or of mice treated with 6-aminonicotinamide (6-AN) are causally related to levels of cerebral constituents or to differences in the rates of consumption of energy reserves in terms of cerebral metabolic rates (CMR). Ischemic anoxia was produced to measure CMR's as originally described by LOWRY et al. (15).

Material and Methods

White male mice (NMRI) fed ad lib. until the time of the experiments were used throughout. Animals weighing 18 to 25g (approximately 5 weeks old) were considered to be young adult (17) while those of 25g and above were rated adult. Hypoxic hypoxia was produced by passing a commercial mixture of $5\%O_2-95\%N_2$ through short pieces of glass tubing housing one animal each (5). Death was noted when the animals stopped gasping. 6-aminonicotinamide (MERCK-Schuchardt, BRD) was given to mice intraperitoneally (35 mg/kg), 6 hours prior to sacrifice or to their exposure to hypoxia.

For the determination of cerebral metabolites animals were frozen whole in liquid N_2. Hypoxic mice were plunged into liquid N_2 directly from their freely movable containers. To obtain total ischemia (15) mice were decapitated and the severed heads allowed to remain at room temperature (25 - 27°C) for 15 or 30 sec., respectively, before being frozen.

Brain hemispheres were chiselled out under liquid N_2 and homogenized by means of a mechanical homogenizer (Ultra Turrax) with 1mM EDTA in 50% ethanol and 0.3M perchloric acid in a sequential manner (6).

*This study was supported by the "Deutsche Forschungsgemeinschaft".

**The skilful technical assistance of Ms. I. Bonsmann and Mrs. N. Blenck is gratefully acknowledged.

Analytical Methods: Free creatine and total creatine and, by difference, phosphocreatine (PC) of acidic extracts were determined colori-
metrically as described (6) whereas neutral extracts were employed
for the spectrophotometric determinations of ATP, ADP, AMP, glucose,
6-phosphogluconate, glycogen, pyruvate and lactate by enzyme methods
(4). All biochemicals were purchased from Boehringer, Mannheim.

Results

Survival times of young adult and adult mice breathing $5\%O_2-95\%N_2$ are
shown in Fig. 1 along with data of animals treated with 6-AN. In
general, young animals were tolerating hypoxic hypoxia much longer
before death occurred than adult animals ($p<0.01$). The two groups of
untreated mice differed in age by 2 to 3 weeks only as the young
adult mice were still in a state of rapid body growth. A profound
prolongation of survival times was found in 6-AN-treated mice; in
particular, 10 out of 16 animals tested were still alive after 30
min. when the experiment was deliberately discontinued.

Cerebral Metabolism and Developmental State

No differences in levels of pertinent cerebral constituents were
found in normal animals of the two age groups (Table 1). To test the
effect of hypoxia a time interval of 2 min. was chosen since it was
to be anticipated from the foregoing experiments (Fig. 1) that even
the more susceptible adult mice would survive that long. Deviations
from normal levels were significant regarding ATP, ADP, AMP, PC, glucose, glycogen and lactate (Table 2). Quantitatively, they were not
uniform however; thus, AMP rose to higher levels in the adult animals than it did in the younger group. The consumption of PC was
significantly less in younger animals too, with ATP showing a similar trend. The energy charge potentials (ECP; 3) are indicating a
greater loss in ECP in adult than in younger animals ($p<0.01$) although they were significantly lowered in both groups compared to
normoxic values (Table 1).

The differences in cerebral metabolic activities were even more
clearly brought out when the metabolic consequences of total cerebral ischemia were examined (Fig. 2). The overall pattern is again
consistent with lower CMR's in young animals. In particular, there
is a striking discrepancy between levels of ATP and AMP by 30 s. of
ischemia in the presence of comparable values of lactate.

Cerebral Metabolism and 6-AN

The administration of 6-AN resulted in significant increases of
cerebral glucose and acid-soluble glycogen while residual glycogen
and lactate fell well below adult control levels (Table 1). 6-
Phosphogluconate whose level rose threefold serves to demonstrate
the effective inhibition of the pentose phosphate shunt by 6-AN.
Hypoxia was not nearly as effective in 6-AN-treated mice as in adult
controls (Table 2) although some response is indicated by significant though lesser changes of PC and lactate.

The response of the 6-AN-group to ischemia was altogether less pronounced than that of the controls (Fig. 3). The breakdown of ATP was
not only much slower but seemed also to level off after 30 s of ischemia, while PC kept falling to approach ischemic control values.

Table 1. Cerebral energy reserves and associated compounds in young adult (< 25 g), adult (> 30 g) and adult mice treated with 6-AN

	Young adult	Adult	Adult, 6-AN-treated
ATP	2.26 ± 0.27	2.39 ± 0.15	2.49 ± 0.31
ADP	0.266 ± 0.083	0.372 ± 0.096	0.415 ± 0.105
AMP	0.042 ± 0.012	0.052 ± 0.013	0.083 ± 0.039[d]
Total AN	2.675 ± 0.342	2.751 ± 0.146	2.988 ± 0.395
ECP[a]	0.914 ± 0.015	0.914 ± 0.018	0.903 ± 0.018
Phosphocreatine	3.56 ± 0.26	3.47 ± 0.26	3.40 ± 0.20
Creatine, free	6.11 ± 0.22[e]	7.02 ± 0.28	5.28 ± 0.26[e]
Glucose	2.13 ± 0.14	1.97 ± 0.21	3.02 ± 0.73 (6)[e]
Glycogen, residual[b]	3.27 ± 0.13 (4)[e]	2.99 ± 0.33 (4)	2.22 ± 0.24 (6)[c,e]
Pyruvate	0.175 ± 0.034 (4)	0.178 ± 0.042	0.129 ± 0.019 (6)[d]
Lactate	2.46 ± 0.30 (4)	2.62 ± 0.21 (4)	0.69 ± 0.38 (6)[e]
6-Phosphogluconate	-	0.342 ± 0.021 (6)	1.033 ± 0.170[e]

Unless otherwise indicated in parentheses values are means ± S.D. obtained from 8 animals, expressed as μmoles/g wet weight except for the dimensionless ECP.

[a]ECP: Energy Charge Potential (3): (ATP) + 0.5(ADP)/(ATP) + (ADP) + (AMP).

[b]Perchloric acid precipitates were dissolved in 1.2 ml 5N KOH for the analysis of residual glycogen (20).

[c]In some instances supernatants were analysed for acid-soluble glycogen as well and found to contain amounts equivalent to 3.49 ± 0.58 (4) in adult mice and 5.03 ± 0.80 (6) μmoles/g wet weight in adult 6-AN-treated mice (p<0.01); however, the means of total glycogen of 6.48 ± 0.87 and 7.25 ± 0.86 μmoles/g wet weight were not significantly different.

[d]p<0.05 according to Student's t-test.   [e]p<0.01.

61

Table 2. Cerebral energy reserves and associated compounds of mice exposed to hypoxic hypoxia for 2 min

	Young adult (8)	Adult (8)	Adult/6-AN (4)
ATP	2.19 ± 0.32	1.82 ± 0.55[a]	2.43 ± 0.18[c]
ADP	0.540 ± 0.076[a]	0.489 ± 0.095[b]	0.542 ± 0.034[b]
AMP	0.078 ± 0.019[a,d]	0.357 ± 0.060[a]	0.078 ± 0.011[d]
Total AN	2.723 ± 0.356	2.615 ± 0.463	3.044 ± 0.186
ECP	0.866 ± 0.035[a,d]	0.780 ± 0.076[a]	0.886 ± 0.007[d]
Phosphocreatine	2.41 ± 0.21[a,d]	1.95 ± 0.30[a]	2.35 ± 0.14[a,c]
Creatine, free	6.21 ± 0.17[d]	7.06 ± 0.59	7.32 ± 0.10[d]
Glucose	0.89 ± 0.15[a]	0.72 ± 0.25[a]	2.34 ± 0.19[d]
Glycogen, residual	2.22 ± 0.19 (5)[a]	2.40 ± 0.21 (5)[a]	1.93 ± 0.32 (5)[c,e]
Pyruvate	0.301 ± 0.030[a]	0.316 ± 0.021 (5)[a]	0.168 ± 0.019[a,d]
Lactate	8.81 ± 1.00[a]	9.04 ± 1.13[a]	5.45 ± 0.38[a,d]
6-Phosphogluconate	–	–	1.123 ± 0.061

Number of animals in parentheses; values are means ± S.D. expressed as μmoles/g wet weight. Levels of significance were calculated according to Student's t-test for differences between normoxia (Table 1) and hypoxia ([a]p<0.01. [b]p<0.05) and for differences between hypoxic results in adult mice compared to those in young adult and 6-AN-treated mice, respectively ([c]p<0.05. [d]p<0.01).

[e]Total glycogen decreased from 7.25 ± 0.86 to 2.93 ± 0.62 μmoles/g in mice treated with 6-AN during hypoxia (p<0.01).

Similarly to ATP, glucose and insoluble glycogen were utilized much less rapidly. Metabolic breakdown products including AMP and lactate accumulated to a much lesser extent, although the increases of lactate from normoxia to anoxia were not as different, i.e. 5.5 μmoles in untreated and 4.0 μmoles/g x 30s in treated animals. Still, when the amount of ~P utilized during ischemic anoxia was calculated from the consumption of ATP, PC, glucose and glycogen (15) clearly different values of 10.6 μmoles in controls and 7.4 μmoles in 6-AN animals were obtained for the first 15s. A somewhat smaller, though still striking difference between CMR's was found when the utilization of soluble glycogen was also taken into account (BERLET, unpublished).

Discussion

From the results, particularly those based on ischemic anoxia, an inverse relationship between hypoxic tolerance and CMR's becomes apparent. In untreated mice the tolerance decreases from a state of young adulthood to full maturity when the available cerebral energy sources are used up most rapidly. Conversely, the increased hypoxia tolerance of animals treated with 6-AN was associated with a distinctly depressed cerebral energy metabolism.

A very rapid increase in metabolic demands of developing brain occurs during the first 10 postnatal days in mice (15, 17, 22), while the ability of newborn mice to withstand anoxia for extended periods of time decreases (11, 21). The activity of cerebral metabolism rises further in mice between 10 days and 6 weeks of age (17, 22), the animals of the latter age group being considered young adult with body weights of 18 - 22g (17).

The results of this study show that the full measure of metabolism is not reached until some weeks later, while the hypoxic tolerance keeps waning. As a practical consequence of this observation it follows that adult animals should be used for metabolic experiments rather than young adult ones or those ranging in body weight from 20 - 30g to obtain reproducible and uniform experimental results.

An atmosphere of $5\%O_2-95\%N_2$ was not consistently found to be fatal to adult mice. LIPPMANN (14) reported a hypoxic threshold of 31.9 torr of O_2 in adult rats, equal to about 4% atmospheric O_2, and mice were found to survive in $5\%O_2$ (9), whereas they failed to do so in the hands of others (2). Adaptation to hypoxia may be rapid (1), and unless care is taken to provide for a sudden switch from normoxia to hypoxia as in the present study the full impact of hypoxia on cerebral metabolism may not be obtained. Since the initial changes of some constituents are more or less reversible as hypoxia continues (9, 18) the immediate metabolic response to hypoxia may be missed.

6-AN is a rather specific inhibitor of 6-phosphogluconate dehydrogenase (10), leading to the accumulation of 6-phosphogluconate in nervous tissue, which in turn is competitively inhibiting the enzyme phosphoglucoisomerase (19). A depressed glycolytic flux should conceivably result from these interactions. In fact, low levels of lactate and slow metabolic rates compared to controls resulting from hypoxia and especially from ischemic anoxia are compatible with that assumption. They also agree very well with data reported recently by KAUFMANN & JOHNSON (12) whereas they are at variance with the previous notion of an increased glycolytic flux (13). Still, the considerably improved hypoxic tolerance of animals treated with 6-AN appears to be due to a reduced demand of energy reserves for cerebral metabolism. This is in accord with the view now prevailing, namely, that energy requirements rather than mere levels of energy reserves or the anaerobic generation of ATP are the critical determinants of hypoxic tolerance of the brain (8, 16, 18, 22).

How 6-AN is bringing about this reduced demand for energy is not entirely clear. Enzyme reactions depending on NAD(P) coenzymes other than 6-phosphogluconate dehydrogenase may also be involved (7). Some of the metabolic effects of 6-AN are certainly attributable to hypothermia since body temperature is lowered in treated animals by 2 -3°C (5).

Summary

Hypoxic survival times of adult mice were shorter than those of young adult mice, and they were much longer in adult mice treated with 6-aminonicotinamide. Rates of cerebral consumption of energy during hypoxia and ischemia anoxia, respectively, were inversely related to hypoxic tolerance. The results are in line with the view that the requirement of the brain for energy is the main determinant of the resistance of animals to hypoxia or anoxia.

REFERENCES

1. ADOLPH, E.F.: Kinetics of the adaptation to hypoxia in infant rats. Amer. J. Physiol. 227, 1030-1032 (1974).

2. ARNFRED, I., SECHER, O.: Anoxia and barbiturates. Tolerance to anoxia in mice influenced by barbiturates. Arch. intern. Pharmacodyn. Thér. 139, 67-74 (1962).

3. ATKINSON, D.E.: The energy charge of the adenylate pool as a regulatory parameter. Interaction with feedback modifiers. Biochem. 7, 4030-4034 (1968).

4. BERGMEYER, H.U.: Methoden der enzymatischen Analyse. 3. Aufl., Bd. II. Weinheim: Verlag Chemie 1974.

5. BERLET, H.H.: Effect of 6-amino-nicotinamide on the tolerance of mice to hypoxic hypoxia. Experientia (Basel) 30, 1065-1066 (1974).

6. BERLET, H.H.: Comparative study of various methods for the extraction of free creatine and phosphocreatine from mouse skeletal muscle. Anal. Biochem. 60, 347-357 (1974).

7. COPER, H., NEUBERT, D.: Einfluß von NADP-Analogen auf die Reaktionsgeschwindigkeit einiger NADP-bedürftiger Oxydoreductasen. Biochim. Biophys. Acta (Amst.) 89, 23-32 (1964).

8. DUFFY, T.E., KOHLE, S.J., VANNUCCI, R.C.: Carbohydrate and energy metabolism in perinatal rat brain: Relation to Survival in Anoxia. J. Neurochem. 24, 271-276 (1975).

9. DUFFY, T.E., NELSON, S.R., LOWRY, O.H.: Cerebral carbohydrate metabolism during hypoxia and recovery. J. Neurochem. 19, 959-977 (1972).

10. HERKEN, H., LANGE, K., KOLBE, H.: Brain disorders induced by pharmacological blockade of the pentose phosphate pathway. Biochem. biophys. Res. Commun. 36, 93-100 (1969).

11. HIMWICH, H.E.: Brain metabolism and cerebral disorders. Baltimore: Williams & Wilkins 1951.

12. KAUFFMAN, F.C., JOHNSON, E.J.: Cerebral energy reserves and glycolysis in neural tissue of 6-aminonicotinamide-treated mice. J. Neurobiol. $\underline{5}$, 379-393 (1974).

13. KELLER, K., KOLBE, H., LANGE, K., HERKEN, H.: Behaviour of the glycolytic system of rat brain and kidney in vivo after inhibition of the glucose phosphate isomerase, II. Substrate concentrations under the influence of ischemia, 6-aminonicotinamide, and 2-deoxyglucose. Hoppe-Seyler's Z. physiol. Chem. $\underline{353}$, 1389-1400 (1972).

14. LIPPMANN, H.G.: Energiereiche Phosphate, Glukose, Laktat und Pyruvat im Hirn der Ratte unter Änderung des pO_2 der Inspirationsluft. Acta biol. med. german. $\underline{27}$, 805-820 (1971).

15. LOWRY, O.H., PASSONEAU, J.V., HASSELBERGER, F.X., SCHULTZ, D.W.: Effect of ischemia on known substrates and cofactors of the glycolytic pathway in brain. J. Biol. Chem. $\underline{239}$, 18-30 (1964).

16. MÄENPÄÄ, P.H., RÄIHÄ, N.C.R.: Effects of anoxia on energy-rich phosphates, glycogen, lactate and pyruvate in the brain, heart and liver of the developing rat. Ann. Med. exp. Fenn. $\underline{46}$, 306-317 (1968).

17. MAYMAN, C., TIJERINA, M.L.: The effect of hypoglycemia on energy reserves in adult and newborn brain. In: Brain Hypoxia (eds. J.B. BRIERLEY, B.S. MELDRUM), p. 242. London: William Heinemann Medical Books Ltd. 1971.

18. NORBERG, K., SIESJÖ, B.K.: Cerebral metabolism in hypoxic hypoxia. I. Pattern of activation of glycolysis: A Re-evaluation. Brain Res. $\underline{86}$, 31-44 (1975).

19. PARR, C.W.: Inhibition of phosphoglucose isomerase. Nature (Lond.) $\underline{178}$, 1401 (1956).

20. PASSONEAU, J.V., GATFIELD, P.D., SCHULTZ, D.W., LOWRY, O.H.: An enzymic method for measurement of glycogen. Anal. Biochem. $\underline{19}$, 315-326 (1967).

21. REISS, M., HAUROWITZ, F.: Über das Verhalten junger und alter Tiere bei Erstickung. Klin. Wschr. $\underline{8}$, 743-744 (1929).

22. THURSTON, J.H., McDOUGAL, D.B., Jr.: Effect of ischemia on metabolism of the brain of the newborn mouse. Amer. J. Physiol. $\underline{216}$, 348-352 (1969).

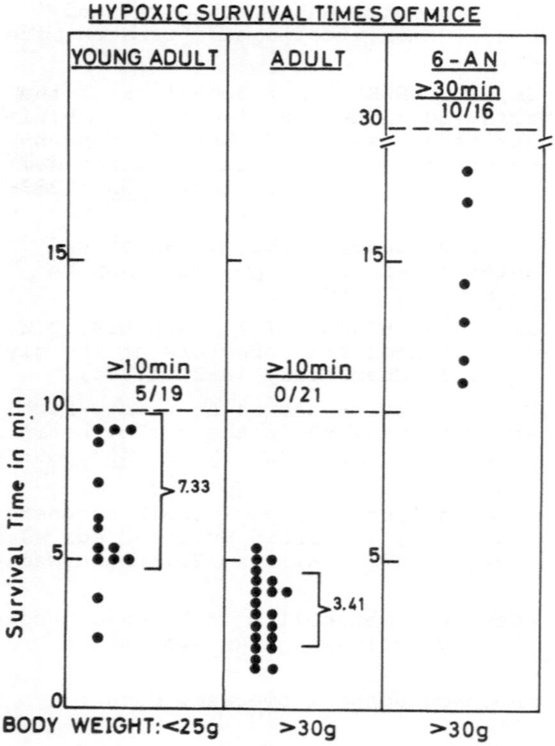

HYPOXIC SURVIVAL TIMES OF MICE

Fig. 1. Survival times of fed young adult (n=19) and adult mice (n=21) exposed to 5%O_2-95%N_2, and of mice treated with 6-AN, 35 mg/kg (n=16), 6 hours prior to hypoxia. Brackets indicate means ± S.D. Hypoxia was discontinued in untreated mice after 10 minutes, in treated mice after 30 min. Animals living beyond these time intervals are shown as fractions of the total number of animals in each group. The difference in survival times between young adult and adult mice was significant (p<0.01, Student's t-test)

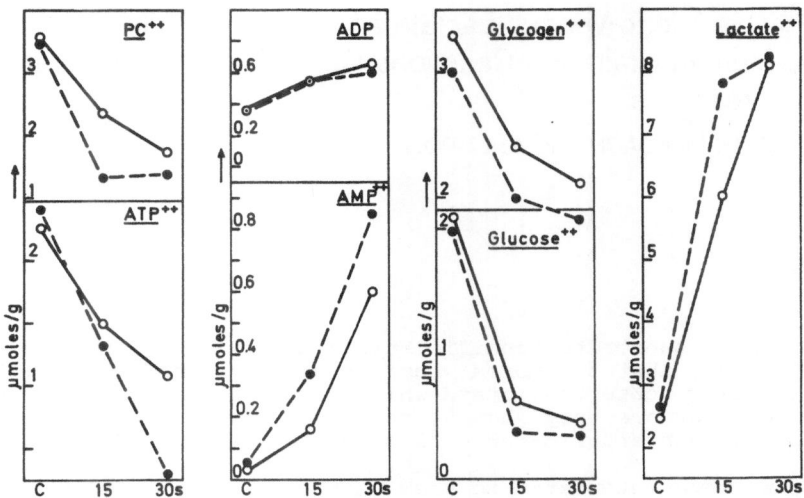

Fig. 2. Ischemic changes of cerebral constituents of young adult
(o————o) and adult mice (• - - - •) in µmoles/g wet weight. C:
Control values of animals frozen whole in liquid N_2 6 (s. Table 1).
Values were submitted to a two-way analysis of variance to test for
differences in rates between the two groups of animals ([+]p<0.05;
[++]p<0.01)

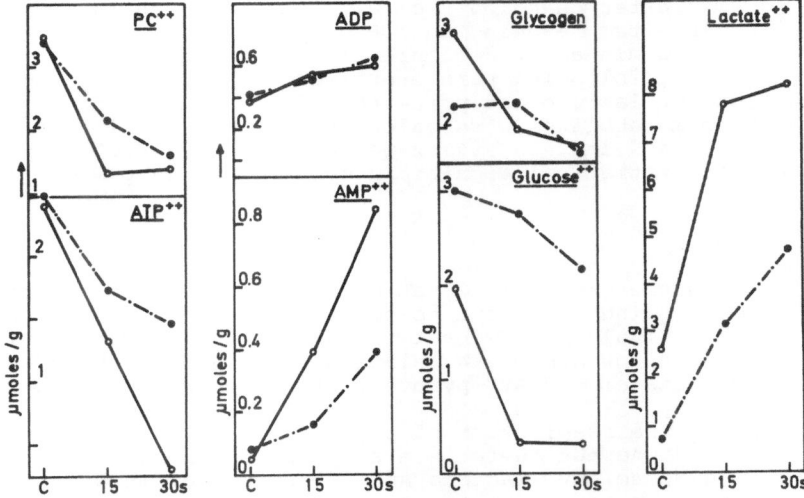

Fig. 3. Ischemic changes of cerebral constituents of mice treated
with 6-AN (o————o) compared to untreated adult controls (•—·—·—•).
Further explanations as for Fig. 1

The Arterio-Venous Lactate and Pyruvate Difference of the Injured Human Brain and Reactions During Different Inspiratory Oxygen Pressures

K. H. HOLBACH and A. CAROLI

Using substrate specific analysing methods GOTTSTEIN et al. (1) found, that the normal human brain converts about 7,6% of the cerebral glucose to lactate which is delivered into the venous blood. Furthermore they showed, that pyruvate is normally excreted, too. The mean arterio-cerebral venous difference (AVD) was 0,1 mg%.

We were interested to know whether the injured human brain takes up or excretes lactate and in how far pyruvate participates in the metabolism of the injured brain, particularly because the extent of brain tissue changes due to hypoxia in the course of brain injury is of vital importance. For this reason we examined simultaneously the influence of different inspiratory oxygen pressures (IOP) upon the AVD-lactate and -pyruvate.

Method

34 examinations were conducted in 34 patients with moderate or severe cerebral lesions. Simultaneously sampling of arterial and cerebral venous blood from the bulbus venae jugularis and also of cerebrospinal fluid (CSF) during the following consecutive periods of each of the examinations was performed: First at inspiring air, second 10 min after changing from air to oxygen, third 10 min and fourth 30 min after reaching an IOP of 1,5 ata in a hyperbaric chamber and fifth 10 min after decompression inspiring oxygen at an IOP of 1,0 ata. The following parameters were measured: PO_2 and the concentrations of lactate and pyruvate and of glucose and oxygen. The AVD of these metabolites were calculated. The significance of the lactate uptake and lactate efflux was analyzed by WILCOXON's pair difference test; statistical significance was given by $p \leq 0,05$.

Results

Within the group of 20 patients suffering from moderate brain injuries being somnolent to stuporous and having moderate EEG-changes with a highly predominant theta-wave activity the initial values showed a low $AVD-O_2$ in relation to a much too high AVD-glucose and AVD-lactate; the AVD-pyruvate still seemed to be in a normal range.

During the respiration of oxygen the $AVD-O_2$ is significantly increased whereas there is a significant and distinct decrease of the AVD-glucose, AVD-lactate and AVD-pyruvate. This inhibition of the glycolysis caused by the respiration of oxygen is best characterized as the "PASTEUR-effect". In the third, fourth and fifth phase of the examination, there is compared with the second phase an almost unchanged AVD-O_2 and an increase of the AVD-glucose; according to that we also find an increase of the AVD-lactate and AVD-pyruvate (Fig. 1).

A totally different behaviour of AVD-lactate and -pyruvate is found in the group with severe brain lesions. These patients were comatous at the time of the examination and had marked EEG-alterations in the form of a predominant delta-wave activity.

At first, we notice that the AVD-O_2 and -glucose are much lower than the corresponding ones of the other group. While in this group with severe cerebral lesions the AVD-O_2 practically remains unchanged during the 5 phases of the examination the AVD-glucose is changed in the same direction as the one of the former group (Fig. 2).

In the initial phase there is in relation to the AVD-O_2 a markedly increased AVD-glucose, which is significantly reduced during the second period of the examination. In the third, fourth and fifth phases the AVD-glucose here also is increased compared to the one of the second phase.

In the group with moderate cerebral lesions the AVD-lactate and -pyruvate reacted likewise. On the contrary, we find in the group with severe cerebral lesions a lactate uptake and simultaneously a pyruvate efflux. Expecially, in the initial phase there is an enormous lactate uptake besides a markedly increased pyruvate excretion in relation to the glucose uptake. In the following periods of the examination under normobaric and hyperbaric hyperoxia the AVD-lactate and -pyruvate distinctly decrease, i.e. the lactate uptake as well as the excretion are reduced.

During the fifth phase we even find a slight lactate efflux. This shows that under the effect of the increased IOP a similarly directed reaction of the AVD-lactate and -pyruvate is established. But the lactate and pyruvate efflux or the AVD-lactate and -pyruvate is in relation to the glucose uptake or to the AVD-glucose very low.

Discussion

The apparently paradoxical situation in which the brain catabolizes lactate and pyruvate while excreting both into the venous blood suggests that the total production of these substances through glycolysis exceeds the amounts that are oxydized by way of the cytrate acid cycle (6). These normal metabolic processes and regulations are also recognized in the group with moderate brain lesions. There we especially notice the hypoxic stimulation of glycolysis resulting in a marked increase of the AVD-glucose, -lactate and -pyruvate. Furthermore we see the effect of the normobaric and hyperbaric hyperoxia in the following phases of the examination in the form of a distinct reduction of AVD-glucose, -lactate and -pyruvate in the presence of a moderate increase of AVD-O_2. This clearly shows the increase of the oxydative glucose metabolism and the reduction of the anaerobic one.

We really must ask now, what kind of pathological mechanism causes the enormous lactate uptake with a simultaneous pyruvate efflux only in the group with severe cerebral lesions. Normally lactate and pyruvate can easily permeate the cell membrane and enter the extracellular fluid of the brain tissue. The next step from the extracellular fluid of the brain to the venous blood is connected with the crossing of the blood brain barrier (BBB). Both lactate and pyruvate readily penetrate the BBB. That this entry is in large part carrier-

mediated was suggested by its concentration dependence and particularly by the stereospecifity of lactate uptake after intra-arterial
injection (4). NEMOTO et al. (2, 3) have shown, in rats and dogs,
that the BBB is sterospecifically 3 times more permeable to L- than
to D-lactate, suggesting facilitated transport, and that the brain
can derive only about 25% of its energy in the form of lactate at
high blood lactate levels, even during hypoglycemia and with CSF
lactate levels rising to 4 mMol. The conclusion was that local metabolism can consume lactate. These findings indicate that lactate
and pyruvate can either be taken up or excreted, i.e. these substances cross the BBB or are transported across the BBB in either direction (in or out of the brain).

The direction in which lactate and pyruvate permeate across the BBB
depends at least to some extent on the concentration gradient, i.e.
if the blood level of these metabolites is higher than the one of
the brain tissue, we find an uptake and vice versa.

Therefore we measured not only the lactate and pyruvate concentrations of the blood (Fig. 3), but also of the CSF (Fig. 4); for the
lactate and pyruvate levels of the CSF correlate closely with their
brain tissue levels (5).

While the blood concentrations of lactate and pyruvate are in the
normal range their CSF concentrations are distinctly increased compared with the mean CSF concentrations of lactate and pyruvate we
have measured in 20 persons with a completely intact CNS:mean CSF
concentrations for lactate 11,8 (s±1.83) mg%, for pyruvate 0,94
(s±0.142) mg%.

According to these values, we should expect a lactate efflux, since
the CSF lactate level is about 3 times higher than the levels in the
arterial blood. We found, however, an enormous lactate uptake against
the direction of the concentration gradient for lactate, which existed between CSF (reflecting brain tissue level) and blood.

On account of these data it really is not possible to find an explanation for this distinct lactate uptake. But it can clearly be
shown that in the group with severe cerebral lesions the typical correlation existing between the AVD-glucose, -lactate and -pyruvate is
lost and that the lactate uptake is not only markedly reduced under
the influence of normobaric and hyperbaric oxygenation but it is even
changed to a minimal lactate efflux.

This effect of the increased IOP on AVD-lactate suggests that the
distinct lactate uptake probably is caused by the more pronounced
hypoxia existing in the group with severe cerebral lesions. For more
severe alterations of the cerebral tissue are accompanied with a
more pronounced hypoxia and tissue acidosis disturbing the functions
of the BBB, of the metabolic processes and also of metabolic regulatory mechanisms.

Summary

In 20 cases with moderate cerebral lesions we found an increased lactate and pyruvate efflux and in relation to the AVD-O$_2$ a markedly increased AVD-glucose. During the following hyperoxic phases an increase of the AVD-O$_2$ and a decrease of the AVD-glucose and of a
corresponding lactate and pyruvate efflux was measured (i.e. PASTEUR
effect). On the contrary, in 14 cases with severe cerebral lesions

we initially found a distinct lactate uptake and a pyruvate efflux. During the hyperoxic phases the AVD-lactate and -pyruvate decreased and we finally even observed a minimal lactate efflux. This effect of the high IOP on this AVD-lactate suggested that the pathological mechanism of the lactate uptake was related to a more pronounced hypoxia and acidosis of the cerebral tissue.

REFERENCES

1. GOTTSTEIN, U., BERNSMEIER, A., SEDLMEYER, I.: Der Kohlenhydrat-stoffwechsel des menschlichen Gehirns. I. Untersuchungen mit substratspezifischen enzymatischen Methoden bei normaler Hirn-durchblutung. Klin. Wschr. 41, 943 (1963).

2. NEMOTO, E., HOFF, J., SEVERINGHAUS, J.W.: Physiolog. 14 (1970).

3·. NEMOTO, E., HOFF, J., SEVERINGHAUS, J.W.: Fed. Proc. 30, 970 (1971).

4. OLDENDORF, W.H.: Blood brain barrier permeability to lactate. Pan. Med. 13, 162 (1971).

5. PLUM, F., POSNER, J.B.: Blood and cerebrospinal fluid lactate during hyperventilation. Amer. J. Physiol. 212, 864 (1968).

6. SACKS, W.: Cerebral metabolism of glucose-3-C^{14}, pyruvate-1-C^{14} and lactate-1-C^{14} in mental disease. J. Appl. Physiol. 16, 175 (1961).

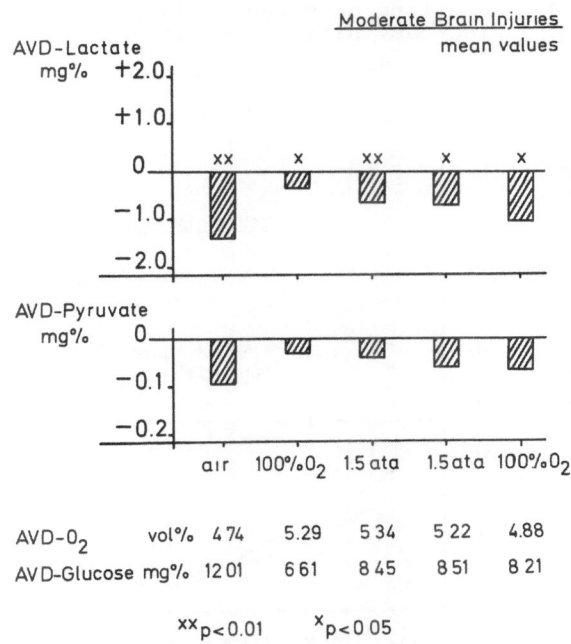

Fig. 1. The mean arterio-cerebral venous differences (AVD) of lactate, pyruvate, oxygen and glucose measured in 20 patients with moderate brain lesions during the initial and different hyperoxic phases of 20 examinations

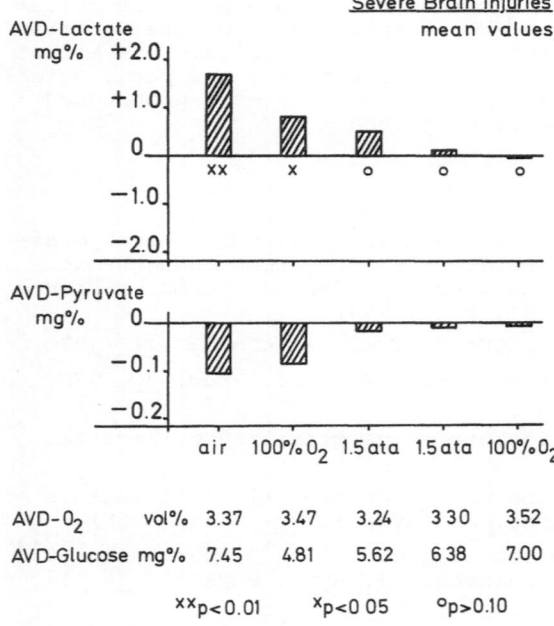

Fig. 2. The mean arterio-cerebral venous differences (AVD) of the metabolites measured in 14 patients with severe cerebral lesions during the initial and different hyperoxic phases of 14 examinations

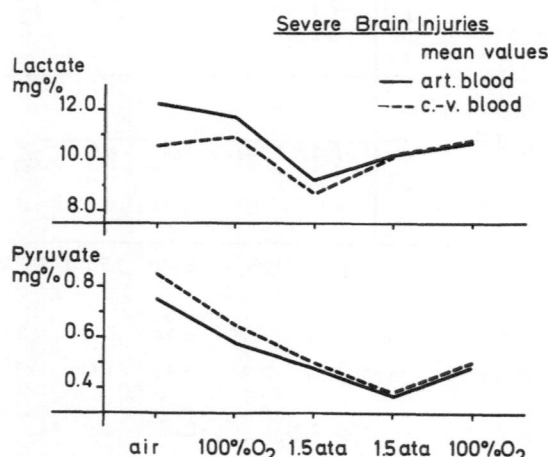

Fig. 3. The mean concentrations of lactate and pyruvate in the arterial and cerebral venous blood measured in 14 cases during different phases of the examinations

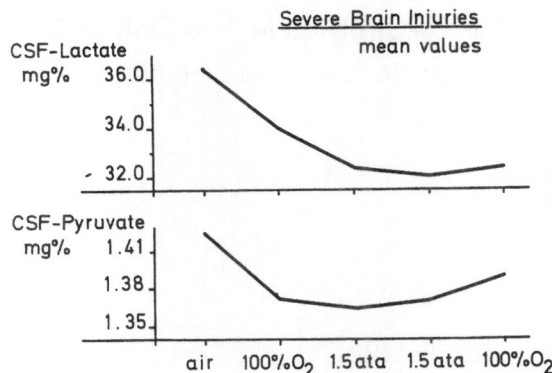

Fig. 4. The mean concentrations of lactate and pyruvate in the cerebro-spinal fluid (CSF) measured in 14 cases during different phases of the examinations

CSF-Electrolytes in Two Different Types of Metabolic Brain Edema*

A. Baethmann, K. Sohler, P. Schmiedek, W. Oettinger, and L. Guggemos

Introduction

The significance of vasogenic brain edema is well understood for a variety of clinical conditions, while this is not true in the case of the cytotoxic form. A lack of knowledge on edema forming mechanisms, on the dynamics of edema development and edema resolution may still impede an appreciation of this type of brain edema. A number of mechanisms may cause the formation of cytotoxic brain edema. Compounds such as e.g. biogenic amines, metabolites (7, 10) etc. could be released into the extracellular compartment increasing the Na-permeability of the plasma membranes. Osmotic activity, which in the intracellular compartment is primarily bound becomes unbound by the process initiating brain edema or by concomitant derangements of the cellular energy metabolism, thus probably dramatically increasing the intracellular osmolarity. In both cases, intracellular swelling would ensue.

Our current concept on the cytotoxic or metabolic brain edema is as follows. Disturbances of energy-producing or -transferring metabolic processes may lead to disturbances of active ion-transport. The sodium pumps fail, leading to a reduction or arrest of the sodium outward transport, while the Na- and water influx remains unchanged or even enhanced. Ion gradients between the extra- and intracellular compartment may be expected to decline. This particular aspect could be studied by analysing electrolyte concentrations in the extracellular, or intracellular compartment.

Cerebrospinal fluid exchanges intimately with the interstitial fluid of brain tissue (5, 11) so that electrolyte concentrations of this fluid may reflect the respective concentrations within the extracellular space.

The current report is concerned with electrolyte measurements in CSF of animals infused with 2.4 dinitrophenol after adrenalectomy. In early experiments it was shown that dinitrophenol causes an intracellular, metabolic type of brain edema as concluded from a decrease in the extracellular fluid space and a lowering of the energy rich phosphate compounds (3, 9). The metabolic nature of the cerebral Na- and water uptake secondary to adrenalectomy may be inferred from changes of the activity of tricarboxylic acid cycle enzymes of cerebral tissue (1) as well as from a reduced cerebral blood flow and glucose consumption (2), while as yet no evidence is obtained that the energy state is affected under those circumstances.

*Supported in part by DFG-Sonderforschungsbereich 51: Medizinische Molekularbiologie und Biochemie, München.

Methods

a) Dinitrophenol Edema

In ether anesthesia, male Sprague Dawley rats (b. w.: 250 - 300 g) were infused into a carotid artery with 4,5 - 5,0 ml of an isotonic glucose solution containing 5,4 mM 2,4 dinitrophenol. Control animals received glucose instead. At termination of the infusion, the carotid artery was clamped, the skin defect was sutured and the animals were allowed to regain consciousness. 6 hours later, the animals were subjected to ventriculo-cisternal perfusion according to PAPPENHEIMER et al. (8) with a mock cerebrospinal fluid in chloralhydrate (360 mg/kg) anesthesia (Fig. 1). The perfusions pressure could be continously controlled. The flow was 0,0375 ml/min. The mock cerebrospinal fluid contained 144,5 meq/l Na, 90 meq/l CI, 54 meq/l thiosulphate, and 53/mM/l glucose, and no potassium. The perfusion periods were in four different groups 60, 90, 120, and 180 minutes, respectively. The outflowing perfusate was collected over an entire experimental period and analyzed for the Na and K concentrations.

The animals were bled then from the carotids and the blood was collected and centrifuged. The plasma Na and K concentrations were determined by flamespectrophonetry in addition after appropriate dilution.

b) Adrenalectomy

Male adult mongrel dogs of 7 - 10 kg b. w. were bilaterally adrenalectomized in pentobarbital anesthesia (25 mg/kg). After surgery, the animals were maintained on a steroid substitution regime consisting of prednisolone and aldosterone until wound healing was complete. Steroid treatment was withheld about 5 days prior to the final experiment which again was conducted in pento barbital anesthesia to measure cerebral blood flow and metabolism. Immediately after induction of anesthesia, CSF was sampled by tapping the cisterna magna. The Na and K concentrations were again measured and the osmolality by freeze point depression in addition. For comparison, the same parameters were determined in plasma samples of blood taken from an arterial catheter.

Results and Discussion

a) Dinitrophenol edema

Animals infused with dinitrophenol reveal a loss of extracellular Na involving the brain tissue as well as the general organism. This is suggested either by the consistently lower plasma Na concentration and by the Na concentrations in the perfusion fluid leaving the ventricle system after perfusion periods of different length when compared with the controls (Fig. 2). Comparing the in- and outflow Na concentration, it is concluded that the cerebral tissue of DNP animals take up Na from the perfusate during the ventricle passage while control animals even appear to loose some Na. Since the brain tissue (on dry weight basis) of DNP-infused animals was found to accumulate Na (3), a decrease of this ion in the extracellular fluid may be indicative for a shift of Na-ions from the extra- into the intracellular compartment in this type of brain edema.

More direct evidence is available supporting this conclusion. Employing thiosulphate distribution measurements to assess the extra- and intracellular cerebral volumes, a significant increase in intracellular space and uptake of intracellular Na at the expense of the extracellular space was found (3). Moreover, a close correlation between the intracellular water content and the intracellular Na concentration was established in these studies.

The plasma and CSF potassium concentrations are seen in Figure 3. In DNP-animals, the plasma concentrations is considerably above that of control animals at a high degree of statistical confidence except the 3 hours values. Two aspects merit particular attention when evaluating the K concentrations in the outflowing mock CSF of both groups. As mentioned in the Methods section, the arterial cerebrospinal fluid was devoid of K ions when entering the ventricular system. However, the perfusate leaving the cisterna magna contained K ions with almost identical concentrations in both controls and experimental animals of about 2,8 meq/l during all perfusion periods.

The CSF-K concentration being unchanged after DNP administration inspite of a rise in plasma K may imply the existence of active mechanisms in the central nervous system maintaining effectively the extracellular K at constant levels as already convincingly demonstrated by DAVSON and BRADBURY (6) in a different experimental model. These authors perfused the ventricle-cisternal system with Ringer's solution containing K concentrations varying from 10 meq/l to zero. In any case, the outflowing perfusion fluid had a constant K concentration of about 2,9 meq/l which is rather similar to that evolving from our own experiments.

b) Adrenalectomy

Basically the same findings were obtained in adrenal insufficient dogs. These animals also develop cerebral edema as already observed in small rodents (1), which in dogs apparently affects the cortical grey matter in particular. Inverse changes of the plasma Na and K are well known and understood in adrenal insufficiency. In our experiments, the mean plasma Na concentration fell from 148,0 $\pm$ 1,0 meq/l in controls to 129,4 $\pm$ 2,5 meq/l in adrenalectomized animals (p < 0,001). Conversely, the mean plasma K rose from 3,96 $\pm$ 0,12 to 6,69 $\pm$ 0,43 meq/l after adrenalectomy (p < 0,001). The marked alterations of both plasma Na and K may be viewed as a measure of how far adrenal insufficiency developed. To our knowledge, respective measurements in adrenal insufficiency have not been performed yet in cerebrospinal fluid.

It may be surmised that the corticosteriod deficiency could affect the processess controlling the liquor production resulting in formation of a CSF abnormally composed. Moreover, the blood-brain-barrier may become more permeable allowing CSF and plasma electrolytes more freely to exchange. This would cause the CSF-Na to fall and the CSF-K to rise as seen in the plasma compartment. Alterations like this could be responsible for the functional derangements of the CNS encountered in adrenal insufficiency, e.g. a lowering of the electroshock seizure threshold as a measure of an increased cerebral excitability (4).

The CSF-Na concentration in fact was found to decrease from 151,7 $\pm$ 1,1 meq/l in controls to 136 $\pm$ 2,0 in adrenalectomized dogs (p < 0,001), although the reduction appeared to be less pronounced than in the plasma compartment. The fall in plasma- and CSF-Na concentration is paralleled by respective changes in osmolality which was observed to decrease from 307 mOsm/kg in plasma or 303 mOsm/kg in the cerebrospinal fluid of controls to 283 (plasma) or 285 mOsm/kg (CSF) in adrenal insufficient dogs. The osmolalities of the plasma liquor compartment being almost identical in the controls or the experimental animals, respectively may suggest that the water exchanges more or less uninhibited between both compartments and that this is not affected by steroid deprivation.

In control dogs the CSF-K concentration was 2,91 ± 0,04 meq/l and fell to 2,65 ± 0,05 meq/l after adrenalectomy (p < 0,001) despite an increase of the plasma-K concentration in opposite direction. The very small standard error of the mean CSF-K concentrations in either experimental models compared e.g. with that of the CSF-Na concentrations or the corresponding plasma electrolytes appears to be noteworthy. The small variability again suggests a very strict control of the extracellular potassium in the CNS, and that the mechanisms involved were still operative after DNP administration of deprivation of corticosteroids.

The small but nevertheless significant decrease of the CSF-K concentration in adrenal insufficiency is difficult to explain. Changes of the pH may be involved as well as an increased binding of K ions to structures on the cell surfaces or intracellulary. Provided the liquor changes reflect changes in the interstitial space, the fall in CSF-K may alternatively be viewed as an adaptation to intracellular losses of K secondary to the steroid deficiency to maintain a constant membrane potential, which, however, would require the tissue K content to decrease.

Summary

Determinations of the Na- and K-concentrations were carried out, (a) in mock cerebrospinal fluid leaving the ventriculo-cisternal system of rats with brain edema induced by 2,4 dinitrophenol, and (b) in natural CSF obtained by tapping the cisterna magna in adrenalectomized dogs left without substitution with corticosteroids who develop also brain edema. The changes of CSF electrolytes were similar in both experimental conditions. After DNP as well as in adrenal insufficiency, the Na- and K-concentrations were found to change inversely, while the CSF potassium concentration remained unchanged in animals with DNP-edema, and was even somewhat reduced in adrenalectomized dogs despite a marked rise in plasma. The decrease in CSF-Na in both types of metabolic brain edema inspite of an accumulation of Na in the cerebral tissue supports the contention that extra- to intracellular Na shifts occur under those circumstances. The CSF potassium remaining constant within a very narrow range suggests that mechanisms were operative strictly controlling the extracellular concentration of this ion very efficiently even in brain edema.

Acknowledgements: The technical assistance of Mrs. R. Hößl and Miss I. Hoffmann is gratefully appreciated.

REFERENCES

1. BAETHMANN, A., VAN HARREVELD, A.: Physiological and biochemical findings in the central nervous system of adrenalectomized rats and mice. In: Steroids and brain edema (eds. REULEN, H.J., SCHÜRMANN, K.), pp. 195 - 202 Berlin - Heidelberg - New York: Springer 1972.

2. BAETHMANN, A., SCHMIEDEK, P., GUGGEMOS, L., OETTINGER, W.: Cerebral water and electrolytes, cerebral blood flow and metabolism in adrenal insufficient dogs. Europ. Surg. Res. 6, (Suppl. 1) 79 - 80 (1974).

3. BAETHMANN, A., SOHLER, K.: Electrolyte- and fluid-spaces of rat brain in situ after infusion with dinitrophenol. J. Neurobiol. 6, 73 - 84 (1975).

4. DAVENPORT, V.D.: Relation between brain and plasma electrolytes and electroshock seizure thresholds in adrenalectomized rats. Amer. J. Physiol. 156, 322 - 327 (1945).

5. DAVSON, H.: The cerebrospinal fluid. Ergebn. Physiol. 52, 20 - 73 (1963).

6. DAVSON, H., BRADBURY, M.: The extracellular space of the brain. Brain Res. 15, 124 - 134 (1965).

7. KLATZO, I.: Pathophysiological aspects of brain edema. In: Steroids and brain edema (eds. H.J. REULEN, K. SCHÜRMANN), pp. 1 - 8 Berlin - Heidelberg - New York: Springer 1972.

8. PAPPENHEIMER, J.R., HEISEY, JORDAN, E.F.: Active transport of diodrast and phenolsulfonphthalein from cerebrospinal fluid to blood. Amer. J. Physiol. 200, 1 - 10 (1961).

9. REULEN, H.J., BAETHMANN, A.: Dinitrophenolödem. Ein Modell zur Pathophysiologie des Hirnödems. Klin. Wschr. 45, 149 - 154 (1967).

10. SACHS, E.Jr.: Acetylcholine and serotonine in the spinal fluid. J. Neurosurg. 14, 22 - 27 (1957).

11. WOODBURY, D.M.: Distribution of nonelectrolytes and electrolytes in the brain as affected by alterations in cerebrospinal fluid secretion. Brain Res. 29, 297 - 312 (1968).

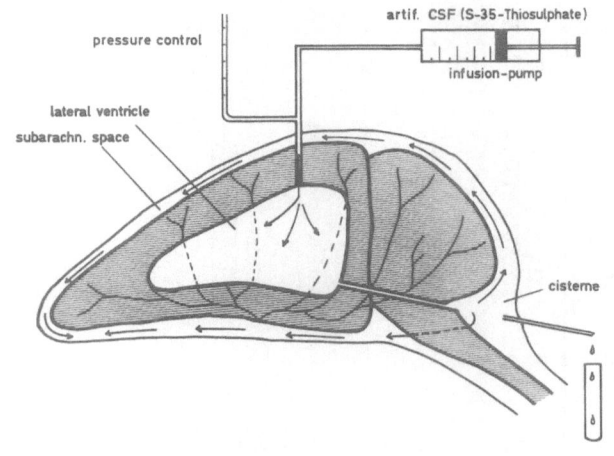

Fig. 1. Schematic illustration of the ventriculo-cisternal perfusion technique. A cannula was inserted into a lateral ventricle by free-hand puncture and connected with an infusion pump allowing to monitor continously the perfusion pressure. The perfusion Flow was 0,0375 ml/min. The atlanto-occipital membrane was incised and a plastic catheter introduced into the cisterna magna in order to collect the outflowing perfusate. Experiments were discarded if the perfusion pressure rose permanently above 100 mm H$_2$O. (From BAETHMANN, A. et al.: Pflüg. Arch. Europ. J. Physiol 316: 51 - 63, 1970)

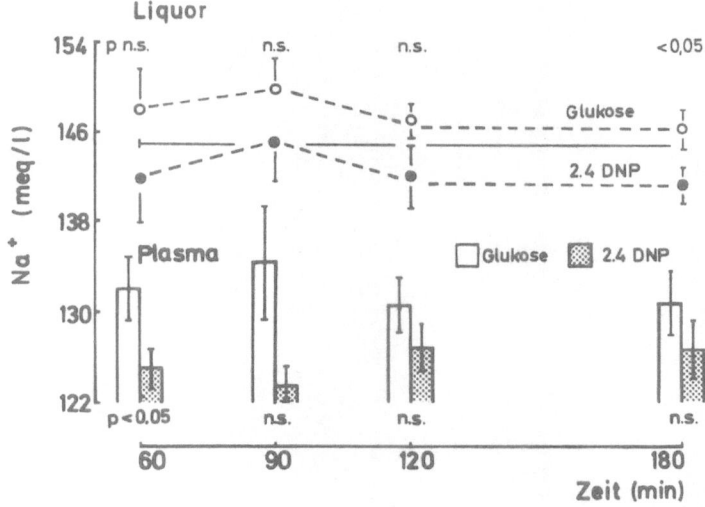

Fig. 2. Na-concentrations of plasma and mock CSF (mean ± SEM) collected after ventricle passage in controls and DNP treated animals at different perfusion periods. The solid line in the upper part of the graph indicates the Na concentration of the perfusate before entering the ventricle, which was 144,5 meq/l. Statistical significances are indicated. n.s. = not significant (from 3)

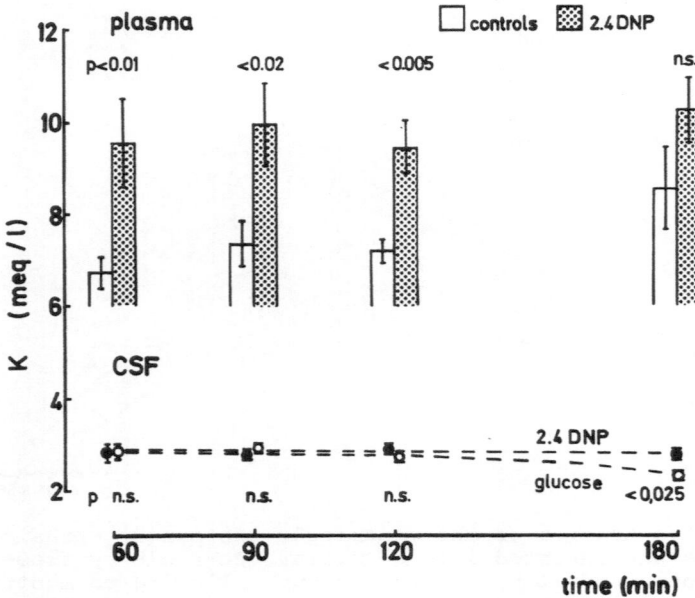

Fig. 3. Plasma and CSF-K-concentrations (mean ± SEM) of controls and animals infused with DNP after various perfusion periods. The small standard error of the mean CSF-K-concentrations is noteworthy. The statistical significances are indicated. n.s. = not significant (from 3)

The Clinical Significance of CSF Acid-Base Determination

P. MARX

The investigation of cerebral spinal fluid (CSF) acid-base parameters
has become increasingly important. The following presentation attempts to summarize the most important principles of CSF acid-base
regulation and to critically evaluate the clinical significance of
CSF acid-base determinations.

CSF secretion at the choroid plexus involves complicated mechanisms
such as active ion transport and different permeabilities for various
anions and cations at the plexus membranes. The most important selective ion transport mechanisms have been attributed to the $Na^+/K^+ATPase$
and the carboanhydrase activities (1, 3, 7, 8).

During circulation of the fluid through the various CSF-channels to
the arachnoid villi, a lively exchange by diffusion of various substances between the extracellular fluid (ACF) of the brain and the
CSF takes place, not only involving O_2 and CO_2 but also Na^+, Cl^-,
HCO_2^-, lactate and pyruvate etc. Therefore changes in brain acid-
base parameters might well be detected in the CSF.

The bulk absorption of the CSF at the arachnoid villi does not seem
to involve selective ion transport mechanisms. The CSF pH follows the
ratio of local concentration of molecular CO_2 (pCO_2) and of bicarbonate according to the Henderson-Hasselbalch equation

$$pH = pK_1' + \log \frac{[HCO_3^-]}{S.P_{CO_2}}.$$

From this formula it might easily be understood that any increase in
CSF pCO_2 decreases CSF pH; whereas a decrease in pCO_2 makes the fluid
more alkaline.

As a result of homeostatic control mechanisms CSF pH is maintained
within narrower limits than that of blood during various states of
systemic metabolic acidosis or alkalosis. This is in part due to the
blood-brain and blood-CSF barrier systems, which are only minimally
or not at all permeable for most acids and bases of the circulating
blood. There is only one exception, and that is CO_2, which is moving
unrestricted through cell membranes and might be converted into carbonic acid.

Additional control of CSF pH stability is achieved by the control of
ventilation by the CSF pH, lowering of which results in forced ventilation with increased elimination of CO_2 out of the fluid. Another
important factor is the chemical control of cerebral blood flow.

Besides these three mechanisms some others also are important, including the intracellular buffer capacity of the brain, adaptation

of the bicarbonate concentration in the brain, the ECF to the actual pCO_2, the potential-difference between CSF and blood and lastly the stimulation of lactic acid production by alkalosis.

The determinations of CSF acid-base parameters includes the measurements of pCO_2, pH, lactate and pyruvate, whereas bicarbonate might be easily calculated by a modified SIGGARD-ANDERSON Nomogram (2). Additionally pO_2 is measured. All these parameters in CSF should be compared to determinations of simultaneously drawn arterial blood samples.

The current understanding of CSF acid-base regulation has influenced general therapeutic measures:

1. We have become more cautious in compensating systemic acidosis by iv. application of bicarbonate solutions. Since CO_2 being released from the bicarbonate, moves much faster through the blood brain and blood CSF barriers than the bicarbonate ion, the CSF pH might temporarily decrease despite a pH increase in arterial blood. This might be accompanied by a deterioration of the patient's condition (4).

2. Since respiratory acidosis is easily transmitted from blood to the brain ECF and to the CSF, inhibition of pulmonary ventilation might be particularly dangerous to patients suffering from a primary metabolic acidosis of the brain. This is the case in cerebrovascular disease or increased intracranial pressure.

3. Since severe hypocapnia stimulates cerebral lactic acid production, hyperventilation as a therapeutical aid in treating increased intracranial pressure should not decrease arterial pCO_2 below 25-30 mm Hg.

Despite these more general applications, CSF acid-base parameters have been correlated to certain clinical conditions. Thereby it could be shown for example that impairment of consciousness in various neurological diseases is accompanied by certain degrees of acid-base deviations in the CSF (5). This is evident also in our material (Fig. 1). Mean CSF lactate and pyruvate values as well as the lactate-pyruvate-ratio were significantly higher in those neurological patients who had lost consciousness as compared to those who had not.

However CSF lactic acidosis is a more general reaction to various noxious stimuli and by no means specific. It may occur in different diseases such as meningitis, head trauma, status epilepticus and many others (Fig. 2).

Correlation between the clinical status of patients suffering primarily from cerebral lesions with certain acid-base parameters in the CSF not only serves a scientific purpose, but also may help in creating a better and more comprehensive understanding of a given patient's situation. However, special care should be given to avoid any non-steady state conditions while the CSF and blood samples are drawn. Since the equilibration of acid-base parameters between brain ECF and CSF takes time, the lumbar cerebrospinal fluid-pH might differ by 0,1 units from the cisternal fluid from some time in changing conditions. Even in ventricular fluid, the adaptation to respiratory changes may take up to ten minutes.

Another source of misleading results might be a massive cisternal herniation with blockade of the cerebrospinal fluid pathways into the spinal column.

Some years ago SEITZ et al. (6) reported that cerebrospinal fluid lactate concentrations of more than 40 mg%, that is about 4,4 mval/1, indicated a bad prognosis in patients with severe head injury. Our data does not agree with this finding. We measured a CSF lactate concentration of 6,5 mval/1 in a patient with severe head injury, whose arterial acid-base parameters were entirely normal.

From a theoretical point of view the simple correlation between CSF lactic acidosis and survival does not seem justified. Such correlation could perhaps hold if the CSF lactate concentration or better yet the lactate-pyruvate-ratio were determined exclusively by the Redox potential of the brain. But this is not true, since lactate can penetrate the blood brain barrier by a carrier mediated transport mechanism. Thus, high lactate concentrations in the blood can be transmitted into the CSF. Such an exogenous lactic acidosis in the fluid of course has another prognostic value than a lactacidosis, which is caused by brain hypoxia.

As could be shown in another patient, an extremely high CSF lactate concentration of 13,2 mEq/1 is compatible with brain stem functions such as spontaneous eye movements, preserved corneal reflexes and spontaneous respiration, at least for some hours.

Summary

The most important mechanisms regulating CSF pH have been briefly summarized and the clinical significance of acid-base determinations in the CSF has been discussed.

REFERENCES

1. DAVSON, H.: Physiology of the cerebrospinal fluid. Boston: Little, Brown and Co 1967.

2. KIENLE, G.: Methodische Hinweise für die Untersuchungen des Säure-Basen-Haushaltes im Liquor cerebro-spinalis. Klin. Wschr. 47, 545-547 (1969).

3. MAREN, T.H., BRODER, L.E.: The role of carbonic anhydrase in anion secretion into cerebrospinal fluid. J. Pharmacol. Exp. Ther. 172, 197-202 (1970).

4. POSNER, J.B., SWANSON, A.G., PLUM, F.: Acid-base balance in cerebrospinal fluid. Arch. Neurol. 12, 479-496 (1965).

5. SCHNABERTH, G., SCHUBERT, H.: Bewußtseinsstörung und Liquormetabolismus. Arch. Psychiat. Nervenkr. 218, 211-222 (1974).

6. SEITZ, H.D., HIRSCHAUER, M., METZEL, E. et al.: Klinische und tierexperimentelle Untersuchungen zum Hirnstoffwechsel und zur Hirndurchblutung beim Schädel-Hirn-Trauma. Neurochirurgia 6, 201-209 (1972).

7. WOODBURY, J.W.: An epilogue. A hypothetical model for CSF formation and blood-brain barrier function. In: Ion homeostasis of the brain (eds. B.K. SIESJÖ, S.C. SØRENSEN), pp. 465-471. Copenhagen: Munksgaard 1971.

8. WRIGHT, E.M.: Mechanisms of ion transport across the choroid plexus. J. Physiol. 233, 327-347 (1973).

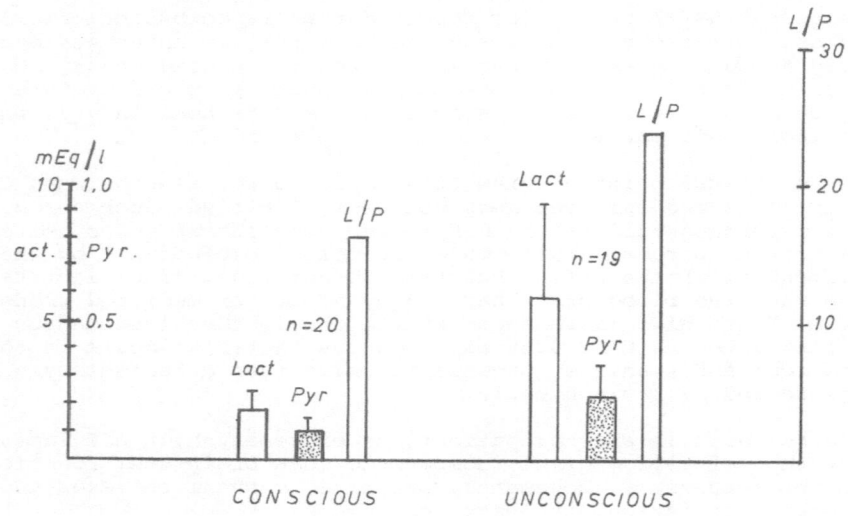

Fig. 1. Comparison between the lactate and pyruvate concentrations in conscious and unconscious patients suffering from cerebral diseases

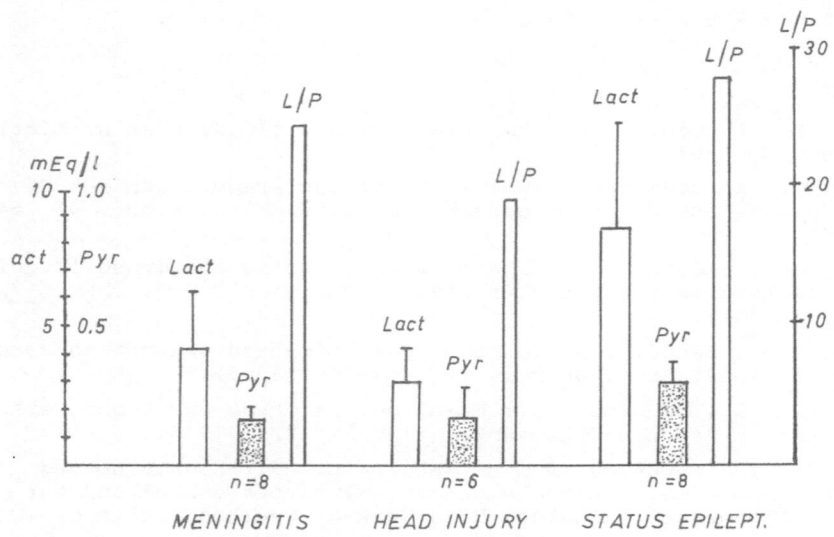

Fig. 2. Lactate and pyruvate concentrations in various cerebral diseases

Clinical Aspects of Cerebral Hypoxia

Th. W. Langfitt

Cerebral hypoxia is the most common cause of disability and death in neurological and neurosurgical patients. It can be divided into hypoxic hypoxia, a reduction in the O_2 content of the circulating blood, and ischemic hypoxia, a reduction in the volume of circulating blood per unit time. The normal value for the partial pressure of O_2 (PaO_2) in circulating blood is approximately 90 torr. A value below the normal range is defined as systemic hypoxemia; but the intact brain can function well at a PaO_2 far below the normal range and does not suffer irreversible damage until the PaO_2 is markedly depressed. Furthermore, in borderline cerebral hypoxia metabolism is deranged, but only in some cells, and the metabolic derangement may not be detectable clinically; vital neurons continue to produce and utilize a normal amount of energy, and the patient is neurologically normal. It is desirable, therefore, to define four levels or categories of systemic hypoxemia: (1) below the normal range of PaO_2; (2) the range of PaO_2 which results in an alteration of metabolism that is not detectable by neurological examination; (3) the range of PaO_2 that depresses neurological function; (4) PaO_2 values that result in irreversible hypoxic brain damage. The same categories are applicable to brain ischemia; mean cerebral blood flow (CBF) ranges from normal to values that result in permanent ischemic brain damage.

A major purpose of many of the techniques that have been developed in the past two decades to diagnose and manage patients with acute brain insults is assessment of the presence and significance of cerebral hypoxia. They include measurements of arterial blood gases, intracranial pressure (ICP), CBF, and the cerebral metabolic rate of glucose and O_2 utilization ($CMRO_2$).

Neurological Status

The clinical diagnosis of cerebral hypoxia is difficult. Cyanosis is clear evidence of systemic hypoxemia but is rare in neurosurgical patients. When present the patient almost always has obvious obstruction within the pulmonary pathways. If the patient improves in response to treatment for systemic hypoxemia (e.g. endotracheal intubation and mechanical ventilation) or cerebral ischemia (e.g. reduction of ICP) then worsens when the treatment is discontinued, this is the best clinical evidence for cerebral hypoxia.

Blood Gases

The quantity of O_2 available to the brain is a function of the O_2 content of the blood, the O_2 affinity of hemoglobin, and the volume of blood flowing through the brain per unit time. Nearly all of the

O_2 in blood is attached to hemoglobin; only a small portion is dissolved in plasma. If hemoglobin is fully saturated, but the patient's hemoglobin is half the normal value, then the O_2 carrying capacity of the blood is reduced by half. Often this factor is not taken into account in attempting to define and treat cerebral hypoxia.

O_2 is released by hemoglobin and diffuses across the vascular wall to supply metabolically active neurons and glial cells. Little is known about the effects of edema, for example, on O_2 diffusion in tissue. In massive focal edema, a neuron that is normally farthest from a capillary and therefore may have barely enough O_2 to function might be further displaced from the capillary by tissue swelling and become hypoxic.

Alterations in arterial CO_2 ($PaCO_2$) can contribute to cerebral hypoxia in two ways. Hypocapnia produces cerebral vasoconstriction, and there is evidence in normal animals and man that hyperventilation to a $PaCO_2$ between 15 and 20 torr can constrict the cerebral vessels sufficiently to produce ischemic hypoxia of the brain. In addition, the respiratory alkalosis produced by hyperventilation shifts the O_2 dissociation curve to the left (BOHR effect). This increases the O_2-hemoglobin affinity, and less O_2 is available to the tissue. Therefore, hyperventilation therapy used so commonly in neurosurgical practice has the potential deleterious effect of critically reducing CBF; at the same time the amount of O_2 released by the blood is diminished because of the shift in the O_2-hemoglobin dissociation curve.

However, when the vasoconstriction produced by the hypocapnia becomes so great as to produce cerebral ischemic hypoxia, the well known hypoxic stimulus to vasodilatation overrides the hypocapnic stimulus to vasoconstriction, and CBF remains constant even though the $PaCO_2$ is reduced further. This is one explanation for the clinical observation that patients with severe hyperventilation and a $PaCO_2$ of 10-15 torr do not have evidence of hypoxic brain damage.

What then are the critical levels of PaO_2 and $PaCO_2$ for adequate oxygenation of the brain? Clearly critical levels vary from patient to patient and within the same patient over time. A patient with multiple injuries who is in peripheral shock from blood loss, is hyperventilating spontaneously, and has reduced CBF because of severe brain edema and intracranial hypertension may suffer cerebral hypoxia despite the fact that his PaO_2 is far above normal. Contrariwise, a healthy young patient with an intact brain and a normal blood pressure who is suffering from pulmonary insufficiency may survive a prolonged period of systemic hypoxemia with a PaO_2 of 40 torr or less without clinical evidence of brain damage.

Intracranial Pressure

Increased ICP appears to produce brain damage only to the degree that it reduces CBF and causes ischemic hypoxia of the brain. CBF may be reduced diffusely or focally, for example within the brain stem in patients with transtentorial herniation. What is a critical level of increased ICP for the production of cerebral ischemic hypoxia that results in disturbed brain metabolism, clinical evidence of ischemia, or permanent ischemic brain damage? When one is recording ICP continuously in a patient with a brain insult, at what level of ICP should treatment be instituted? Again there are guidelines but no rules. The interpretation of the data and the management of the patient must be individualized. A patient with an essentially normal brain and intact cerebral autoregulation will tolerate marked intracranial hypertension well, whereas a patient with diffuse cerebral damage, defective autoregulation, and brain edema will exhibit signs of cerebral ischemia with only moderately increased ICP.

Fig. 1 illustrates a young woman with a cerebellar hemangioblastoma and obstructive hydrocephalus. ICP was recorded from a cannula in a lateral ventricle and systemic arterial pressure (SAP) from a catheter in the radial artery. The patient was alert and well oriented, and the only neurological deficit was a mild truncal ataxia from the tumor. For prolonged periods of time mean ICP approached mean SAP; the cerebral perfusion pressure was only 7-10 torr. Yet she remained neurologically normal. ICP fell to normal in response to brief periods of voluntary hyperventilation, demonstrating that the vasoreactivity of the cerebral vessels was also normal. In contrast, we have observed many patients with diffuse brain damage and cerebral edema who deteriorated neurologically when ICP exceeded 25-30 torr, then improved when ICP was reduced by hyperventilation or hypertonic mannitol.

Cerebral Blood Flow and Metabolism

In intact animals and man the level of CBF required to maintain normal metabolism appears to be 40-45% of the normal value of approximately 50 ml/100gm/min. When CBF falls below that level cerebral hypoxia is manifested by slowing in the EEG and metabolically by anaerobic glycolysis and a decline in high energy phosphates in brain tissue. But this level of CBF is critical only if brain metabolism of O_2 and glucose is normal. If for any reason metabolism is reduced, then less O_2 and therefore less blood flow are required to maintain normal (aerobic) brain metabolism. For example, a reduction in body temperature from normal to 30°C halves brain metabolism and therefore halves the brain requirement for O_2.

To date most studies of the energy state of the brain have depended on measurements of the concentration of high energy phosphates such as adenosine triphosphate (ATP) in brain tissue. Critical levels of PaO_2, SAP, and CBF for oxidative phosphorylation (production of ATP) in mitochondria have been defined in experimental animals. Since the brain is dependent on a constant production of ATP for its energy needs, the brain machinery runs down as ATP falls, and when ATP is depleted neuronal and glial function ceases. After the brain has been deprived of O_2 for a period of time that is still controversial, irreversible damage ensues.

Measurements of the tissue concentration of ATP provide accurate information on the amount of ATP available for metabolic needs; but they do not measure the *rate* of metabolism of ATP. In deep hypothermia the subject is comatose, indeed may have all the clinical signs of brain death. Both production and utilization of ATP are reduced to a fraction of normal; but production equals utilization, and therefore the *concentration* of ATP in brain tissue will be normal even though the *rate* of turnover of ATP is greatly reduced.

The rate of utilization of ATP in man can be estimated by measuring $CMRO_2$ according to the equation:

$$CMRO_2 = \frac{\text{mean CBF x A-VDO}_2}{100}.$$

Where the mean CBF is determined for whole brain and A-VDO$_2$ is the arterio-venous difference of O$_2$ content across the brain measured from samples of arterial and jugular bulb blood. The normal value of CMRO$_2$ in awake man is approximately 3.5 ml/100gm/min. In brain damaged patients CMRO$_2$ is reduced, and in deeply comatose patients CMRO$_2$ may be 1/10 the normal value.

Hypoxia reduces brain metabolism of O$_2$ (and increases the metabolism of glucose), but when O$_2$ metabolism is reduced the need for O$_2$ is less. The major issue, however, is not the amount of O$_2$ required to maintain a normal metabolic rate, but the amount of O$_2$ required to prevent irreversible neuronal damage. Teleologically the decrease in metabolism produced by hypoxia might be considered a compensatory mechanism to prevent irreversible damage. The problem with this hypothesis is that the cellular substrates of irreversible hypoxic injury are unknown.

Fig. 2 illustrates a patient who was comatose following a head injury. A left cerebral angiogram demonstrated marked swelling of the temporal lobe. CBF was reduced throughout the hemisphere, and PaO$_2$ was normal. PaCO$_2$ was reduced from spontaneous hyperventilation. Cerebral autoregulation, tested by intravenous injection of angiotensin, was defective adjacent to the mass only. Following administration of hypertonic mannitol elevated ICP fell, and CBF rose to normal or nearly so throughout the hemisphere. CMRO$_2$ was markedly depressed, but as CBF improved, focally after angiotensin and diffusely after mannitol, CMRO$_2$ increased from 1.15 to 1.26 to 1.58 ml/100gm/min. Table 1 illustrates a series of patients with unilateral post-traumatic masses and Table 2 a group a patients without a mass lesion, as determined by cerebral angiography. In 10 of the 13 patients in the two groups, mean CBF in the hemisphere examined increased from 10 to 35 ml/100gm/min. The response of CMRO$_2$ varied greatly, but in two patients (J.L. and C.D.) there was a marked increase, and in one patient (H.M.) CMRO$_2$ returned to normal. The implication of the data is that CMRO$_2$ was reduced in these patients because of ischemic hypoxia secondary to reduced CBF. When CBF was increased by administration of mannitol, CMRO$_2$ also increased demonstrating that the hypoxic insult was reversible. Unfortunately for this hypothesis, patient J.L. had a normal CBF prior to administration of mannitol.

Conclusion

It is unfortunate that the alterations in intracranial dynamics and brain function produced by acute brain insults are so complex. The practicing neurosurgeon wishes to have as firm guidelines as possible in the management of his patients, and few neurosurgeons have available the full array of special techniques described in this report.

The most important criterion for initiating treatment or changing from one form of therapy to another is deterioration in the patient's neurological status, and the best evidence that the therapy has been effective is clinical improvement. Increased ICP, for example, is significant mainly in terms of brain function. When a rise in ICP results in neurological deterioration, it is clear that the intracranial hypertension should be treated. A more difficult decision is when to treat elevated ICP prophylactically, and that is a matter of clinical judgment. As an example, spontaneous pressure waves of increasing frequency and magnitude are an ominous sign, because experience has taught that even though there are no neurological signs in association with the pressure waves, a "terminal" pressure wave may

Table 1. CBF, ICP, and CMRO$_2$ before and 30 minutes after administration of a bolus of intravenous mannitol in patients with a unilateral mass lesion following head injury

	Mannitol. Unilateral mass						
	Control			Post-mannitol		
	CBF	ICP	CMRO$_2$	CBF	ICP	CMRO$_2$
B.E.	35	39	1.15	50	16	1.58
H.M.	35	41	1.96	68	35	3.54
J.N.	18	47	0.39	38	48	0.48
R.W.	44	56	1.01	69	19	1.79
M.F.	32	21	0.87	34	18	1.28
R.Wa.	52	10	1.63	62	6	1.26

Table 2. Same as Table 1 in patients without a mass lesion

	Mannitol. No mass						
	Control			Post-mannitol		
	CBF	ICP	CMRO$_2$	CBF	ICP	CMRO$_2$
J.G.	31	22	1.61	50	23	1.63
J.L.	52	23	1.76	87	17	2.59
C.D.	38	14	1.65	57	9	2.34
E.D.	62	16	1.42	76	11	.81
B.J.S.	111	29	0.98	130	18	1.27
G.A.	31	0	1.65	36	2	1.80
J.B.	39	10	1.11	40	5	1.35

follow and lead to rapid deterioration and death of the patient before treatment can be instituted.

The ultimate value of measurements of CBF and brain metabolism in patient management remains to be determined. Certainly a reliable non-invasive technique for measurement of CBF is required. There is much information still to be learned from this relatively new technology, but the final test will be whether that information can be used to better diagnose and treat the patient who is in danger of dying from an acute brain insult.

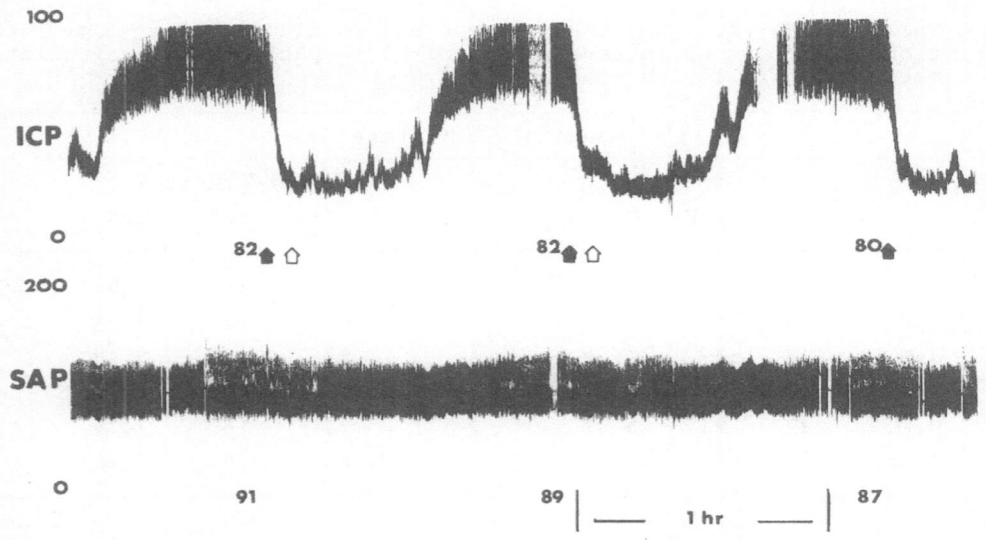

Fig. 1. ICP and SAP recorded continuously in a patient with a cerebellar hemangioblastoma. ICP varies with the onset (black arrow) and
cessation (white arrow) of voluntary hyperventilation. The numbers
along the horizontal axis are mean pressures for ICP and SAP. All
pressures in torr

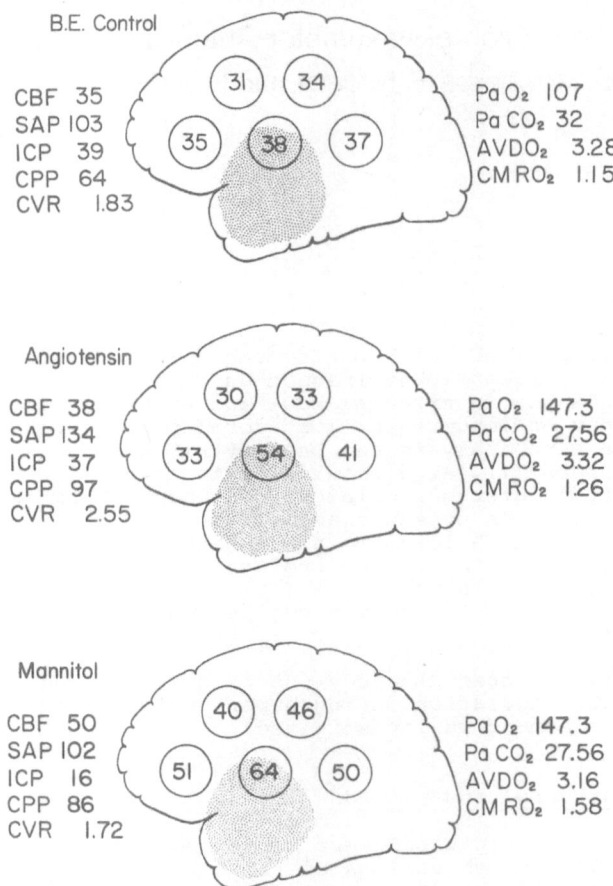

Fig. 2. Patient with a left temporal lobe contusion. Numbers in the circles are regional CBF values determined by height/area analysis of the clearance curves of 133 Xenon injected into the left internal carotid artery. CPP = mean SAP - mean ICP. CVR = CPP/CBF

Restitution of Vasomotor Autoregulation by Hypocapnia in Brain Tumors

A. HADJIDIMOS, F. FISCHER, and H. J. REULEN

In patients with brain tumors regional cerebral blood flow (rCBF) is significantly diminished and the physiological regulation of rCBF to changes in arterial pCO_2 and arterial blood pressure (*autoregulation*) may be impaired or lost focally or globally (2, 4). This tendency to a vasoparalysis has been attributed to tissue acidosis in edematous areas (1). As a result, acute arterial hypertension may be followed by deleterious clinical consequences by abnormally increasing tissue perfusion pressure as well as rCBF in areas with impaired vasomotor tone which leads to a break-through of pressure in the capillary system with further production of perifocal edema and increase of intracranial pressure (ICP). Dexamethasone was proved to substantially restore vasomotor regulation and increase rCBF in brain tumors (4, 6).

In the present study the role of induced *hypocapnia* on the impaired autoregulation during hypertension before and after dexamethasone treatment is investigated.

Material and Methods

9 investigations were performed in patients with supratentorial brain tumors with various degree of malignancy. All patients were submitted to rCBF measurements before and 3 of them after 6 days of dexamethasone treatment. Only the diseased hemisphere was investigated. Investigation was always performed under neuroleptic anesthesia, relaxation and control respiration. Mean arterial blood pressure (MABP in mmHg) was continuously monitored. Global and regional vascular regulation mechanisms were studied by means of functional tests: normotension-normocapnia, normotension-hypocapnia, hypertension-normocapnia and hypertension-hypocapnia.

For rCBF measurements the intra-arterial Xe^{133}-clearance technique (2, 4, 5) was used ("two-minutes-flow index" in ml/100 g.min). Values obtained during rest and hypertension were corrected to a "standard $paCO_2$" of 40 mmHg. Cerebro-vascular resistance (CVR) was calculated as the ratio of MABP and MrCBF in mmHg/ml/100 g.min.

Results

Global Hemispheric Effect of Hypocapnia During Impaired Autoregulation

a) Before Dexamethasone Administration: (Table 1, Fig. 1) According to previous results (2, 4) mean hemispheric rCBF at *normocapnia-normotension* (rest-state) was significantly reduced as compared to normal (about 55 ml/100 g.min). Interchannel coefficient of variation (ICV) as well as cerebro-vascular resistance (CVR) were markedly increased suggesting the presence of tissue perfusion pressure gradients still at the resting state (4).

Following induction of *hypocapnia* under *normal* arterial blood pressure, hemispheric blood flow decreased in all cases, except cases 7 and 8 (Table 1), but a partial CO_2-regulation defect was almost always present. CVR changed in the opposite direction indicating a diminished but still active vasoconstriction. During *hypertension at normocapnia*, autoregulation was found to be impaired in all cases, at least regionally. Average hemispheric flow increase was observed in 6 out of 9 instances, and CVR did not increase sufficiently (Fig. 1, a) in order to maintain the flow at the values observed during the resting state.

Following induction of *hypertension during hypocapnia*, blood flow was found significantly decreased in relation to hypertension during normocapnia and CVR increased more as in either one or the two previous tests (Fig. 1 c>a+b) indicating a restoration of the autoregulation and an astonishing active vasoconstriction.

b) *Following Dexamethasone Administration:* (Table 1, patients I, II and III) Autoregulation was completely restored in case I and CBF did not change. In the two other cases hemispheric rCBF increased and CO_2-regulation as well as autoregulation were significantly improved. The beneficial effect of hypocapnia upon the autoregulation can here be observed only regionally.

Regional effect of hypocapnia during impaired autoregulation. Table 2 quantifies the regions with abnormally increased rCBF during *hypertension at normocapnia* in contrast to *hypertension and hypocapnia*; the regional increases in rCBF during hypocapnia at normotension ("inverse steal syndrome") are also presented. It is clear that as well before as after dexamethasone administration the number of pathological increase in rCBF markedly decreases in hypocapnia-hypertension as compaired to normocapnia-hypertension.

Two examples shall be illustrated in order to demonstrate the *regional* beneficial effect of hypocapnia by impaired autoregulation in brain tumors.

The *first example* (Fig. 2, case 6 of Table 1) illustrates a *complete* restoration of the autoregulation disturbances observed during hypertension at normocapnia (low left) at the perifocal as well as the more remote areas of the hemisphere following hypertension and hypocapnia (low right).

The *second example* (Fig. 3, case 2 of Table 1) shows a remarkable but only *partial* beneficial effect of hypocapnia on the severely impaired autoregulation at the periphery of a highly vascularized malignant brain tumor.

Following dexamethasone treatment and reinvestigation of the same patient autoregulation at normocapnia is remarkably improved mainly at the remote perifocal areas (Fig. 4, case II of Table 1). Hypocapnia restores almost completely autoregulation (lower right) and *potentiates* the beneficial effect of dexamethasone.

Table 1. Test of Autoregulation at normocapnia and hypocapnia in the diseased
hemisphere of patients with brain tumors. Individual hemispheric values

| PATIENT | NORMOCAPNIA | | | | | | | | | | HYPOCAPNIA | | | | | | | | | |
| | NORMOTENSION | | | | | HYPERTENSION | | | | | NORMOTENSION | | | | | HYPERTENSION | | | | |
	$PaCO_2$	MABP	MrCBF	ICV	MrCVR	$PaCO_2$	MABP	MrCBF	IVC	MrCVR	$PaCO_2$	MABP	MrCBF	ICV	MrCVR	$PaCO_2$	MABP	MrCBF	ICV	MrCVR
1	46	80	45.6	17	2.0	43	140	40.2	24	3.8	29	83	20.9	15	4.0	29	145	22.3	18	6.2
2	40	107	29.6	23	3.6	39	155	34.0	49	4.4	30	97	25.6	38	3.8	25	153	27.4	37	5.6
3	41	82	19.2	50	4.4	41	140	18.5	35	7.7	27	82	11.7	42	7.0	27	142	15.2	38	9.3
4	40	100	13.4	31	7.5	46	125	19.9	40	6.2	29	108	11.3	29	9.6	29	135	11.8	34	11.4
5	40	90	29.4	16	3.0	38	133	29.9	21	4.2	30	88	19.9	17	4.4	25	133	22.5	18	5.9
6	45	80	31.4	16	2.9	39	135	33.2	23	3.9	26	80	19.9	15	4.0	27	137	19.3	18	7.1
7	39	105	26.5	21	3.8	41	130	37.6	14	3.5	28	100	27.4	13	3.6	29	138	23.6	11	5.8
8	40	80	15.8	12	5.0	40	125	19.3	7	6.5	29	78	14.6	9	5.3	27	115	16.2	11	11.0
9	42	110	26.1	15	4.4	41	140	33.0	18	4.5	27	112	20.5	10	5.5	27	147	19.0	19	7.8
I	44	95	41.2	17	2.5	46	145	35.0	21	4.7	31	93	21.8	17	4.3	30	145	23.0	19	6.3
II	43	95	33.5	22	3.0	43	155	29.6	21	5.4	28	100	15.2	18	6.6	32	195	17.1	28	11.4
III	41	93	28.6	14	3.3	41	140	28.8	13	4.9	29	90	19.8	19	4.5	31	147	22.1	20	6.7

$PaCO_2$ (mmHg) - MABP (mmHg) - MrCBF (ml/100 g.min) - ICV % - MrCVR (mmHg/ml/100 g.min).

Table 2. Regional evidence of restoration of the autoregulation by hypocapnia before and after dexamethasone treatment. Potentiation of the dexamethasone-effect

| CASE | DIAGNOSIS | REGIONS (n) | HYPERTENSION | | NORMOTENSION HYPOCAPNIA (n) |
			NORMOCAPNIA (n)	HYPOCAPNIA (n)	
1	Small brain metastasis	16	3	O	O
2	Brain metastasis	15	11	O	O
3	Brain metastasis	15	12	O	O
4	Glioblastoma	14	9	O	O
5	Brain metastasis	15	15	2	4
6	Brain metastasis	15	12	2	2
7	Glioblastoma	14	13	7	2
8	Oligodendroglioma	16	10	7	3
9	Astroblastoma	15	8	6	O
I	Case 1 + Dexameth.	16	O	O	O
II	Case 8 + Dexameth.	15	4	1	O
III	Case 9 + Dexameth.	16	7	1	O

Discussion

It is well known that the clinical state of patients with brain lesions and perifocal brain edema may severely decompensate following an acutely developing phase of hypercapnia and/or acute arterial hypertension. Since it is known that autonomic regulation of CBF is considerably disturbed in peritumoral edematous areas and sometimes even throughout the whole hemisphere an increase in arterial blood pressure will be passively followed by an increase of CBF in all areas with impaired autoregulation. Globally the cerebral blood volume will increase with subsequent increase of ICP. Due to vasoparalysis the arterial pressure head will break through into the capillaries, thus conspicuously increasing the formation of vasogenic brain edema. A predominantly unilateral increase in tissue volume may then aggravate an already existant brain shift and induce structural brain herniation.

For neurosurgeons the question is of utmost importance of which therapy would be efficient in the management and prevention of this dangerous situation.

The use of *hypertonic solutions* does not influence autoregulation and further it could induce a supplementary increase in interhemispheric pressure difference thus complicating the vicious circle.

Dexamethasone treatment during 4 to 6 days is followed by a remarkable alleviation of the clinical state of patients with brain tumor.

Although its genuine mechanism of action is not completely understood, dexamethasone was shown to reduce brain edema and restore the vasomotor regulation of the cerebral vessels (4, 6).

However, during an acute phase of arterial hypertension the efficient therapy would be to rapidly try to counteract tissue acidosis in the capillary level and restore autoregulation of CBF.

The role of *hypocapnia*, induced by apparative hyperventilation, in the reduction of increased ICP is well established (3, 6). Diminution of ICP results from a decrease in blood flow and volume in regions of the brain with preserved CO_2-response. The condition for this effect is the existence of sufficient regions of relatively healthy brain able to respond by means of the vasoconstriction to the hyperventilation, i.e. a state of so called "dissociated vasoparalysis" (5). In addition, LASSEN and PAULSON have demonstrated that a globally impaired autoregulation in the controlateral to the space occupying lesion hemisphere could be efficiently restored by means of hyperventilation. Since, however, the disturbances of autoregulation as well as CO_2-reactivity usually are much more pronounced in the tumor-bearing hemisphere, particularly in the perifocal areas, the question arises whether hypocapnia induced by hyperventilation may also restore the autoregulatory capacity and the hemodynamic situation in these areas.

The present results show that during acute systemic hypertension in patients with brain tumor and severe perifocal as well as homolateral global impairment of autoregulation the induction of hypocapnia through hyperventilation significantly improves and frequently completely restores (case 1, Fig. 2) autoregulation of CBF in the peritumoral brain tissue. The efficiency of this treatment may also be demonstrated in cases with very depressed cerebral blood flow at rest and severely impaired vasomotor response to $PaCO_2$ changes provided that "dissociated vasoparalysis" is regionally still present (case 4, 7 and 8, Tables 1 and 2).

It may be assumed that hyperventilation might induce by means of respiratory alkalosis an increase of bicarbonate, thus counteracting the tissue acidosis by increasing the pH in the capillary wall and the extracellular space.

The marked increase of CVR during hypocapnia and hypertension might indicate that following a diminished tissue acidosis, a *potentiation* of the vasoconstrictive effect is occurring by means of the individual differential reestablishment of the autoregulation as well as the CO_2 regulation of the brain capillaries.

In the cases treated with *dexamethasone* it is further shown that the marked improvement of autoregulation obtained by means of this drug is further supported (Fig. 4, case II) under hypocapnia even at high systemic arterial pressure.

It can be suggested that as well pre-, as postoperatively in patients with brain space-occupying lesion and acute brain edema the combination of dexamethasone administration with the induction of a moderate hypocapnia may optimally be used to prevent as well as to treat an acute state of impaired autoregulation and thus control cerebral edema and increased ICP.

Fig. 2. Report of a case with complete restoration ▷
of autoregulation at hypocapnia

Summary

Patients with cerebral tumor and perifocal edema may severely decompensate following acure hypertension. This is due to the impairment of the autoregulation at the peritumoral edematous areas and attributed to tissue acidosis. It is shown that the induction of moderate hypocapnia during acute arterial hypertension remarkable restores the autoregulation in the hemisphere bearing the tumor. Respiratory alkalosis is thus assumed to counteract metabolic tissue acidosis on the capillary wall. The beneficial effect of dexamethasone upon the autoregulation is potentiated by hypocapnia.

REFERENCES

1. BETZ, E., HAUSER, D.: Cerebral cortical blood flow during changes of acid-base equilibrium of the brain. J. Appl. Physiol. 23, 726-733 (1967).
2. BROCK, M., HADJIDIMOS, A., DERUAZ, J.P., SCHÜRMANN, K.: Regional cerebral blood flow and vascular reactivity in cases of brain tumor. In: Brain and blood flow (ed. R.W.ROSS RUSSEL), pp.281-284. London: Pitman 1971.
3. GORDON, E.: The effect of controlled ventilàtion on the clinical course of patients with severe traumatic brain injury. In: Brain and blood flow (ed. R.W.ROSS RUSSEL), pp.365-369. London: Pitman 1971.
4. HADJIDIMOS, A., STEINGASS, U., FISCHER, F., REULEN, H.J., SCHÜRMANN, K.: The effect of dexamethasone on rCBF and cerebral vasomotor response in brain tumors. Europ. Neurol. 10, 25-30 (1973).
5. PAULSON, O.B.: Restoration of autoregulation by hypocapnia. In: Brain and blood flow (ed. R.W. ROSS RUSSEL), pp.313-321. London: Pitman 1971.
6. REULEN, H.J., HADJIDIMOS, A., SCHÜRMANN, K.: The effect of dexamethasone on water and electrolyte content and on rCBF in perifocal brain edema in man. In: Steroids and brain edema (eds. H.J. REULEN, K. SCHÜRMANN), pp. 239-252. Berlin-Heidelberg-New York: Springer 1972.

Fig.1. see page 98

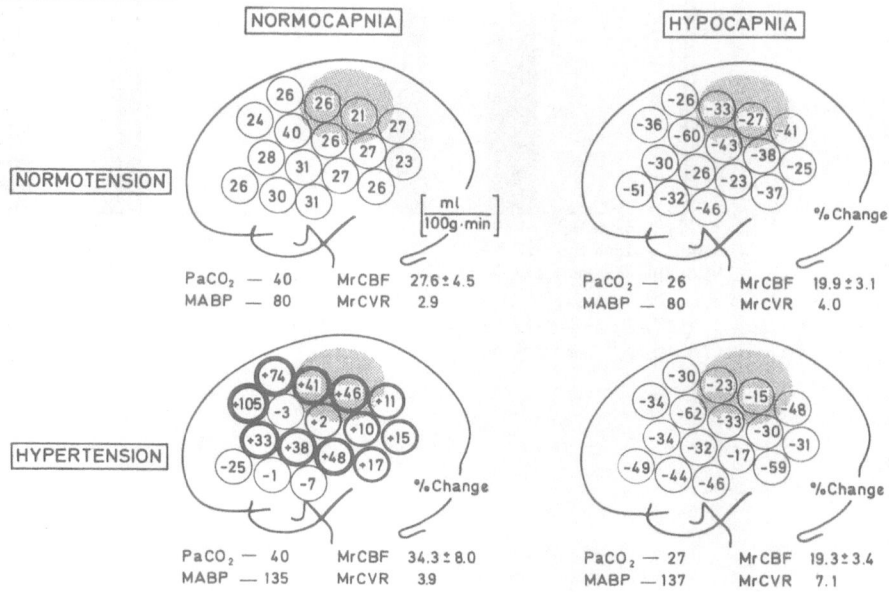

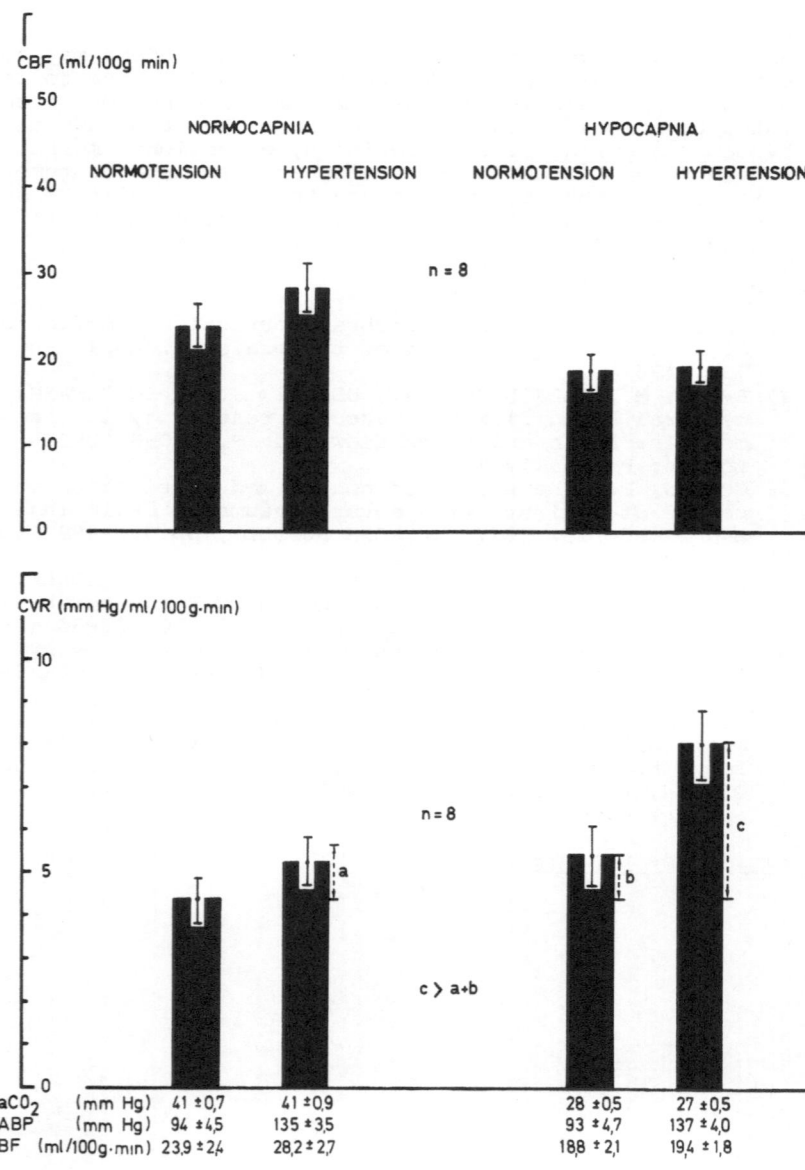

Fig. 1. Loss of autoregulation at normocapnia and its restoration at hypocapnia. *Mean of hemispheric values*

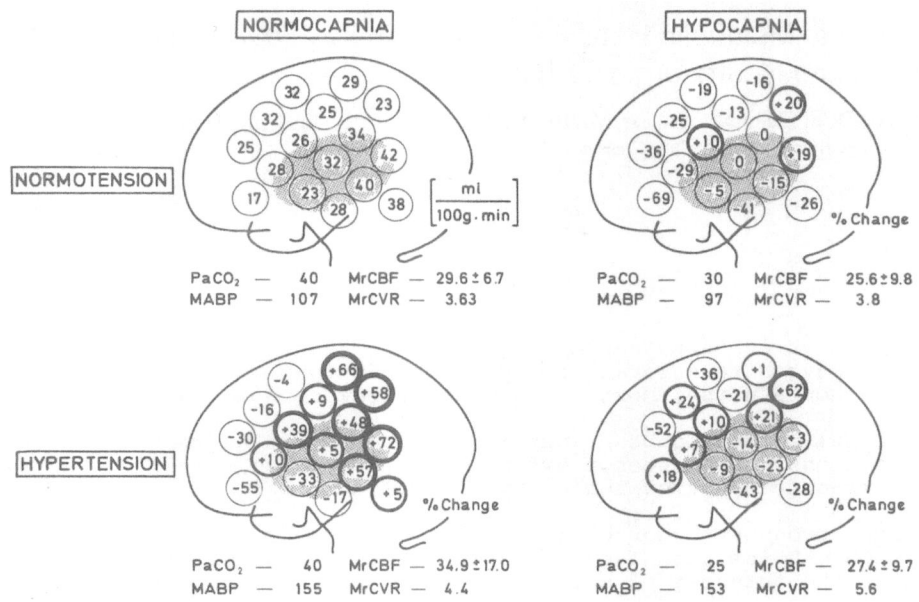

Fig. 3. Report of a case with significant but *partial* restoration of autoregulation at hypocapnia

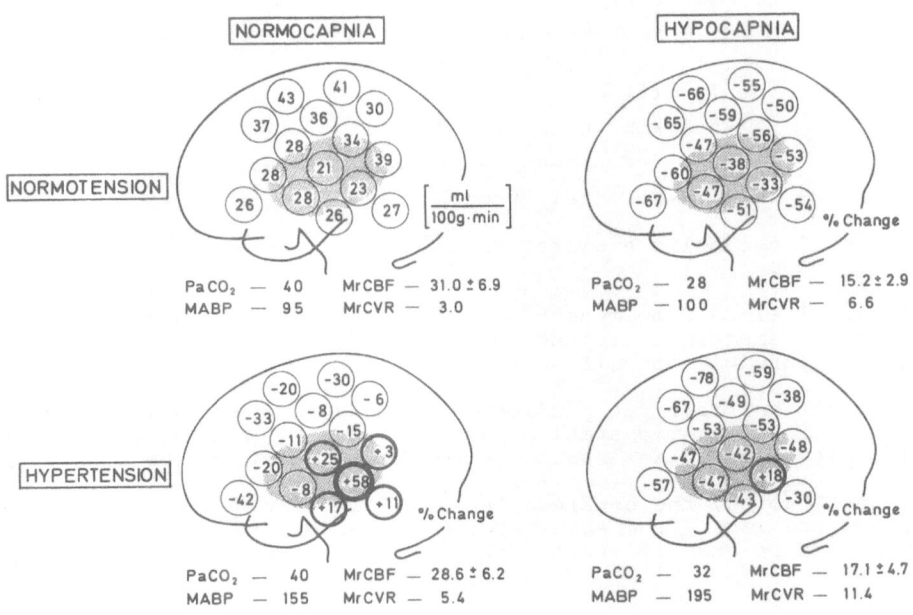

Fig. 4. Report of the same case as in Fig. 3 showing the *potentiation* of the beneficial effect of dexamethasone on the impaired autoregulation by hypocapnia

Cerebral Metabolic Behaviour in Relation to Oxygen in Comas During the Acute Neurosurgical Phase

B. ROQUEFEUIL, M. BALDY-MOULINIER, E. VIGUIE, E. ESCURET, A. CALLIS, F. FREREBEAU, and CL. GROS

This paper concerns cerebral blood flow values and cerebral metabolic oxygen rate levels found in thirty four neurosurgical patients in an acute phase, most of them after severe head injury.

Cerebral metabolic behaviour is analysed first in the steady state conditions, then after a dynamic modification obtained either by hypercapnic hypertension or by an aramine induced hypertension.

A real prognostic correlation can be deduced from steady state condition studies and also from dynamic state studies, which clearly shows the interest of metabolic exploration in patients in deep coma.

I. Material and Method

Our 34 patients are divided as follows:

- 28 coma patients with severe head injuries, of which:
    - 9 have predominant brain stem disease;
    - 18 have either unilateral hemispheric contusion (6) or diffuse contusion (12);
    - 1 with bilateral chronic subdural hematoma.
- 5 with cerebrovascular disorders.
- 1 with cerebral tumor.

Cerebral metabolic exploration takes place between the third and the tenth day.

Cerebral Blood Flow measurement (CBF) is accomplished by the intra-arterial carotidian injection of X_e 133, in the injured side in unilateral predominant ailments disease, either side with other ailments.

Each patient is first studied in a steady state condition then, afterwards, in a dynamic state obtained either by a $PaCO_2$ level increase (16 cases) or by an aramine intravenous injection (18 cases).

Under Aramine, the obtained tensional increase is about 50 to 100 mmHg, and lasts from about 10 to 15 minutes, sufficient time to take CBF measure and different metabolic samples.

II. Results

1. Cerebral Blood Flow (CBF) and cerebral metabolic rate for oxygen (CMRO$_2$) in a steady state condition

A. Cerebral Blood Flow (Table 1)

The average of the 34 hemispheric CBF measures is 35,15 $\pm$ 13,01 ml/100g/mn, that is to say a mean value clearly inferior to the normal CBF value (50 ml/100g/mn).

Relative to the depth of the comas the lowest mean CBF values are found in the most serious cases (C$_3$: 33,16 $\pm$ 11,95).

The mean CBF value equally shows an interesting prognostic meaning:

- 15,3% of survivals in the patients (13 cases) with a mean CBF lower than 30 ml/100g/mn;
- 61,9% of survivals in those (21 cases) with a mean CBF higher than 30 ml/100g/mn.

Table 1. Mean CBF and mean CMRO$_2$ in steady states conditions

Average of	Mean CBF in ml/100 g/mn			Mean CMRO$_2$ in ml O$_2$/100 g/mn	
Average of 34 measures	35,15 $\pm$ 13,01			1,80 $\pm$ 0,94	
Related to the depth of coma	C$_1$ (7 patients) : 38,57 $\pm$ 16,97			2,44 $\pm$ 1,15	
	C$_2$ (10 patients): 36,16 $\pm$ 12,53			1,67 $\pm$ 0,77	
	C$_3$ (17 patients): 33,16 $\pm$ 11,95			1,58 $\pm$ 0,86	
		< 30	> 30	< 1,50	> 1,50
	Patients	13	21	15	19
Prognostic Value	Deaths	11	8	10	7
	Survivals	2	13	5	12
	% survey	15,3%	61,9%	33,33%	63,15%

B. Cerebral metabolic rate for oxygen (CMRO$_2$)   Table 1

Mean CMRO$_2$ (the average of 34 measures) is equally lowered, 1,80 $\pm$ 0,94 ml O$_2$/100g/mn (normal value : 3,30 ml/100g/mn).There also seems to be a good correlation between the mean CMRO$_2$ and the depth of the coma, the lowest mean CMRO$_2$ - 1,58 $\pm$ 0,86 - being found in the most severe cases (C$_3$). Likewise the level of CMRO$_2$ seems to have a prognostic signification:

- 33,33% of survivals in the patients (15 cases) with a CMRO$_2$ lower than 1,30 ml/100g/mn;
- 63,15% fo survivals in those (19 cases) with a mean CMRO$_2$ higher than 1,50 ml/100g/mn.

2. Metabolic brain behaviour after a dynamic change ($PaCO_2$ increase or Aramine induced hypertension)

A. Cerebral reactivity to $PaCO_2$ (Table 2)

After having induced a moderate hypercapnic increase, in 16 patients, the results permitted us to separate 2 groups:

- the first (G_1 : 8 cases) where the mean CBF reactivity to $PaCO_2$ is high. A $PaCO_2$ increase of 1 mmHg gives us a mean CBF increase of about 2,65 ± 1,91 ml/100g/mn;
- a second group (G_2 : 8 cases) where the mean CBF reactivity to $PaCO_2$ is very low (0,35 ± 0,26 ml/100g/mn/1 mmHg $PaCO_2$ increase).

The mean $CMRO_2$ variation is nearly identical in both groups and can not be interpreted. The survival rate is almost the same in both cases, therefore without evident prognostic correlation.

On the contrary, $PaCO_2$ reactivity seems clearly linked to the depth of the comas:

- lowered in severe comas (C_3), 0,80 ml mean CBF increase per one mmHg $PaCO_2$ increase;
- higher in the less severe comas (C_1 and C_2), 2,06 ml mean CBF increase per one mmHg $PaCO_2$ increase.

B. Brain response to Aramine induced hypertension (Table 3)

With Aramine, mean CBF and $CMRO_2$ variations permit us to classify 3 groups:

- a first group (8 cases) where a systolic arterial pressure (SAP) increase of about 63 mmHg shows practically no mean CBF (+ 2,5 ml) and mean $CMRO_2$ (- 0,26) changes (0,45 ml mean CBF increase per 10 mmHg SAP increase - autoregulation);
- in the second group (4 cases) an identical SAP increase - 70 mmHg - diminishes the mean CBF (- 15 ml/100g/mn) and the mean $CMRO_2$ (- 0,90 ml/100g/mn), that's to say a mean CBF reduction of about (-2,01 ml per 10 mmHg SAP increase).
- in the third group (6 cases), the SAP increase - + 88 mmHg - raises distinctly the mean CBF (+ 29,1 ml/100g/mn) and the mean $CMRO_2$ (+ 1,09 ml/100g/mn), that's to say a mean CBF variation of about + 2,83 ml/10 mmHg SAP increase (loss of autoregulation).

In the same manner, the brain response to Aramine shows:

- a prognostic relationship, 58,3% of survivals in groups I et II (autoregulation present) and 16,66% of survivals in group III (loss of autoregulation);
- and then a clinical relationship, the CBF increase is clearly higher in severe comas.

C. $CMRO_2$ change related to CBF change (Table 4)

The $CMRO_2$ change - in per cent of initial value - related to CBF change (equally in per cent of I.V.) permit us to separate three patients groups:

Table 2. Cerebral behaviour to PaCO$_2$ increase - (16 studies - 16 patients)

	Group I (8 patients)			Group II (8 patients)		
	- a - Control values	- b - PaCO$_2$ increase	- c - Mean change	- a -	- b -	- c -
Me PaCO$_2$ (in mmHg)	31,12 ± 8,39	42,75 ± 15,09	+ 11,63	32 ± 8,60	48,88 ± 9,28	+ 16.8
Me CBF (in ml/100g/mn)	43,08 ± 18,17	70,76 ± 33,41	+ 27,68	28,64 ± 8,70	33,96 ± 8,69	+ 5,58
Me CMRO$_2$ (in ml/100g/mn)	2,16 ± 1,01	2,18 ± 1,03	+ 0,02	1,35	1,03	- 0,32
PaCO$_2$ response related to prognosis.	+ 2,65 ml MCBF ↗ / 1 torr PaCO$_2$ ↗ ± 1,91			+ 0,35 ml MCBF ↗ / 1 torr PaCO$_2$ ↗ ± 0,26		
Patients	8			8		
Survivals	5			4		
Deaths	3			4		

Average of 16 studies : 1,50 mean CBF ↗ / 1 torr PaCO$_2$ ↗

PaCO$_2$ response related to coma depth.	Comas level C$_2$ (9 cases) : 2,06 ± 2,23 MCBF ↗ / 1 torr PaCO$_2$ ↗
	Comas level C$_3$ (7 cases) : 0,80 ± 0,56 MCBF ↗ / 1 torr PaCO$_2$ ↗

Table 3. Cerebral behaviour to induced aramine hypertension

(equal $PaCO_2$ level in the 3 groups)

	G1 (8 cases)			G2 (4 cases)			G3 (6 cases)		
	- a - Initial values	- b - SAP ↗	- c - Mean change	- a -	- b -	- c -	- a -	- b -	- c -
Me SAP	125 ±20	188 ±14,58	+63,75	127,5 ±22,17	200 ±33	+72,5	100 ±22,57	188 ±31,89	+88
Me CBF	33,15±12,52	36,09±12,20	+2,93	40,35 ± 6,90	25,85 ±10,01	-14,48	32,5 ±10,01	61,6 ±23,36	+29,11
Me $CMRO_2$	1,83± 0,94	1,57± 0,86	-0,24	2,21 ± 1,16	1,31 ± 0,97	-0,90	1,52 ± 0,80	2,67 ± 1,51	+ 1,09
Me CBF change/ 10 mmHg SAP increase	G1 : normal autoregulation + 0,45			G2 : excessive autoregulation - 2,01			G3 : loss of autoregulation + 2,83		
Prognosis related to	Patients: : 12 Deaths : 5						6 5		
Aramine response	Survivals : 7 ----> 58,3%						1 ----> 16,66%		

Aramine response related to coma depth	CBF change per 10 mmHg SAP ↗		$CMRO_2$ change
	Levels C1 + C2 (8 patients) :	- 2,85	- 0,40
	Level C3 (10 patients) :	+ 23,34	+ 0,40

- a first group - 10 cases - where, for each one, the $CMRO_2$ shows an identical change to CBF; in that group, the survival rate is high: 70%.
- a second group - 14 cases - where the $CMRO_2$ is lowered while the CBF increases - luxury perfusion syndrome - and for them a poor prognostic : 21,2% of survival rate.
- a third group - 10 cases - where the $CMRO_2$ increase is higher than the CBF increase (insufficient perfusion).

Table 4. Prognostic value of hemodynamic and metabolic behaviour

A. Severe comas (C_3)

	Initial values	CO_2 reactivity	Aramine response
Mean CBF	↘ +++	↘ ++	↗ +++
Mean $CMRO_2$	↘ ++	# 0	↗

B. Survivals rate in %

Mean CBF	< 30 : 15,3%	> 30 : 61,9%
Mean $CMRO_2$	<1,50: 33,3%	>1,50 : 63,15%
Autoregulation to hypertension	Lost : 18,66%	Normal or : 58,3% excessive

C. Prognostic incidence of mean $CMRO_2$ change related to mean CBF change $(CO_2O_2$ Aramine hypertension)		Patients	Survivals rate in %
	— Mean $CMRO_2$ change (Δ) = mean CBF change (Δ) in % and scale : + or -	10	70%
	— Mean $CMRO_2$ Δ < MCBF Δ (luxury perfusion syndrom)	14	21,2%
	— Mean $CMRO_2$ Δ > MCBF Δ (insufficient perfusion)	10	50%

Discussion

Brain metabolic study is important in the acute phase where it is often very difficult to make a prognosis. The mean CBF value - 35,15 ml/100g/mn - that we find is identical to that claimed by other authors (3, 8) in acute traumatic comatose patients with low $PaCO_2$ values.

Certain (9) find much lower CBF values - 23,5 ml/100g/mn - but do not precisely state the mean $PaCO_2$ level... In vascular comatose patients (6) it seems that, for the same $PaCO_2$ and identical coma levels, the mean CBF lowering is more important.

The mean $CMRO_2$ value in our study is nearly the same as that claimed by different above mentioned authors. For them, the relation is clear between the clinical state (therefore the prognosis) and mean CBF and $CMRO_2$ values, but they compare comatose patients, awake patients with a neurologic deficit and normal patients...

In our study - comatose patients only - such relation still exists but less pronounced; it is not found in vascular comas (6) with different levels.

Thus, without overestimating the data, we can assume that a mean $CMRO_2$ higher than 1,50 ml/100g/mn and a mean CBF higher than 30 ml/100g/mn actually are rational survival criteria.

Mean $PaCO_2$ cerebral reactivity is low - 1,50 ml/mmHg $PaCO_2$ - but identical to that stated by others, much lower than $PaCO_2$ reactivity found in normal experimental animals - 2,5 ml/mmHg - (8).

If we admit that (7) $PaCO_2$ cerebral reactivity presume the vascular brain capacity in response to an eventual need increase, we assume the importance of the exact relation existing between the coma levels and the $PaCO_2$ response. There is no significant $CMRO_2$ increase in the hypercapnic state and perhaps this fact can be related (8, 10) to a possible metabolic cerebral rate decrease when under the carbon dioxyde tension influence.

The Aramine induced hypertension study states still better the brain behaviour; the autoregulation to hypertension is lost in 30% of our comas, those which are the most serious and those which have the poorest prognosis.

Fortunately, the loss of autoregulation is not a rule, since 60% of our cases have a normal or an excessive autoregulation. While this fact - present autoregulation as a response to hypertension - has been advanced in ischemic cerebral areas (1), the mechanisms are still poorly understood. But above all the dynamic changes (CO_2 or Aramine hypertension) permit us to establish the usefulness of circulatory change.

A $CMRO_2$ level which exactly corresponds to the CBF evolution indicates that (7) brain ischemic suffering does not increase - this brain behaviour is evident in ten of our patients, and for them the prognosis is rather good - .

The "Luxury Perfusion Syndrome" is present in 14 cases and these have the poorest prognosis; so for them, the usual reanimation therapies - all trying to reduce this unuseful perfusion - seem logical.

On the other hand, the insufficient perfusion syndrome - ten cases - only revealed by dynamic studies, can signify a cerebral metabolic need unsatisfied by circulatory conditions. From this we presume that in these cases the usual therapies (mechanical ventilation, neuroplegic drugs) must be strictly discussed, because they all decrease the mean CBF; this also reminds us that hypertensive drugs have equally been proposed in the treatment of vascular cerebral disorders (1, 2, 4, 5).

So in the traumatic comatose patients the CBF and $CMRO_2$ values, as the $PaCO_2$ and the Aramine response, seems well correlated to the clinical state. The prognostic importance of the brain metabolic study is evident, chiefly because the brain need for oxygen varies with each patient.

Summary

Concerning 34 CBF and $CMRO_2$ measures in 34 acute neurosurgical patients, the author find a quite good relationship between the CBF and $CMRO_2$ values, in steady states conditions, and either the level coma or the prognosis. With an hypercapnic change, the $PaCO_2$ reactivity is found low in the most severe comas. Under Aramine induced hypertension, 30% of the cases show a loss of autoregulation. The $CMRO_2$ change related to CBF permits them to separate those who have a good metabolic autoregulation from those who have a loss of metabolic autoregulation, either under the category of "luxury perfusion syndrome" or under the category of "insufficient perfusion". For these, the authors chiefly discusses the therapy attitude.

REFERENCES

1. AGNOLI, A.: Troubles de l'autorégulation dans les foyers de ramollissements cérébraux. (Autoregulation disturbances in brain infarct areas). In: Journées Internationales de Circulation Cérébrale. Toulouse: L'ischémie cérébrale dans le territoire carotidien.(eds. J. GERAUD, G. LAZORTHES, A. BES), pp. 297 - 303 (1972).

2. AGNOLI, A.: Dérangement de l'autorégulation dans les foyers ischémiques cérébraux: possivilité thérapeutique des médicaments hypertenseurs. (Autoregulation disturbances in brain infarct areas: possible use of hypertensive drugs). In: Symposium International sur la Circulation Cérébrale.Paris, 15 - 16 octobre. pp. 114-120. Paris: Editions Sandoz 1966.

3. BALDY MOULINIER, M., FREREBEAU, Ph.: Cerebral blood flow in cases of coma following severe head injury. In: Cerebral blood flow (eds. M. BROCK, C. FIESCHI, D.H. INGVAR, N.A. LASSEN, K. SHURMAN), pp. 216 - 218. Berlin - Heidelberg - New York: Springer 1969.

4. FAZIO, C.: Autoregulation of brain circulation. J. Sandoz of Med. Sci. II, 93 - 98 (1971).

5. FIESCHI, C., AGNOLI, A., BOZZAO, L., BATTISTINI, N., PRENCIPE, M.: Discrepancies between autoregulation and CO_2 reactivity of cerebral vessels. In: Cerebral Blood flow (eds. M. BROCK, C. FIESCHI, D.H. INGVAR, N.A. LASSEN, K. SHURMANN). Berlin - Heidelberg - New York: Springer 1969.

6. GERAUD, J., BES, A., ESCANCHE, M.: Cerebral blood flow and metabolism in coma due to stroke. Research on the cerebral circulation, Proc. 4th int. Salzbourg Conference (eds. J.S. MEYER, M. REIVICH et al.), pp. 237 - 248. Springfield/Ill.: Charles C. THOMAS 1970

7. HARP, J.R., WOLLMAN, H.: Cerebral metabolic effects of hyperventilation and deliberate hypotension. Brit. J. Anaesth. 45, 256 - 262 (1973).

8. HOYER, S., PISCOL, K., STOECKEL, H., HAMER, J., KONTOPOULOS, B., WOLF, P., WEINHARDT, F.: CBF and metabolism in patients with acute brain injury with regard to autoregulation. In: Cerebral blood flow and intracranial pressure. Proc. 5th Int. Sympo. Roma-Siena, 1971. Part. II. Europ. Neurol. 8, 174 - 180 (1972).

9. KAMRAN TABBADOR, M.D., BHUSHAN,C., M.D., PEVSNER, D.H., M.D., WALKER, A.E., M.D.: Prognostic value of cerebral blood flow (CBF) and cerebral metabolism rate of oxygen ($CMRO_2$) in acute head trauma. J. Trauma 12, 1053 - 1055 (1972).

10. MACMILLAN, V., SIESJÖ, B.K.: Cerebral energy metabolism in hypoxemia. In: Cerebral blood flow and intracranial pressure. Proc. 5th Int. Sympo., Roma-Siena, 1971, Part. I. Europ. Neurol. $\underline{6}$, 66-72 (1972).

11. HARPER, A.M., DESMUKH, V.D., SENGUPTA, D., ROWAN, J.O., JENNET, W.B.: The effect of experimental spasm on the CO_2 response of cerebral blood flow in primates. Neuroradiol. $\underline{3}$, 134 - 136 (1972).

Influence of CSF-Resorption Pathways on Intracranial Capacitance

M. Brock, M. Furuse, M. Hasuo, and H. Dietz*

Knowledge on the intracranial pressure/volume (P/V) relationship and its changes under various influences is of practical and theoretical importance (1-6). However, among the several factors possibly responsible for the intracranial spatial buffering capacity the role of CSF resorption has merited only little attention to date.

SCHULMAN and MARMAROU (3) demonstrated a reduced intracranial capacitance in hydrocephalic children. LÖFGREN et al. (7) suggested that obstruction of CSF resorption pathways in the course of repeated experimental subarachnoid hemorrhage progressively reduces the ability to tolerate increases in intracranial volume.

These data indicate that the pressure/volume response might not be entirely "due to an interaction between the elastic properties of the spinal dural sac and the resistance of the vascular bed to compression and distension" (8). Other variables, such as fast changes in CSF absorption could also influence the response of ICP to an increase in intracranial volume.

In the present study a model of acute malresorptive hydrocephalus was used to evaluate the influence of CSF resorption on intracranial P/V relationship.

Material and Methods

Seven adult apparently healthy mongrel cats of both sexes weighing 2.3 to 3.5 kg were studied under intraperitoneal Nembutal anesthesia (35 mg/kg body-weight). The femoral vessels on one side were catheterized for continuous recording of systemic arterial pressure (Statham P 23 Db), blood sampling and administration of drugs as needed. All animals were tracheostomized, immobilized and mechanically ventilated under normocapnic conditions (PaCO$_2$: 27-35 mmHg) with a Sterling pump. Following fixation of the prone animal's head in a stereotactic frame, one polyethylene catheter (outer diameter: 1.0 mm) was inserted into each lateral ventricle through small symmetrical frontal burr-holes. CSF leakage was avoided and the burr-holes were sealed with dental cement. One catheter was used to measure CSFP (Statham P 23 Db) while the other was employed for intraventricular infusions as described below. Infratentorial tissue pressure was recorded from one cerebellar peduncle (6, 9, 10). The animals were divided into two groups:

---

*The authors are indebted to Miss Irma BUSCHE, Miss Gudrun HEINE and Miss Elvira RIECHERS for their valuable technical help.

Group I (n=5): The influence of intraventricular infusion of 2.0 ml of saline at a constant rate of 0.5 ml/min on intracranial compliance was studied prior to, as well as 1 h and 3 h following intraventricular administration of 2 ml of a neutral soot dispersion (containing 10% soot, 9.5% gelatin and 1.3% phenol).

Group II (n=2): These animals were subjected to repeated intraventricular infusion of saline after 1 h and 3 h as in group I, but were not given soot dispersion. They served as controls for group I.

At the end of the experiment the animals were sacrificed by intravenous administration of saturated KCl solution. The brain and spinal cord were carefully removed and the distribution of soot particles studied.

Results

The method here described for producing an acutely progressive malresorptive hydrocephalus has proven to be simple and reliable. It differs from the procedure applied by WEED (11) in that the amount of particles is sufficient to impair CSF resorption. In no instance have we noticed obstruction of the aqueduct or the basal cysterns. The injected soot particles have always propagated throughout the entire subarachnoid space.

The usual pressure-course following the administration of soot particles into the CSF compartment consists in a progressive rise in ICP leading to death of the animal within a few hours.

Prior to intraventricular soot administration the constant-rate infusion of saline into one lateral ventricle leads to a significant average ICP increase from the resting value of 7.8 (±0.7 SE) mmHg to 42.3 (±6.4 SE) mmHg at the end of the second minute (=1ml), followed by a non-significant decrease to 38.5 (±6.2 SE) mmHg at the end of the infusion period (4 min, i.e. 2ml). When the soot infusion is discontinued, pressure promptly returns to levels only slightly higher than control values (Table 1, Fig. 1).

At the end of the first hour following soot administration, resting CSFP has risen to 18.0 (±1.4 SE) mmHg. Intraventricular infusion of 2 ml of saline then leads to a steady and steep pressure increase to values of 89.6 (±14.1 SE) mmHg, significantly different from the controls. When the soot infusion is discontinued, pressure promptly decreases but remains significantly above the pre-infusion value (Table 1, Fig. 1).

At the end of the third hour following soot administration, resting CSFP is 32.1 (±4.8 SE) mmHg and intraventricular infusion of 2 ml of saline causes an even steeper increase of CSFP to values of 140.8 (±21.7 SE) mmHg. These values are significantly higher than those obtained 1 h after soot administration. When the soot infusion is discontinued, pressure again sharply decreases, remaining, however, significantly higher than the pre-infusion values (Table 1, Fig. 1).

In the animals of group II (no administration of soot) no difference was noted between the P/V curves obtained after 1 h and 3 h (Fig. 2).

Tissue pressures in the cerebellar peduncle follow CSF pressures but remain at lower levels. The transtentorial pressure gradients amounted up to 30 mmHg and were more marked at high CSFP levels.

Table 1. CSFP changes to intraventricular saline infusion (0.5 ml/min) before and after soot administration

Time (minutes)	Infusion Period					Post-infusion Period			
	0	1.0	2.0	3.0	4.0	5.0	6.0	7.0	8.0
Infusion volume (ml)	0	0.5	1.0	1.5	2.0	–	–	–	–
Pressure changes prior to soot administration (mmHg)	7.8 (0.7)	34.1 (6.8)	42.3 (6.4)	39.5 (5.8)	38.5 (6.2)	19.2 (2.2)	15.2 (1.5)	13.8 (1.8)	12.6 (0.9)
Pressure changes 1 hour after soot administration (mmHg)	18.0 (1.4)	52.5 (7.4)	77.8 (11.3)	86.2 (13.8)	89.6 (14.1)	51.2 (6.4)	39.8 (3.3)	35.8 (1.9)	31.0 (1.9)
Pressure changes 3 hours after soot administration (mmHg)	32.1 (4.8)	94.8 (30.5)	136.4 (23.1)	142.2 (23.6)	140.8 (21.7)	87.0 (10.0)	71.0 (8.0)	56.0 (5.0)	49.0 (4.0)

( ) = SE

111

Comments

The increase in resting ICP following soot administration as performed in the present study is an expression of impaired CSF resorption, since it seems improbable that the presence of soot might lead
to an "irritative" increase in CSF production - another possible
cause of rised ICP (12, 13).

Thus, it becomes apparent that soot particles, by obstructing the CSF
resorption pathways, cause an imbalance of intracranial fluid dynamics leading to a progressive increase in resting CSFP. The fact that,
in the normal animal, prior to soot administration, ICP returns to
control values within a few minutes following intraventricular infusion of 2 ml of saline solution can not be explained by an increased
CSF resorption rate alone (12, 13). It is probable that this adaptation occurs partly at the expenses of a decrease in available reserve
capacitance. In other words, there is a concomitant displacement of
the system towards the steep limb of the P/V curve. This situation
is aggravated in the presence of a progressive obstruction of the
CSF pathways by the soot particles. From our results we conclude that
changes in CSF resorption strongly influence the intracranial pres-
sure/volume response. Although neither the elasticity of the container (craniospinal compartment) nor that of the contents (CNS,
blood and CSF) are altered, the pressure-response of the system to an
increase in volume is markedly altered in the presence of a deficient
CSF-resorption. It follows that the P/V response in a biological system such as the craniospinal is dependent on two components: the
first of these is given by the elastic properties of the container
and of the contents, while the second is determined by the fluid dynamics within the system.

REFERENCES

1. LANGFITT, T.W., WEINSTEIN, J.D., KASSELL, N.F.: Vascular factors
   in head injury: contribution of brain swelling and intracranial
   hypertension. In: Head injury, pp. 172-194. Philadelphia: Lippin-
   cott 1966.

2. MERREM, B.: Intraventrikuläre Druckvolumenregulation des Ver-
   schlußhydrocephalus. Zbl. f. Neurochir. 32, 35-52 (1971).

3. SCHULMAN, K., MARMAROU, A.: Pressure-volume considerations in
   infantile hydrocephalus. Develop. Med. Child. Neurol. 25 (13),
   90-95 (1971).

4. NAKATANI, S., OMMAYA, A.K.: A critical rate of cerebral compression. In: Intracranial pressure (eds. M. BROCK, H. DIETZ), pp.
   144-148. Berlin-Heidelberg-New York: Springer 1972.

5. MILLER, J.D., PICKARD, J.D.: Intracranial volume/pressure studies
   in patients with head injury. Injury 5, 265-268 (1974).

6. FURUSE, M., BROCK, M., WEBER, R., HASUD, M., DIETZ, H.: Intracranial pressure/volume relationship in acute experimental water
   intoxication. In: Intracranial pressure II (eds. N. LUNDBERG, U.
   PONTEN, M. BROCK), pp. 101-106. Berlin-Heidelberg-New York:
   Springer 1975.

7. LÖFGREN, J., STEINER, L., ZWETNOW, N.: Intracranial pressure
   course in repeated subarachnoid hemorrhage. In: Intracranial pressure II (eds. N. LUNDBERG, U. PONTEN, M. BROCK), pp. 113-117.
   Berlin-Heidelberg-New York: Springer 1975.

8. LÖFGREN, J.: Mechanical basis of the CSF pressure/volume curve. In: Intracranial pressure II (eds. N. LUNDBERG, U. PONTEN, M. BROCK), pp. 79-81. Berlin-Heidelberg-New York: Springer 1975.

9. BROCK, M., WINKELMÜLLER, W., PÖLL, W., MARKAKIS, E., DIETZ, H.: Measurement of brain tissue pressure. Lancet 2, 595-596 (1972).

10. PÖLL, W., BROCK, M., MARKAKIS, E., WINKELMÜLLER, W., DIETZ, H.: Brain tissue pressure. In: Intracranial pressure (eds. M. BROCK, H. DIETZ), pp. 188-194. Berlin-Heidelberg-New York: Springer 1972.

11. WEED, L.H.: Studies on cerebro-spinal fluid. No. III: The pathways of escape from the subarachnoid spaces with particular reference to the arachnoid villi. J. Med. Res. 31, 51-91 (1914).

12. LORENZO, A.V., PAGE, L.K., WATTERS, G.V.: Relationship between cerebrospinal fluid formation, absorption and pressure in human hydrocephalus. Brain 93, 679-692 (1970).

13. RUBIN, R.C., HENDERSON, E.S., OMMAYA, A.K., WALKER, M.D., RALL, D.P.: The production of cerebrospinal fluid in man and its modification by acetazolamide. J. Neurosurg. 25, 430-436 (1966).

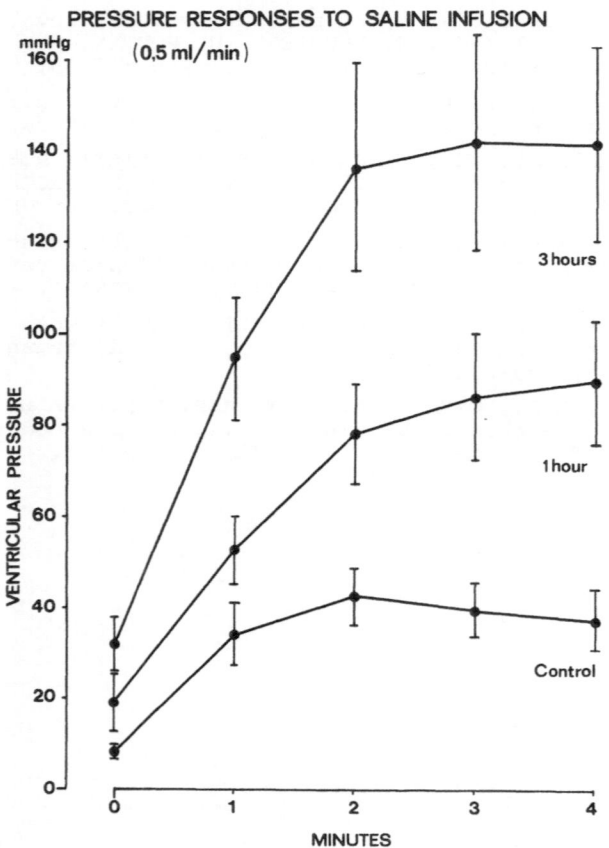

Fig. 1. P/V curves obtained by intraventricular infusion of physiologic saline (0.5 ml/min) before and after administration of 2 ml of
neural soot dispersion into one lateral ventricle

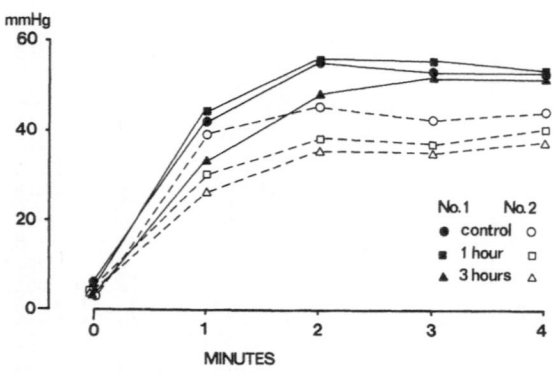

Fig. 2.
P/V curves in control
animals (no administra-
tion of soot)

Five Year Follow-Up of 65 Patients Treated With Extra-Intracranial Arterial Bypass for Cerebral Ischemia

O. GRATZL, P. SCHMIEDEK, and H. STEINHOFF

The purpose of the microvascular anastomosis between an extracranial and a cortical arterial vessel (2, 8) is to supply additional collateral blood flow to an ischemic cortical region of the brain. A major benefit may be derived from the by-pass in preventing or postponing further ischemic lesions and improving local blood flow. Based on our own clinical material the attempt is made in this study, to assess the therapeutic effect of this operation.

The report covers a five year period during which 65 patients received an extra-intracranial bypass procedure (EIAB).

Clinical Material

The clinical material consisting of 65 patients, 50 men and 15 women with a mean age of 50.1 years is divided into 4 separate groups according to the preoperative diagnosis: transient cerebral ischemic attacks (TIA), prolonged reversible ischemic neurological deficits (PRIND), stroke in evolution (SIE) and completed stroke (CS).

- TIA group: 10 patients showing an average of 3.7 attacks of focal neurological deficits lasting not longer than 24 hours prior to hospitalization.
- PRIND group: 19 patients presenting with mild focal neurological deficits lasting longer than 24 hours, however, showing a tendency to improve thereafter.
- SIE group: 7 patients with neurological deficits developing over a period of more than 6 hours and with more than 24 hours duration.
- CS group: 29 patients presenting with moderate (8 pat.) to severe (21 pat.) neurological deficits of less than a 6 hour evolution period and more than 24 hours duration.

The patients were studied pre- and postoperatively by serial cerebral angiography and regional cerebral blood flow (rCBF) measurement using the xenon-133 clearance with a 16 detector apparatus (4, 6, 7). The preoperative angiographical findings were as follows: occlusions of one or more cerebral vessels in 46 cases, stenoses in 11 and generalized arteriosclerosis of small vessels in 8 cases.

Preoperative rCBF was found to be uniformly reduced in 6 patients out of the CS-group. In the remaining CS- and the TIA-, PRIND-, and SIE-patients focal changes of CBF alone or a pattern of general moderate flow reduction with an additional focus of relative ischemia were detected.

A detailed description of the operative procedure used for EIAB is published elsewhere (2, 5, 8). The operation consists in the dissection of the superficial temporal artery, a small temporal craniectomy and an end-to-side anastomosis of the superficial temporal artery to a cortical branch of the middle cerebral artery with 10 to 12 single sutures of 10/0 monofilament nylon using the operating microscope.

Follow-up Studies

The follow-up assessment includes a period from 6 to 60 months postoperatively with an average of 20 months. The following results were obtained:

- TIA group: none of these patients has experienced another episode of cerebral ischemia postoperatively.
- PRIND group: following EIAB the neurological condition remained stable in 15 and improved in 4 patients.
- SIE group: in these 7 cases a further inaffected deterioration of the neurological condition was noted.
- CS group: eight patients showed postoperative neurological improvement, 20 patients remained unchanged and one patient died from an unrelated cause (glioblastoma of the contralateral, non-operated hemisphere).

Using cerebral angiography (Figs. 1, 2) and measurement of rCBF, graft patency could be established in 80%. A significant increase in rCBF was documented in 18 patients as a result of the operation. On repeated studies 10 months after EIAB a secondary occlusion of the bypass was seen in 3 patients, whereas a further increase in rCBF was noted in the remaining cases when compared with the first postoperative measurement. This finding is supported by angiographic studies showing a subsequent dilatation of the feeding extracranial artery as well as an increased brain area supplied by the anastomosis.

Table. Indication for EIAB according to a five year follow-up period in 65 patients based on clinical findings and rCBF studies (+ indication for EIAB. - no indication for EIAB. ( ) unusual coincidence of clinical and rCBF findings.)

		rCBF		
		focal ischemia	relative focal ischemia	uniform reduction
clinical	TIA	+	+	( )
	PRIND	+	+	( )
	SIE	-	-	-
	CS (moderate deficit)	+	+	-
	CS (severe deficit)	( )	+	-

Discussion

There is clear evidence that EIAB results in an increase of nutritional blood flow within an ischemic cortical region of the brain, as demonstrated by a comparison of pre- and postoperative rCBF studies (4, 5, 7). An adaptable increase of the anastomosis over time occurred primarily in the younger age group (3) which is also supported by an experimental study reported by BANNISTER (1). The clinical effectiveness of the surgical procedure is particularly encouraging in cases with TIA's, but also in patients with PRIND's and CS with moderate neurological deficits, when compared with the natural history of these cerebrovascular disease states (5). On the contrary the clinical condition was unaffected postoperatively in cases with SIE. A poor result, no change of the clinical status and a reduction of the function of EIAB was seen in those patients presenting CS revealing a uniformly decreased flow in the preoperative rCBF study.

Summary

This report covers a five year period during which 65 patients received an EIAB for cerebral ischemia. During the follow-up period the therapeutic effect was assessed by the evaluation of the clinical condition, angiographical findings and changes in rCBF.

From our results it is suggested that EIAB represents a promising approach to the treatment of CVD in properly selected patients of the TIA-, PRIND-, and CS-group.

REFERENCES

1. BANNISTER, C.: Anastomoses of small vessels in growing animals. Proceedings of the first International Symp. Microneurosurgical Anastomoses for Cerebral Ischemia. Loma Linda/Ca. 1973 (in press).

2. DONAGHY, R.M.P.: What's new in surgery. Neurologic surgery. Surg. Gynec. Obstet. 134, 269-271 (1972).

3. GRATZL, O., SCHMIEDEK, P., STEINHOFF, H.: Extra-intracranial arterial bypass in patients with occlusion of cerebral arteries due to trauma and tumor. In: Microneurosurgery (ed. J. HANDA). Tokyo: Igaku Shoin (in press).

4. GRATZL, O., SCHMIEDEK, P., STEINHOFF, H., ENZENBACH, R.: Quantitative and regional effects of microneurosurgical extra-intracranial vascular anastomosis in patients with cerebral ischemia. Europ. Surg. Res. 6, 27 (1974).

5. GRATZL, O., SCHMIEDEK, P., SPETZLER, R., STEINHOFF, H., MARGUTH, F.: Clinical experience with extra-intracranial arterial anastomoses in 65 cases (in press).

6. INGVAR, D.H.: Regional cerebral blood flow in cerebrovascular disorders. Progr. Brain Res. 30, 57-61 (1968).

7. SCHMIEDEK, P., STEINHOFF, H., GRATZL, O., STEUDE, U., ENZENBACH, R.: rCBF measurements in patients treated for cerebral ischemia by extra-intracranial vascular anastomosis. Europ. Neurol. 6, 364-368 (1971/72).

8. YASARGIL, M.G.: Microsurgery applied to Neurosurgery. Stuttgart: Georg Thieme 1969.

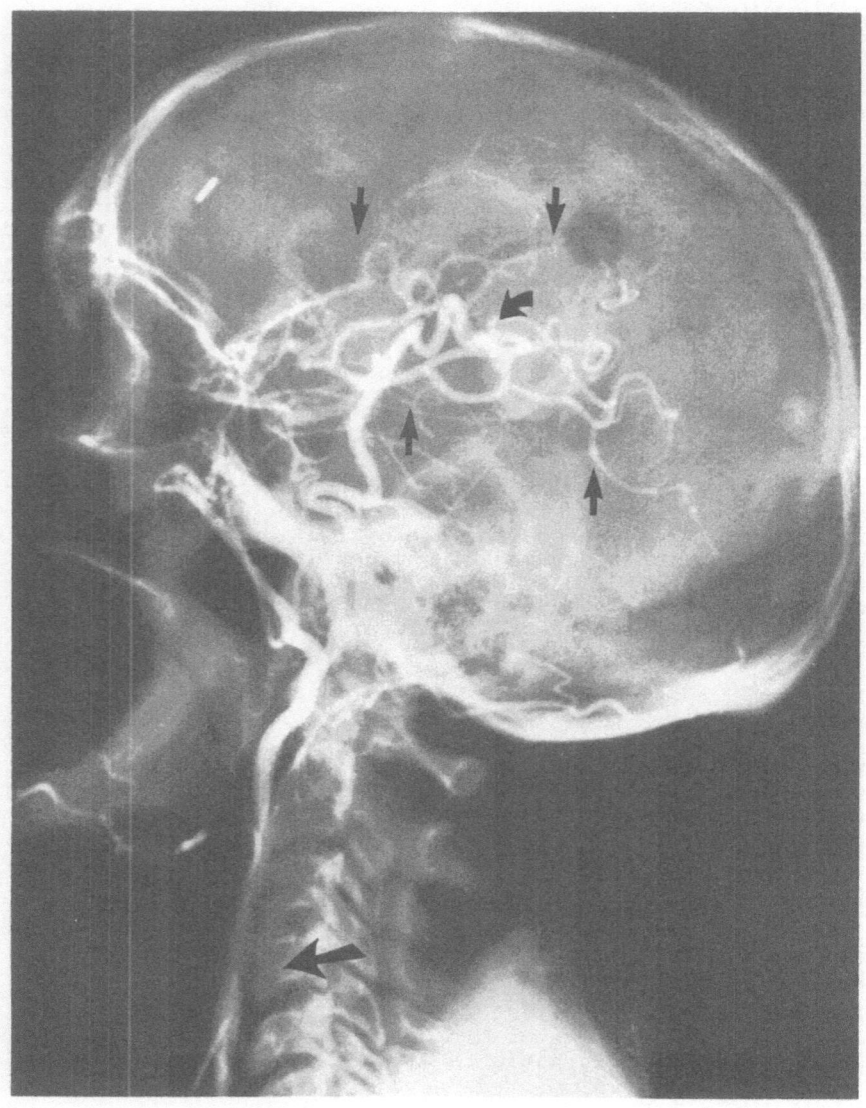

Fig. 1. Angiogram - 10 months following EIAB - shows left internal carotid artery occlusion (↙), site of the anastomosis (↶), enlarged superficial temporal artery and extend of filling through EIAB (↑↓)

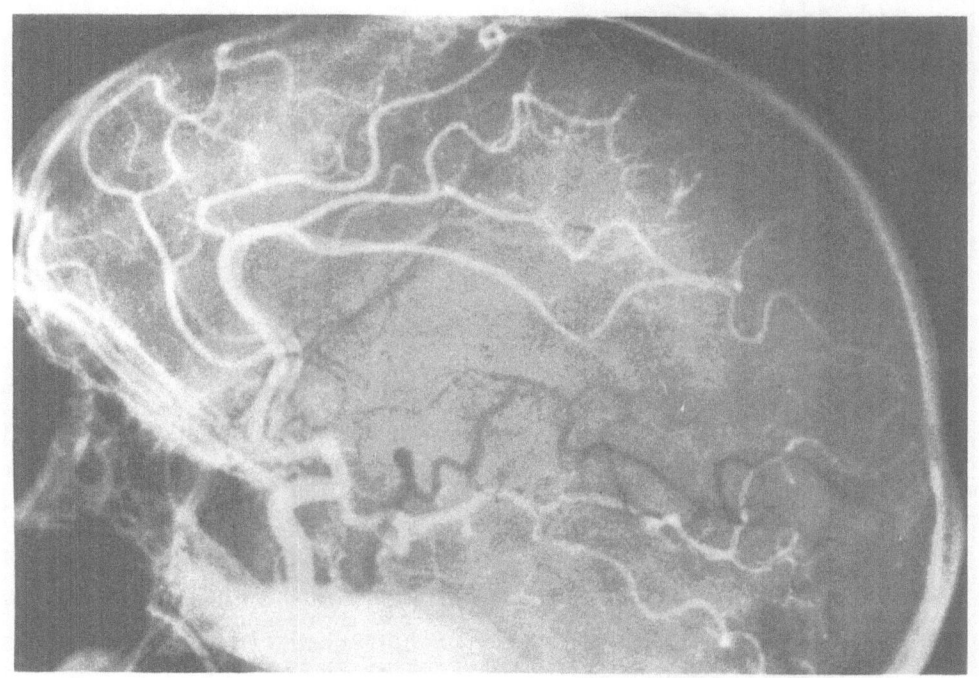

Fig. 2. Preoperative angiogram (white vessels) revealing middle cerebral artery occlusion added to a postoperative external carotid angiogram illustrating superficial temporal artery and extend of filling
of middle cerebral artery branches through EIAB (black vessels)

The Response of Human Cerebral Blood Flow to Anaesthesia With Thiopentone, Methohexitone, Propanidid, Ketamine, and Etomidate

H. HERRSCHAFT, H. SCHMIDT, F. GLEIM, and G. ALBUS

Summary

The effects of methohexitone, thiopentone, propanidid, ketamine and etomidate on regional cerebral blood flow (rCBF) were studied in 122 normal subjects under light halothane, nitrous oxide-anaesthesia (inspired halothane concentration of $0,1 - 0,4$ Vol.%). Cerebral blood flow was determined from the clearance of ^{133}Xenon, following the intra-arterial injection of the isotope. Baseline values for rCBF under N_2O/O_2/halothane anaesthesia were 15% greater than values in conscious subjects. Autoregulation and CO_2-responsiveness were preserved in the patients studied. A single intravenous injection of thiopentone (4 mg/kg) decreased rCBF by 45% when measured at 30 sec., 5 min and 10 min after termination of the intravenous injection. Propanidid (5 mg/kg) and methohexitone (1 mg/kg) reduced rCBF by 45% and 46% resp. 30 sec after the intravenous injection, by 24% and 22% resp. at 5 min and to 2% and 6,4% resp. (start of measurements at 10 min). Ketamine (2 mg/kg) reduced rCBF by 28% at 30 sec and by 15% at 5 min rCBF was reduced to baseline values by 10 min. The least decreasing effect on cerebral blood flow was caused by etomidate. The reduction of rCBF very rapidly subsided from 31% (start of measurements 30 sec after termination of i.v.-injection) through 19% (start of measurements at 3 min) to 1,8% and 0,9% (start of measurements at 5 and 10 min).

Introduction

Although the effects of thiopentone on cerebral blood flow (rCBF) have been quantified in humans and in animal experiments by DUNDEE (1956); KETY et al., (1948); PIERCE et al., (1962); SOKOLOFF (1959) and WECHSLER, DRIPPS and KETY (1961), few studies (TAKESHITA, OKUDA and SARI, 1972) have been made of the influence of other intravenous anaesthetic agents, e.g. methohexitone, propanidid, ketamine and etomidate on cerebral blood flow in man.

However, a knowledge of the effects of such drugs on cerebral blood flow may be of clinical importance. The increasing number of elderly patients and patients with pre-existing cerebral blood flow disturbances submitted to surgery may present problems for the anaesthetist.

In such patients autoregulation may be defective and, as a result, their ability to compensate for reductions in arterial blood pressure is limited.

Reductions in cerebral blood flow induced by agents could increase the extent of cerebral ischemia in such patients. Thus a knowledge of the magnitude and of the duration of the effect of intravenously administered anaesthetic drugs on cerebral blood flow is necessary for an accurate assessment of the risk of anaesthesia.

Methods

The quantitative measurement of local cerebral blood flow is effected by the intra-arterial ^{133}Xenon-clearance-method, using a ten-detector-equipment which has been described in detail elsewhere (HERRSCHAFT, SCHMIDT, and DUUS, 1972).

a) Anaesthesia

Thirty minutes prior to the induction of anaesthesia, adult patients received 0,5 atropine sulphate. Anaesthesia was induced with propanidid (5 mg/kg body weight) injected over 30 - 45 sec. Following the injection of succinyl choline (50 mg) the patients were intubated and I.P.P.V. was maintained, using a semi-open system and an Ambu-E valve, the latter to keep rebreathing to a minimum. Maintenance of anaesthesia was by means of a N_2O (6 l/min), O_2 (4 l/min) halothane (0,1 - 0,4% by volume) mixture. No incidence of awareness was noted under this light anaesthetic technique. Relaxation was maintained with a continous drip infusion of 0,2% succinyl choline chloride. During anaesthesia the end-expired CO_2 concentration was monitored, using an Uras M infra-red analyser. In addition, peripheral arterial blood pressure and pulse rate were measured. The rate and volume of ventilation were adjusted as required to maintain an end-tidal CO_2 concentration of 5,2 - 5,6%. Arterial pCO_2, pO_2 and pH were determined using direct reading CO_2 and O_2 electrodes. Blood samples were drawn directly from the internal carotid artery immediately prior to, and then 3 and 5 min after the injection of the ^{133}Xenon. The mean value obtained from the three pCO_2-results was used for correction of the blood flow.

b) rCBF-measurements

Regional cerebral blood flow was determined from the clearance of ^{133}Xenon. 3 - 5 mc of ^{133}Xenon, dissolved in 0,9% saline solution at body temperature was injected into the internal carotid artery. Clearance of the isosope was measured over 10 discrete regions. Each clearance curve was followed for 10 min. The first measurement of rCBF (at least 10 min after the induction of anaesthesia) was termed the "resting value". Five min after completion of the first rCBF determination, the anaesthetic drugs under study were administered by intravenous injection. A second measurement of rCBF was then carried out. In each case, 2 mg of methohexitone and 0,2 mg of etomidate per kg of body weight were administered. The rCBF values were calculated by a computer programme, which delivers the following data for each scintillation detector: rCBF of grey and white matter and the mean weighted flow value, calculated by compartmental analysis; also, the mean rCBF value for a period of 10 min, and extrapolated to infinity, estimated by stochastic analysis.

Following the administration of the anaesthetic drug under study, as a rule rCBF was determined at 30 sec, 5 min and 10 min after the end of the intravenous injection. In addition rCBF was measured at 3 min after the application of etomidate. A total of 122 patients were studied. The patients had been admitted to hospital to exclude organic neurological disease and underwent carotid angiography.

The numerical distribution over the 16 different measurement series, broken down according to the 5 anaesthetics, was as follows:

Ketamine: 30 sec - n = 10; 5 min - n = 8; 10 min - n = 8.

Propanidid: 30 sec - n = 12; 5 min - n =10; 10 min - n = 8.

Table 1. Response of cerebral blood flow to different intravenous
Start of measurement: 30 sec after completed i.v. injection
of single dose customary for induction
of anesthesia

Anaesthetic	Parts of Brain	Substance	CBF Resting Value	S.D.	(ml/100 g/min) Anaesthesia Value	S.D.
I Etomidate	gray	a)	107.2	16.8	67.5	12.6
(0,2 mg/kg)	white	b)	21.6	3.2	16.4	2.6
n = 6	total	c)	54.2	5.9	35.8	3.8
		d)	49.4	4.7	33.9	5.7
II Ketamine	gray	a)	124.2	16.40	79.56	15.40
(2 mg/kg)	white	b)	30.16	6.30	19.91	5.80
n = 10	total	c)	63.19	14.90	42.27	11.40
		d)	55.07	17.20	38.51	11.20
III Propanidid	gray	a)	125.25	19.00	70.74	14.55
(5 mg/kg)	white	b)	30.16	7.67	17.73	5.03
n = 12	total	c)	72.19	14.96	38.54	9.26
		d)	64.61	14.56	35.64	9.97
IV Metho-hexitone	gray	a)	111.77	10.8	59.58	14.8
(1 mg/kg)	white	b)	27.37	4.0	17.79	4.8
n = 6	total	c)	67.06	7.0	37.25	5.8
		d)	60.83	7.4	34.58	6.0
V Thiopentone	gray	a)	114.33	18.26	65.08	11.33
(4 mg/kg)	white	b)	27.16	5.09	15.75	5.30
n = 10	total	c)	66.84	12.71	36.09	7.78
		d)	58.96	12.10	33.03	6.56

c)   = calculation according to 2-compartment-analysis
d)   = calculation according to stochastic analysis
n   = number of cases
S.D.   = standard deviation
CBF   = Cerebral blood flow (average of the mean values calculated
           per group)
$APCO_2$ = arterial carbon dioxide pressure (mm Hg)
APO_2 = arterial oxygen pressure (mm Hg)
MABP   = mean arterial blood pressure (mm Hg)
Paired T-Test: Significance: x = 5%, xx = 1%, xxx = 0.1%
                Ø = no significance

anesthetics in man

Decrease in %	Statistical Significance	APCO$_2$ Rest. Anaesthesia value		APO$_2$ Rest. Anaesthesia value		MABP Rest. Anaesthesia value	
37.0	xxx						
24.1	xxx	37.0	38.5	110	112	106.6	106.6
33.9	xxx						
31.4	xxx						
26.38	xxx						
33.98	xxx	39.3	38.0	110.6	109.8	89	95
33.22	xxx						
30.07	xxx						
43,52	xxx						
41,22	xxx	39.1	38.9	125.6	124.6	96	95
46.62	xxx						
44.84	xxx						
46.4	xxx						
34.5	xxx	35.5	36.0	141.0	128.3	108	105
45.5	xxx						
42.5	xxx						
43.08	xxx						
42.02	xxx	38.2	37.6	127.0	125.4	107	103
46.02	xxx						
43.98	xxx						

Thiopentone: 30 sec - n = 10; 5 min - n = 10; 10 min - n = 8.

Methohexitone:30 sec - n = 6; 5 min - n = 7; 10 min - n = 7.

Etomidate: 30 sec - n = 6; 5 min - n = 6; 10 min - n = 3.

The results obtained were evaluated from two different points of
view. In the first place, a comparison was made between the mean values, obtained before and after the administration of the anaesthetic
drugs in one and the same patient and within a group of patients,for
blood flow through the grey and white matter and for mean blood flow.
Secondly, the effect on blood flow through the grey and white matter
and on mean regional blood flow in 10 different regions was determined for a group of patients before and after the administration of
the anaesthetic drugs.

Results

The changes in cerebral blood flow produced by etomidate, ketamine,
propanidid, methohexitone and thiopentine 30 sec after the end of the
injection of the drug are shown in Table 1. Thirty seconds after the
end of the injection, ketamine (2 mg/kg) and etomidate (1 mg/kg)
caused a similar reduction of cerebral blood flow. The decrease in
blood flow through the cerebral cortex amounted to 24,1% and 37% respectively, the decrease in the white matter flow was 24% and 23,9% (2-
compartmental-analysis) and 22,8% and 31,4% (stochastic analysis)
resp. in mean blood flow. Propanidid, methohexitone and thiopentone
produced greater reductions in cerebral blood flow 30 sec. after the
termination of the injection. Cerebral cortical blood flow was reduced by 43,5% after propanidid (5 mg/kg), by 46,4% after methohexitone (1 mg/kg) and by 43,1% after thiopentone (4 mg/kg). Propanidid
reduced mean blood flow by 46,6% (2-compartmental-analysis) or
44,8% (stochastic analysis) and methohexitone by 45,5% (2-compart-
ment-analysis) and 42,5% (stochastic analysis) respectively, while
thiopentone decreased mean blood flow by 46,0% (2-compartmental-analy-
sis) and 43,9% (stochastic analysis). Thus 30 seconds after the
intravenous injection of the anaesthetic drug propanidid, thiopentone
and methohexitone reduced cerebral cortical blood flow and mean blood
flow by a similar degree, a decrease in cerebral cortical and mean
blood flow twice as great as that observed with ketamine and etomidate.

Table 2 depicts the response of the cerebral blood flow to etomidate,
ketamine, propanidid, methohexitone and thiopentone 5 min after the
completion of the intravenous injection of the individual drug.
Following thiopentone administration, the blood flow values obtained
for grey and white matter and the mean.blood flow did not differ from
the values observed at 30 seconds. Blood flow through the cerebral
cortex was reduced by 40,7%, blood flow through the white matter by
31,7% and mean blood flow by 46,6% (2-compartment-analysis) and 43,9%
(stochastic analysis) respectively. In contrast to the changes noted
with thiopentone, the reduction of cerebral blood flow under propanidid
and methohexitone was considerably smaller when compared with the
reading at 30 seconds. Five minutes after the injection, the cerebral
cortical blood flow was reduced by 17,9% and 26,0% resp., blood flow
through the white matter by 17,7% and 24,7% resp. and mean blood flow
by 22,3% and 25,3% resp. (2-compartment-analysis) and 23,9% and 22,3%
(stochastic analysis) resp.. In comparison with the value at 30 sec,
this means a diminution of the propanidid-or methohexitone-induced
reduction of cerebral blood flow by nearly one-half. Five minutes
after the end of an injection of ketamine, cerebral cortical blood
flow was reduced by 12,1% and mean blood flow by 10,8% (2-compartment
analysis) and 12,9% (stochastic analysis). After etomidate at 5 min

there was no longer a significant difference from the resting value. Three minutes after the end of an injection of etomidate, cerebral cortical blood flow was reduced by 19,8%, blood flow through the white matter by 15,6% and mean blood flow by 19,1% (2-compartment-analysis) and 19,1% (stochastic analysis).

Table 3 show the changes in rCBF 10 minutes after the intravenous injection of the anaesthetic drugs.At this time cerebral cortical blood flow was still markedly decreased with thiopentone. The decrease of cerebral cortical blood flow amounted to 35,0%, while blood flow through the white matter was decreased by 36,9% and mean blood flow by 42,3% (2-compartment-analysis) and 45,1% (stochastic analysis). After propanidid and methohexitone, on the other hand, there was no longer a significant difference from the resting value. Likewise with ketamine and etomidate, cerebral blood flow no longer differed significantly from the resting value. In Fig. 1 the results of the investigations are summarized. The decrease of the rCBF in percentage following a single injection of the different intravenous anaesthetics is plotted against time.

Discussion

The fact that a study on the effects of intravenously administered anaesthetics drugs on cerebral blood flow has been made in patients who were already in a state of anaesthesia raises the question as to what effect basal anaesthesia may have on the results.

A change in cerebral blood flow due to the *premedication* can be ruled out since no drug other than 0,5 mg of atropine sulphate had been given.

Anaesthesia was induced with propanidid, a drug which is very rapidly broken down to hypnotically inactive metabolites and which, as we were able to show only altered CBF significantly for a period of at most 10 minutes after the administration of a single dose of 5 mg/kg. In as much as the first measurement of cerebral blood flow is not made until.at least 10 minutes after the induction of anaesthesia, an effect of the anaesthesia-inducing agent on the measured results can be almost completely ruled out. The baseline values for the measurement of CBF conform to the conditions of a very light nitrous oxide-halothane analgesia.

The results of investigation into the effect of halothane on cerebral blood flow have been reported by a number of authors. WOLLMAN et al. (1964), ALEXANDER et al. (1964) and COHEN et al.(1964) have reported an increase of cerebral blood flow during halothane anaesthesia despite a simultaneous decrease in cerebral oxygen consumption. McDOWALL and HARPER (1967), LASSEN, HØEDT-RASMUSSEN and CHRISTENSEN (1969), McHENRY and SLOCUM (1965) and we ourselves (HERRSCHAFT, 1972) have confirmed these findings. WOLLMAN et al (1964) and HERRSCHAFT (1972) further demonstrated that anaesthesia with halothane does not essentially alter the reactivity of the cerebral vessels to CO_2 when compared with the waking state. The studies on the effect of halothane on cerebral blood flow in humans and animals were carried out with 1 - 2% by volume concentrations of halothane. There have been no reports regarding a change in cerebral blood flow after the administration of 0,2 - 0,4% halothane. Since cerebral blood flow increase under halothane to an approximately proportional degree at constant blood pressure and constant arterial pCO_2 and pO_2 levels, and 1,0 - 1,2% by volume halothane leads to a 25% increase of the cerebral

Table 2. Response of cerebral blood flow to different intravenous

Start of measurement: 5 min after completed i.v. injection of
single dose customary for induction of
anaesthesia

Anaesthetic	Parts of Brain	Substance	CBF Resting Value	S.D.	(ml/100 g/min) Anaesthesia Value	S.D.
I Etomidate	gray	a)	92.9	9.3	92.9	10.1
(0.2 mg/kg)	white	b)	23.8	1.9	23.5	2.1
n = 8	total	c)	53.9	4.4	53.0	4.4
		d)	49.9	3.7	48.9	4.1
II Ketamine	gray	a)	125.38	21.2	110.15	16.6
(2 mg/kg)	white	b)	28.93	3.7	24.79	4.1
n = 8	total	c)	68.24	11.2	60.85	10.5
		d)	61.15	10.6	53.23	11.3
III Propanidid	gray	a)	130.71	18.97	107.59	19.01
(5 mg/kg)	white	b)	28.26	5.17	26.07	4.79
n = 10	total	c)	72.98	13.32	56.74	11.41
		d)	64.61	11.61	49.15	10.76
IV Metho-hexitone	gray	a)	88.21	15.0	65.20	13.3
(1 mg/kg)	white	b)	19.71	4.7	14.77	3.8
n = 7	total	c)	48.35	9.7	35.92	8.0
		d)	41.23	7.2	31.93	7.1
V Thiopentone	gray	a)	128.69	20.94	76.24	16.31
(4 mg/kg)	white	b)	30.42	5.14	20.78	4.40
n = 10	total	c)	77.35	13.08	41.27	9.80
		d)	68.27	11.73	38.29	9.26

c) = calculation according to 2-compartment-analysis
d) = calcualtion according to stochastic analysis
n = number of cases
S.D. = standard deviation
CBF = cerebral blood flow (average of the mean values calculated per group)
$APCO_2$ = arterial carbon dioxide pressure (mm Hg)
APO_2 = arterial oxygen pressure (mm Hg)
MABP = mean arterial blood pressure (mm Hg)
Paired T-Test: Significance: x = 5%, xx = 1%, xxx = 0.1%
Ø = no significance

Decrease in %	Statistical Significance	$APCO_2$ Rest. Anaesthesia value		APO_2 Rest. Anaesthesia value		MABP Rest. Anaesthesia value	
0.7							
1.1		38.0	39.0	98	94	120	117.6
1.6							
1.9							
12.15	x						
14.32	x	39.5	38.9	112.6	110.0	97	101
10.38	x						
12.96	x						
17,69	xx						
7.75	x	41.7	40.2	109.2	114.5	109	107
22.36	xx						
23.93	xx						
26.0	xx						
22.7	xxx	40.0	38.5	108.3	115.5	110	108
25.3	xx						
22.3	xx						
40.76	xxx						
31.69	xxx	41.1	38.9	117.4	120.6	107	102
46.65	xxx						
43.92	xxx						

Table 3. Response of cerebral blood flow to different intravenous

Start of measurement: 10 min after completed i.v. injection of
single dose customary for induction of
anaesthesia

Anaesthetic	Parts of Brain Substance		CBF Resting Value	S.D.	(ml/100 g/min) Anaesthesia Value	S.D.
I Etomidate	gray	a)	117.5	12.4	114.0	11.8
(0.2 mg/kg)	white	b)	20.8	1.8	20.2	1.5
n = 4	total	c)	51.2	7.3	50.8	7.2
		d)	48.6	6.2	48.0	6.0
II Ketamine	gray	a)	118.74	20.15	113.44	20.94
(2 mg/kg)	white	b)	30.82	5.45	31.04	4.81
n = 8	total	c)	57.57	17.72	55.21	13.76
		d)	50.42	15.04	50.47	12.92
III Propanidid	gray	a)	107.75	21.67	109.28	22.69
(5 mg/kg)	white	b)	24.16	5.78	24.76	5.96
n = 8	total	c)	61.77	14.11	62.66	15.95
		d)	54.92	13.40	56.04	14.53
IV Metho-hexitone	gray	a)	103.17	14.4	90.63	10.3
(1 mg/kg)	white	b)	24.87	2.7	23.32	2.1
n = 7	total	c)	60.48	5.3	54.29	3.6
		d)	53.87	5.1	49.64	3.3
V Thiopentone	gray	a)	126.61	23.60	82.20	17.91
(4 mg/kg)	white	b)	32.28	5.76	20.34	5.50
n = 8	total	c)	75.38	14.94	43.33	13.33
		d)	69.05	12.51	37.91	10.44

c)   = calculation according to 2-compartment-analysis
d)   = calculation according to stochastic analysis
n   = number of cases
S.D.   = standard deviation
CBF   = Cerebral blood flow (average of the mean values calculated per group)
$APCO_2$ = arterial carbon dioxide pressure (mm Hg)
APO_2 = arterial oxygen pressure (mm Hg)
MABP   = mean arterial blood pressure (mm Hg)
Paired T-Test: Significance: x = 5%, xx = 1%, xxx = 0.1%
                            ∅ = no significance

anesthetics in man

Decrease in %	Statistical Significance	APCO$_2$ Rest. Anaesthesia value		APO$_2$ Rest. Anaesthesia value		MABP Rest. Anaesthesia value	
− 2.9							
− 0.9		37.5	39.0	110	115	112	107
− 0.8							
− 0.8							
− 4.47							
+ 0.71		38.9	38.4	130.7	133.0	113	116
− 7.57							
+ 0.09							
+ 1.40							
+ 2.48		38.8	38.7	122.0	116.2	99	97
+ 1.44							
+ 2.04							
13.1							
3.0		40.6	41.2	125.8	129.8	104	103
9.7							
6.4							
35.08	xxx						
36.98	xxx	39.8	37.8	114.1	123.5	108	104
42.31	xxx						
45.10	xxx						

blood flow on the average, a 15% increase of the cerebral blood flow may be expected with the use of 0.5% by volume halothane. The increase presumably approaches 10% with the inhalation of 0.2 - 0.4% halothane.

As WOLLMAN et al. (1965) and PIERCE et al. (1962) and SMITH et al. (1947) were able to show, the administration of muscle relaxants in the usual doses for anaesthesia does not affect cerebral blood flow. WOLLMAN et al. (1965) showed, in addition, that a 7 : 3 mixture of N_2O and O_2 given simultaneously with muscle relaxants does not significantly alter cerebral blood flow relative to waking values.

Any change in cerebral blood flow due to marked arterial blood pressure fluctuations or to changes in the arterial partial pressures of oxygen or carbon dioxide can be ruled out in the present study. These parameters were kept nearly constant (Table 1 - 3). Although the evaluation program we used, permits correction of the calculated cerebral blood flow values to an arterial pCO_2 of 40 mm Hg (using the correction method described by ALEXANDER et al. 1964), we took care to make certain that the arterial pCO_2 in one and the same patient did not vary by more than 4 mm Hg before and after the administration of the anaesthetic drugs. Similarly, the arterial oxygen tension, which always exceeded 80 mm Hg, was kept very constant in one and the same patient.

In all the cases in the thiopentone, methohexitone, etomidate and propanidid series, the mean arterial blood pressure was 5 - 8 mm Hg below the waking values at most and it was never lower than 90 mm Hg. In the ketamine series, a small blood pressure rise averaging 5 mm Hg, invariably occurred after the adminstration of the anaesthetic.

Previously, KETY et al. (1948), WOLLMAN et al. (1965), PIERCE (1962), SOKOLOFF (1959), DUNDEE (1956), WECHSLER et al. (1951) and PICHLMAYR et al. (1970) using different experimental techniques found a decrease in cerebral blood flow after the adminstration of thiopentone of approximately 50% using the nitrous oxide method. These results agree very well with the values we obtained (45% decrease of CBF) by the intra-arterial isotope clearance method.

With respect to the influence of propanidid and methohexitone on cerebral blood flow, the only studies reported have been animal experiments by PICHLMAYR et al (1970), who noted a 20% decrease of blood flow through the cerebral cortex 45 seconds after the intravenous injection of propanidid (7 mg/kg body weight) and a 20.6% decrease after methohexitone (3 mg/kg). The reduction of human cerebral blood flow which we found in our series following the i.v. administration of propanidid (5 mg/kg) and methohexitone (1 mg/kg) was twice as great at identical times (45%).

The comparatively small effect exerted on cerebral blood flow by ketamine in the usual anaesthesia-inducing dose of 2 mg/kg body weight conforms to the results of animal experiments published by KREUSCHER and GROTE (1967). In dogs under light nitrous oxide anaesthesia, they found that the intravenous injection of ketamine (2 mg/kg) was followed by a decrease of timed cerebral blood volume from 76.4 ml/100 g/min to 69.5 ml/100 g/min. after 2 minutes and to 52.6 ml/100 g/min. after 10 minutes. These values correspond to a reduction of cerebral blood flow by approximately 10% after 1 min and by approximately 32% after 10 min. These study results are in close agreement with our finding of a decrease of cerebral blood flow by nearly 25% over a measurement period of 10 minutes.

They contrast with the data published by TAKESHITA and co-workers (1972) showing an increase in cerebral blood flow in man following the intravenous administration of ketamine (2 mg/kg). Their studies, carried out with the N_2O-method according to KETY-SCHMIDT, were done in patients breathing spontaneously; under these circumstances the maintenance of constant experimental conditions over a measurement period of 15 min cannot be positively assured. Accordingly, the authors also noted an average increase of the arterial CO_2 level by 6 mm Hg during the measurement of cerebral blood flow under ketamine as compared with the control values. The first arterial pCO_2 value was not determined until 3 - 4 min after the completed injection of ketamine. As we were able to show in our measurement, the decrease of cerebral blood flow by ketamine is already markedly diminished 5 min after the end of the i.v. injection. In contradiction to our study, the patients were ventilated with pure oxygen for 15 min. prior to the examination and with a 1 : 9 mixture of N_2O and O_2 hereafter. The mean arterial oxygen content was 492 and 478 mm Hg, respectively. These O_2 values are several times higher than the normal arterial pO_2 values, and it is not known whether and to what extent such high arterial oxygen levels alter cerebral blood flow.

With respect to the effect of etomidate on cerebral blood flow, no studies have been reported to date. In comparison with the other intravenously administered anaesthetics, this drug caused the least decreasing effect on human cerebral blood flow in our series of investigations.

REFERENCES

1. ALEXANDER, S.C., WOLLMAN, H., COHEN, P.J., CHASE, P.E., BEHAR, M.: Cerebrovascular response to aPCO_2 during Halothane anaesthesia in man. J. Appl. Physiol. _19_, 561 (1964).

2. BERNSMEIER, A., GOTTSTEIN, U.: Die Sauerstoffaufnahme des menschlichen Gehirns unter Phenothiazinen, Barbituraten und in der Ischämie. Pflügers Arch. ges. Physiol. _263_, 102 (1956).

3. BETZ, E., OEHWIG, H., WÜNNENBERG, W.: Die Wirkung verschiedener Narkotika auf die lokale Gehirndurchblutung bei der Katze. Z. Kreisl.-Forsch. _54_, 503 (1965).

4. COHEN, P.J., WOLLMAN, H., ALEXANDER, S.C., CHASE, P.E., BEHAR, M.: Cerebral carbohydrate metabolism in man during Halothane anaesthesia. Anesthesiol. _25_, 185 (1964).

5. DUNDEE, J.W.: Thiopentone. London: E. & S. Livingstone 1956.

6. GOTTSTEIN, U., BERNSMEIER, A., LEHN, H., NIEDERMAYER, W.: Hämodynamik und Stoffwechsel des Gehirns bei Schlafmittelvergiftung. Dtsch. med. Wschr. _86_, 2170 (1961).

7. HERRSCHAFT, H., SCHMIDT, H., DUUS, P.: Cerebral blood flow in man under general anaesthesia with regard to several narcotics. Europ. Neurol. _6_, 373 (1971).

8. HERRSCHAFT, H., SCHMIDT, H.: Die quantitative Messung der örtlichen Hirndurchblutung in Allgemeinnarkose unter Normo-, Hypo- und Hypercapnie. Anaesthesist _22_, 422 (1973).

9. HERRSCHAFT, H., SCHMIDT, H.: Das Verhalten der globalen und regionalen Hirndurchblutung unter dem Einfluß von Propanidid, Ketamine und Thiopental-Natrium. Anaesthesist _22_, 486 (1973).

10. HIMWICH, W.A., HOMBURGER, E., MARESCA, R., HIMWICH, H.E.: Brain metabolism in man, unanesthetized and in pentothal-narcosis. Amer. J. Psychiat. _103_, 689 (1947).

11. HOMBURGER, E., HIMWICH, W.A., EPSTEIN, B., MARESCA, R., HIMWICH, H.E.: Effect of pentothal anaesthesia on canine cerebral cortex. Amer. J. Psychiat. 104, 765 (1948).

12. KETY, S.S., WOODFORD, R.B., HARMEL, M.H., FREYMAN, F.A., APPEL, K.E., SCHMIDT, C.F.: Cerebral blood flow and metabolism in schizophrenia - the effects of barbiturate semi-narcosis, insulin and electroshock. Amer. J. Psychiat. 104, 765 (1948).

13. KREUSCHER, H., GROTE, J.: The effect of the phencyclidine derivate ketamine (CI 581) on blood flow and oxygen uptake of the brain in the dog. Anaesthesist 16, 10, 304 (1967).

14. LASSEN, N.A., HØEDT-RASMUSSEN, K., CHRISTENSEN, M.S.: Halothane, A cerebral vasodilator drug. In: Pharmakologie der lokalen Gehirndurchblutung (Hrsg. E. BETZ, R. WÜLLENWEBER), S. 111. München: Dr. E. BANASCHEWSKI: 1969.

15. LEHMANN, Ch.: Das Ultrakurznarkotikum Methohexital. Anaesthesiologie und Wiederbelebung. Berlin-Heidelberg-New York: Springer 1972.

16. McDOWALL, D.G., HARPER, A.M.: Cerebral oxygen uptake and cerebral blood flow during the action of certain anesthetic agents. In: Pharmakologie der lokalen Gehirndurchblutung (Hrsg. E. BETZ, R. WÜLLENWEBER). München: Dr. E. BANASCHEWSKI 1969.

17. McHENRY, I.C.,Jr., SLOCUM, H.C.: Hyperventilation in awake and anesthetized man. Arch. Neurol. 12, 270 (1965).

18. PICHLMAYR, I., DROST, R., SOGA, D., BEER, R.: Response of cerebral blood flow in the dog to anesthesia with propanidid and methohexital sodium. Anaesthesist 19, 144 (1970).

19. PIERCE, E.C., LAMBERTSEN, C.J., DEUTSCH, S., CHASE, P.E., LINDE, M.W., DRIPPS, R.D., PRICE, H.L.: Cerebral circulation and metabolism during thiopental anesthesia. and hyperventilation in man. J. Clin. Invest. 41, 1664 (1962).

20. SMITH, S.M., BROWN, H.O., TOMAN, J.E., GOODMAN, L.S.: The lack of cerebral effects of d-tubocurarine. Anaesthesist 1, 8 (1947).

21. SOKOLOFF, L.: The action of drugs on the cerebral circulation. Pharmacol. Rev. 11, 1 (1959).

22. TAKESHITA, H., OKUDA, Y., SARI, A.: The effects of ketamine on cerebral circulation and metabolism in man. Anesthesiol. V. 36, 69 (1972).

23. WECHSLER, R.L., DRIPPS, R.D., KETY, S.: Blood flow and oxygen consumption of the human brain during anaesthesia produced by thiopental. Anesthesiol. 12, 308 (1951).

24. WOLLMAN, H., ALEXANDER, S.C., COHEN, J.P., SMITH, T.C., CHASE, E.P., VAN DER NOLEN, R.A.: Cerebral circulation during general anaesthesia on hyperventilation in man. Thiopental induction to notrous oxide and d-tubocurarine. Anesthesiol. 26, 329 (1965).

25. WOLLMAN, H., ALEXANDER, S.C., COHEN, P.J., CHASE, P.E., MELMAN, E., BEHAR, M.G.: Cerebral circulation of man during halothane anaesthesia. Anesthesiol. 25, 180 (1964).

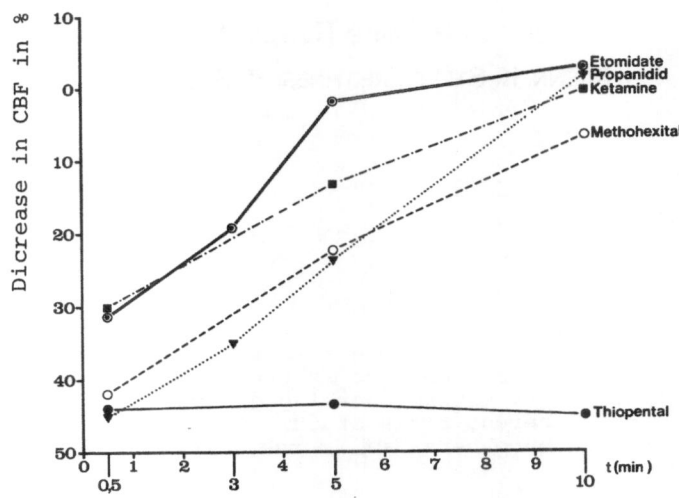

Fig. 1. Change in cerebral blood flow in man under the influence of
thiopentone (4 mg/kg), methohexitone (1 mg/kg), propanidid (5 mg/kg),
ketamine (2 mg/kg) and etomidate (0,2 mg/kg) in relation to time
after i.v.-injection of a single dose (resting value = 100%)

The Value of Routine Respirator Treatment in Severe Brain Trauma

J. KRENN, K. STEINBEREITHNER, P. SPORN, V. DRAXLER, and C. WATZEK

In recent years long term respirator treatment (with hyperventilation) has been recommended as *the* optimal management of severe brain injuries by several working groups (1, 3, 4, 5, 12 etc.). Pointing out the inherent risks of this technique, such treatment has been criticized by others (cf. survey given by GORDON, 4, 8, 16).

In an attempt to contribute to the solution of this rather important question, we tried to analyse all cases treated up to now in our own ICU; since most of the results published hitherto were gained retrospectively, we additionally started a prospective study. In this paper data of this prospective study as well as the results of the retrospective analyses will be given in order to allow some conclusions as to the usefulness of routine "prophylactic" respirator treatment in severe cerebral trauma.

Material and Selection Criteria

a) *Prospective Study:* Patients admitted to the ICU because of severe brain injury were treated at random either by mechanical ventilation or by insufflation with oxygen under spontaneous respiration. In order to warrant rather homogeneous selection conditions, the requirements to be fulfilled were as follows:

(1) Age range between 5 - 50 years.

(2) Patients with concomitant chest or abdominal injuries (polytrauma) were excluded, whereas cases with simple extremity fractures without signs of severe shock were allotted to the study.

(3) Only cases admitted directly to our casualty-department were allotted, patients transferred because of deterioration of clinical status and/or later than 24 h after the accident were excluded.

(4) Every case of primary respiratory insufficiency was excluded.

After intracranial interventions (trepanation because of (suspected) subdural or epidural haematoma, etc.), assisted respiration (CPNPB), triggered by the patient was used for about 12 h, continuing at random with artificial ventilation or spontaneous breathing with oxygen. The additional therapeutic regime corresponded to our usual management of severe brain trauma:

Artificial ventilation: use of pressure cycled ventilators (BENNET, BIRD) with negative pressure applied during expiratory phase in order to avoid venous congestion; weaning from the respirator not before the 5th day of treatment with change to oxygen insufflation under spontaneous breathing. Blood gas controls twice a day (p_aCO_2 30-40 Torr, p_aO_2 in the range of 120-140 Torr); hypocapnia caused by hyperventilation was corrected by adding a dead space (14) and/or by administration of sedatives.

Spontaneous breathing: oxygen insufflation 6-8 l/min under continuous humidification.

Routine tracheobronchial toilet and periodical manual hyperinflation in order to prevent atelectases (intervals of 2-4 h) were done in both categories of patients.

Sedation: Diazepam (80-100 mg/day) as basic medication, additional "lytic cocktail" according to requirements. Prophylactic osmo- and onkotherapy: Human albumin 20% alternating with Sorbitol 40% and/or Mannitol at intervals of 2-4 h for about 10 days. No corticoids were given. The decision, whether prolonged intubation or tracheostomy were to be preferred, was taken according to the individual course (facial cranium injury, difficulties in tracheobronchial suction etc. favouring tracheostomy). All other measures of intensive care (parenteral nutrition, use of antibiotics, treatment of hyperthermic attacks, general nursing care etc.) corresponded to accepted guidelines.

b) *Retrospective Analysis:* All patients with brain injuries admitted to the ICU since its opening in 1963 were included, irrespective of age, sex, severity of lesions, and type of treatment.

Results

A survey of the prospective study group is given in Table 1. It includes (since 1969) 44 patients fulfilling the conditions outlined above. Age distribution and duration of treatment are identical in both groups; the same holds true approximately for most of other criteria (intubation, or tracheostomy, additional fractures of extremities), the number of trepanations in both groups also shows only a small difference. The influence of peripheral irritation on the evolution of a midbrain syndrome (2,9) as well as the effects of intracranial interventions, therefore, may be excluded from discussion.

There is, however, a distinctive difference in mortality between the two groups: 4 ventilated patients died, whereas only one case in the non-ventilated group expired.

Results obtained in 383 patients (divided into two equal periods of years) are presented in Table 2. There is a decrease in the number of patients treated during the period 1969-75 due to a more strict selection before admission. It is to be seen furthermore, that, whereas initially respirator treatment was used only exceptionally, the indication for long term respirator treatment (starting in 1967, cf. 15) did increase steadily.

Discussion

A comparison of the overall mortality during the periods 1963-69 and 1969-75 reveals a decrease in mortality from 56,2 to 27,9%. That this fact cannot be ascribed to the more frequent use of respirator treatment - the number of ventilated cases during the second period being practically doubled - may easily be seen by comparing the results in respirator treated to those in nonventilated patients, the decrease of mortality in the latter group being much more pronounced than in

Table 1. Severe brain injury - prospective study group

	artificial ventilation (n = 24)	spontaneous breathing (n = 20)
Mean age, years	28,1 ± 13,9	28,0 ± 12,0
Mean range of intensive treatment, days	25,5 ± 18,0	25,0 ± 17,1
Severe brain damage only	17 (70,8%)	13 (65,0%)
Severe brain damage + fractures of extremities (without signs of shock)	7 (19,2%)	7 (35,0%)
Trepanation	11 (45,8%)	9 (45,0%)
Prolonged intubation	8 (33,3%)	9 (45,0%)
Tracheostomy	16 (66,6%)	11 (55,0%)
Mean duration of respirator treatment, days	8,5 ± 5,8	
Patients expired	4 (16,7%)	1 (5,0%)

Table 2. Mortality rate in severe brain injury (all ICU-patients)

	1963-1969 (%)		1969-31.3.1975 (%)	
Number of cases	222		161	
patients expired	125	(56,2)	45	(27,9)
Respirator treatment	82	(37,0)	106	(65,8)
expired	52	(63,5)	37	(34,9)
Spontaneous breathing (with oxygen)	140	(63,0)	55	(34,2)
expired	73	(52,2)	8	(14,5)
Significance of difference in mortality	n.s.		n.s.	

the ventilated collective. (The statistical evaluation of difference in both treatment-periods as well as in the study group does not reveal any significance; when dividing the cases treated during the period 1969-75 into the entire study group and the rest of cases, there a statistically significant difference may be obtained for the latter group, cf. Table 3.) In our opinion the decrease in mortality is mainly due to growing experience and improvements in management as well as to better defined selection criteria. The point of view is corroborated by similar results in other groups of cases treated in our ICU.

The lower overall mortality in the study group (cf. Table 3) seems to justify the conclusion, that some additional factors - which were excluded by the "selection rules" (higher age, polytrauma, insufficient initial treatment etc.) might be determinants of survival in severe

Table 3. Mortality rate of severe brain injury (period: 15.6.1969 – 31.3.1975)

	study group (%)		rest of cases analysed (%)	
Total number of cases	44		117	
Expired	5	(11,4)	40	(34,2)
Respirator treatment	24	(54,6)	82	(70,1)
Expired	4	(16,7)	33	(40,2)
Spontaneous breathing (with oxygen)	20	(45,4)	35	(29,9)
Expired	1	.(5,0)	7	(20,0)
Significance of difference in mortality	n.s.		$p < 0,05$	

cerebral trauma. (Thus, e.g. the association of brain trauma with major chest injuries led to an increase in mortality up to 70% in our material even in most recent years.)

Obviously there are definitely *much poorer results to be seen in ventilated cases in all groups* investigated when compared to spontaneously breathing patients. In our opinion this may be caused by a variety of factors, which are summarized in Table 4.

Table 4. Factors possibly responsible for an increase in mortality during artificial ventilation in severe brain injury

(1) Primary indication (hypoventilation, increase in p_aCO_2, extensor spasms)

(2) Aspiration

(3) Polytrauma ("shock-lung"?), chest injury etc.

(4) Pulmonary "shock equivalents" (starting with "fluid lung") secondary to increase in intracranial pressure (cf. MOSS et al., 10)

(5) Sequelae of respirator treatment
   a) hyperventilation (not or corrected too late) with impairment of CBF with secondary increase of lactate-levels in CSF (13)
   b) venous obstruction
   c) unrecognized hypercapnia (PAUL et al., 11)
   d) general complications of respiratory care (hypoxia, infections, etc.)

It might be argued that our study was not suitable for a comparison with results obtained by other groups under deliberate hyperventilation. An analysis of the data given by CROCKARD et al. (1), however, reveals even a higher mortality rate (38,7%) in hyperventilated cases than in our own group of ventilated patients 1969-75 (34,9% cf. Table 2). The therapeutic value of hyperventilation may furthermore be questioned because of various reasons: As PAUL et al. (11) have demonstrated, an efficacious decrease in intracranial pressure cannot be achieved by lowering p_aCO_2 to values less than 30 Torr. On the other hand, these measures additionally cause a lowering of cerebral blood flow with resulting local hypoxia and promotion of cerebral edema. Our own investigations demonstrating a steep increase in CSF-lactate levels under hyperventilation (13) are pointing in the same direction.

Conclusions

What are the clinical implications to be derived from the results presented here?

(1) For survival in severe brain injury as well as for the extent of (partial) recovery, the following factors - rated according to their respective significance - may be responsible: Extent of trauma, severity of brain edema, additional traumatic lesions and their sequelae, and - finally - the experience and quality of management achieved in the ICU.

(2) The primary indication for artificial ventilation emerges from the vital risks of hypoxemia and hypercapnia, caused by the brain trauma itself, by concomitant injuries, or by sequelae of therapeutic measures (heavy sedation, relaxation etc.).

(3) Adequate oxygen supply, unimpaired ventilatory conditions and stability in circulation being secured, a decisive influence of "prophylactic" respirator treatment on the course and outcome of patients with severe brain injury cannot be expected. As our results demonstrate, long term respirator treatment has certain inherent risks. Artificial ventilation on prophylactic reasons, therefore, cannot be recommended, this holding true especially under unsatisfactory conditions (lack of experienced personnel, etc.).

(4) Whether continuous monitoring of intracranial pressure combined with systematic release in pressure by CSF-withdrawal, "temporary" hyperventilation, and osmotherapy according to instant needs (7) might force a revision of therapeutic attitudes in the near future, cannot be decided at this moment.

Summary

Various working groups have recommended routine long term respirator treatment in severe cerebral trauma. Contrary to this widely accepted opinion, the analysis of almost 400 cases treated in our ICU from 1963 to 1975 revealed a higher mortality in respirator cases. Results obtained in a prospective study comprising carefully selected cases treated at random with respirator treatment or simple oxygen insufflation were similar. Though there are, of course definite indications for respirator treatment in cerebral trauma, "prophylactic" ventilation does not justify too optimistic expectations, since the final outcome in ventilated cases is - at least - not better than in patients, where adequate oxygenation is secured by other appropriate measures.

REFERENCES

1. CROCKARD, H.A., COPPEL, D.L., MORROW, W.F.K.: Evaluation of hyperventilation in treatment of head injuries. Brit. Med. J. 4, 634-640 (1973).

2. EULER, J., GERSTENBRAND, F., KRENN, J., LEHFUSS, H.: Frühversorgung von Extremitätenfrakturen bei schweren Schädelhirntraumen. Mschr. Unfallheilk. 75, 45-54 (1972).

3. GORDON, E.: Controlled respiration in the management of patients with traumatic brain injuries. Acta anaesth. scand. 15, 193-208 (1971).

4. GORDON, E.: The acid-base balance and oxygen tension of the cerebrospinal fluid, and their implications for the treatment of patients with brain lesions. Acta anaesth. scand. Suppl. 39, 1-36 (1971).

5. GORDON, E., BERGVALL, V.: The effect of controlled hyperventilation on cerebral blood flow and oxygen uptake in patients with brain lesions. Acta anaesth. scand. 17, 63-69 (1973).

6. GORDON, E., ROSSANDA, M.: Importance of cerebrospinal fluid acid-base status in treatment of unconscious patients with brain lesions. Acta anaesth. scand. 12, 51-73 (1968).

7. JOHNSTON, I.H., JOHNSTON, J.A., JENNET, B.: Intracranial pressure changes following head injury. Lancet 2, 433-436 (1970).

8. KRENN, J., SPORN, P.: Indikation und Durchführung apparativer Beatmung beim Schädel-Hirnverletzten. Anaesthesiol. Informat (in press).

9. LEHFUSS, H., GERSTENBRAND, F., EULER, J., KRENN, J.: Ergebnisse der Frühversorgung von Extremitätenfrakturen bei akuter traumatischer Hirnstammschädigung. Acta Chir. Austr. 4, 16-19 (1972).

10. MOSS, G., STAUNTON, C., STEIN, A.A.: The centrineurogenic etiology of the acute respiratory distress syndromes. Amer. J. Surg. 126, 37-41 (1973).

11. PAUL, R.L., POLANCO, O., TURNEY, St.Z., CRAWFORD, Mc., ASLAN, T., ADAMS COWLEY, R.: Intracranial pressure responses to alterations in arterial carbon dioxide pressure in patients with head injuries. J. Neurosurg. 36, 714-720 (1972).

12. ROSSANDA, M., DI GIUGNO, G., CORONA, S., BETTINAZZI, N., MANGIONE, G.: Oxygen supply to the brain and respirator treatment in severe comatose states. Acta anaesth. scand. Suppl. 23, 766-774 (1966).

13. STEINBEREITHNER, K., BEHNE, H.J., KOLB, R., MÜLLER, E., WISCHIN-KA, E.: Untersuchungen zum Verhalten von Blutgasen und sauren Metaboliten im Liquor bei schweren Schädel-Hirn-Traumen. Proceedings of the 5th International Anaesthesia Postgraduate Course, 6.-10. Sept. 1971, p. 179-192. Wien: Wiener Medizinische Akademie 1971.

14. SUWA, K., GEFFIN, B., PONTOPPIDAN, H., BENDIXEN, H.H.: A nomogram for dead space requirements during prolonged artificial ventilation. Anesthesiol. 29, 1206-1210 (1968).

15. STEINBEREITHNER, K., KUCHER, R.: Schädel-Hirn-Trauma. Hirnoedem. In: Intensivstation, Intensivpflege, Intensivtherapie (Hrsg. R. KUCHER, K. STEINBEREITHNER), pp. 423-438. Stuttgart: Georg Thieme 1972.

16. STOECKEL, H., HOYER, S., HAMER, J., ALBERTI, E.: Der Einfluß verschiedener Ventilationsformen auf Stoffwechsel und Durchblutung des Gehirns bei schweren Schädel-Hirn-Traumen. In: Jahrestagung 23.-26. Nov. 1972 Hamburg. Deutsche Ges. Anaesth. Wiederbel. (Hrsg. P. LAWIN, U. STRATHMANN), pp. 561-572. Berlin-Heidelberg-New York: Springer 1974.

Pain

Central Interactions of the Systems of Rapidly and Slowly Conducted Pain

R. Hassler

Pain is always a manifestation of consciousness, a subjective phenomenon, an experience. This is often forgotten by those medical men
who are orientated predominantly to somatic aspects. Pain exists only
in conjunction with an experiencing or sensitive subject. There is
no such thing as an unconscious pain. The easiest way to induce the
absence of pain sensation is by administering general anaesthesia,
since this cuts out consciousness. Thus, pain is a phenomenon of the
central nervous system. Peripheral processes, which can be recorded
during painful stimulation, are able to trigger off the pain experience, but if the impulse is prevented from reaching the central nervous system, there is no pain experience. Neural impulses triggered
by painful stimuli lead to the experience of pain only if they are
conducted further into the central nervous system and, somewhere
within the brain, pass over the threshold of consciousness.

These few sentences are not merely an indisputable introduction, but
also have a clinical significance in the evaluation of whether a pain
is psychogenic; on the part of the physician, the consideration of
possible malingering almost always being involved. Pain is not an objective phenomenon which can be recorded as such, but a conscious reaction of the individual to a variety of stimuli which have in common
the fact that they can all lead to damage to the body of a person. As
with any phenomenon of consciousness, with pain, too, the experience
also includes an evaluation appropriate to the mental (psychological)
situation of the moment. Since pain is a conscious experience, the
identical painful stimulus does not trigger the same pain experience
in such widely varying and greatly differing constellations, in which
an individual can live at any particular moment of time. The physiological processes that trigger off the pain experience are, more than
in other somatic sense systems, transformed before being, as it were,
visualized on a monitor and finally projected to the periphery as a
sensation. There is no justification for denying any conscious experience of pain claimed by another person unless this person can be
convicted to swindle.

Not only is the identical noxious impact on the skin variously experienced as pain by different individuals, but also one and the same
person experiences the identical noxious effect on the skin in different situations to varying degrees of tolerability right up to the
unbearable or, he may experience nothing at all. In a highly exciting
situation, for example, during a battle, the identical noxious stimulus on the skin is experienced in a different way than if it is presented in a calm, pleasant atmosphere. Many painful war wounds are
often not experienced as painful at all at the moment they are received during the battle. Similar remarks also apply in the sphere of
sexual experiences. If there is no "focussing" on the noxious experience, or if no attention is paid to the noxious experience, the noxious effects on the skin can remain completely unnoticed.

Despite this, the word pain should not be used for every unpleasant or disagreeable experience. Only phenomena that are experienced in a localized area can be described as pain. This information we owe to none less than Spinoza. What is not experienced as being localized is, for Spinoza, melancholia, but not pain. If the problem of pain is to be understood, in a terminologically narrow sense, only localized or localizable phenomena may be described as pain, not the *Weltschmerz* or the pain "experienced by the soul", which are merely linguistic metaphors. The widespread opinion that pain exists only during the time when painful stimuli influence the skin or mucosae, which is, unfortunately, also held by some physicians, is certainly wrong. Even with such a small thing as an insect sting or a small cut in the skin, a burning, "radiating" pain is experienced, long after the sting or the cut itself has ceased to be effective as a stimulus! (second pain see below)

The pain experience is not restricted in time to the duration of the peripheral noxious impact and not always due to such an appropriate stimulus to the skin. The corresponding excitatory processes take place, both under normal and pathological conditions, after several amplifications, in discrete diencephalic systems of the brain, and the experience is then projected outwards to the surface of the skin, secondarily. Such excitatory processes in the central pain systems can also occur when the conduction pathways from the peripheral pain fibres are interrupted and, as a result, a peripheral, noxious effect can no longer be experienced as pain.

If the central pain-conducting and pain-processing neural systems themselves are damaged, they can be excited without any noxious peripheral stimulus, so that they give rise to pain experiences which are independent of any noxious impact to the skin, such as occur in anaesthesia dolorosa or in spontaneous pain, for instance due to a thalamic malacia. This type of pain, too, is experienced as projected onto the skin, where no painful stimulus has occurred.

Physicians who, themselves, are inexperienced in intractible pain, will probably suspect that a spontaneous pain in regions of the skin that are hypalgetic or anaesthetic to pain, is psychogenic. This also applies to pain experiences in diseases of the pain-processing systems in the midbrain and basal ganglia. There are many neurosurgeons, psychiatrists and even neurologists who believe that it is impossible for a "phantom-pain" patient to feel pain in parts of the body which he no longer possesses, although painful experiences can no longer be triggered from the amputated stump and its nerve stumps.

This "phantom feeling", irrespective of whether it is painful or without pain, is a fact that in most cases has nothing to do with a desire for compensation and is not an expression of an inability to come to terms with the experience of losing a limb. Every person, irrespective of whether he still has his limbs or whether he has lost one, has a pain experience which depends upon the fact that the central representation system for the experience of pain in definite parts of the body is in an excited state.

Since pain is basically a phenomenon of consciousness, I shall begin my explanations on the neurobiological fundamentals of pain with aesthesiophysiological experiments. Already 85 years ago, GOLD-SCHEIDER and, following him, THUNBERG, demonstrated that one and the same short-lasting, painful stimulus applied to distal parts of the skin, leads to two separate and distinct pain experiences: the first (fast) pain which stops immediately, with the stimulus, and a second (slow) pain which "radiates" in an unpleasant way and which outlasts the causal effect.

For demonstration, a needle can be used which is jabbed into the area between the thumb and the index finger. When I do this for a fraction of a second, I have an initial sensation, virtually without any latency period, simultaneous with the action of pinprick, locally and temporally exactly circumscribed and exactly localizable, perhaps a little alarming but certainly not very unpleasant. After a pause of about half a second, without any further stimulus, a slow, radiating, burning pain is experienced which long outlasts the painful stimulus. The "first pain", the sensation of pain, can easily be differentiated in intensity and quality (epicritical) (Figs. 1a and b). Biologically, perhaps, it is a warning system which "announces" the second slow, spreading pain that is always experienced as disagreeable and burning. Considered psychologically, the second pain is protopathic, a disagreeable ego-state, since the subject experiencing the sentiment of pain or the pain feeling is involved and reacts with the attempt to eliminate this pain by scratching or rubbing. The second pain, therefore, is a feeling of pain. We must thus state: a single rapid mechanical effect on the skin is experienced twice, in each case differing locally and with respect to the quality of the experience.

The receptors of the second pain are unmyelinated free nerve endings which, in the receptor cells of the epidermis give rise to unmyelinated fibres, less than 1 μ thick, the so-called C-fibres which have a conduction velocity of less than 1 m per second. The first pain originates in the mechano-receptors in the skin and is conducted by myelinated $A\delta_2$ fibres, which have a diameter of about 2-5 μ and a conduction velocity of 10 to 25 metres per second. The conduction velocity is, therefore, 20 to 30 times higher than that of the C fibres. This is the explanation for the fact that the first pain is experienced much earlier than the much more slowly conducted, delayed "second pain". ZOTTERMAN (39) has demonstrated this fact electrophysiologically.

The pain stimulus cannot be defined physically or chemically. What is common to pain stimuli is the circumscribed damage done to the skin which, initially, deforms a formed receptor somewhat (first pain) and leads to the passage of fluid and ions, in particular potassium ions, out of the cells. Through interaction of chemical processes, the free, unmyelinated nerve endings are excited - a fact which makes the considerable delay in the "second pain" more understandable.

Pain under which a person suffers, always has a longer duration and points to a change in the ego state, to a feeling or emotion. Such pain is always based on an uninhibited C fibre excitation. The C fibre type of pain is most marked in causalgia, the intolerable, burning pain in the palm of the hand or the sole of the foot in the case of chronic mechanical damage to the median or tibial nerve.

The $A\delta_2$ and the C-fibres have their neurons in the spinal ganglia. The axons leading away from these latter form the posterior roots. In them, the finest fibres are collected together in the lateral part of the Obersteiner-Redlich root entrance zone, while the thicker, myelinated fibres reach the spinal cord via the medial root entrance zone. For the past 60 years, since BILLINGSLEY and RANSON (1916), it has been known that a stimulation of the medial part of the root entrance zone gives rise to rapid pressure sensations or a tingling parasthaesia, while the stimulation of the lateral root entrance zone, with the C fibres, gives rise to a long-lasting burning pain, which is accompanied by an increase in blood pressure. If the lateral root entrance zone is severed or constricted as a result of chronic meningeal inflammatory processes as in tabes dorsalis, peripheral stimulation no longer triggers long-lasting burning pain, or an increase in blood pressure. The destruction of the rapidly conducting myelinated nerve fibres in the lateral root entrance zone, on the other hand, leads to chronic spontaneous pain. From this it may be concluded that, in the region of the posterior horn of the spinal cord, an antagonistic effect occurs between the rapidly conducting and slowly conducting pain systems - as was supposed by FOERSTER. The first place where the rapid and slow pain systems converge and influence each other is the posterior horn of the spinal cord.

The numerous small nerve cells in the substantia gelatinosa of the posterior horn with their non-myelinated axons which branch immediately, form a large inhibition and control apparatus for the sensory messages from the periphery. Here, we also have the site of the "gate control", the input control predominantly for the slow, second pain from the periphery. The interaction between the sensory impulses from the periphery that are conducted at varying velocities ($A\beta$; $A\delta_2$ and others) and the C-fibre pain is, however, not the only control mechanism for pain. Rather, the excitations of the sensory fibres are also under the inhibiting influence of the reticular formation of the midbrain, of the red nucleus and also of the fields of the somatosensory region in the cerebral cortex.

In the posterior horn the descending influences from the brain stem and cortex predominate even the ascending sensory inflow from the periphery. In addition, the posterior horn and, in particular its substantia gelatinosa, is the first location in which such a strong convergence of excitation from the periphery and from the brain centres is possible, that the threshold of consciousness may be crossed. As a result of the destruction of the grey matter of the posterior horn, for example in syringomyelia and syringobulbia, a state of permanent spontaneous pain can arise.

A disturbance in the relationship between the rapidly conducting and slowly conducting and adapting pain systems also forms the basis for sensory hyperpathias. In hyperpathia, a hypaesthesia for various qualities of stimulus usually present in addition to the unpleasant painful sensation that outlasts its stimulus. The preferential damage of the large-diameter, rapidly conducting myelinated sensory fibres, including the rapid pain system, for example by chronic pressure damage caused to peripheral nerves, gives rise to a hyperpathia. It is usually associated with a hyperaesthesia, so that, although peripheral stimuli are less well perceived, after their effect has ceased they trigger a long lasting, unpleasant burning sensation which the majority of patients describe as pain. The hyperpathia is due to a disproportion between the myelinated sensory nerve fibres, including the $A\delta_2$ fibres on the one hand and the C fibres of the slow pain feeling on the other, so that the latter, as in the normal case, are no longer inhibited by the more rapidly conducting epicritical sensations.

The secondary fibres of the pain-conduction pathways originate in the neurons "embedded" in the substantia gelatinosa, or in the large fascicular cells of the posterior horn and from the nucleus proprius of the posterior horn. After crossing in front of the central canal, they ascend towards the brain stem in the ventrolateral column of the contralateral side. It has long been known that in the ventrolateral column, the diameter of the fibres is not uniform throughout, but becomes smaller from dorsal to ventromedial. 60% of the fibres of the spinothalamic tract have a diameter of less than 2 μ; in addition, there are many C fibres, i.e. non-myelinated fibres, in the spinothalamic tract.

With the aid of integrated leads from 16 various individual pathways in the ventrolateral column, MANFREDI and CASTELLUCCI established that, on strongly supramaximal stimulation in the periphery, two differentiable waves can be measured in the spinothalamic tract, too, that is potentials of the rapidly conducting and slowly conducting pain systems, separately.

When the rapid pain systems are blocked by means of tetanic (high-frequency) stimulation of the peripheral nerves, the same peripheral skin stimuli trigger only a slow wave in the spinothalamic tract which corresponds exactly with the C fibre wave.

In Fig. 2 it can be seen that the two waves from the rapid and the slow pain system are formed in the spinothalamic tract and that they are less clearly differentiated in the thoracic spinal cord than in the cervical spinal cord, where, in consequence of the length of the conduction pathway, the slowly conducted wave is more markedly separated and delayed. In various regions of the brain stem, in particular in sections of the paramedian reticular formation, it has been demonstrated that only C-fibre excitations of the slow pain system have an effect on these nuclei. As in the peripheral neuron, so in the first central neuron, too, a slow and a rapid pain conduction can be differentiated, the slow pain conduction being associated with an unpleasant painful feeling, that is, mediating the protopathic emotional C fibre pain.

The same separation into a slow and a rapid pain system is also possible in the rostral region of the midbrain and in the region of the diencephalon. The sparsely myelinated or non-myelinated fibres with their slow conduction velocity from the spinothalamic tract run medially in the base of the thalamus and end in the nucleus limitans, perhaps in parts of the nucleus centromedianus and in the intralaminary nuclei of the thalamus. This is shown in pictures of experiments on baboons with a cordotomy at the level with C4/C5 (Figs. 3 and 7). The thick nerve fibres of the spinothalamic tract, with their gross degeneration products, also with the Nauta-Gygax method, lie in the ventral nuclei of the thalamus, in particular, in the small-celled caudal ventral nucleus (V.c.pc), where the nerve ending degenerations achieve their greatest density. The ventral nuclei supplied by the rapidly conducting fibres of the spinothalamic tract, project to the cerebral cortex and the small-celled ventral nucleus of the thalamus, in particular to area 3b, to the sensory konio-cortex in the post-central gyrus.

On the border between midbrain and thalamus, a dichotomy of the pain conduction occurs, into a cortical pain pathway for the sensation of pain, and a subcortical pain pathway for the feeling of pain. For the nuclei which receive the slow pain fibres, such as the nucleus limitans and the intralaminar nuclei, have their outflow not to the cerebral cortex but to parts of the basal ganglia, in particular to the outer segment of the pallidum. This can be demonstrated by the fact that, after isolated destruction of the outer part of the pallidum, e.g. in stereotactic operations for Parkinson's disease, a retrograde nerve cell atrophy and cell destruction occurs in the intralaminar and limitans nuclei of the thalamus months, or even years, later. If, on the other hand, the pathways from the thalamus to the cerebral cortex are interrupted, the nerve cells of all the ventral nuclei (V.c.pc), including the small-celled ventral nucleus for the rapid cortical pain-conducting pathway, degenerate.

The cortical pain-conducting pathway is the anatomical substrate for the discriminating pain perception. Damage to the cortical pain pathway in the region of the cerebral white matter or in the area 3b of the post-central gyrus, result in a hypalgesia, i.e. reduced sensibility towards painful stimuli. The various degrees of intensity of pinprick stimuli can scarcely be differentiated; nevertheless they elicit subsequently unpleasant radial feelings that are referred to as hyperpathia. Despite the reduction otherwise found in the perception of the painful stimulus, these slower pain feelings are mediated by the subcortical pathway of the slow (C-fibre) pain feeling. After the destruction of the cortical pain pathway, a painful stimulus is perceived as less painful than on the other side of the body, but, at the same time, it is also experienced as a particularly prolonged and unpleasant feeling.

The extreme case of a dissociation between the perception of the pain and pain feeling can be observed in conditions of thalamic pain and also of spontaneous pain of other location (Figs. 4 and 5). The patients manifest an insensitivity to pain on one side of the body, but, nevertheless, also experience, even without an external painful stimulus, a feeling of pain, a spontaneous pain, on this analgetic side. This is a central form of anaesthesia dolorosa. The anaesthesia is due to an interruption of the cortical pain pathway, the experience of the "dolorosa" is dependent upon the subcortical pathway for pain feeling being intact. Since the latter is normally under the inhibitory influence of the cortical pathway for pain perception, the systems for the (slowly conducted) pain feeling are disinhibited under the condition of a thalamic syndrome with spontaneous pain. This can be unequivocally demonstrated in post-mortem studies of spontaneous thalamic pain patients. They regularly have destroyed the most important nucleus of the cortical pain-conducting pathway, namely the small-celled caudal ventral nucleus (V.c.pc), which projects to the area 3b, as Fig.7 shows. In accordance with this, the patient was analgetic on the opposite side of the body. The softening foci did not, however, destroy the medial slow-conducting pathway for the pain feeling or its terminal nucleus; the limitans and the intralaminary thalamic nuclei remain intact. They are disinhibited by the antagonistic effect of the rapid cortical pain-conducting pathways and thus give rise to agonizing, burning spontaneous pain.

On the basis of this concept, we have developed a new type of stereotactic pain operation, both for vascular cases of thalamic pain and also for other forms of otherwise intractable pain, such as phantom pain and anaesthesia dolorosa in the trigeminal nerve. When the patient suffers from a disinhibition and an overactivity of the slow subcortical pathways for pain feeling, the nuclei of the subcortical pain pathways, in particular the nucleus limitans at the boundary of the midbrain and the thalamus (and also the nucleus parafascicularis) are disconnected by stereotactic coagulation. In this way, it is possible to relieve the patient from his intolerable pain, that is intractable to any other kind of treatment. The foci that make this possible can be seen in Figs. 4 and 6. Fig. 4 is a case of thalamic pain and Fig. 6 is a case of a Pancoast tumor with intolerable shoulder and neck pain. If the nuclei of the subcortical system of pain feeling are selectively disconnected, as was first done by MARKS with a different rationale, the relief of intolerable pain can be obtained without causing hypalgesia or analgesia for pain perception.

Thus, it seemed that selectively inactivating the slow system for pain feeling did not give rise to any functional loss phenomena in the somatosensory system. This is, however, not the case. If, in these patients, in accordance with aesthesiophysiological methods, the experience of the first and second pain is investigated on the sound and on the operated sides of the body, it is found that the patients with an inactivated subcortical pain system no longer perceive the second slow, burning, irradiating pain, although they are able to have this experience on the uninfluenced side of the body. At the same time, the dermatographism is strongly diminished and much less widespread than on the healthy side in the areas of skin, the central representation of which in the subcortical pain pathway have been disconnected. Thus, the inactivation of the central components of the slow pain system leads, as does the functional loss of the C fibres in the peripheral pain-conduction, to a loss of the second, slow unpleasant pain feeling and to the loss of dermatographism.

I am of the opinion that the observations described here demonstrate that the pain systems from the receptors in the skin to their terminals in the basal ganglia and cortex are divided into two systems, namely, a rapidly conducting and rapidly adapting and a slowly conducting and poorly adapting system. Each system has separate conduction pathways and separate nuclei, in the periphery, in the spinothalamic tract, in the nuclei of the brain stem and in the diencephalon. The rapid pain system is responsible for feeling of pain perception and the pain discrimination, as has already been postulated by FOERSTER. The slow pain system is a system for pain sensation, a protopathic pain system, which is not able to reflect the effective pain stimuli accurately with respect to time and location. The patients, however, suffer only under the excitations of the slow pain system. It must be the intention of the neurosurgeon, not to relieve the patient of every experience of pain, but only to inactivate the protopathic, slow system of pain feeling, both in the periphery and centrally, in order to free the patient from his sufferings.

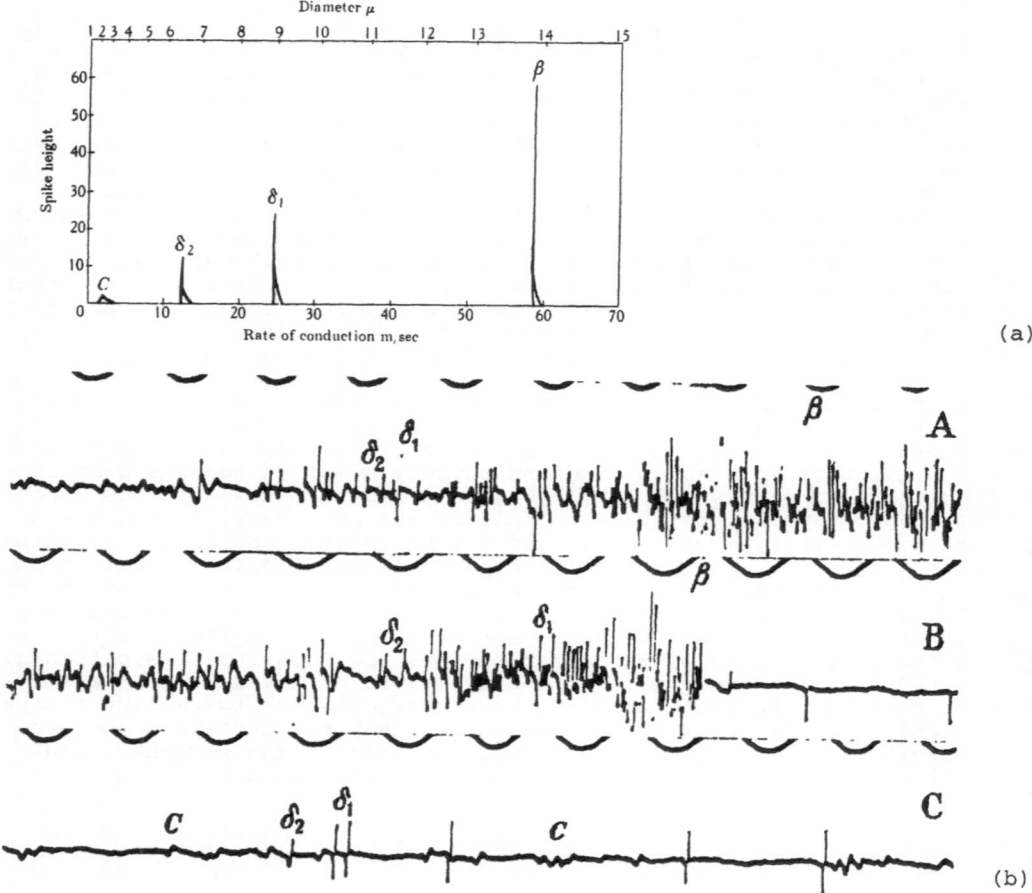

(a)

(b)

Fig. 1 a. Diagram of the relationship between the spike height, the conduction rate and the caliber of different types for somato-sensory fibers, namely, the Aβ, Aδ₁, Aδ₂ and C fibers

Fig. 1 b. Action potentials of peripheral nerves to be read from right to left. A: during the end of a firm stroke to the skin with afterwards afterpotentials. B: during needle prick to the skin starting at βδ₁, δ₂ potentials are recorded during and after the needle prick whereas β spikes are of very short duration. C: the same preparation 3 sec later showing C potentials at irregular frequencies intermingled by some δ₁ and δ₂ potentials. Time 1/50 sec (after ZOTTERMAN, 1939)

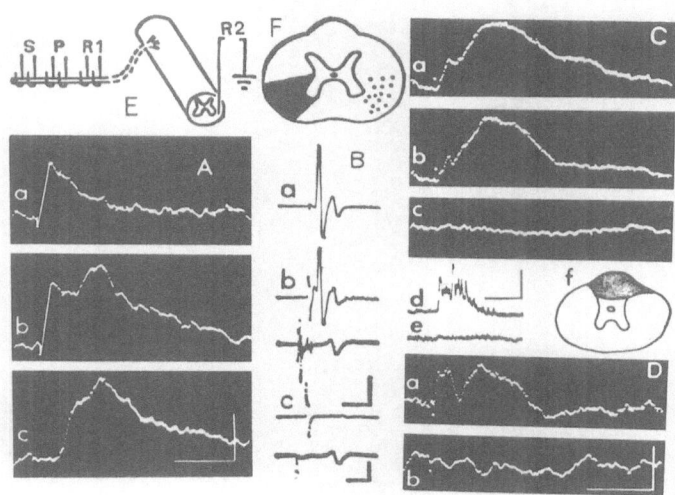

Fig. 2. Integrated discharges (A) recorded from 16 individual spots, as illustrated in F under the experimental conditions shown in E, demonstrate the excitation of the anterolateral column better than the simple conventional recording in B. Aa shows the reaction with a stimulation intensity ten times greater than the Aβ fibre threshold registered from the lead R_1 on the dorsal root in the lumbar level; only the myelinated Aβ and Aδ fibres were excited. Ab: During stimulation intensity 200 times greater than the Aβ fibre threshold there is in the dorsal root recording a much slower C fibre-potential (under Bb) in addition to the Aβ and Aδ potentials. The pertinent integrated response (Ab) clearly shows a second slower elevation due to C fibres, which also continue to conduct the excitations in the anterolateral column. Ac: After polarisation of the nerves, which blocks all fibres except the C fibres, the same stimulus intensity elicits an integrated response (Ac) in which the C fibre response is increased, whereas the myelinated fibre (Aβ and Aδ) responses are missing. Diagram Bc illustrates that the myelinated fibre reactions were intercepted by polarisation. Ca: The integrated discharges from the anterolateral column of the mid-thoracic cord, recorded as a result of stimulating the peripheral nerve, which produced a myelinated wave and a C-fibre wave, shows a small fast and a large slow impulse wave due to longer spinal cord conduction. Cb: After severing the posterior columns (Cf) the fast component has been reduced, but the large wave is almost unchanged. Cc: After severing the whole spinal cord below the recording spot (R_2), there is no more response to sensory stimulation. D: The integrated discharge in the anterolateral column transmitted from the cervical part of the cord, in response to a series of impulses from myelinated and non-myelinated fibres, shows two elevations which now differ even more from one another because the C-fibres conduct the impulses more slowly along the anterolateral column than the myelinated fibres. After transection of the spinal cord, the integrated impulses in the cervical part of the medulla fail to respond to the same stimulation (Db) (after MANFREDI and CAS-TELLUCCI, 1969)

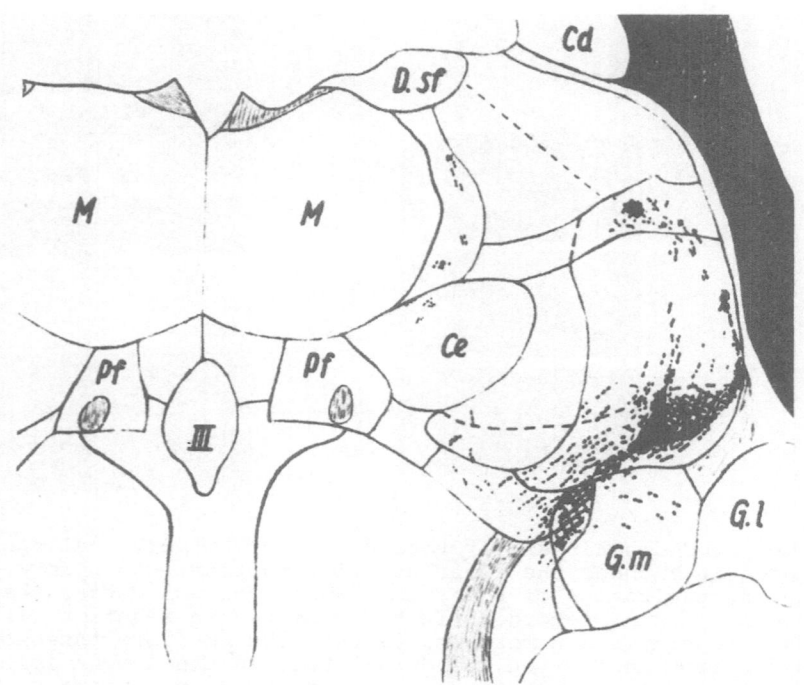

Fig. 3. Degeneration of spino-thalamic fibres after left chordotomy, at the level of the fifth cervical segment in the baboon. The Nauta-Gygax method shows degeneration, firstly in the large-cell part of the medial geniculate (G.m.mc), secondly in the small-celled caudal ventral nucleus, that is in its lateral part (V.c.pc.e), and thirdly in the lateral part of the caudal ventral nucleus (V.c.p.e) and in the caudal inter-mediary nucleus (Z.c.e). Finer medial degenerations can be seen in the intralaminar nuclei (i.La) after passage through the center median (Ce) and in limitans (Li) (HASSLER, 1972, after experiments with IMAI, KUSAMA and WAGNER)

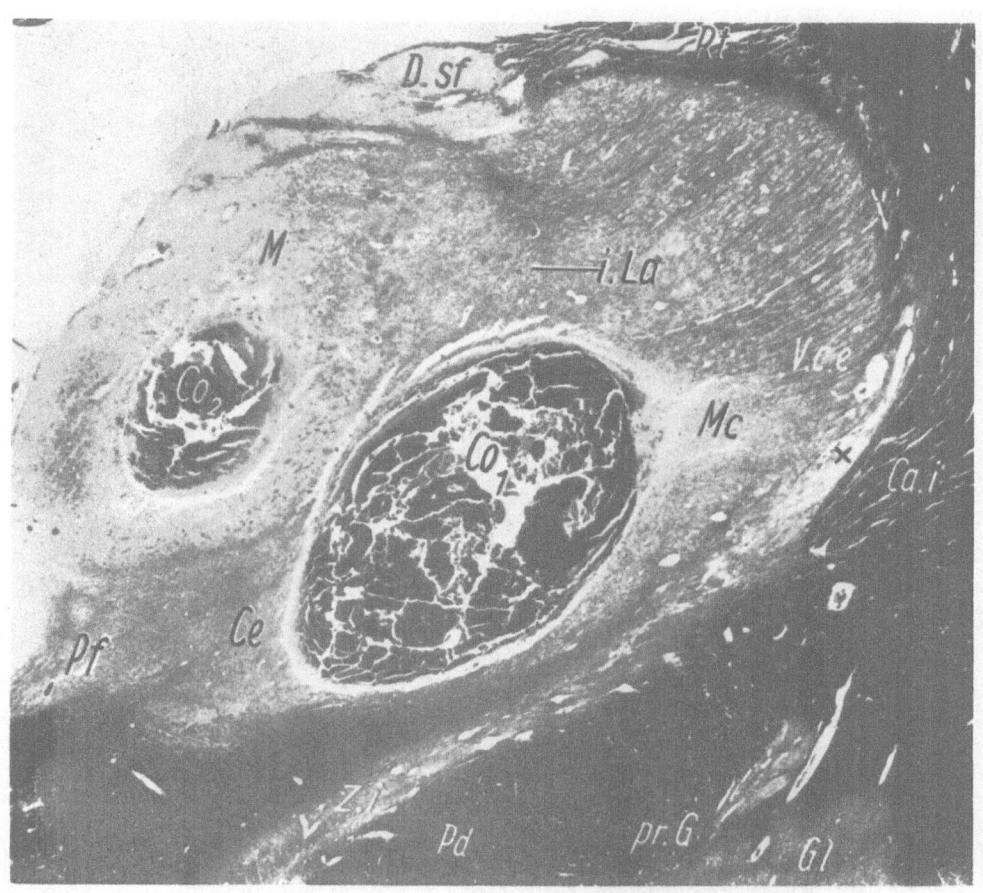

Fig. 4. Thalamic cross-section in a case of spontaneous thalamic pain,
treated successfully with stereotactic coagulation. Occlusion of the
thalamogeniculate artery produced softening around the sensory ventral nucleus (V.c.e) of the thalamus. There is demyelination (Mc) in
the area described as V.c.e. as well as in the neighbouring portion
of the nucleus reticulatus thalami, marked with an x. The medial part
of the sensory ventral nuclei, in particular its base with the small-
celled ventral nuclei, has been destroyed by a large area of coagulation (Co_1). This extends medially to the edge of the center median
(Ce). A second area was coagulated (Co_2) in the medial nucleus (M),
in order to reduce psychological reaction to spontaneous pain. (Fibre
straining according to HEIDENHAIN-WOELCKE; 6:1 magnification) (HASS-
LER, 1972)

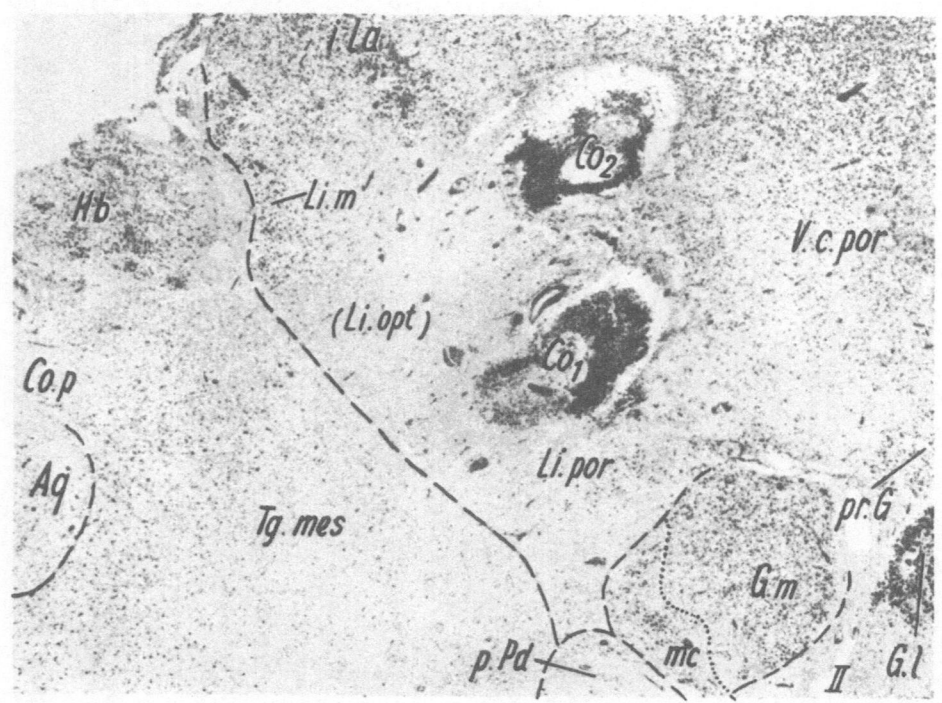

Fig. 5. Cross-section through the thalamus-midbrain border in the
same case, 1.6 mm further on caudally. The midbrain-thalamus border
is illustrated as a broken line, where the ganglion habenulae was
separated from the thalamus. Normally the midbrain-thalamus border is
taken up by the Nc. limitans, but in this case only its medial section (Li.m) is preserved. The limitans opticus and limitans portae
have lost most of their nerve cells, due to the two coagulation areas
induced by a string electrode (Co_1 and Co_2) placed into the lateral
part of these nuclei. The geniculatum mediale with its large cells
(mc) has not been coagulated and there is no cell destruction. As a
result of these two coagulation areas and degeneration of the Nc.
limitans, the patient remained free from pain during the last seven
weeks of life (HASSLER, 1972)

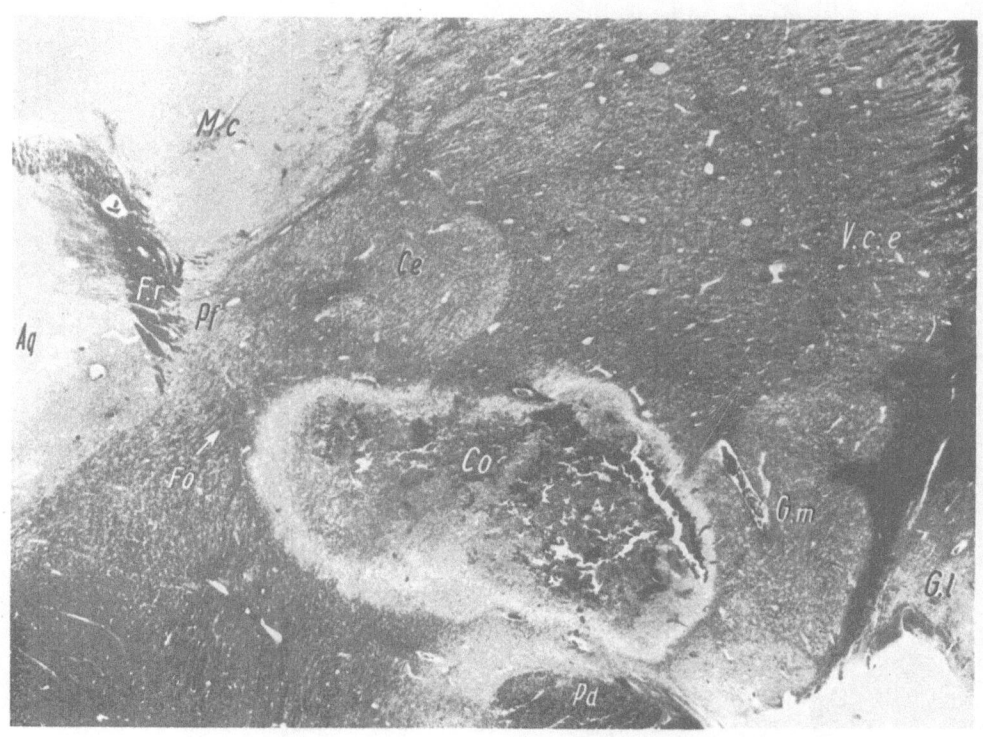

Fig. 6. In the case of Pancoast tumor the second coagulation has destroyed all parts of the limitans nucleus and also the magnocellular part of the medial geniculate body (G.m), which receives dense terminals of spino-thalamic fibres. The clinical effect was a complete relief of both spontaneous and evoked pain for life and a contralateral hemianesthesia. Magnification 6:1 (HASSLER, 1970)

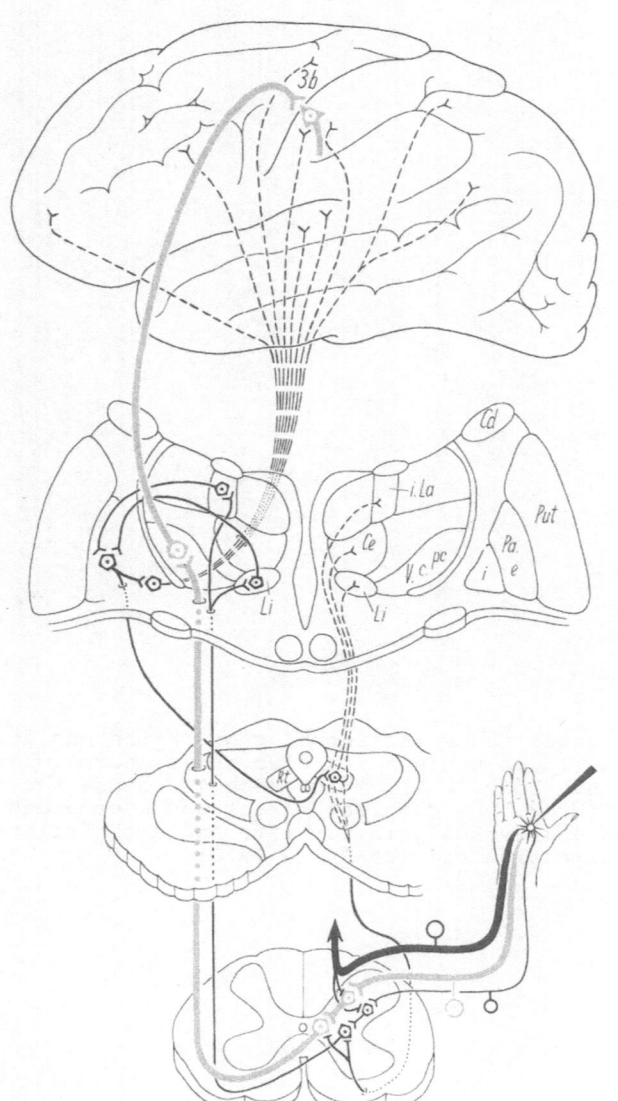

Fig. 7

Open Spinal Surgery for (Intractable) Pain

K. PISCOL

The task of presenting a paper on the "open" spinal operations for
the relief of pain, that is, the longest-known neurosurgical measures
for combatting pain, has, to an equal degree, both its advantages and
disadvantages. One of the advantages is, without a doubt, the fact
that the basic problems, the techniques and their results in their
trend significance can be assumed to be known; in particular since
the writer of this paper has just contributed a handbook article on
this topic (PISCOL, 1974). The disadvantages put in an appearance
when, from these cold ashes, an attempt is made to rekindle the fire.

It can immediately be stated that, in the meantime, no new open methods have been developed and that the trend of the results of the individual groups has not changed. The purpose of this paper is, therefore, an attempt to determine the position of these methods in the
present-day situation of neurosurgical pain therapy and to clarify
their usefulness. Under these circumstances, three methods might be
mentioned: posterior rhizotomy, commissural myelotomy and anterolateral cordotomy.

Posterior Rhizotomy

In the case of posterior rhizotomy, the decision as to whether the
intradural or the extradural approach should be selected is of importance. In the case of processes involving the ganglion or the
root, the intradural approach should always be selected, in the case
of other peripherally located lesions, the extradural intervention
can be selected. Within the framework of intradural rhizotomy, the
attempt, formerly propagated by KUHN and by RANSON, to section selectively the laterally located fine fibres in the posterior roots,
has been reintroduced, now admittedly, employing micro-neurosurgical
techniques (for example SINDOU in Lyon). The question as to whether
a laminectomy, a hemi-laminectomy, a fenestration or the technique of
SCOVILLE or FRYKHOLM should be employed is, of course, dependent upon
the location of the planned root section, and also on the technique
of the surgeon and the physical condition of the patient. It has been
shown that in the case of segmental pain in the trunk and the cervical region, the best results can be obtained when the afferent fibres
are divided, not only the segments involved, but also the neighbouring segments - that is, that in monosegmental or bisegmental pain,
three to six roots are sectioned. In the regions of the extremities,
this is usually not possible on account of subsequent impairment of
function.

Let us now take a look at some typical results (Table 1). The table
presents two large, thoroughly evaluated and thus representative,
groups of patients from hospitals with considerable experience in

157

providing pain therapy. The three smaller groups cannot be dealt with in detail here.

Table 1. Rhizotomy

Author	Indication	Number	Success Rate
ECHOLS	Malignant diseases	31	81%
	Ischialgias, postop.	62	60%
	Headaches	3	66%
	Leg pain	3	66%
	Intercostal neuralgias	19	79% (63%)
		118	68% (66%)
WHITE	Malignant diseases, cervic.	33	58%
	Brachial plexus neuralgias	3	66%
	Ulnar lesions	5	60%
	Ischialgias, postoperative	12	75%
	Intercostal neuralgias	6	83%
	Meralgia	5	60%
	Abdominal scars	5	60%
	Specific intestinal pain	10	100%
	Non-malignant diseases		66%
SCOVILLE	Malignant and non-malignant diseases	12	good 6 pats. satisf. 6 pats.
PISCOL	Radicular pains thoracic and lumbar	5(6)	4 pats.
PIERI	Zoster	4	3 pats.

At first sight, the percentage data might appear problematical. They have, however, been incorporated in the table since, only in this way is a comparison possible, and also since they have been confirmed within the framework of larger surveys.

I am sure that there is no need to emphasize that, in particular in the case of malignant lesions, the patients are strictly selected and present with particularly circumscribed pain patterns. On the basis of these prerequisites, the success rate is considerable: in WHITE's group 58% and in ECHOLS as many as 81% of the cases were relieved of their pain. In this connection, of course, the shortened life expectancy of the patients also has a certain significance.

In the case of non-malignant processes, it can be assumed that 65% to 68% of the patients are helped. It is certain that the so-called uncomplicated peripheral nervous and radicular pain conditions represent the indications which promise the greatest success. The table provides information on further details.

As was to have been expected, the selection of the patients is of considerable significance for the overall results in the case of coccygodynia. In the meantime, it has been established that coccygeal pain in the case of carcinoma or cicatricial conditions in the true pelvis can be extremely refractory. So-called spontaneous coccygodynias, said to be due to chronic microtraumatization, are, on the other hand, much more amenable to surgical treatment; the adequate technique being rhizotomy involving S4 - CO bilaterally and S3 unilaterally. The different composition of the groups of patients is probably the reason for the discrepancy between the results obtained by ECHOLS and those of other workers (Table 2).

Table 2. Coccygodynia

Authors	1:Number	2:Pain-free	3:Pain	2+3
BOHM and FRANKSSON	15	14	–	14
PENZHOLZ	4	2	2	4
PISCOL	7	4	1	5
WHITE and SWEET	1	(1)	1	1
ECHOLS	26	12	–	12
Total	53	32	4	36
	100%	60%	8%	68%

The advantage of posterior rhizotomy is, without question, to be seen in the fact that the patient has only a slight sensory loss - even after extensive operation. Surprisingly, after rhizotomy operations, the agonising dysaesthesias which can occur after other operations to relieve pain, are not observed. For this reason, in particular WHITE, but also ECHOLS, MATSOU and SHILLITO, PAILLAS and PELLET, PENZHOLZ, SCOVILLE et al., have advocated the increased use of this method. At the present time, however, the successes achieved with neurostimulation techniques in cases of extremity pain, have narrowed the indications for this method.

There is general agreement that the results are better and more permanent when, in addition to the segments involved, one to two neighbouring segments in the cranial and caudal directions are "knocked out", too.

As an explanation for this, we must assume that, in the case of chronic changes to the peripheral neurons, for example taking the form of a pathological fibre spectrum (see NOORDEN-BOS, WEDDELL) or a permanent pathological formation and conduction of excitation impulses (see BARNES, FLECKENSTEIN, STÄMPELI), changes in the appropriate posterior horn structures also occur which, according to HASSLER, represents the substrate which is "able" to give rise to a "painful sensation of a pain experience" (Fig. 1). Although the division of a single root can interrupt the direct pathological excitation inflow, it does not "knock out" the simultaneous stimulation of the changed posterior horn zone by irradiation from the neighbourhood, in particular through vertical interactions. This can be abolished only by supplementary root sectioning.

Since the number of sectioned roots is limited, the upper limit is, in accordance with the table, probably six posterior roots, only monosegmentally to oligosegmentally-limited processes can be considered for posterior rhizotomy.

Commissural Myelotomy

The technique of commissural myelotomy, advocated by GREENFEELD, AMOUR, LERICHE, has not found particular acceptance in Germany as a method for combating pain. The information provided by WERTHEIMER and LECUIRE (1953) reflects the results following thoraco-lumbar interventions in the first phase of application - mainly in France - quite reliably. Convincing results were obtained in only about one-third of the patients so treated (Table 3); PUTNAM carried out this operation, under the designation "mediolongitudinal chordotomy" also in the cervical spinal cord.

Table 3. Commissural Myelotomy

Authors	Level	Number	Indication		Results
WERTHEIMER & LECUIRE	thoraco-lumbar	100			very good 33% improvement 32% 4 deaths
LEMBCKE	cervical	12	Stump pain	(2)	
			Brachial plexus lesion	(3)	pain-free (6-10 years)
			Phantom pain	(1)	
			MS	(1)	recurrent pain
			Malignant tumours	(5)	4 pain-free 1 improvement
GRUNERT et al.	thoraco-lumbar	10	Malignant tumours	(9)	pain-free
			Benign processes	(1)	pain recurrence

In the USA, the technique was abandoned. Elsewhere, too, the literature on this subject dried up until LEMBCKE reported, in 1964, on 12 patients, on whom he had carried out the intervention in the cervical region employing the old technique. The indications can be seen in Table 3. Myelotomy was usually carried out between C3/C4 and C8/T1, in one instance even from C2 (!) to C5, without any deaths being reported. In one instance (case with MS), recurrent pain occurred. In a patient suffering from a malignant disease, only an improvement was achieved. All the remaining patients became pain-free; the cases presenting with non-malignant processes remaining pain-free, even after 6 to 10 years.

Later, the opportunity presented itself of carrying out the intervention employing the surgical microscope. In 1970, GRUNERT, SUNDER-PLASSMANN and GESTRING reported on 10 cases in whom they had carried out commissural myelotomy from T9/T10 - T11/T12 and from T10 - L1 or T12 - L4. During the - admittedly short - follow-up period, 9 patients with malignant disease remained pain-free, while, in the case with a benign process, recurrent pain occurred (Table 3). We, ourselves, have carried out the operation in the thoraco-lumbar region, in a female patient presenting with bilateral pain in the pelvic and perineal regions, the operation being carried out applying strictly microneurosurgical techniques. With regard to the technical and sur-

gical-aesthetic considerations, the operation was more impressive
than a chordotomy, but otherwise more complicated, difficult and
more stressful for the patient. The neuropathologist confirms that,
even after micro-neurosurgical operations, more extensive damage to
the spinal cord can certainly be found (JELLINGER). For these reasons,
we are, at present, adopting a wait-and-see attitude.

An advantage of the method is considered to be the fact that only the
decussating fibres - that is those for pain and temperature - are divided. The result should, therefore, be a pure analgesia and thermo-
anaesthesia in the area supplied, admittedly, bilateral. In the 23
cases of the last few years particularly considered here, however,
temporary paralyses were observed and, in one case, a bladder disorder was indicated by the patient.

Even without these complications, there still remains a number of
questions to be discussed, which we shall only be able to answer after long-term follow-up observations.

The advantage of the method of involving only the decussating fibres,
can also become a disadvantage in patients with long survival times.
It is known - and this will be discussed in more detail when we deal
with chordotomy - that, particularly in the case of the course of the
pain-conducting fibres, considerable variations can be found. Here
we would simply mention the reports of FOERSTER, FRENCH and PEYTON,
VORIS, SWEET and AMASSIAN. In addition, attention must be drawn to
the multi-synaptic-afferent system which, according to investigations
carried out by SHEALY, can also effect homolateral pain conduction.
And finally, it remains to be mentioned that the level of cross-over
of pain-conducting fibres to the contralateral side is subject to
appreciable individual variations.

Accordingly, the results obtained in the last few years are really
better than they ought to be. Of course, it should be remembered that,
initially, the diaschisis effect probably also played a not-inconsid-
erable role, which was particularly positive in the case of patients
suffering from malignant diseases and having only a short survival
time. The Vienna working group has collected further experience
which it will present in a discussion contribution. The results obtained by LEMBCKE are surprising.Unfortunately, however, in his report he made no mention of whether other forms of pain or whether
dysaesthesia occurred and how the patients with sensory disorders in
the previously healthy arm, managed to cope.

The intervention is certainly interesting - in particular when carried out as a micro-neurosurgical intervention. Despite the positive
results mentioned, however, it cannot be said that it entails no
risks. Applied to the cervical region and for use with benign processes, it can be considered, at the present time, only in exceptional
cases. All in all, further reports must be awaited before a final
assessment can be made.

Anterolateral Cordotomy

And now we finally come to the procedure which for decades "ruled"
surgical therapy for pain - anterolateral cordotomy. Since its introduction by SPILLER/MARTIC and FOERSTER/TIETZE in the years 1911/
1912, it has been subjected to modifications and supplementations
and is carried out with a variety of different approaches. Laminec-
tomies, hemilaminectomies, fenestrations can all be selected, in the

cervical regions also the elegant and patient-sparing SCHWARTZ technique and the ventral approach of CLOWARD. Of greater importance, however, is the procedure involving the anterolateral column itself. In this connection, in addition to the endeavours to divide - either completely, partially or selectively - only the spinothalamic tract, the view is also held that only as radical a separation of the anterolateral column as possible has any prospects of providing long-lasting success. In order to ensure an improved orientation and to protect blood vessels, a number of workers make use of the operating microscope or magnifying glasses.

We have tried, elsewhere, on the one hand to represent the difficulties attached to the statistics of success while, on the other hand, providing at least a survey of representative results obtained with the various basic diseases (PISCOL, 1974). Let us recapitulate on a few remarks as a basis for discussion. In the case of malignant processes, the success rate is 72% to 88%, in benign processes 30% to 60% (Table 4). The reason for this is not merely the shorter life expectancy of patients with malignant disease, but also the fact that a number of non-malignant painful pictures are particularly resistant to chordotomy and that in otherwise healthy people, there is a greater reluctance to undergo radical sectioning of the spinal cord. In the malignant processes, pain in the lower half of the body can be influenced more positively and more long-lastingly than that localized at a higher level (Table 5). This also applies to benign processes (Table 6) and the reason is to be seen in the difficulty of attaining and retaining an adequately high level of analgesia. Surprisingly good initial results gradually revert to the former state with time (RÖTTGEN), (Table 7). A repetition of an open cordotomy has markedly lower chances of success than the initial intervention (Fig. 2). The slightly better results following bilateral cordotomy hardly outweigh the disadvantages in unilateral pain. Worthy of mention is, however, the fact that in all the more recent publications, where necessary, *bilateral* procedures are given preference (RASKIND). In the case of pain involving the lower half of the body, cervical chordotomy carried out employing the SCHWARTZ technique, can prove of advantage with respect to the short and sparing character of the intervention, but the results with respect to freeing the patient from pain are not significantly better.

On the other hand, there can be no doubt that, as experience has shown, the number and duration of successes increase with the depth and extent of the section. In particular the results obtained by WHITE and SWEET, SCHWARTZ, OGLE et al., but also our own experiences, are proof of this. Individual successes with selective measures (for example HYNDMAN or JENKNER) are not incompatible with this observation. Here, it is the statistical probability that is decisive.

In this connection, we must deal with our own idea of the organization of the anterolateral column. SHEALY once called into question the justification of cordotomy since he denied the existence of ordered pain tracts in the anterolateral column, favouring rather the multisynaptic afferent system and a diffuse course of the fibres. This opinion certainly goes too far. In hundreds of unilateral chordotomy operations, a complete contralateral analgesia has been observed, but a homolateral analgesia in only a few cases. In the awake patient, the level of the analgesia can be controlled by the extent of the section; a limited number of specific experiments has even shown that it is possible to "knock out" the sensation of pain in localized regions of the body. In this connection, the stimulation and "knock out" results obtained with percutaneous cordotomy may be

Table 4

Authors	Surgical Results				Number of Cases	Mortality (%)
	pain-free (%)	good (%)	mod-erate (%)	unsuc-cessful (%)		
FOERSTER, GAGEL (1932)	50 (73)	23	27		29	7
GRANT (1941)	64 (79)	15	7 (21)	14	109	10
KAHN (1933)	(80)		(20)		(78)	
PEET (1948)	75		10 (25)	15	96	
RIECHERT (1960)					69	3
FRANKEL, PROKOP (1961) Malignant processes	67	27		3	59	11
Inflammatory	11	77		11	9	
Degenerative	100	0		0	3	
Traumatic	25	75		0	4	
SCHWARTZ (1962)	52 (72)	25	16 (28)	7	120	9
NATHAN (1963)	77		23		104	3
BISCHOF, SCHÜTTE (1965) Overall results	69	23	3	8	65	7
Malignant processes	83	12,5	15	4,5	48	
Benign processes	30	53		17	17	
DIEMATH (1967)	67 (88)	21	12		144	4
WHITE (1968) Malignant processes	72		28		318	11
Benign processes	63		37		56	0
RASKIND (1969) Overall results	45 (81)	36	12	7	237	3,4
Benign processes	(60)		19 (40)		(30)	
PISCOL (1972) Immediate result / Overall results	91 / 62 (76)	4 / 14	3 / 15 (24)	2 / 9	202 / 103	5
Malignant processes	80		12 (20)	8	80	
Benign processes	48 (61)	13	30 (39)	9	23	

163

Table 5

Site of the primary tumor	Number of patients	Successes No. =	Successes %	Early failures	Late pain recurrence	Remaining success rate (%)
Mamma	19	14	74	5	7	37
Lungs	21	11	52	10	2	43
Upper gastro-intestinal tract	9	5	56	4	2	33
Lower gastro-intestinal tract	63	53	84	10	3	80
Kidneys	8	6	75	2	–	75
Bladder	17	13	77	4	2	65
Prostate, testes, penis	15	13	87	3	1	80
Ovary, uterus, cervix, vagina	101	76	75	25	10	65
Bones	29	18	62	11	2	55
Other soft parts	18	16	89	2	2	78
Total	300	225	75	75	31	65

Table 6

		Cases	Successes early (%)	Successes late (1-20 years) (%)
Stump pain	leg	8	100	63
Phantom pain	leg	18	94	67
	arm	4	100	25
Peripheral nerve pain	leg	8	100	63
	arm	2	100	50
Tabetic crises		9	88	77
Pain after zoster (thorax or abdomen)		7	85	57
Non-malignant process, total		56	95	63

Table 7

	Freedom from pain after 2 weeks (%)	2 to 12 weeks (%)	3 to 6 months (%)	6 to 12 months (%)	1 to 12 years (%)
Primary thoracic cordotomy (46 cases)	95	83	71	51	47
Secondary and tertiary thoracic cordotomy (8 cases)	36	36	36	27	18
Primary cervical cordotomy (14 cases)	93	86	64	54	46
Secondary cervical cordotomy (6 cases)	66	17	17	0	0

mentioned (TAREN). The number of "counter examples" from FRENCH, VORIS, SWEET, AMASSIAN or OSACAR is small. Although the analytical studies of fibres carried out by HÄGGQVIST and VAN BEUSEKOM, the modern structural and functional conception which HASSLER had developed and special neuro-physiological results (see ECCLES, ZIMMERMANN and others) should be taken into account, the neurosurgeon should not forget his own experience and knowledge. Rather, he must try and find a synthesis for his activity and then orientate the measures he undertakes accordingly. This orientation should serve our working scheme which contains not only pain-surgical, but also general neurological aspects (Fig. 3). The boundaries with respect to topical organization must be understood to be fluid (right-hand side of the cross-sectional scheme) the organization of the modalities-to-be in the sense of a varying fibre concentration (left-hand side). The individual range of fluctuation is considerable and extends right up to the "runaways" mentioned (PISCOL). This scheme shows where targetted partial or selective "knock out" attempts have the greatest chance of success - today the domain of percutaneous cordotomy - but also that the attempt to achieve a complete "knock out" must take into account the entire anterolateral column. In such a case, NOORDENBOS's term "spinal leucotomy" is apt.

In establishing indications, however, not only the success rate and the surgical technical fundamentals are to be considered, but, to an equal extent, also the complications and postoperative discomfort. In the case of unilateral interventions, disorders of the bladder (5% to 10%) and pareses (0% to 8%) are, as a rule, only of a temporary nature or slight. In more recent work, permanent defects are rarely reported. In the case of bilateral operations, the complication rate increases considerably and, in a larger percentage, remains permanent: disorders of the bladder, longer-lasting or persistent in 15% to 30%, pareses in 1% to 24% (severe or permanent in 0% to 5%) of the cases. Here we cannot discuss in detail the problems involving disorders of respiratory function after bilateral high-cervical chordotomies. These disorders usually disappear within 24 to 48 hours and surprisingly rarely give rise to insoluble problems. A particular stress for the patient are, however, the postoperative complaints, in particular allachaesthesia, agonizing dysaesthesias and cincture sensations (zonaesthesia). These are reported in 3% to 20% of all cases.

If we compare the successes in relieving pain with the complications and dysthaesias, and if we then compare the results with other presently available possibilities of treating pain, the technique of open anterolateral cordotomy as an initial surgical intervention remains to be considered only in cases with malignant primary disease. In this latter case, however, we feel that it is still indicated. Basically, open cordotomy is, for a practised surgeon, a short operation and with the more modern, less heroic approach, one that is not too demanding of the patient. Of advantage are the good view of the cord, the possibility of effecting a thorough-going division of the anterolateral column - if required - and the greater possibility of not having to repeat the operation at some future date. Carried out in the thoracic region, it also has the advantage over the percutaneous technique that the arms will, with certainty, remain intact.

In the case of non-malignant diseases, cordotomy should be considered only when the other methods have failed, that is, it should be a last resort. Pain in the lower half of the body has a greater chance of being influenced than pain in the upper half. In view of the postoperative disturbances mentioned previously, in the case of pain in the lower half of the body, we again prefer to employ thoracic cordotomy and for unilateral pain, the unilateral version. In our experience, the informed patient would prefer to be re-operated on on the contralateral side rather than to put up with initially unnecessary deficiencies.

Evaluation

An evaluation of open spinal surgery for the treatment of pain in the present situation of neurosurgical therapeutic possibilities, in particular in comparison with percutaneous cordotomy and neurostimulation procedures, may not only serve as an orientation, but it must, of necessity, also lead to recommendations. Table 8 represents the attempt to deduce such recommendations from appropriate comparisons and to represent them in a clear manner. They are put up for discussion in the hope that they will provoke some critical and "corrective" suggestions. It might be said at this point that we, ourselves, in all painful conditions of a non-malignant nature, first make use of the various neurostimulation procedures since, here, no neurological deficits need to be accepted. Until a final clarification of effectiveness has been obtained, we try, at least transcutaneous neurostimulation, even in patients with malignant diseases and pain in the extremities.

In Table 8, open cordotomy is listed as being extensively used only in the case of malignant processes involving the lower half of the body and as the method of choice in bilateral pain or pain in the midline; admittedly, however, only in the thoracic version, in order reliably to avoid negative results in the arms. On account of the monosegmental to oligosegmental painful conditions in the region of the trunk, rhizotomies are given three crosses in the group of benign processes. Double markings are also employed for situations in which other methods have failed or cannot be effected. Our views on commissural myelotomy have already been presented in the appropriate section. A single cross indicates that we should like to retain the option for special cases, the cross in brackets means that this indication is advocated by some authors.

Instead of a summary, I should like to make a topical comparison. If the new methods and techniques of combatting pain be compared with a modern sports coupé provided with lots of electronic equipment, the open methods might then be seen as old timers which simply do not attract any attention in the year 1975, and which do not dominate the pain-therapeutic street scene. Basically, they still run reliably and can, occasionally, carry us to our destination when the road has become too uneven for the newer models.

Table 8. Recommendations for pain therapy with spinal operations

Indication / Pain site	Rhizotomy	Commissural myelotomy	Open cordotomy				Percutaneous cordotomy		TNS → DCS
			Unilat. thorac.	Bilat. thorac.	Unilat. cervic.	Bilat. cervic.	Unilat. cervic.	Bilat. cervic.	
Benign diseases									
Upper extremity, unilateral	(+)	?			+		++		+++
Upper extremity, resist./recur.	+	+			++		+++	+	
Lower extremity, unilateral	(+)	?	+		(+)		++		+++
Lower extremity, resist./recur.	+	(+)	++	(+)	+		+++	+	
Trunk (and bilateral radiation)	+++	+	+	++	+	(+)	++	+	+
Phantom pain, zoster pain, etc.	+	?	+	?	(+)		+	(+)	++
Malignant diseases									
Only upper half of the body, unilateral	+	(+)			++		+++	+	+++
Up to the upper half of the body, unilateral	(+)				++		+++	+	+++
Up to the upper half of the body, bilateral						++		+++	+
Up to the upper half of the body, resist./recur.					+	++	+	+++	
Only trunk (mostly lower half)	+	++	?	+++			?	+	+
Lower half of the body, unilateral	?		+++	+	+		++	+	+++
Lower half of the body, bilateral		+		+++		+		++	+
Lower half of the body, resist./recur.		+		+++		+	+	++	

167

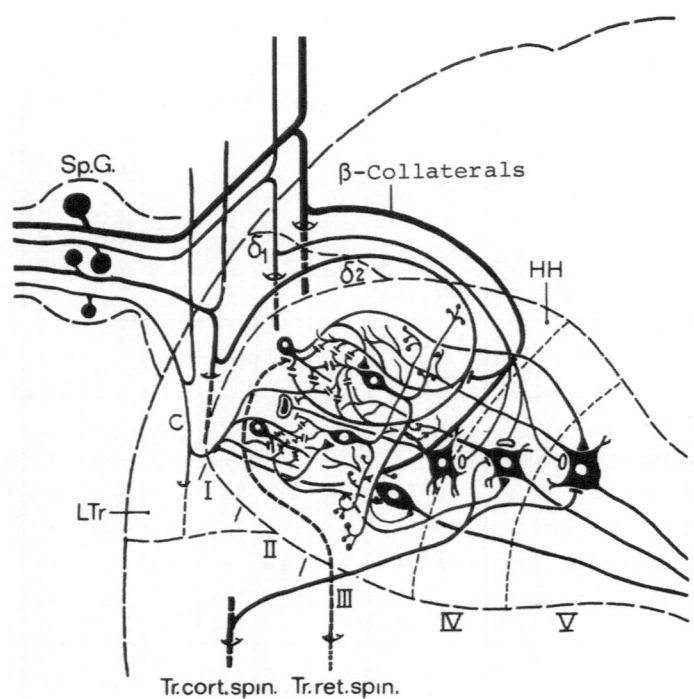

Fig. 1. Schematic representation of the relationships between the posterior root fibres and complicated posterior horn structures (see also PISCOL, 1974). Although a division of the posterior root between the spinal ganglion (Sp.G.) and the spinal cord interrupts the direct inflow of impulses via this root, it does not interrupt irradiations or interactions via the ascending and descending collaterals in the root inflow zone (for example LISSAUER tract) and in the posterior horn column itself (see also text)

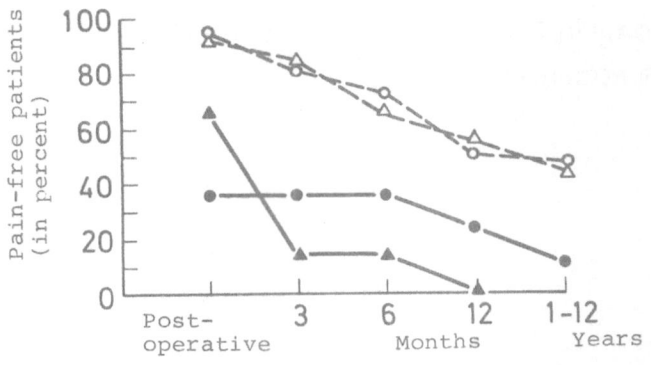

Fig. 2. In second and third interventions, the chances of success are markedly lower than with first operations (after WHITE and SWEET, 1969)

○--○ 46 high-thoracic cordotomies in 34 patients followed over 1 year (primary operation)

△--△ 14 high-cervical cordotomies in 13 patients followed over 1 year (primary operation)

●——● 11 high-thoracic cordotomies in 9 patients followed over 1 year (secondary and tertiary operation)

▲——▲ 6 high-cervical cordotomies in 6 patients followed over 1 year (secondary and tertiary operation)

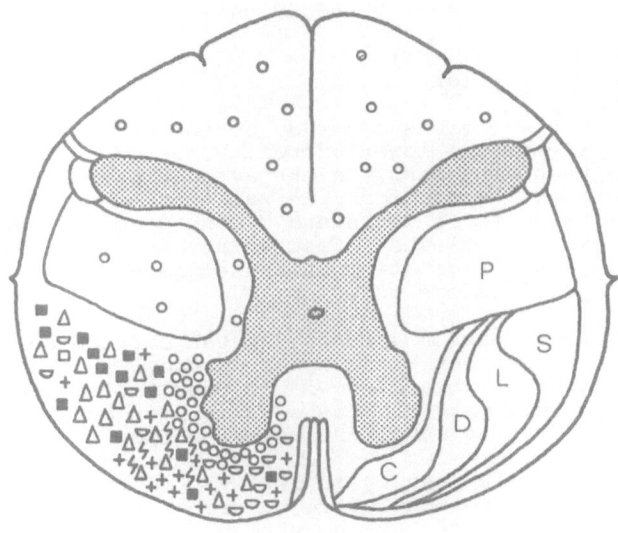

Fig. 3. Scheme of the organization in the anterolateral column from the point of view of the surgeon operating for pain relief (PISCOL, 1973, 1974) (see also text)

△ Pain (Tr.spth)
○ Pain (MAS?)
□ Temperature
+ Touch
  Pressure
  Respiration

C = Fibres from the cervical segments
D = Fibres from the thoracic segments
L = Fibres from the lumbar segments
S = Fibres from the sacral segments
P = Pyramidal tract

Anterolateral Cordotomy in Cases of Phantom Limb Pain

A. PERNECZKY and M. SUNDER-PLASSMANN

Introduction

The surgical treatment of phantom limb pain is a problem which has
not been solved so far. On account of the special pathophysiology of
this phenomenon, most authors (1, 4, 5, 7, 8) disapprove of a surgical treatment of phantom limb pain. This opinion, however, is opposed by publications of some other authors (3, 6, 9). As we observed surprisingly good results after cordotomy in some of our patients suffering from phantom limb pain, we decided to check the
effectiveness of anterolateral cordotomy in so far as it influences
phantom limb pain.

Material and Method

In the period from 1965 to 1974 anterolateral cordotomy was carried
out at the Neurosurgical Department of the University of Vienna in
14 patients suffering from phantom limb pain. The patients treated
were 13 men and one woman. At the time of the operation, the patients
were between 25 and 72 years old with an average age of 57.

Description

Table 1 gives a survey of the indications for amputation. In 13 patients one lower extremity, in one patient an upper extremity had
been amputated. On the average phantom limb pain had occured 12 years
after amputation. The patients had been suffering from phantom limb
pains for 8 years and 3 months on the average. Four of the cordotomised patients showed an abuse of analgetics. In addition Table 1
gives information on those therapeutic measures which had been applied before cordotomy.

In 13 patients, cordotomy was carried out as an upper thoracic, in
one patient as an upper cervical section of the spinothalamicic
tract. Table 2 shows the results immediately after the operation
with regard to phantom limb pain and phantom limb sensation. Postoperative complications are also to be found in Table 2.

The late results in twelve cordotomised patients are shown in Table
3. The postoperative observation period was five and a half years on
the average. At the time of the last examination two patients had no
pain. Six patients complained about bearable phantom limb pain and
the administration of analgetics was not necessary. The remaining four
patients complained about strong phantom limb pain, which would be
relieved to a certain extent only by regular alkaloid medication. All
patients, also those without pain, stated that they had phantom limb
sensation. Thus, 12 patients (66.7% of the cases) had either no pain
or less pain by the time of the last examination.

Table 1. History of 14 cases of phantom limb pain

Indication for amputation	case No	pain in the limb before amputation	beginning of phantom limb pain after amputation	duration of phantom limb pain before cordotomy	abuse of drugs	other operations before cordotomy
trauma	1	no	21 years	4 years	no	twice revision of the stump
	2	no	2 years	20 years	no	one revision of the stump
	3	no	14 years	6 years	no	no
	4	no	2 months	20 years	no	twelve revisions of the stump
	5	no	1 year	20 years	no	sympathectomy, revision of the stump
	6	no	19 years	6 years	no	sympathectomy
	7	no	23 years	1 year	alkaloids	no
	8	yes	3 months	$1^1/2$ years	no	no
osteomyelitis	9	no	10 years	4 years	phenacetin	no
	10	yes	27 years	12 years	no	three revisions of the stump
	11	no	4 years	14 years	no	operation at level D11(?), E-shock
vascular disease	12	yes	8 years	4 years	alkaloids	no
	13	yes	39 years	1 year	no	no
	14	yes	2 months	$1^1/2$ years	alkaloids	no

The effectiveness of the interruption of the spinothalamic tract is especially obvious immediately after the operation, as 13 of 14 patients (92%) had no pain or less pain. The method of treatment was not the reason why the operation was unsuccessful in case 4. In this case it was demonstrated that the crossing of the spinothalamic tract was missing (2). Our results, therefore, have to be considered to be good, as only three late failures occurred in eleven patients (case 4 not calculated) at the time of the last examination.

We could not find any relation between the duration of phantom limb pain and the effectiveness of the cordotomy nor between an abuse of drugs and the change of pain brought about by operation.

As the rate of complications occurring as irreversible neurological failures is low (cases 2 and 10), anterolateral cordotomy is recom-

Table 2. Postoperative results of cordotomy in 14 cases of phantom limb pain

case No	phantom limb pain no pain	improved	no change	phantom limb	complications temporary	permanent
1	x			no		
2		x		yes		dysfunction of the bladder
3		x		yes		
4			x	yes		
5	x			no	bladder atony	
6	x			no		
7		x		yes		
8		x		yes	extremity weakness	
9	x			no		
10		x		yes		dysfunction of the bladder
11	x			no	extremity weakness	
12	x			yes		
13		x		yes		
14		x		yes		
total	6 = 42,8%	7 = 50%	1 = 7,2%			

mended for the elimination of phantom limb pain with a relatively high rate of success.

Summary

The authors report on the effectiveness of anterolateral cordotomy in eliminating phantom limb pain in 14 patients. Immediately after the operation 13 patients stated that they had either no pain or less pain. In one patient, in whom the character of pain did not change, although cordotomy on the homolateral side had a good effect, the crossing of the spinothalamical tract was demonstrated to be missing. At the time of the last examination, late failure was diagnosed in 3 of 11 patients (above-mentioned case not calculated). Anterolateral cordotomy is recommended for the elimination of phantom limb pain as the complication rate is low and the operative effect satisfying.

Table 3. Late results of cordotomy in 12 cases of phantom limb pain

case No	duration of follow up after cordotomy	phantom limb pain no pain	bearable	unbearable	phantom limb
1	6 years	x			yes
2	9 years			x	yes
4	9 years			x	yes
5	9 years		x		yes
6	4 years		x		yes
7	5 years			x	yes
8	6 years			x	yes
10	2 years		x		yes
11	1 year	x			yes
12	3 years		x		yes
13	3 years		x		yes
14	9 years		x		yes
total		2 = 16,7%	6 = 50%	4 = 33,3%	

REFERENCES

1. BAILEY, A.A., MOERSCH, F.P.: Phantom limb. Canad. Med. Ass. J., 45, 37 - 42 (1941).

2. BRENNER, H., PENDL, G.: Ipsilateraler Chordotomieeffekt. - Ein seltener Fall einer ungekreuzten Schmerzbahn. Wr. Med. Wschr. 116, 1041 (1966).

3. FALCONER, M.A.: Surgical treatment of intractable phantom limb pain. Brit. Med. J. 1, 299 - 304 (1953).

4. GULEKE, N.: Die Eingriffe am Gehirnschädel, Gehirn, an der Wirbelsäule und am Rückenmark. In: Allgemeine und spezielle chirurgische Operationslehre, Bd. II. Begr. v. M. KIRSCHNER. Berlin-Heidelberg-New York: Springer 1950.

5. LIVINGSTON, W.K.: Pain Mechanismus: A Physiologic Interpretation of Causalgia and its Related States. New York: MacMILLAN 1943.

6. RIDDOCH, G.: Phantom limbs and body shape. Brain 64, 197 - 222 (1941).

7. SCHÜRMANN, K.: Die operative Schmerzbehandlung aus der Sicht des Neurochirurgen. In: Schmerz und Schmerztherapie (Hrsg. D. GROSS, D. LANGEN). Stuttgart: Hippokrates 1971.

8. STROHECKER, J., KOLLAR, W.A.F.: Phantomschmerz und Stumpfneurom. 13. Neuropsychiatrisches Symposium, Pula (Jugoslawien) 1973.

9. WHITE, J.C., SWEET, W.H.: Pain and the Neurosurgeon. Springfield/III.: CHARLES C. THOMAS 1969.

Results After Open Cordotomy

W. PIOTROWSKI and C. PANITZ

The first patient being treated in a new neurosurgical clinic usually does not have a meningioma or an arterial aneurysm. This was
also the case in Mannheim, where we had to care first for a 70-year-
old man suffering from severe pain in his lower extremities due a
rectum carcinoma. He was paraplegic and had lost all control of bladder function. He was obtunded due to a high dosage of alkaloids,
which had to be given many times a day.

After unilateral open cordotomy at the level of D 4, he was immediately free of pain so that the medication of alkaloids could be with-
drawn. He felt much better than before operation but died 24 days
later due to the carcinoma. The postoperative degeneration of the
spino-thalamic tract is shown in Fig. 1.

Over a period of 2 years we treated 15 patients, 6 males and 9 females, by open cordotomy, all of them suffering from malignant tumors (Table 1).

Table 1. Primary diagnosis in 15 patients treated by open anterolateral cordotomy

Mannheim 1973 - 1974	
Rectum Carcinoma	5
Genital Carcinoma	3
Mamma Carcinoma	2
Unknown Carcinoma	2
Bronchus-Ca	1
Hypernephroma	1
Synovialoma	1

The cordotomy was done in 13 patients at an upper thoracic level, in
11 cases the incision being made bilaterally at different segments.
Only in two cases did we use the cervical cordotomy (Table 2). 9 patients suffered preoperatively from paresis of one or both lower extremities and 8 of these patients had lost control over their bladder function. Postoperatively only one additional patient became
paraplegic.

The results of the cordotomy were good or excellent in 12 patients,
some of them being completely free of pain. The remaining 3 patients
had only minor relief.

Table 2. Open anterolateral cordotomy in malignant tumors (n = 15)

age and sex	incision C	D	paresis	bladder function	hypalgesia from	analgesia from	good relief	minor relief	recurrence of pain
					postoperative symptoms				
55 m		1;3	→	+		D_6bil	+		∅
19 m		2;4	→	→		D_{12}bil	+		∅
53 m		1;3	+	→		D_{11}bil		+	∅
70 m		4	→	→		D_{11}	+		∅
51 w		1;3	→	→		L_1bil		+	∅
48 m	2		∅	∅	C_5	D_{12}	+		∅
55 w		1;3	∅	+	D_{11}bil		+		R
40 w		1;3	∅	∅		L_1bil	+		R
27 w		1;3	→	→		D_8bil	+		R
46 w		1;3	→	→	D_4 D_6	D_{12}bil	+		R
64 w		1;3	→	+	D_8	D_8 L_5	+		R
73 m		1;3	→	→		?		+	R
55 w		2	∅	∅		D_{12}	+		R
61 w		1;3	→	→		D_{12}	+		∅
46 w	1		∅	∅		D_{11}	+		R

→ preoperative lesion

All patients died within 1 - 13 months after the operation (Fig. 2). In 8 cases pain recurred some days or weeks before they died, so that alkaloid medication had to be restored. However, in almost all cases, the open cordotomy had given some or even complete relief of pain, thereby improving the patients' situation. In agreement with the results of SCHWARTZ (1962), DIEMATH (1967), and WHITE (1968) the open cordotomy can be recommended as a still valuable method in treating the unbearable pain of patients, suffering from malignant tumors.

REFERENCES

1. DIEMATH, H.E.: Zur neurochirurgischen Schmerzbekämpfung bei Malignomen. Wien. klin. Wschr. 78, 309 - 310 (1967).

2. SCHWARTZ, H.G.: High cervical cordotomy. Technique and results. Clin. Neurosurg. 8, 282 - 293 (1962).

3. WHITE, J.C.: Operations for the relief of pain in the torso and extremities: Evaluation of their effectiveness over long periods, p. 503 - 519. London - New York: Academic Press 1968.

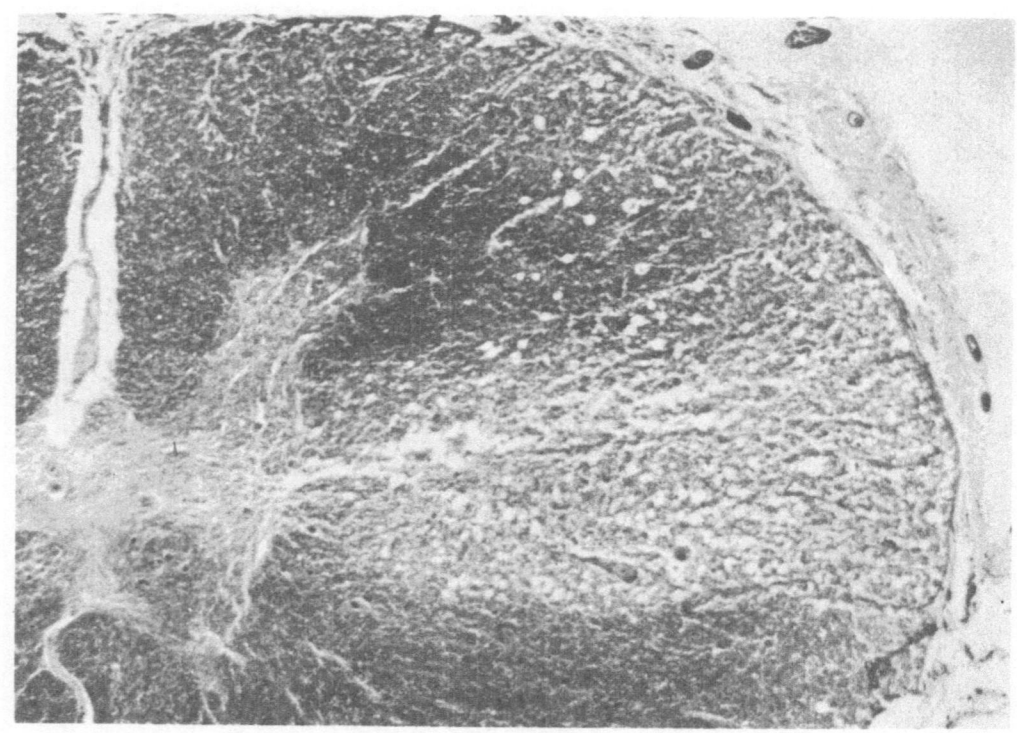

Fig. 1. Postoperative degeneration of the spino-thalamic tract at the level of D 4.
We want to express our thanks to Prof. P.W. HOER (Frankfurt/M.) for the permission to use this slide

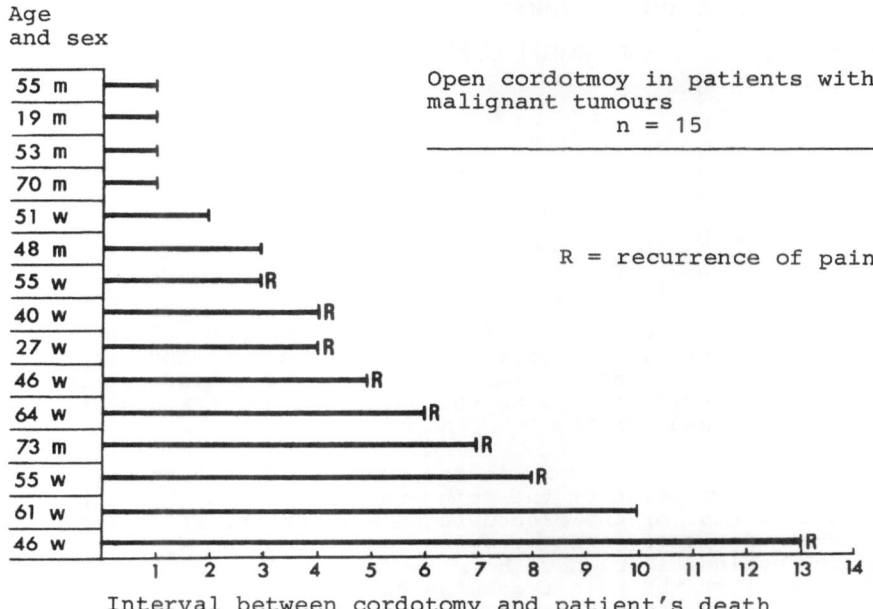

Fig. 2. Open anterolateral cordotomy in patients with malignant
tumors (n = 15)

177

Percutaneous Cordotomy

R. LORENZ, TH. GRUMME,H.-D. HERRMANN, H. PALLESKE, A. KÜHNER, U. STEUDE, and J. ZIERSKI

Interruption of the anterior lateral quadrant of the spinal cord, the spino-thalamic tract, has been used for many years for the relief of intractable pains. Cordotomy was introduced in the USA in 1912 by MARTIN following the advice of SPILLER and in Germany by FOERSTER and TIETZE.

Percutaneous cordotomy is the youngest of the techniques used for the interruption of the spino-thalamic tract. Principally the requirements for the procedure as well as its effects are similar to that of classic open cordotomy and depend on whether all pain-conducting fibers have been severed at the level of interruption and on whether the pain transmission from the area involved does not take place through other systems. HASSLER (1975) reported extensively on the present state of anatomical and functional knowledge of a pain transmitting system. Position and distribution of pain-conducting fibers in the spinal cord have not been fully clarified as yet. There is some evidence that pain is transmitted not only through the spino-thalamic tract, and it seems that the concept of somatotopic distribution will have to be altered at least in some aspects (PROCACCI, ZOPPI, and MARESCA, 1973).

The report deals with the present state of percutaneous cordotomy and its results. The data of the literature (approximately 2,600 cordotomies) for this report were kindly supplied by ·the Neurosurgical Departments in Berlin-Westend, Giessen, Heidelberg, Homburg/ Saar, Hull/Great Britain and Munich (approximately 224 cordotomies).

Percutaneous Cordotomy Technique

The procedure was originally described by MULIAN, HARPER and HEKMAT-PANAH et al. in 1963. They used a radioactivate-tipped needle, but changed to electrolytic coagulation in 1965. At the same time ROSO-MOFF et al. reported first 268 radiofrequency percutaneous cordotomies in 177 patients.

Both MULLAN et al. as well as ROSOMOFF et al.used the lateral approach at the C 1/C 2 level (Fig.1). The needle is advanced under X-ray check and aims at the junction between the anterior one-third and posterior two-thirds of the spinal canal. ALKSNE in 1966 and LIN, GILDENBERG and POLAKOFF (1966) used the anterior approach with the hope of avoiding the lesion of the reticulo-spinal tract. Their technique was percutaneous, and the needle had to penetrate the cervical disc. Correction of the position of theneedle sometimes required many repeated punctures. In 1964 CLOWARD described (see also

HARDY and LECIERQ in 1974)the open anterior approach to cervical cordotomy. CRUE, TODD and CARPEGAL in 1968 chose the posterior approach. This approach necessitates the puncture of the spinal cord and advancing the electrode forward in order to reach the spino-thalamic tract.

Whatever approach to the spinal cord is used, fixation of the head is necessary, the patient lying supine for lateral and anterior cordotomy, and prone for posterior cordotomy. The procedure is performed in local anesthesia.

Spinal lesion was produced by isotopes (MULLAN et al. 1963), unipolar coagulation (electrolytic lesion, MULLAN et al. in 1965), "bipolar" coagulation (radiofrequency lesion ROSOMOFF et al. 1965) and with cold (cryocordotomy, RAND et al. 1965).

The technique most frequently used is thatof the lateral approach and radio-frequency lesion (MULLAN 1951 and ROSOMOFF 1971, TAREN 1971, ROTHBARD 1972, MATTMANN 1972, ONOFRIO 1971, TASKER, ORGAN and EVANS 1973, LIPTON 1972 and others).

Checking the Placement of the Needle

After the subarachnoid space has been punctured, there is a free outflow of CSF, displacement of the needle is possible and careful check of the position of its tip in relation to the spinal cord is, therefore, necessary. For this purpose the cord is outlined either with air (ROSOMOFF 1965) or with positive contrast-medium (Panto-paque) (MULLAN and coll. 1965). SMITH (1973) advocated the injection of Tantalum-powder. Placement checked by radiological markings of the cervical spine alone is insufficient.

The majority of the authors performed cervical myelography with an emulsified contrast-medium (Pantopaque, Duroliopaque). The important factor is the position of the needle in relation to the denticulate ligaments. This is practically impossible to realize with air myelography, but can be seen relatively well at Pantopaque myelography. If the position of the tip of the needle is correct, it should project just in front of the denticulate ligaments and for lesions aiming to interrupt pain conduction from the upper extremity, the electrode can be introduced slightly more ventral. It can happen that the resistance of the pia mater is such that penetration of the cord is difficult, and it tends to be pushed over to the other side or to rotate. This situation can be very easily recognized with a positive contrast medium used to visualize the denticulate ligaments.

Penetration of the cord is checked by measurement of impedance introduced by ORGAN, TASKER and MOODY in 1968. Change of the impedance between CSF, pia mater and spinal cord can be checked optically or acoustically while advancing the electrode.

Final check of the correct position of the electrode is done by stimulation (MULLAN 1971). Stimulation with rectangular impulse of higher frequency (75 - 100 Hz) with 0.1 - 0.25 volts produces a feeling of warmth (100 Hz) or cold (75 Hz) as well as paresthesia in the contralateral parts of the body, suggesting that the tip of the needle is placed within the spino-thalamic tract. Stimulation with 2 Hz current at 1 - 2 volts produces ipsilateral twitching of trapezius and neck muscles. These are the ideal values for the position of the electrodes.These differ, of course, if the needle is placed at some distance from the center of the spino-thalamic tract.

X-ray check and visualization of denticulate ligaments, impedance measurement, and stimulation provide a high degree of certainty about the correct position of the tip of the electrode. Impedance measurement and stimulation are now mandatory and considerably diminish the risk of the procedure, originally stressed by ROSOMOFF at a time when radiological check only was used. On the other hand, cordotomy series with a low complication rate were reported by surgeons who did not use impedance measurement and stimulation for checking the position of the electrode (UIHLEIN 1969).

Coagulation

Another check is done during the coagulation itself, which is performed in steps. Careful neurological examination after each coagulation will possibly reveal undesired effects thus preventing irreversible damage. In cases in which information received from the stimulation of the spinal cord is insufficient or bizarre, even after correction of the placement of the electrode, coagulation should, if at all indicated, be performed in steps.

Often an unavoidable lesion of the reticulo-spinal tract may manifest itself after the operation or at sleep. The fact that the reticulo-spinal tract becomes damaged during cordotomy has been known for a long time (WHITE, SWEET, HAWKINS, NILGES, 1950). This notion became important with the increase of high cervical percutaneous procedures performed particularly with bilateral cordotomies. Respiratory disturbances and cases of death in sleep following cervical cordotomy directed LIN, GILDENBERG, and POLAKOFF to choose the anterior approach. Anatomical relations of the reticulospinal tract were described in detail by HITCHCOCK and LEECE in 1967. In patients with normal respiratory function, the risk of respiratory distrubances after cervical cordotomy is relatively low. Patients with reduced pulmonary function e.g. patients at an advanced age with pulmonary diseases and low pO_2 (MATTMANN 1972) are a much higher risk. Such patients after having their reticulo-spinal tract damaged usually control their respiration when awake, but do not do so when asleep, in other words, they "forget to breathe".

Indications for Percutaneous Cordotomy

Indications for percutaneous cordotomy as far as pain and choice of patients is concerned, are principally the same as for an open procedure. However, there is a whole series of factors, which influence the indications and tend to favour the choice of the percutaneous procedure. These include, first of all, the relative simplicity of percutaneous cordotomy, its rapidity, and lack of such phenomena as blood-loss or disturbances in wound-healing, which may accompany an open procedure. Moreover, it must be stated that percutaneous cordotomy can be performed in patients in a markedly reduced general state, in which an open procedure will certainly be too risky. The immediate sequelae of the procedure must also be taken into account. Meningeal irritation following percutaneous cordotomy occurs only rarely and bed rest, providing the loss of CSF had been kept to a minimum, does not exceed 2-3 days.

This relative simplicity and low risk of the percutaneous procedure directed several surgeons to extend the domain of cordotomy, reserved so far for patients with intractable pain due to carcinoma or other malignancy, onto patients with phantom-limb pains, neuralgia, causalgia, and nerve-root pains (ROSOMOFF, 1972). These broader indications are, however, under discussion.

Results

Results of percutaneous cervical cordotomy compiled from the review of the literature and our collected statistics from 6 centers are shown in Table 1.

Table 1. Results of 2840 cordotomies

	Review of literature[a]		Collected statistics[b]
Number of cordotomies	2616		224
Early results good	80	– 96 %	85 %
Late results good	42	– 75 %	60 %
Mortality	O	– 4,6%	3 %
Respiratory disturbances	O	– 4,6%	3,5%
Bladder dysfunction	1,5	– 15 %	7,6%
Transient hemiparesis	4	– 17 %	7,6%
Permanent hemiparesis	O	– 3 %	1 %
Ataxia	seldom	– 28,3%	4 %
Dysasthesia		– 5 %	
Horner's Syndrome		– 50 %	
Depression of blood pressure		– 3,3%	2,2%

[a]Series of ACOSTA et al. 1969, CLOUGH et al, 1969, GILDENBERG et al. 1967/1969, LIPTON 1973, MATTMANN 1972, MUEKE 1973, MULLAN 1966, ROSOMOFF 1965, TASKER et al. 1973, VAILATI et al. 1965.

[b]Series of Berlin-Westend, Giessen, Heidelberg, Homburg/Saar, Hull/ Great Britain, Munich.

Early results of percutaneous cordotomy are usually good. Failures are caused by difficulties arising from patients' uncooperativeness, impossibility to achieve correct positioning of the needle, or less frequently, failure to penetrate the spinal cord. As an early result we defined patients' complaints about pain at leaving the Neurosurgical Unit. In our series failures and bad results were mainly due to difficulties in achieving complete abolition of pain arising from the brachial plexus and not sufficiently high level of anesthesia. Analysis of late results was rendered difficult, mainly because the main indication for percutaneous cordotomy was pain connected with malignancy and accordingly survival following the procedure is usually short. So far the best analysis was reported by ROSOMOFF in 1971, who reported late results after 350 coagulations. With the prolongation of the follow-up period, the results are getting worse. He reported 90% of good results 6 months after the procedure, but only 24% after 36 months following cordotomy. In our collected statistics the follow-up period was usually too short in order to draw certain conclusions. The majority of patients in whom percutaneous cordotomy was performed, died in peripheral hospitals and no reliable postmortem findings were available. In those few cases, in which the spinal cord was sectioned, histological examination showed complete interruption of the spino-thalamic tract. The recurrence of pain in previously anesthetized areas has to be explained either by incomplete interruption of the spino-thalamic tract or pain transmission through another way.

The mortality after cervical percutaneous cordotomy is relatively high: 4,6% (literature data) and 3% (collective statistics) respectively. This is due to respiratory disturbances which occurred in patients with primarily reduced respiratory function. It has to be said that in the majority of patients in our series, death occurred after a period of prolonged artificial respiration and was due to the sequelae of artificial respiration. However, not every patient who shows respiratory disturbances after percutaneous cordotomy dies because of it. According to LIN et al. there are less respiratory disturbances following cordotomy by the anterior approach. However, the number of patients and the frequency with which percutaneous cordotomy was performed through the ventral approach is small. These authors do not mention complications arising from the multiple puncturing of the cervical intravertebral space. Data concerning urinary disturbances due to cervical cordotomy are not uniform. Some authors have seen no bladder disturbances even after bilateral cordotomies, others reported that every sixth patient submitted to cervical cordotomy had micturition troubles.

The percentage of transient motor weakness is relatively high. In some of our cases motor weakness developed with a certain delay. Transient character and delayed appearance of these signs would suggest hemodynamic sequelae or accompanying oedema. Since introduction of an impedance measurement and stimulation into our practice, we had no case of immediate motor weakness occurring during cordotomy.

Limb ataxias were sometimes noted, reflecting accompanying lesion of the spino-cerebellar tract. In a few cases, paresthesias were reported in the area which has been rendered analgetic.

ACOSTA and GROSSMAN (1969) reported a Horner-syndrome in more than 50% of their patients due to the lesion of pupillodilatory fibers running in the vicinity of the anterior lateral tract.

Meningeal reactions were rare. Some authors reported occipital neuralgias. These are due to the irritation of the C2 root, and according to our experience are quite frequently observed in the first hours or days after percutaneous cordotomy. There was no case of persistent occipital neuralgia.

Attention should be drawn to the usually transient but sometimes resistent depression of blood pressure mainly after bilateral cordotomies. This blood pressure depression is of the orthostatic type and in a few cases the application of an antigravity suit was necessary.

Finally we would like to briefly mention the risk of bilateral percutaneous cordotomy. In our collected statistics, there were 24 patients in whom cordotomy was performed on both sides. 5 of them developed respiratory disturbances, 3 of them died after a prolonged period of artificial respiration. 2 patients had transient hemiparesis, 6 of them micturition disturbances, and 3 blood pressure depression. The risk of bilateral cordotomy is therefore quite considerable, particularly as far as respiratory disturbances are concerned.

Conclusion

In the last 12 years, since the introduction of the percutaneous cordotomy by MULLAN, the method has been developed and now has a solid
place in the neurosurgical management of pain problems. A review of
the literature and collective statistics of six centers showed that
the lateral approach at the C 1/C 2 level with X-ray check, visualization of the spinal cord by means of positive contrast myelography,
impedance measurement, and stimulation is the most widely used and
the least complicated method. Early results are good, analysis of
late results shows that in 50% of cases the pain recurs. This fact
should be kept in mind when considering the indications for cordotomy.
There is uniform opinion that percutaneous cordotomy should be mainly
used in the management of intolerable pain in patients with malignancy. The number of failures can be markedly reduced if other forms of
pain are excluded.

In comparison with classic open cordotomy, the percutaneous procedure
has the advantage of avoiding a major surgical procedure with operative wound and opening of the CSF space. It can be performed in patients at an advanced age and in poor general condition. As far as
the neurological complications are concerned, the difference between
an open and a percutaneous procedure (WHITE and SWEET) is not significant.

REFERENCES

ACOSTA, C., GROSSMAN, R.G.: Relief of intractable pain by percutaneous
anterolateral radiofrequency cordotomy. Texas. Med. (Austin) 65, 36-40
(1969).

ALKSNE, J.F.: Percutaneous anterior cordotomy. Pacif. Med. Surg.
(Seattle) 74, 192-195 (1966).

CLOUGH, G.A., MAXWELL, J.A.: Relieving intractable pain. The use of
percutaneous cordotomy in the management of pain. J. Kansas Med. Soc.
70, 117-119 (1969).

CLOWARD, R.B.: Cervical cordotomy by the anterior approach. J.
Neurosurg. 21, 19-25 (1964).

CRUE, B.L., TODD, E.M., CARREGAL, E.J.A.: Posterior approach for high
cervical percutaneous radiofrequency cordotomy. Confin. Neurol.
(Basel) 30, 41-52 (1968).

FOERSTER, O.: Vorderseitenstrangdurchtrennung im Rückenmark zur Be-
seitung von Schmerzen. Berl. Klin. Wschr. 50, 1499-1500 (1913).

GILDENBERG. P.L.: Percutaneous cervical cordotomy for relief of
intractable pain. Cleveland clin. Quart. (Ohio) 36, 183-188 (1969).

GILDENBERG, P.L., LIN, P.M., POLAKOFF II., P.P.: A sterotaxic
approach to the spinal cord. Confin. Neurol. (Basel) 29, 252-255
(1967).

HITCHCOCK, E., LEECE, B.: Somatotopic representation of the respiratory pathways in the cervical cord of man. J. Neurosurg. 27,
320-329 (1967).

HARDY, J., LECLERCQ, T.A.: Microsurgical selective cordotomy by the
anterior approach. Vortrag: 1974 Joint Meeting of the American Association of Neurological Surgeons, and the Society of Neurosurgical
Anesthesia and Neurologic Supportive Care. St. Louis (Missouri)
22.-25. 4. 1974.

HASSLER, R.: Central interactions of the systems of rapidly and slowly conducted pain. In: Advances in Neurosurgery, Vol. 3 (eds. H. Penzholz, M. Brock, J. Hamer, M. Klinger, O. Spaerri), pp. Berlin-Heidelberg-New York: Springer 1975.

LIN, P.M., GILDENBERG, P.L., and POLAKOFF II, P.P.: An anterior approach to percutaneous lower cervical cordotomy. J. Neurosurg. 25, 553-560 (1966).

LIPTON, S.: Percutaneous cervical cordotomy. Proc. R. Soc. Med. 66, 607-609 (1973).

MATTMANN, E.: Die perkutane hochzervikale Chordotomie zur symptomatischen Schmerzbehandlung. Schweiz. Arch. Neurol. Neurochir. Psychiatr. (Zürich) 111, 341-352 (1972).

MUEKE, R.: Eine verbesserte Möglichkeit zur Ausschaltung der Schmerzbahn – die perkutane zervikale Chordotomie. Z. Prakt. Anaesth. 105-108 (1973).

MULLAN, S.: Percutaneous cordotomy. J. Neurosurg. 35, 360-366 (1971).

MULLAN, S., HARPER, P.V., HEKMATPANAH, J., TORRES, H., DOBBEN, G.: Percutaneous interruption of spinal-pain tracts by means of a Strontium-90 needle. J. Neurosurg. 20, 931-939 (1963).

MULLAN, S., HARPER, P.V., HEKMATPANAH, J., BECKMAN, F., DOBBEN, G.: Radiological aspects of percutaneous cordotomy. Acta Radiol. Ther. (Stockholm) 40-47 (1966).

MULLAN, S., HEKMATPANAH, J., DOBBEN, G., BECKMAN, F.: Percutaneous, intramedullary cordotomy utilizing the unipolar anodal electrolytic lesion. N. Neurosurg. 22, 548-553 (1965).

ONOFRIO, B.M.: Cervical spinal cord and dentate delineation in percutaneous radiofrequency cordotomy at the level of the first to second cervical vertebrae. Surg. Gynecol. Obstet. 133, 30-34 (1971).

ORGAN, I.W., TASKER, R.R., MOODY, N.F.: Brain tumor localization using an electrical impedance technique. J. Neurosurg. 28, 35-44 (1968).

PROCACCI, P., ZOPPI, M., MARESCA, M.: Recent advances in the anatomy and physiology of pain. J. Neurosurg. Sci. 17, 115-145 (1973).

RAND, R.W., BAUER, R.O., SMART, C.R., JANNETTA, P.J.: Experiences with percutaneous sterotaxic cryocordotomy. Bull. Los Angeles Neurol. Soc. 30, 142-147 (1965).

ROSOMOFF, H.L.: Vortrag: 39th Meeting of the American Association of Neurological Surgeons, Houston/Texas 1971.

ROSOMOFF, H.L.: Vortrag: Congress of the American College of Surgeons, New York 1972.

ROSOMOFF, H.L., CARROLL, F., BROWN, J., SHEPTAK, P.: Percutaneous radiofrequency cervical cordotomy:technique. J. Neurosurg. 23, 639-644 (1965).

ROSOMOFF, H.L., SHEPTAK, P., CARROLL, F.: Modern pain relief: percentaneous chordotomy. JAMA 196, 482-486 (1966).

ROTHBARD, M.J., KOTSILIMBAS, D.G., JACOBSON, S.A., SALL, S.: Relief of intractable pain in cervical carcinoma with percutaneous radiofrequency cordotomy. Obstet. Gynecol. 40, 50-55 (1972).

SMITH, R.: Outlining the cervical spinal cord with Tantalum-powder: application to percutaneous cordotomy. Technical note. J. Neurosurg. 38, 257-260 (1973).

SPILLER, W.G., MARTIN, E.: The treatment of persistent pain of organic origin in the lower part of the body by division of the anterolateral column of the spinal cord. J. Amer. Med. Assoc. <u>58</u>, 1489-1490 (1912).

TAREN, J.A.: Physiologic corroboration in stereotaxic high cervical cordotomy. Confin. Neurol. (Basel) <u>33</u>, 285-290 (1971).

TASKER, R.R., ORGAN, L.W., EVANS, R.J.: Experience with percutaneous cordotomy. Canad. J. Surg. <u>16</u>, 112-114 (1973).

UIHLEIN, A., WEERASOORIYA, L.A., HOLMAN, C.B.: Percutaneous electrical cervical cordotomy for the relief of intractable pain. Mayo Clin. Proc. <u>44</u>, 176-183 (1969).

VAILATI, G., MULLAN, S.: Cordotomia percutanea mediante isotopi radioattivi. Tecnica e risultati in 66 pazienti. Minverva Neurochir., 118-123 (1965).

WHITE, J.C., SWEET, W.H.: Pain. Its mechinsms and neurosurgical control. Springfield/Ill.: Charles C. Thomas 1955.

WHITE, J.C., SWEET, W.H., HAWKINS, R., NILGES, B.G.: Anterolateral cordotomy: results, complications and causes of failure. Brain <u>73</u>, 346-367 (1950).

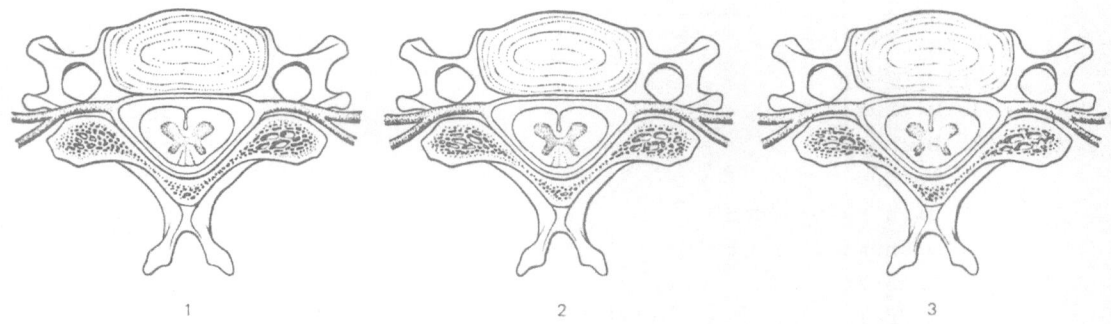

Fig. 1. Schematic drawing of the different approaches to the spinal cord. 1. MULLAN et al. 1963; 2. ALKSNE 1966; 3. CRUE et al. 1968

Pain Treatment of Advanced Malignant Diseases by High Cervical Percutaneous Cordotomy

W. Bettag, H. Wandt, and K. Roosen

The authors performed 73 high cervical percutaneous cordotomies on 55 patients, aged from 21 to 74 years. They all suffered from intractable pain caused by malignant tumors. Table 1 demonstrates the painful disorders.

Table 1. List of pain-causing malignant tumors

	Solitary Tumors	Metastasizing Tumors
A. Carcinomas		
1. uterus	2	13
2. breast	1	11
3. rectum	2	11
4. urinary bladder		2
5. bronchial tract		2
6. prostate		2
7. thyroid		1
8. testis		1
9. stomach		1
B. Other neoplasms		
10. sarcoma - lumbar vert. spine	1	
11. chondroma - lumbar vert. spine	1	
12. Hodgkin's disease		1
13. melanoblastoma		2
14. vertebral metastases of an unknown primary tumor		1
	7	48

This study is based upon the pre- and postoperative neurological check-ups, and on the results of answered questionnaires sent to the patients, the hospitals and the practitioners.

49 unilateral and 12 bilateral cordotomies were done in 41 cases on the right side of the neck and 32 times on the left side. The time in

between two operations on the same patient at the same level of the spinal cord between the first and the second cervical vertebra varied from 7 days to 6 months.

Because of intolerable pain during the spinal puncture, the operation had to be stopped in 5 cases, before the spino-thalamic tract could be coagulated.

Having visualized the denticulate ligaments, the anterolateral tract of the spinal cord is punctured under continuous measurement of the impedance. By electrical stimulation the intramedullary position of the needle can be determined; if necessary it is corrected according to the sensations described by the patient. Coagulation time is 15 seconds; at each cordotomy we perform two coagulations with 30 mV.

In Table 2 the proximal level of analgesia after cordotomy may be seen. Above that, the correlation between the area of the radiating pain and the postoperative neurological deficits. Through further experience, we may be able to reduce the area of analgesia and thermanaesthesia to those regions of the body the pain is radiating to. In 36 cordotomies we achieved analgesia in selected parts of the contralateral body half.

In 47 cases the neurological status was not changed except by the operative effect. Immediately after the operation all patients were without pain. 7 of them suffered from recurrent pain after a symptom-free period ranging from 12 hours up to 3 months. In 3 cases this

Table 2. Postoperative neurological status

Proximal analgetic segment	Patients
C1 - C3	27
below C^4	10
Th1	4
Th3	1
Th4	5
Th5	3
Th6	2
Th8	5
Th10	5
Th12	5
L1	6

Areas of pain	Complete hemianalgesia	Partial analgesia
shoulder-arm	21	-
thorax	4	2
abdomen + lumbar vertebral spine	3	9
sacrum	5	10
leg	4	15

phenomenon resulted from further growth of the neoplasm causing painful pressure on nervous structures above the line of analgesia. Four times this level sank because of the decreasing edema around the coagulation necrosis. This symptom was stated by 8 patients; the deficit of analgesia was about 3 to 6 segments. Recurrent pain made us to repeat the cordotomy in 7 cases.

Table 3 demonstrates the complications. The pareses improved through antiedematous therapy. The subarachnoid hemorrhage caused headaches and nuchal rigidity. Unfortunately it was not possible to single out the cause of the convulsions. A 63-years-old female patient was suffering from a carcinoma of the breast. Retrospectively it is very likely that there was an intracerebral metastasis causing the seizures. The urinary and fecal incontinence, once observed, did not improve.

Table 3. Complications

1. Pareses	4
ipsilateral, motor hemipareses	
2. Cysto- and proctoparalysis	1
3. Subarachnoid hemorrhage	1
4. Grand mal convulsions	2
a) intraoperative (1)	
b) 1st postop. day (1)	

A 59-year-old male patient had an extensive bronchial carcinoma. He died two days after cordotomy was performed. Cause of death: hypostatic pneumonia. It was not clear whether this complication resulted from the primary disease or from the cervical cordotomy causing a paralysis of the respiratory muscles.

The incidence of postoperative complaints is shown on Table 4. The cordotomy was regarded positively by 17 patients or relatives - at the time of our catamnestic inquiry 36 out of 55 patients had already died - and by 20 physicians.

8 patients objected to percutaneous cordotomy: 3 because of the painful operative procedure; five other patients did not observe a decisive relief of pain in spite of the fact that analgesia and thermanaesthesia could be proved by neurological examination. The answers which demonstrated the personal, clinical and psychological problems in describing and interpreting pain, have to be evaluated with special regard to the psychopathological background of the malignant diseases.

The possibility of an ambulant treatment and of a selective elimination of pain, the fact that this operative procedure can be tolerated by cachectic cancer patients, the relatively few risks, the prevention of an abuse of analgetics and the relief of pain during the final days of life are the decisive advantages of this method of pain treatment.

Table 4. Postoperative symptoms

1. Subjective complaints			
a) headaches	22	ca.	30%
b) giddiness	8		11%
c) nausea	14		19%
d) vomiting	4		6%
2. Abstinence symptoms after withdrawal of analgetics	12		16,5%
3. Burns because of thermanesthesia	5		7%
4. Paresthesias in the area of analgesia	4		6%

Experience with Percutaneous Cordotomy

W. Entzian and D. Linke

Since FOERSTER (1912) and SPILLER and MARTIN (1912) described and performed the section of the spino-thalamic tract (STT), this method had become a neurosurgical standard procedure in patients suffering from pain not treatable by other means. MULLAN (1965), ROSOMOFF (1965) and HITCHCOCK (1969), developed a simpler semi-stereotactic method, by which means the STT and the level of C 2/3 is encountered percutaneously with a needle and interrupted by thermocoagulation.

We shall describe our experience with this method which we applied 75 times in 62 patients since Sept. 1973.

Patients

Table 1 shows the indications for cordotomy with a predominance of patients with pain from malignant tumors. Patients with stump-neuralgia were treated after local surgical and orthopedic means had been performed exhaustively. One patient suffered from a stump neuralgia, two others from additional phantom pains. There was no patient treated who had described a phantom pain alone. Another group of patients had pain from cicatricial compression either of neural roots after spinal operation or traumatic transversal lesion or of peripheral nerve origin after traumatic lesions. Finally a 70-year-old lady describing a perineal pain was cordotomized unilaterally.

Method

Using an image intensifier, the spinal canal is tapped through a lateral puncture between C_1 and C_2. The denticulate ligament is demonstrated by positive contrast media and the spinal cord tapped ventrally under the control of impedance measurements. The usual stimulation of sensation allows the localisation of the tip of the needle in the spinothalamic tract, motoric stimulation is done to recognize the distance to the pyramidal tract. Thermocoagulation is performed with a radiofrequency of 30 mA and up to 60-120 sec in general until analgesia is achieved.

Results

The results are shown in the same Table 1. On an average the result was excellent or good in 80% of the patients; that means, the pain had disappeared completely or that there remained a negligible rest. These patients did not need further analgetic drugs. Approximately 10% of the cases described the pain to continue in a lesser degree than preoperatively, however, the result was considered just partial or even insufficient. Some patients needed analgetic drugs. In a final group of 10% of all the cases, no effect at all was achieved.

Concerning the localisation, approximately 20% of the patients suffered from pain in the region of arm and shoulder, approximately 80% described their pain in hip and leg. The result of the therapy seems to be equal for both groups. Sometimes it was possible to restrict the area of analgesia to the painful leg or arm respectively, though such an result cannot be predicted positively.

Table 1. Number and indications for percutaneous cordotomy. Definite relief on an average in 80% of the patients within 20 months observation time

75 Percutaneous cordotomies, 62 patients

Pain from	Relief		
	Definite	Partial	No
Malignant, unilat. tumor	39	2	2
— , bilat.	5	1	
[— , midline accent'd]	6	1	
Stump neuralgia	} 2 1	} 1	} 1
Phantom			
Radicular, neural (causalgia)	3	2	2
Perineal	—	—	1
Arm, shoulder	11	3	2
Leg, hip	39	3	3
62 Pat.:	~ 80%	~ 10%	~ 10%

Discussion

The reasons for inadequate effects of therapy seemed to be of a mechanical-technical nature in some cases, whereas in others neuroanatomical and local peculiarities impaired the operative procedure or the therapeutic result:

In four patients the first session was discontinued before the spinothalamic-tract (STT) was encountered. This occurred among the first 20 patients possibly because of beginning experience of the neurosurgeon. There was an unusual and unexplainable experience in two patients, in whom the stimulation of sensation through the STT was performed typically, however, thermocoagulation produced no analgesia at all.

Variations in the neuroanatomy is the reason for another experience: In 3 cases uncrossed fibers of the STT were encountered homolaterally at the typical site ventral to the denticulate ligament.

Patients reported a complete hemi-analgesia intraoperatively, however, they were found to have normal algesia and undiminished intensity of pain some hours later. Obviously the fibers of STT in some patients may run less narrowly bundled, what might be the reason for incomplete coagulation.

Late recurrences of remarkable intensity occurred after an interval of days or weeks in 9 patients (15%). There is no definite correlation between recurrence and decrease in primary analgesia, because numerous patients show partial return of algesia, but no recurrence. On the other hand we observed two patients complaining of pain localized in the joints of their arms though they had a complete analgesia of the skin of all the upper quadrant.

One complained of new pains contralaterally to operative hemianalgesia very shortly after the cordotomy. In this single case we did not feel that new metastases were the reason for the new pains, however, some phenomenon of pain-shifting had occurred.

Among the problems of laterality it is to be mentioned that in some cases after unilateral cordotomy the result is optimal because of unilateral dominating pain: the pain may vanish on both sides. This phenomenon may depend on the varying homolateral and contralateral supply of algesia and on the varying localisation of the analgetic boderline, which may run at some distance paramedian to the anatomical midline.

Because of immediate or late recurrence or because the STT was missed, a reoperation was done in 6 cases, most of these were performed successfully. In one patient an open thoracic cordotomy was added.

Obviously the result of the surgery on pain-conducting structures depends on the psychic situation of the patients. We feel, that among those patients with insufficient effects after percutaneous cordotomy there is a number who seemed to be noticeable concerning their reaction to their pain. However, no psycho-pathological studies were done on this problem.

The risks of the percutaneous cordotomy (Table 3) can be kept within small limits because of the chance of electrophysiological control intraoperatively:

Homolateral transient paresis was produced in five patients, a permanent one in no case.

After unilateral and after bilateral percutaneous cordotomy, micturition was disturbed - one patient in each group - because the feeling of intravesical pressure is missed. A similar disturbance of control of the bowel, however, of a lesser degree, was reported by one patient.

Patients very often complain of occipital neuralgia after percutaneous cordotomy, which is probably produced by the needle touching the C_2 root. In six patients (8% of operations) this complaint persisted long and intensively.

Three patients reported paraesthesia in the supplying region of the incompletely interrupted STT, however, the complaints were of moderate importance.

Burns or similar severe complications because of the loss of the protective function of analgesia have not been reported by any patient yet, though a number of physically active patients are observed. It should be mentioned, that even intelligent patients though informed pre- and postoperatively, need the experience of the hot bath before realizing the loss of analgesia and thermesthesia.

Table 2. Problems during the procedure of percutaneous cordotomy and recurrence incidence. The difficulty of encountering the spino-thalamic tract stands in the foreground

75 Percutaneous cordotomies, 62 patients

	Pat.
I. Mechan., technical problems	
1. Spino-thal. tract not encountered	4
2. Tract - stimulated, not coagulable	2
II.Physio., anatomic. problems	
3. Homolat. stimulation (localisation) of spi.-thal. tr.	3
4. 1st session without effect (immediate)	3
5. 2nd session without effect (immediate)	1
6. Late recurrence	9
7. Pain shifting	1
8. Reoperation performed	6

Table 3. Percutaneous cordotomy, operation risks

75 Percutaneous cordotomies, 62 patients

III. Op.-Risks	Pat.
1. Homolat. hemiparesis, transient	5
2. - - , permanent	O
3. Cystoplegia, unilat. P. Ch. (Sens)	1
4. - , bilat. P. Ch.	1
5. Potency deficit, unilat. P. Ch.	1
6. Defecat. deficit, unilat. P. Ch.	1
7. Burns	O
8. Occip. neuralgia, permanent	7
9. Parasthesia	3
10. Mortality (1st, 2nd, 8th postop. day)	3

The known phenomenon of hypotonia after bilateral percutaneous cordotomy was observed just once - in a patient with traumatic paraplegia.

The mortality within the first 8 days reveals a relatively small number of 3 patients, i.e. 4% among 75 cordotomies. The first patient, being in very bad condition, developed a circulation collapse intra-operatively and died 20 hours later. The second patient probably died from pulmonary metastatic complications. The third patient was in very good condition and died suddenly at home eight days after the second session of a bilateral percutaneous cordotomy. Unfortunately no autopsy could be done.

Results and summary

Percutaneous cordotomy was proven to be a useful routine method for the therapy of severe pain caused by malignant tumors and otherwise untreatable radicular or neural neuralgia. Until now no patient has been treated exclusively because of phantom pain or causalgia. However, there seems to be a reasonable indication for patients with combined stump neuralgia and phantom pain.

Unilateral and bilateral percutaneous cordotomy is followed by a moderate mortality (4%), and the burden of typical complications such as homolateral paresis and functional disturbances of bowel and bladder is smaller than in open thoracic or cervical cordotomy. Additionally, the operative stress and the length of hospital care have been reduced markedly.

For these reasons there are very few limitations for the indication of percutaneous cordotomy concerning the patients' age or general condition. Even as far as the underlying disease is concerned, the indication for percutaneous cordotomy might be put on a larger scale.

Potentials and Limits of Percutaneous Cervical Cordotomy

R. MÜKE and A. CORREIA

Without doubt percutaneous cordotomy represents a certain improvement
in the possibilities of pain surgery. Of course there are limits to
it, due to its very nature.

The critical evaluation of percutaneous cervical cordotomy has to be
based on two parameters: what are the advantages, and, on the other
hand, are there disadvantages as compared to open cordotomy.

Results

From 1971 to 1975, 226 percutaneous cervical cordotomies were performed on 178 patients in our department in Hamburg. Out of these,
24 were done on both sides and 21 had to be repeated once. In 75% of
the patients the procedure was required for malignant disease, 25%
of the patients suffered from pain due to benign origin. A great number of the patients complained of severe pain in the upper half of
the body (tumors of the lung, carcinoma of the breast etc.).

Elimination of pain in the intended area was achieved in 159 out of
the 178 patients, equalling 89,3%; 12 or 6,5% improved. In 7 patients
or 3,9% the method failed.

The following complications were observed:

4 fatal outcomes in connection with cordotomy, that is 2,2%.

6 further fatal outcomes, due to the underlying disease while the
patients were still hospitalized.

7 respiratory difficulties, 4 of which were severe, requiring artificial respiration.

5 persistent pareses of 2,8%, of which 2 were severe, one of medium severity and two minor ones, consisting of impaired gross
power.

In 27 further cases we observed transient impaired motility of one
or only a few days duration.

The urinary bladder was permanently affected in 5 patients or 2,8%;
transient bladder disturbances were observed in 10 patients.

As can be expected, the rate of complications decreased with increasing experience and methodological improvement. In *1971*, the first
year in which percutaneous cervical cordotomy was performed in our
department, we had to cope with 3 fatal outcomes in the 17 patients
we operated on. They were due to respiratory difficulties. Moreover,
we observed 3 persistent pareses and one persistent urinary bladder

disturbance. At that time we were not yet able to measure electrical resistance and to perform electrical stimulation. However, during *1974 and 1975* there were no casualties and no persistent pareses in 73 patients operated on, although a number of those were in very bad general condition due to far advanced carcinomas. In the latter cases we almost certainly would have abstained from open cordotomy.

We want to point out, that the burden to be taken by the patient is comparatively small in percutaneous cervical cordotomy. From 1973 onward we timed the operation. In 152 cordotomies on 122 patients a mean of 39 minutes was recorded. During only a few minutes of those 39 the patients experience some discomfort; that is during local anaesthesia, during the needle puncture through dura and pia and during the actual coagulation. Moreover, there were no minor complications following cordotomy, like disturbances in wound healing, pains from the wound etc. Usually, the patients were able to ambulate the following day and we did not observe any problems such as pneumonia, thrombosis or embolic phenomena. Once there was urinary tract infection, once asthma occurred and in five more patients the course following operation was impaired by the advanced underlying disease. Only once in 152 cordotomies did hypotension result following the operation. In one-fifth of these cases there were mild headaches for about one to three days, due to spinal tap and air insufflation. In 25 cases we observed very mild transient ataxia, not preventing early mobilization at all. In half the cases, an incomplete HORNER syndrome developed which often vanished already during the time of hospitalization and remained almost unrecognized by the patients themselves.

The time of hospitalization for percutaneous cordotomy is very short; it is even shorter than demonstrated by our figures since many of the patients had to stay on the ward longer than necessary due to social or organizational reasons. Our figures show a distinct decrease from a mean of 13,8 days hospitalization time in 1971 to 4 days in 1975. We never operate on out-patients. In high unilateral or bilateral cordotomies we even believe this practice to be dangerous.

Due to its very nature, percutaneous cervical cordotomy is not apt to result in less relapses than open cordotomy. The only question is, whether the number of relapses is increased. We had the impression, that in most patients with pain from malignant disease this pain was eliminated until they died. Unfortunately we are not able to produce exact figures of all our patients due to lack of cooperation of the patients' relatives.

28 out of the 41 patients with pain from benign disease could be reexamined or they answered our questionnaire. Of these we accounted for 15 relapses, equal to 53% and for 13 without relapse, equal to 47%. 7 out of the 15 patients having relapsed were still analgetic in the initially intended area as checked by pin prick. In 3 patients the level of analgesia had dropped and in 5 we do not have the result of reexamination but only the questionnaire. 3 patients or 10,7% had painful dysaesthesia after cordotomy; they belong to those with relapses. Dysaesthesias of some other variety, like itching, irritability and sensation of warmth were seen in 8 patients; they were either transient or described as very mild and insignificant. Out of the patients without relapses 4 reported with mild dysaesthesia. Interestingly enough, all relapses occurred within the first 5 months following operation, while all patients without relapses are free from pain, partly for years (3,6 years - 1,9 - 0,5 - 0,6 - 1,5 - 1,6 - 2,9 - 2,9 - 2,1 - 2,2 - 1,5 and 6 weeks).

Discussion

The paramount advantage of the percutaneous versus the open cordotomy is the decreased stress for the patient. The rate of pain elimination is at least equally high (89,3% in addition 6,7% improvement), complications are less on the average (2,8% persistent pareses, 2,8% persistent urinary bladder disturbances). Another advantage of percutaneous cervical cordotomy lies in the certainty of rendering the patient painless up to very high cervical segments. In about 90% we achieved the analgetic effect desired. Pains in the shoulder-arm area are treated successfully as well. A segmentally limited cordotomy, for instance analgesia of isolated thoracic or cervical dermatomes, has in our hands proven to be impossible in most cases and does not seem advisable due to the higher rate of recurrences.

Because of decreased time of hospitalization a more effective utilization of hospital beds can be expected. With the same capacity more patients can be operated on.

The method of percutaneous cordotomy is easy to perform and has the advantage of equally simple re-operation if required: In 21 patients this re-operation was successfully performed.

As compared to open cordotomy there is a disadvantage: percutaneous cordotomy cannot be performed on both sides in one session. On the other hand, we often achieve very effective diminution of the pain, which often is more severe one one side than the other, by cordotomy on one side only. Thus, waiting for the second operation is not at all as troublesome as one might think. Besides, if the patients are operated on in two sessions, complications, especially urinary bladder disturbances, are less common.

It is not our opinion to disapprove of double percutaneous cordotomy on principle. There were 4 fatal outcomes in the first year where we performed this operation. However, in the following 20 percutaneous cordotomies on both sides there was not one casualty. This may be due to an interval between operations of 3 to 4 weeks, to a better electrode position with electrical stimulation and to abstaining from bilateral high cervical analgesia levels.

One might argue, that relapses are more frequent after coagulation of the nerve tracts than after surgical separation, since the lesion in a percutaneous coagulation cannot be seen and is only estimated by its effect; and this effect might be transitory due to the heat of coagulation and the developing edema. However, comparing our results and those in the literature, quoting particularly for open cordotomy the experiences of WHITE and SWEET, there are apparently no substantial differences in the relapses after open versus percutaneous cordotomy.

As an absolute figure, relapses are high if viewed on a long term basis. This, however, is the case in all operations aimed at rendering a patient painless. Therefore one has to remain very critical of a pain-eliminating operation for pain syndromes of benign origin. This is not at all a novelty, it has been proclaimed over and over again.

In these benign cases we had expected a positive effect from transcutaneous or dorsal column stimulation. Unfortunately these methods did let us down in about one-half of the cases. We are not attempting anything new, demanding special attention to the psychological situa-

tion of the patient with pain of benign origin, before any pain eliminating operation is taken into consideration.

Summary

The potentials and limits of percutaneous cervical cordotomy are discussed in this paper. It is based on 226 cordotomies in 178 patients,
which were performed from 1971 to 1975. Complete pain elimination
was achieved in 89,3%; mortality was 2,2%; there were 2,8% persistent
pareses and 2,8% persistent urinary bladder disturbances. Relapses
were about equal to those following open cordotomy. The burden to be
taken by the patient is considerably smaller in percutaneous than in
open cordotomy; hospitalization following the percutaneous procedure
was remarkably shorter.

Neurophysiological Models for Nociception, Pain, and Pain Therapy

M. ZIMMERMANN

Already in 1943 MARTINI, GUALTIEROTTI and MARZORATI (18) observed an
anesthetic effect of repetitive electrical current application to the
cat's spinal cord. There has been renewed interest in this phenomenon
recently, when electrical stimulation of the spinal cord (e.g. the
dorsal columns) and of peripheral nerves was used in man for the relief
from chronic pain (c.f. the clinical reports to this meeting). What
is the neurophysiological basis of this beneficial therapeutic method?

Unfortunately, unlike in other sensory systems in the realm of pain,
a coherent neurophysiological description has not been established as
yet. There is still much debate about the fundamentals of a theory of
pain perception (e.g. see the controversy about the gate control hypothesis (19, 29, 4, 10, 20)). This should be kept in mind when reading
the following statements, summarizing some recent findings of experimental neurophysiology, which possibly might be related to electroanalgesia or to hypalgesia in man.

1. Nociceptors as Encoders for Pain Stimuli, and Peripheral Effects of Electrical Nerve Stimulation

Nociceptors

There is much evidence that in the periphery, noxious stimuli are
transmitted via the activation of specific receptors, which have a
high threshold of excitation, e.g. by mechanical or/and thermal stimuli (1, 2, 3). These nociceptors have non-myelinated (C, or Group IV)
or small myelinated (Aδ, or III) afferent fibers. Recently, recordings have been made in man of single C-fibers, which did not respond
to skin stimuli unless these had a painful intensity (14, 27).

An example of a heat nociceptor, the cat's foot is shown in Fig. 1.
In this experiment we recorded from single C-fibers separated by mi-
crodissection from the nerve to the foot. The high correlation (Fig.
1B) between discharge frequency and skin temperature during the heating by thermal radiation provides information conveyed in these afferents on the intensity of the noxious stimulus. About 30% of the
afferent C-fibers from the foot belong to this population of nociceptors. Behavioural and electrophysiological findings suggest that
there are virtually no sensitive warm receptors in the cat's hind
foot. Therefore noxious radiant heat to the foot might be considered
as a rather selectively noxious stimulus, thus providing a favourable
condition for studies in the central nervous system on nociception
(see Figs. 3 and 4).

Peripheral Effects of Electrical Nerve Stimulation

It has been suggested that the pain relief achieved by electrical
stimulation of nerve trunks might be, at least in part, a peripheral
interference with nociceptive afferents. This was found when studying
experimental neuromas in rats (28). Ongoing discharges initiated within the neuroma were observed in small myelinated afferents (III-
fibers). Repetitive electrical stimulation of these fibers silenced
the spontaneous discharges, this intermission outlasting the period
of stimulation by several minutes (Fig. 2). The silencing is claimed
to be due to changes effected by the antidromic action potentials in
the pathological generator region of the sprouting nerve endings.
The mechanism might be an electrogenic ion transport as will be described in the text on Fig. 6.

The association of this finding with pain relief in man is, however,
complicated by the dilemma that high frequency stimulation of the
presumably pain-producing afferents is required to silence them for
a while. Thus, the electrical stimulus itself might be painful. In
spite of this obvious difficulty, research should be continued along
this line, to clarify more quantitatively the effects of electrical
currents on nociceptive afferents, including the C-fibers.

On the other hand a peripheral interference of the kind suggested
above must be excluded in the case of dorsal column stimulation (DCS),
which excites the collaterals of large myelinated (I- and II-) afferents only, coming from sensitive mechanoreceptors. Nociceptive fibers
are absent in the dorsal columns, and therefore cannot be stimulated
antidromically by DCS.

2. Inhibitory Actions in the Spinal Cord

Types of Spinal Neurons Responding to Noxious Stimuli

In the spinal cord two basic types of neurons have been found onto
which the afferent fibers from cutaneous nociceptors terminate:

a. Units in the marginal layer of the grey matter of the dorsal horn
   respond *specifically* to various types of noxious stimuli (7),
   which are transmitted via III- and C-afferents. They have been
   identified histologically as the large WALDEYER cells; it is estimated that this population consists of less than 1% of dorsal horn
   neurons. Some of them project to the anterolateral tract. Thus far
   no experiments have been made on whether inhibitory influences
   upon these neurons are exerted by stimulation of the dorsal columns or of peripheral nerves.

b. *Polymodal neurons* which are excited by both noxious and non-noxious
   skin stimuli. These polymodal units constitute the bulk (70%) of
   neurons encountered in our systematic microelectrode penetrations
   of the dorsal horn (9, 12). They have excitatory convergence of
   afferents ($A\beta$ or II) from low threshold cutaneous mechanoreceptors,
   and of afferents from nociceptors ($A\delta$ or III, and C or IV). Some
   of them have an axon ascending in the anterolateral tract, or in
   the spino-cervico-lemniscal pathway. We used radiant heat to the
   skin as a selective noxious stimulus to excite these neurons (Fig.
   3A), and to demonstrate inhibitory influences upon them, as will
   be shown in the subsequent paragraph. Part of these polymodal
   units exhibit convergence of somatic and of visceral afferents
   (24), and mutual inhibition of these two inputs (25). These neurophysiological findings might be of relevance for the phenomena, in
   man, of referred pain and of somato-viscero counter-irritation.

In other brain regions, which are assumed to be important for pain (13), it is still not clear whether neurons exist which have an exclusively nociceptive input. Recently it has been claimed that all the information on noxious stimuli appears in polymodal units (21). Therefore, the polymodal dorsal horn neurons might be neurophysiological models for the processing of pain messages in higher brain centers.

Inhibition of Spinal Neurons by Electrical Stimulation

In Fig. 3A the discharge of a polymodal neuron of segment L_1 is shown during noxious heating of the skin. The response is suppressed or even abolished by electrical stimulation of the dorsal columns at L_2, depending on the frequency of the DCS. The dorsal columns consist of the ascending collaterals of large myelinated afferent fibers, therefore many of the II-afferents of cutaneous nerves are excited antidromically by DCS. In most of our polymodal neurons these afferent impulses will eventually set up excitation; however, particularly at higher frequencies of DCS (e.g. 50 Hz) the competing inhibitory influence prevails over the excitation. Similar inhibitions were found during electrical stimulation of the II-fibers in the plantar nerves, which innervate the heated skin region. The inhibition observed might have pre- or/and postsynaptic components; it never outlasted the period of DCS or nerve stimulation by more than about 100 msec.

Supraspinal Inhibitory Control of Spinal Neurons

An inhibitory control of supraspinal origin was revealed by locally cooling the spinal cord at L_1 (Fig. 4A). By this procedure axonal conduction was blocked reversibly, thus releasing the spinal neurons from any descending influences. In Fig. 4B, C, the modification of the responsiveness to noxious heat is shown in two polymodal units. When the cord was blocked reversibly, both units responded vigorously to the noxious stimulus. The response to an identical stimulus was reduced (Fig. 4B) or completely suppressed (4C) after the withdrawal of the cold block of the descending pathways, thus indicating a tonic inhibitory influence by the supramedullary CNS.

There are various regions in the brain which are known to modulate spinal neurons. Recently electrical stimulation in the periaqueductal grey matter in the midbrain has been reported to yield a powerful analgesia, which at least in part might be due to descending inhibition in dorsal horn cells (22).

Thus the inhibition of spinal neurons during DCS might have 3 components: a. segmental, b. ascending activation of suprasegmental descending systems, c. direct stimulation of descending tracts. There are hints that the inhibition of nociceptive neuronal responses also occurs in other brain regions. The neurophysiological findings reported here therefore might be regarded as models of inhibitory effects upon nerve and dorsal column stimulation.

3. Other Potential Mechanisms Contributing to Pain Relief

Pain relief in man by DCS and nerve stimulation has been reported to outlast the stimulation period often by minutes or even hours. On the other hand, the synaptic inhibitions evoked by a stimulus in the CNS do not last for longer than about 100 msec beyond that stimulus.

Therefore we have to ask for other neuronal interactions, having longer time courses. In the subsequent paragraphs we will speculatively discuss two mechanisms, which might also be involved in pain phenomena.

Long-term Changes in Synaptic Connectivity

Evidence is accumulating rapidly now that in the CNS, plastic changes do occur (e.g. 11). Two main mechanisms are thought to contribute to this plasticity: a. sprouting of new terminals, which eventually form synaptic connections to other neurons; b. alterations in the efficiency of a synapse.

Apart from their normal role in the developing and mature nervous system (e.g. in learning), both mechanisms are probably involved in the restitution of function after lesions or other pathological alterations in the nervous system.

For example, partial denervation of the spinal cord will induce collateral sprouting of the persisting terminals (8), and denervation supersensitivity, a phenomenon particularly well-investigated in neuromuscular junctions and in the autonomic nervous system (5, 26): the postsynaptic region develops an increased sensitivity to its transmitter when all or part of the presynaptic terminals degenerate (Fig. 5).

On the other hand, morphologically existing synapses might be functionally ineffective. Such ineffective synapses could be turned on when other synapses on the same neuron are silenced by losing their normal synaptic drive, e.g. after a lesion of the afferents. Examples have been reported of such turning-off and on (repression and depression) of neuromuscular synapses during competitive innervation of a muscle by different motor nerves (6). Some or all of these mechanisms might be involved in the enhanced responsiveness of central neurons after deafferentation (Fig. 5): following such manipulations an increase in firing frequency to a stimulus, or an increased spontaneous discharge have been observed (15, 16).

It is very tempting to hypothesize that some states of chronic pain have to do with denervation supersensitivity, or with depression of synapses, e.g.: thalamic pain; aggravation of pain following temporary relief by a cordotomy; persistence of phantom limb pain after dorsal rhizotomy; dermatome border hyperalgesia after dorsal rhizotomy. Could electrical stimulation interfere with such pathological enhancement of synaptic connectivity? Experiments on the model synapse, the neuromuscular junction, indeed revealed, that both supersensitivity and the turning-on of ineffective synapses could be prevented by electrical stimulation of the silent presynaptic afferents, or even of the postsynaptic elements (17). Thus far, however, experimental evidence is rather indirect that such synaptic plasticity could be involved in pain. Experiments using quantifiable noxious stimuli should be performed to test this hypothesis.

Effects on Neuronal Metabolism

It is well known that longlasting repetitive stimulation gives rise to a pronounced hyperpolarization of neurons, or of nerve fibers, by which they are rendered less excitable. This hyperpolarization is produced by the active transport of Na^+ ions out of the cells; since there is a surplus positive charge transfer in the outward direction by this Na^+ transport, it is called an electrogenic pump. As a consequence, the membrane hyperpolarizes, decreasing the neurons' excitability to the synaptic drive, and the probability of spontaneous discharges.

The details of this electrogenic transport of Na^+ ions subsequent to stimulation have been studied particularly in non-myelinated or C-fibers (23), which might be considered as a model for central neurons in this respect. A feature which might be of importance in the context of pain is shown in Fig. 6. In Fig. 6A several records of hyperpolarizations are superimposed after stimulations at increasing durations. The hyperpolarizations last several minutes, and the time constant of recovery increases in proportion to the duration of the stimulus train (Fig. 6B).

Such a process could well contribute to a longlasting decrease in responsiveness to noxious stimuli. Any means of repetitive stimulation of the neuron (direct, by antidromic invasion from the axon, or transsynaptic) would be good to initiate the hyperpolarization. In addition, it was observed that an increase in extracellular K^+ concentration will activate the electrogenic Na^+ pump; thus it should be expected that even K^+ release induced by the stimulation of neighbouring cells could yield some hyperpolarization.

Direct neurophysiological tests for a potential role of postsynaptic hyperpolarization by an electrogenic Na^+ pump on nociceptive responses in central neurons have not yet been performed. Therefore the hypothesis stressed above must be considered as highly speculative.

4. Concluding Remarks

The term "pain" is used for a great variety of sensations, ranging from those evoked by well-defined stimuli under laboratory conditions to the excruciating chronic pain of the thalamic syndrome. It would be a comparable situation if we used the expression "brightness" to subsume all our sensations in the visual system. Thus semantic problem will arise when asking for *the* neurophysiological correlates of pain, since obviously these might be different for different types of pain.

Therefore our experimental search for the neuronal basis of pain should be restricted to specified situations of experimental stimuli or of distinct pathological disorders, instead of comparing incommensurable subjects. In order to succeed in this task, neurobiologists and clinicians should come to a serious cooperation: the clinicians to demonstrate intricately the various pain syndromes, enabling the physiologists to develop and to study experimental models of certain pain situations, which, in turn, could provide results to yield new therapies.

Summary

Four mechanisms are discussed as potential neuronal correlates of the phenomenon of pain relief by electrical stimulation of afferent nerves or the dorsal columns:

1. Suppression of ongoing discharges initiated in peripheral endings of regenerating nociceptive afferents

2. Pre- or postsynaptic inhibition of spinal neurons involved in the processing of noxious stimuli

3. Repression of denervation supersensitivity of neurons in the CNS

4. Longlasting hyperpolarization by postexcitatory active transport of ions

Acknowledgements. Our investigations have been supported by the Deutsche Forschungsgemeinschaft. The help in bibliographic work and the typing of the manuscript by Mrs. U. Nothoff is gratefully acknowledged.

REFERENCES

1. BECK, P.W., HANDWERKER, H.O., ZIMMERMANN, M.: Nervous outflow from the cat's foot during noxious radiant heat stimulation. Brain Res. 67, 373-386 (1974).

2. BESSOU, P., PERL, E.R.: Response of cutaneous sensory units with unmyelinated fibers to noxious stimuli. J. Neurophysiol. 32, 1025-1043 (1969).

3. BURGESS, E.R., PERL, E.R.: Myelinated afferent fibres responding specifically to noxious stimulation of the skin. J. Physiol. 190, 541-562 (1967).

4. BURKE, R.E., RUDOMIN, P., VYCKLICKY, L., ZAJAC III, F.E.: Primary afferent depolarization and flexion reflexes produced by radiant heat stimulation of the skin. J. Physiol. 213, 185-214 (1971).

5. CANNON, W.B., ROSENBLUETH, A.: The supersensitivity of denervated structures. New York: MacMillan 1949.

6. CASS, D.T., SUTTON, T.J., MARK, R.F.: Competition between nerves for functional connexions with Axolotl muscles. Nature 243, 201-203 (1973).

7. CHRISTENSEN, B.N., PERL, E.R.: Spinal neurons specifically excited by noxious or thermal stimuli: marginal zone of the dorsal horn. J. Neurophysiol. 33, 293-307 (1970).

8. GOLDBERGER, M.E., MURRAY, M.: Restitution of function and collateral sprouting in the cat spinal cord: the de-afferented animal. J. Comp. Neurol. 158, 37-54 (1974).

9. GREGOR, M., ZIMMERMANN, M.: Characteristics of spinal neurones responding to cutaneous myelinated and unmyelinated fibres. J. Physiol. 221, 555-576 (1972).

10. GREGOR, M., ZIMMERMANN, M.: Dorsal root potentials produced by afferent volleys in cutaneous Group III fibres. J. Physiol. 232, 413-425 (1973).

11. GUTH, L.: Axonal regeneration and functional plasticity in the central nervous system. Exp. Neurol. 45, 606-654 (1974).

12. HANDWERKER, H.O., IGGO, A., ZIMMERMANN, M.: Segmental and supraspinal actions on dorsal horn neurons responding to nocuous and non-nocuous skin stimuli. Pain 1, (in press).

13. HASSLER, R.: Die zentralen Systeme des Schmerzes. Acta Neurochirurgica, Vol. 7, 354-423 (1960).

14. HEES, J. VAN, GYBELS, J.M.: Pain related to single afferent C fibers from human skin. Brain Res. 48, 397-400 (1972).

15. KJERULF, T.D., LOESER, J.D.: Neuronal hyperactivity following deafferentation of the lateral cuneate nucleus. Exp. Neurol. 39, 70-85 (1973).

16. LOESER, J.D., WARD, A.A., Jr.: Some effects of deafferentation on neurons of the cat spinal cord. Arch. Neurol. _17_, 629-636 (1967).

17. LØMO, T., ROSENTHAL, J.: Control of ACh sensitivity by muscle activity in the rat. J. Physiol. _221_, 493-513 (1972).

18. MARTINI, E., GUALTIEROTTI, T., MARZORATI, A.: Die Rückenmarkelektronarkose. Pflügers Arch. ges. Physiol. _246_, 585-596 (1943).

19. MELZACK, R., WALL, P.D.: Pain mechanisms: A new theory. Science _150_, 971-979 (1965).

20. NATHAN, P.W., RUDGE, P.: Testing the gate-control theory of pain in man. J. Neurol. Neurosurg. Psychiat. _37_, 1366-1372 (1974).

21. NYQUIST, J.K., GREENHOOT, J.H.: A single neuron analysis of mesencephalic reticular formation responses to high intensity cutaneous input in cat. Brain Res. _70_, 157-164 (1974).

22. OLIVERAS, J.L., BESSON, J.M., GUILBAUD, G., LIEBESKIND, J.C.: Behavioral and electrophysiological evidence of pain inhibition from midbrain stimulation in the cat. Exp. Brain Res. _20_, 32-44 (1974).

23. RANG, H.P., RITCHIE, J.M.: On the electrogenic sodium pump in mammalian non-myelinated nerve fibres and its activation by various external cations. J. Physiol. _196_, 183-221 (1968).

24. SELZER, M., SPENCER, W.A.: Convergence of visceral and cutaneous afferent pathways in the lumbar spinal cord. Brain Res. _14_, 331-348 (1969).

25. SELZER, M., SPENCER, W.A.: Interactions between visceral and cutaneous afferents in the spinal cord: reciprocal primary afferent fibre depolarization. Brain Res. _14_, 349-366 (1969).

26. STAVRAKY, G.W.: Supersensitivity following lesions of the nervous system. Toronto: Univ. of Toronto Press 1961.

27. TOREBJÖRK, H.E., HALLIN, R.G.: Identification of the afferent C units in intact human skin nerves. Brain Res. _67_, 387-404 (1974).

28. WALL, P.D., GUTNICK, M.: Properties of afferent nerve impulses originating from a neuroma. Nature _248_, 740-743 (1974).

29. ZIMMERMANN, M.: Dorsal root potentials after C-fiber stimulation. Science _160_, 896-898 (1968).

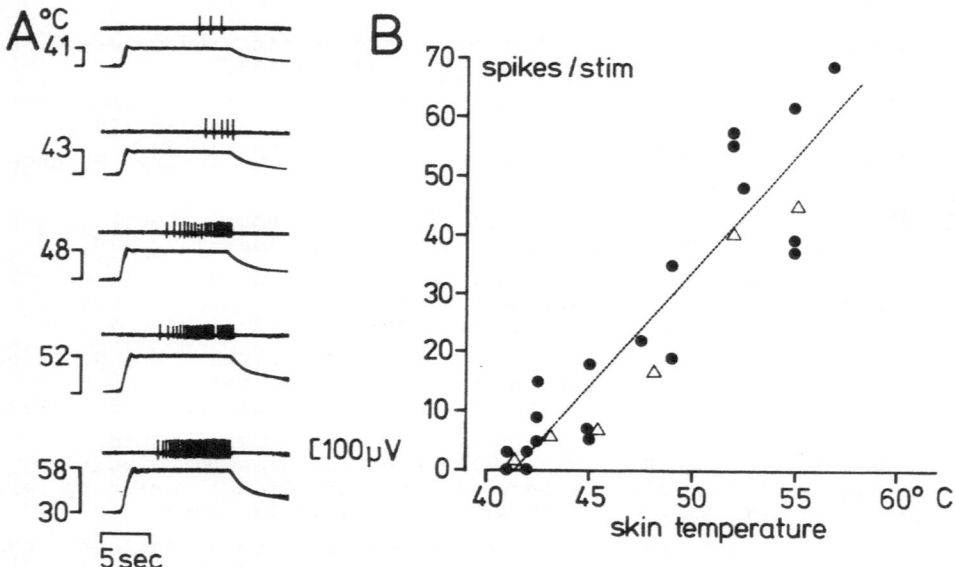

fibre 2572 - C14

Fig. 1. Discharges of a "C-heat-receptor" in the cat's footpad at different skin temperatures. A: Nerve impulses (upper traces) during 10 sec heating; time course of temperature recorded with a thermocouple (lower traces). B: Total number of impulses per stimulus (•) plotted versus skin temperature. Receptor located in hairy skin of second toe. Conduction velocity of fiber 0.6 m/sec. From (1)

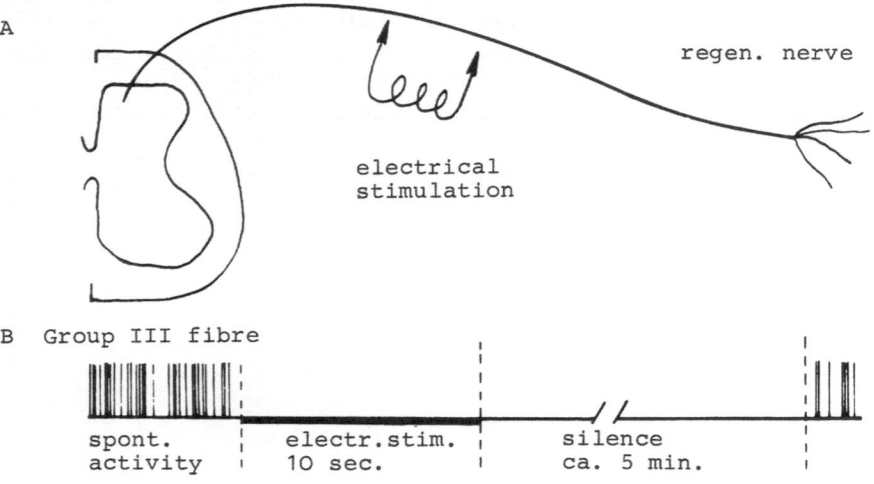

Fig. 2. Effect of electrical nerve stimulation (arrangement shown in A) on spontaneous discharges from regenerating nerve sprouts in an experimental neuroma (schematic). B: Ongoing discharge in a Group III-fiber is silenced for several minutes after a 10 sec train (100 Hz) of electrical nerve stimulation. According to (28)

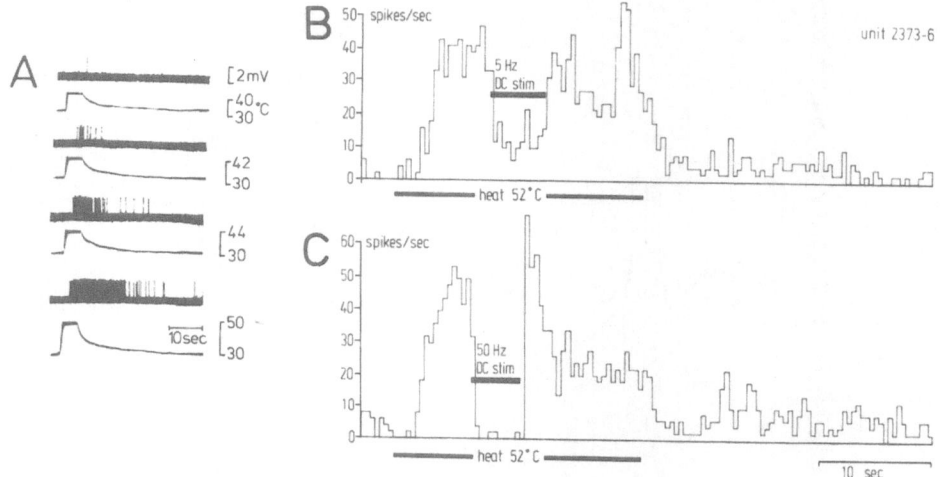

Fig. 3. Responses in polymodal dorsal horn neurons of the cat upon
noxious heat stimulation of the foot skin. A: Impulses (upper traces)
evoked by heating the skin to various temperatures (lower traces).
B: Time course of discharge frequency of another unit during heating
of the skin to 52°C, and concurrent dorsal column stimulation at 5
Hz. C: Same unit as in B, dorsal column stimulation, however, at 50
Hz. Animal was anesthetized with pentobarbital-Na; spinal cord tran-
sected at L_1 level. From (12)

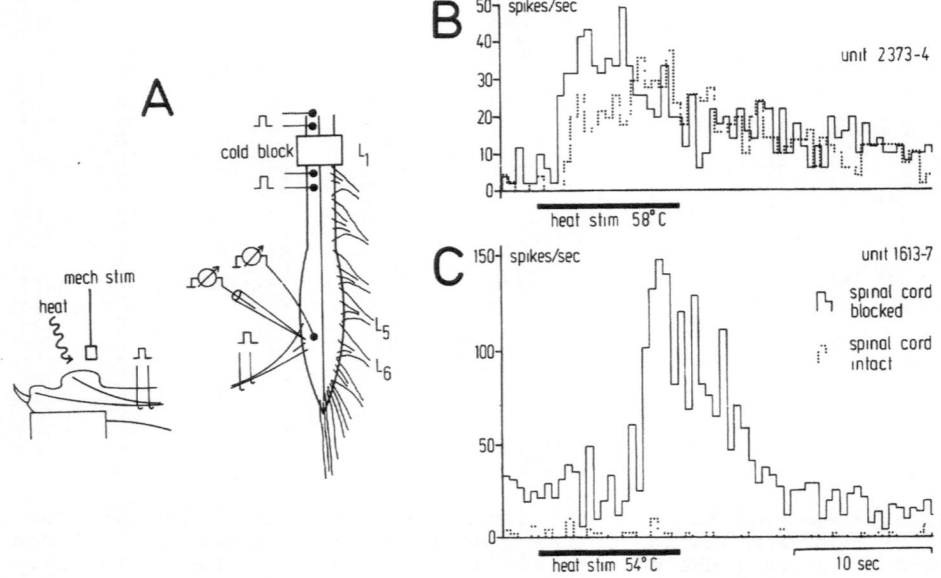

Fig. 4. Effect on dorsal horn neurons of cold block of the spinal cord. A: Schematic diagram of sites of electrical and adequate stimuli, of recording electrodes on and in spinal cord, and of thermode for local cold block of the spinal cord. B: Effect of cold block on the discharge induced in a polymodal dorsal horn neuron by heating the foot skin to 58°C. Time course of discharge frequency when cord is blocked at L_1 (solid line histogram), and with cord intact (dotted line histogram). C: Same procedure as in B, different unit in another animal. Pentobarbital-Na anesthesia. From (12)

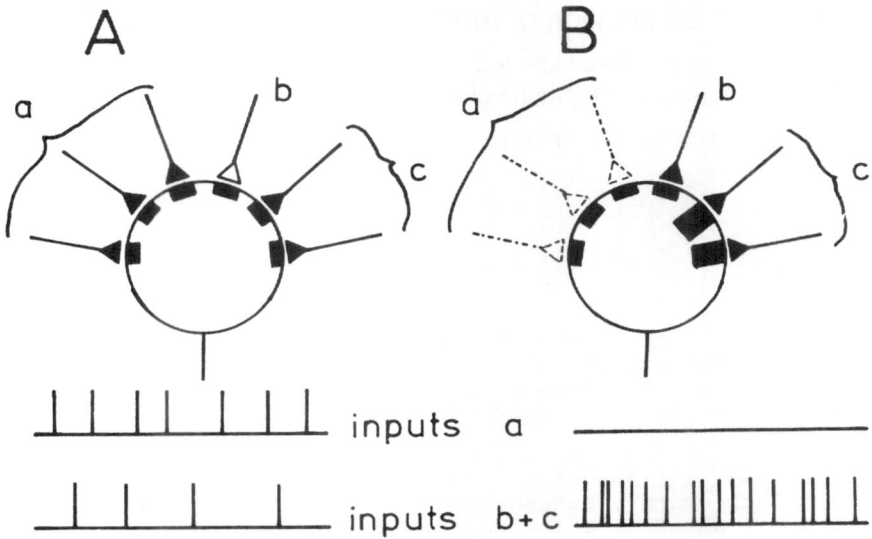

Fig. 5. Effect of denervation on responsiveness of neurons. A: Schematic hypothetical neuron with 5 normal synapses (a, c) and one functionally ineffective synapse (b). Below, the hypothetical normal responses of the neuron are shown to a standard stimulation of either inputs a or b+c. B: Same neuron as in A, however the afferents a have either become silent by peripheral interruption, or have degenerated. Synapse of afferent b is indicated to be derepressed, and those of afferents c to be supersensitive. The discharge of a neuron upon the standard stimulus to b+c is enhanced, as is indicated below

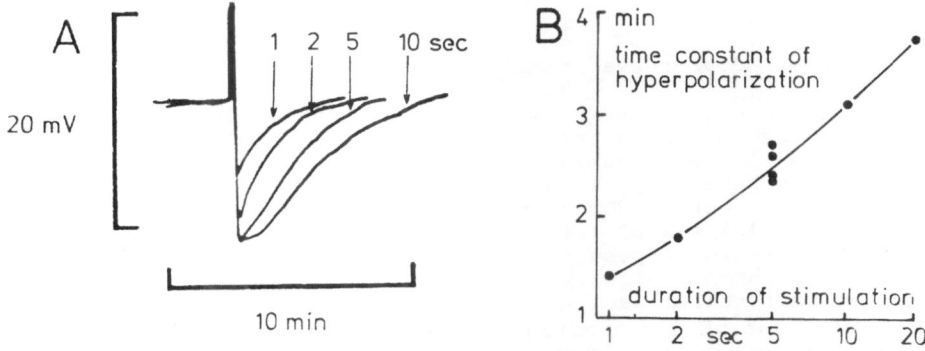

Fig. 6. Poststimulation hyperpolarization by electrogenic active transport. A: Time course of hyperpolarization in non-myelinated nerve fibers after repetitive stimulation (30 Hz) at 4 different durations. B: Relation between duration of stimulation and the time constant of recovery of hyperpolarization recorded under slightly different conditions than in A. From (23)

Electrical Stimulation of the Spinal Cord for the Relief of Pain*

Method – Patient Selection and Clinical Results (Based on the Results of the Freiburger „Arbeitsgespräche über elektrische Schmerzhemmung", October 1974)

J.-U. KRAINICK and U. THODEN

The first description of electrical pain therapy was given by the Roman physician SCRIBONIUS LARGUS (9) in 47 B.C., who gave a report on a man who happened to get in contact with an electric torpedo fish with resulting pain relief in his arthrotic knee.

During the Middle Ages, the application of this electrical stimulation was recommended for various diseases and pain etiologies. In the 17th century acupuncture was already known in all details in Europe. SALANDIÈRE (8) published a book recommending a combination of the original needle acupuncture with the application of electrical current for treatment of pain. During the 18th century there was an increasing interest in the application of electrical currents for cure purposes with a development of electrostatic pulse generators. At the beginning of the 20th century this interest in electrical stimulation diminished due to the rapid development of pain controlling drugs in the pharmaceutical industries.

Since MELZACK and WALL (4) published their gate control theory as a new concept of pain in 1965, various electrical stimulation methods to control pain have been clinically evaluated. All methods were aimed at the stimulation of large rapidly-conducting afferent fibers to inhibit the transmission of pain stimuli in the small A-Delta and C-fibers. Besides the non-invasive transcutaneous stimulation of peripheral nerves (TNS), SWEET and WEPSIC (13) implanted electrodes on peripheral nerves and later SHEALLY (10) on the dorsal columns of the spinal cord.

Transcutaneous nerve stimulation (TNS)

Transcutaneous nerve stimulation, originally developed as a screening procedure for patients selection prior to a DCS implant, rapidly developed into a valuable therapy for chronic and acute pain. The apparatus we have been using consists of a battery pulse generator (weighing approx. 300 g) cables and skin electrodes. SHEALLY and MAUERER (12) saw 80% of good pain relief in 125 patients with acute postoperative or post-traumatic pain. Trying TNS on 625 patients with various chronic pain etiologies, the success rate of achieving excellent pain relief was in the neighbourhood of 25%.
During the pain symposium in Freiburg on electrical pain inhibition in October 74[1], reports were presented on a total of 206 patients

*Supported by Bundesministerium für Arbeit und Sozialordnung and Sonderforschungsbereich Hirnforschung (SFB 70) der DFG, Bonn/W. Germany.

[1]Active participants: J.A.V. Bates, London; D. Bowsher, Liverpool; H. Dietz, Hannover;   Fischer, Homburg/Saar; H. Gerbershagen, Mainz;

treated with TNS. Fair to good results have been reported in 43% of these cases. This relatively high rate of success has to be seen in the light of a different pre-selection group and different grading criteria.

It became apparent how difficult it is to compare results of different authors. To achieve a more uniform description in the grading system, we made the attempt to develop a standardized pain evaluation form and a pain profile form during this symposium. Pain symdromes that responded well to TNS were postherpetic neuralgia, stump pain, low back pain (in the U.S.), while phantom pain showed only unsatisfactory results. This safe and easily applicable method should be recommended as a first treatment for pain, as no major side effect have been reported yet (14).

Dorsal Cord Stimulation with Implantable Systems

The system consists of an implantable electrode - lead - receiver combination and an externally worn radio-frequency transmitter with antenna. By means of inductive coupling, the energy is transmitted to the electrode. Amplitude is variable from 0 to 14 volts, pulse width from 0,1 to 1 msec and the frequency from 8 to 250 Hertz using a biphasic rectangular pulse shape.

Operation Technique

SHEALLY (10), NASHOLD et al. (5) recommended implanting the electrode subdurally or subarachnoidally and fixing it to the dura to have the electrode in close contact with the dorsal cord. Implantation level depends on the segmental distribution of the pain and should be some segments higher than the last segment with pain input. Complications of CSF leakage and CSF cysts have been reported.

We place the electrode endodurally between two layers of the dura, trying to dissect out the inner layer as thinly as possible to avoid high tissue resistance (7, 2).

The *advantages of the endodural approach* are as follows: No opening of the subdural space, time-saving, *no radicular pain caused by direct contact of the electrodes with the dorsal roots*, and fewer postoperative arachnoidal reactions.

The following disadvantages have been seen with this technique: Higher stimulation threshold, sometimes needing the maximum amplitude of the device (special high out-put devices had to be supplied to those patients). Unpleasant radicular stimulation which *rather could be controlled by changing the pulse width*.

---

[1] cont.: J. Gybels, Loewen; E. Hauglie-Hanssen, Oslo; R. Hassler, Frankfurt/M.; H.J. Hufschmidt, Bonn; R. Jung, Freiburg i. Br.; J.-U. Krainick, A. Kühner, Heidelberg; R. Lorenz, Gießen; B. Meyerson, Stockholm; J. Miles, Liverpool; Muhtaroglu, Kiel; J.M. Mumford, Liverpool; H. Penzholz, Heidelberg; E. Perret, Zürich; K. Piscol, Bremen; C.D. Ray, Minneapolis; T. Riechert, Freiburg i. Br.; F. Schönberg, Hamburg; J. Siegfried, Zürich; J. Spierdijk, Leiden; A. Spring, Günzburg; Steude, München; A. Struppler, München;, U. Thoden, Freiburg i. Br.; W. Winkelmüller, Hannover; M. Zimmermann, Heidelberg.

Patient Selection

Preoperative careful patients selection has a major influence on a good success rate. A multi-disciplinary approach is therefore recommended. The first step should be a general neurological exploration to assure that there is no causal cure for the pain syndrome. In a psychiatric interview we try to define the psycho-pathological personality traits, as it has been demonstrated that a low rate of success can be expected in seriously disturbed patients, as well as in drug addicts.

Additional personality tests like MMPI recommended by some American pain clinics are certainly valuable but did not find acceptance in Europe because of their extremely time consuming nature. Evaluations of different authors have demonstrated that the physician's opinion about his patient correlates in most cases with the findings of a MMPI (6).

Against our *initial* selection criteria, we now tend to treat even drug addicted pain patients in cooperation with the psychiatrist, if the electro-stimulation is accompanied by a withdrawal treatment.

Patient Selection with Electrical Stimulation Methods

Initial neurological exploration of the pain patient is followed by the application of transcutaneous peripheral nerve stimulation. Does the patient benefit from TNS, then he will be discharged with a TNS. In case that the patient seriously disliked the paresthesias of TNS he is no longer considered a candidate for electrical stimulation. In case TNS shows only a partial success or electrodes cannot be applied for other reasons, for example leg amputees, we try *percutaneous DCS* (1). Via a Dattner-canula, a 300 u steel electrode is inserted into the subdural space above the pain segment. The stimulation is performed with a battery powered pulse generator. We try to verify whether or not the induced paresthesias are tolerated (10% of our cases do not tolerate these paresthesias), and pain relief is achieved. The value of this procedure is limited to chronic pain syndromes with consistent pain, or if the patient can trigger a pain attack during the testing procedure. The variation of the acute pain threshold has no significant correlation with the postoperative success and cannot be used as a selection criterion.

This *percutaneous short-term DCS* is certainly a stress situation for the patient. The procedure is uncomfortable for him and he tends to give unprecise answers in order to terminate the testing procedure as soon as possible. During the last year we started using flexible *floating electrodes* which can be inserted either in the lumbar or high cervical area C1/C2 from the side into the subdural space under X-ray control. The advantages of this technique are that the electrodes can remain in place for about 2 to 3 days and the postoperative situation is simulated for this period of time. We have seen a very good correlation between good testing results and good postoperative results (3).

This screening procedure has been tried on 25 patients and we excluded about half of this group from implantation often on the patient's own request. Beside insufficient pain relief some patients have major difficulties in operating the technical device. Complications from cerebral spinal fluid leakage are considerable due to the spring coil construction of the electrode which includes a potential risk of infection which we, however, have not experienced yet.

With the above described screening methods we exclude altogether about 90% of all patients coming for DCS.

Clinical Results

DCS systems have been implanted in 98 patients. 73 of them have been implanted for more than 1 year up to 3 years ago.

To judge the operative success we use the subjectively percentage-wise estimated pain relief of the patient and the reduction of drug intake.

Statistics (Table 1)

In the group with amputational pain we saw a fair to excellent result in 62%. A 25% pain reduction or less was considered to be a failure. The two other groups are too small to show any statistical significance.

The reduction of drug-intake (Table 2) with 73% is significantly higher than the estimated pain reduction. Among those patients who reduced their drug intake considerably, we found patients who claimed to get no pain relief from stimulation, however they discontinued their regimen with anagesics.

Table 1. Post-operative results vs. pain relief

Diagnosis		Pain relief				
	N	0	1	2	3	4
post amp. pain	52	10	10	10	11	11
peripheral, rad., spinal lesions	16	7	3	2	1	3
other pain syndromes	5	2	0	1	1	1
	73	19	13	13	13	15
		44%		56%		

Table 2. Post-operative drug intake vs. pain relief

Drug intake		Pain relief					
	N	0	1	2	3	4	
no drugs afterwards	25	4	1	4	6	10	73%
less than before	28	2	8	6	7	5	
same as before	15	8	4	3	0	0	27%
more than before	5	5	0	0	0	0	
	73	19	13	13	13	15	

Essential for pain relief is that the induced paresthesias are felt in the area of pain. No pain relief can be generally expected if the paresthesias do not cover the painful area.

Table 3. Masking of pain area and post-op. DCS results

masking of pain areas and electrical paresthesias	Pain relief					
	N	0	1	2	3	4
masking	40	2	4	10	11	13
no masking	33	17	9	3	2	2
	73	19	13	13	13	15

With percutaneous DCS as well as with permanent implantable systems, we observe a *correlation between the pulse width and the distribution of paresthesias*. With unipolar systems and a small pulse width of 0,1 msec we saw a more segmental distribution of the paresthesias, some segments above and below the implantation site, while with a larger pulse width of 1 msec duration, they were felt much stronger in the lower part of the body. This phenomenon is independent of the frequency and has not been seen with bipolar systems. For pain in the upper part of the body we preferred to implant unipolar systems, thus avoiding the distribution of paresthesias in the lower extremities.

During the Freiburg Symposium on electrical pain inhibition in October 74, the participants reported on 206 cases with implantable systems. The follow-up period was three months to 3 years. Though it seems to be impossible to compare the results of the different groups, an overall rate of 60% fair to excellent results was shown.

A 60% success rate for the treatment of chronic pain syndromes is relatively satisfactory, however, long-term results have to be awaited.

Development of percutaneous chronic implantable systems, improvement of screening procedures and apparatus shows a promising future for this mode of pain treatment.

REFERENCES

1. HOSOBUCHI, Y., ADAMS, J.E., WEINSTEIN, P.R.: Preliminary Percutaneous Dorsal Stimulation Prior to Permanent Implantation. Meeting of the American Association of Neurologia Surgeons, April 1971.

2. KRAINICK, J.-U., THODEN, U., RIECHERT, T., TENSCHERT, G.: Elektrische Hirnstrangreizung bei chronischen Schmerzen. Klinische Erfahrung über zwei Jahre. Neurochirurgia 17, 162 (1974).

3. KRAINICK, J.-U., THODEN, U., RIECHERT, T.: Spinal Cord Stimulation in Post Amputation Pain. Surg. neurol. (in press).

4. MELZACK, R., WALL, P.D.: Pain Mechanisms: A New Theory. Science 150, 971 (1965).

5. NASHOLD, B.S., FRIEDMAN, H.: Dorsal Column Stimulation for Control of Pain. Preliminary Report on 30 Patients. J. Neurosurg. 36, 597 (1972).

6. PERRET, E.: Methoden der Patientenselektion. Arbeitsgespräch über elektrische Schmerzhemmung, Freiburg i. Br., Oktober 1974.

7. RIECHERT, T., KRAINICK, J.-U., THODEN, U.: Experience with DCS, especially in Pantom and Stump Pain. Pain Seminar Minneapolis, Minnesota 1973.

8. SALANDIÈRE, J.B.: Mémoires sur l'electro-puncture. Paris 1825.

9. SCRIBONIUS LARGUS: De compositone medicamentorum liber. CLXII.

10. SHEALLY, C.N.: Dorsal Column Electrohypalgesia. Headache 9, 2, July 1969.

11. SHEALLY, C.N.: Dorsal Column Electroanalgesia. A 5 1/2-year experience. Vortrag in Freiburg i. Br. (19. 9. 1972).

12. SHEALLY, C.N., MAUERER, D.: Transcutaneous Nerve Stimulation for Control of Pain. A Preliminary Technical Note. Surg. Neurol. 2, 45 (1974).

13. SWEET, W.H., WEPSIC, J.G.: Treatment of Chronic Pain by Stimulation of Fibers of Primary Afferent Neuron. Trans. Amer. Neurol. Ass. 93, 103 (1968).

14. THODEN, U., KRAINICK, J.-U.: Ambulante Schmerzbehandlung durch transkutane Nervenstimulation. Dtsch. med. Wschr. 99, 1962 (1974).

Control of Pain by Electrical Stimulation
A Clinical Follow-Up Review

CH. D. RAY

Introduction

Clinical results of electrical stimulation therapy for acute and
chronic pain are continuing to accumulate. While the mode of action
remains the subject of theory, successes obtained with both cutaneous
and implanted stimulating devices lead to a better understanding of
the mechanisms involved and better use of these techniques. The collective clinical data reported here were obtained from over 25 neurosurgeons cooperating in pain-treatment study groups. Cases were
collected and analyzed by follow-up correspondence to determine the
lasting results of transcutaneous, dorsal column, peripheral nerve
and direct brain stimulation devices. The patient-scoring criterion
form used is presented and results are reported for each of the four
techniques used in this study. These findings and their implications
are, therefore, a composite of the present state of the art of pain
control by electrical stimulation as practiced by a number of neurosurgeons in North America.

Method of Study

The management of acute and chronic pain is a decidedly important
phase, and a very difficult one, of medical care. There have evolved
a number of materials and methods for the medical, surgical and psychiatric management of patients having acute or chronic pain. Electrical stimulation may now be added as an additional method. Although
the concept and practice of electrical stimulation for pain control
is rooted in history, it is only since the development of the "gate
control theory" by MELZACK and WALL in 1965 that a new and refreshing
look at the potential use of electrical stimulation for pain control
has occurred (1). Following the first clinical implantation of a dorsal column stimulation device in 1967 by SHEALY (2, 3), new techniques and devices utilizing this mode of therapeutic management have
emerged at an ever-increasing rate. The results have ranged from
spectacular to disappointing. There is now accumulating a considerable
evidence fo the neurophysiological basis of electrical stimulation in
pain control, but much physiological and anatomical mystery persists.
Nonetheless, this concept has provoked more intensive study of the
anatomy and physiology of sensory mechanisms in the spinal cord than
any other clinical therapeutic mode (with the possible exception of
the older destructive techniques for pain control). One of the most
attractive aspects of electrical stimulation for pain control lies in
its non-destructive and reversible nature. If good results are not
obtained either in a short or prolonged period of time, the removal
of the device will in all cases (with the exception of rare complications resulting from pressure exerted on nerve or spinal cord by
electrodes) return the patient to his pre-implantation state. Further,

electrical stimulation may indeed somehow "re-train" or "modulate" the nervous system so that, in due time, the pain disappears without the need for further treatment.

This report contains the collective experiences of 25 neurosurgeons in North America who have utilized various modes of electrical stimulation for the control of acute and chronic pain. Four reports are included here: transcutaneous nerve stimulation, dorsal column stimulation, peripheral nerve stimulation, and direct brain (thalamic or internal capsular) stimulation. This work was done by study groups formed and supported by Medtronic, Incorporated, in order to further evaluate both the concept and the specific application of devices. The study group method brings together expert clinicians who may share experiences relevant to patient selection, screening criteria and methods, surgical techniques, problems, follow-up results, indications and contraindications, device and electrode design improvements, comprehensive pain management programs, drug detoxification, third party payment for devices and fees, etc. In the early stages of the development and application of new devices, there is a limited quantity of instruments available; the study group helps to "ration" the devices. Further, study groups help insure that the well controlled clinical studies are subjected to review by peers.

A number of patient evaluation forms have been developed but the most representative appears to be a series of questions which permit the scoring of a pain profile relative to five major criteria.[1] The scoring matrix shown in Table 1 was developed principally by PICAZA aided by SHEALY and RAY. In the questionnaires developed by Medtronic, Inc., to be filled out by the physician and by the patient, responses are arranged according to five criteria into grades ranging from 0 to 4. Since pain is a subjective, conscious process, and since the responses of patients to inquiry regarding their pains will always be highly loaded with subjective impressions, this pain profile and the associated questionnaires make a maximum attempt at objectifying (and quantifying) the very subjective nature of most pain syndromes.

At intervals, beginning prior to implantation or cutaneous stimulation treatment, and following therapeutic use of the corresponding devices, patients are asked to complete questionnaires from which the profile could be drawn each time. In many cases physician interviews and impressions were reduced to a scoring of the profile for comparative purposes. In conducting a post-therapeutic follow-up by mail, a great number of patients will not respond. Therefore, direct patient surveys must often be supplemented by having a member of our staff (a registered nurse skilled in the techniques of patient interview and follow-up analysis) contact the non-responding patients by telephone in order to urge their completion of the form or, in order to obtain oral information sufficient to complete the scoring of the profile. All such subjective follow-up techniques may cast some doubt as to the reliability of results, but since the same group of people evaluated all the responding patients, and since these clinical assistants were not associated with the operating surgeon or treating physician, it is felt that this might have helped to remove some patient bias (where he might have desired to satisfy his clinician as to good results when there might not have been any).

---

[1]Forms available from Medtronic, Inc.

Table 1. Pain profile scoring matrix

Grade	Daily duration of pain	Intensity of pain	Activity level	Drugs	Behavior
0	No pain	None	Normal	None	Normal – alert, cheerful, cooperative
1	Having pain up to 25% of time	Mild	Slightly restricted activity	Aspirin	Slightly disturbed – irritable, disagreeable, complaining, moody
2	Up to 50% of time	Discomforting	Moderately restricted	Sedatives tranquilizers	Moderately disturbed – dull, unhappy, anxious, uncooperative
3	Up to 75% of time	Distressing	Severely restricted	Hypnotics Darvon	Quite disturbed – quite depressed, moderately withdrawn, bitter, desperate
4	Up to 100% of time	Horrible or excruciating	Incapacitated	Narcotics	Asocial – severely withdrawn, belligerent, combative, asocial, panic state

Table 3. Transcutaneous nerve stimulation for relief of chronic pain

Amount of pain relief reported after:	7 months of therapy 394 patients		12 months of therapy 78 patients	
	N	% of total	N	% of total
Complete relief (100%)	26	7%	7	9%
Major relief (75–99%)	68	18% } 63%	8	10% } 55%
Significant relief (50–74%)	147	38%	28	36%
Minor relief (25–49%)	62	16%	15	19%
Minimal relief (1–24%)	55	14%	16	21%
No relief (0%)	26	7%	4	5%
Total	394	100%	78	100%

Transcutaneous Nerve Stimulation

In this collective study, 396 chronic pain patients were followed. Their average age was 48 years, ranging from 18 to 80.

The results of the average seven-month duration of use for various pain etiologies is presented in Table 2.

Table 2. Transcutaneous nerve stimulation for the relief of chronic pain. 396 patients: 7 month average time device used (direct patient survey)

Etiology	N	Successful % (50-100% relief)		Unsuccessful % (0-49% relief)	
Low back syndrome	29	19	66%	10	34%
Multiple op-low back	125	69	55%	56	45%
Post trauma-low back	18	11	61%	7	39%
Post trauma-thoracic	5	2	40%	3	60%
"Other" - upper back	4	3	75%	1	25%
Multiple op-cervical	6	5	83%	1	17%
Post trauma-cervical	8	7	88%	1	13%
Degenerative spine	14	9	64%	5	36%
Arthritis	14	10	71%	4	29%
Cancer	3	3	100%		
Headache	5	4	80%	1	20%
Causalgia	5	4	80%	1	20%
Postherpetic	5	3	60%	2	40%
Neuroma	3	3	100%		
Amputation/phantom	10	8	80%	2	20%
Unknown	72	44	61%	28	39%
Other	53	37	70%	16	30%
Total	379	241	64%	138	36%

Seventy-eight patients who were using the device at the end of 12 months responded to a follow-up questionnaire. The comparison of overall results between these two groups are given in Table 3, where it may be noted that patients showing 50% or better pain relief comprise 63% of the patients in the seven-month group and 55% of the patients in the twelve-month group. Since TNS is a very simply applied external device, it is indeed important that in this collective study the success was quite high, considering the nature of the pain and the fact that a great number of cases had pain over long periods of time, even years, prior to treatment by electrical stimulation.

In general, patients who show significant, major or complete relief of pain, also show improvement in nearly all of the other criteria of the pain profile. Indeed, PICAZA (4) has found that when patients show improvements in all elements of their profile with the exception of 1 or 2, then the validity of their results may be questioned. (The only possible exception to this lies in the use of drugs where one may find a disproportionately high percentage of patients having major relief of pain who, nevertheless, continue to use drugs in grades 3 or 4.)

Nonetheless, the technique is so innocuous and easily applied that the method is worthy of trial in a great number of pain cases, not only as a method of screening for subsequent implantation, but also as the sole mode of therapy. TNS is often combined with other therapeutic means in a comprehensive pain program and a number of clinics have reported series ranging up to as many as 3,000 cases whose overall results appear to be similar to those given here (5, 6, 7).

Further, a very large population of patients exist who have been treated for *acute* pain by transcutaneous nerve stimulation but no firm statistics are available at this time.

In general, the acute applications show an overall efficacy as high as 80% (8) as compared to approximately 25% efficacy for chronic pain cases over a long term period (9). The acute applications include traumatic pain in limbs and joints, postoperative pain management following abdominal or thoracic procedures, acute episodes of headache, rehabilitation (such as in range of motion exercises) and as an adjunct to local anesthesia for various surgical and dental procedures.

Of course, we can assume that a large number of patients who initially had tried the treatment, dropped out before seven months and an even larger number by 12 months; they did so because of receiving little or no relief of their pain.

Dorsal Column Stimulation

The patients reported in this collective series, as shown in Table 4, comprise a large number of pain etiologies. Two hundred and sixty-six patients are reported in a follow-up period having an average of 18 months implantation. These patients were divided into two groups. The first group was an earlier collection of 481 cases in which only 39% of the questionnaires were returned completed. The majority of the cases either did not return their questionnaires or they were returned incomplete. A second group of 119 cases returned 66% (78) of the questionnaires. This represents a combined total of 266 patients who responded out of a total of 600 cases sent questionnaires. Since the time of collection of these data, a number of the patients have been followed by telephone and by additional correspondence and it appears that the non-responding patients probably fall fairly equally divided between those patients who have not been adequately relieved and those patients who have (This will be the subject of a subsequent publication). In general, the results show that approximately 50% of the cases had 50% or better pain relief over 18 months of average implantation time. More recently, the use of acute and relatively chronic indwelling electrodes, mostly placed extradurally for longer term screening, has resulted in an overall improvement in patient selection. It is anticipated that this may well result in an elevation of the general efficacy of this technique (10, 11).

Peripheral Nerve Stimulation

In Table 5, one finds the combined results of 75 patients who responded. In general, this technique appears to have an efficacy similar to that of dorsal column stimulation for selected cases. It is most often used for low-back syndromes with pain radiation into one leg. The large number of sciatic implants reflects this principal application.

Table 4. DCS implant survey of U.S. study group members. Average follow-up period of 18 months, total of 266 patient respondents

Diagnosis/Etiology	Successful (50-100% pain relief)		Unsuccessful (0-49% pain relief)		Total
	N	(%)	N	(%)	
Low back pain described as:					
1. Low back syndrome	27	(45)	33	(55)	60
2. Unsuccessful disc surgery	39	(53)	34	(47)	73
3. Adhesive arachnoiditis	25	(45)	30	(55)	55
4. Degenerative disc disease	4	(50)	4	(50)	8
Subtotal low back	95	(48)	101	(52)	196
Trauma	6	(35)	11	(65)	17
Cancer	0	(0)	3	(100)	3
Paraplegia	1	(50)	1	(50)	2
Post-amputation	2	(40)	3	(60)	5
Peripheral nerve syndrome	1	(50)	1	(50)	2
Neuroma	1	(100)	0	(0)	1
Postherpetic neuralgia	0	(0)	2	(100)	2
Multiple sclerosis	2	(100)	0	(0)	2
Other	7	(44)	9	(56)	16
Unknown	2	(50)	2	(50)	4
Total	117	(47)	133	(53)	250

Table 5. PNS patient survey of U.S. study group members. 75 patient respondents

Electrode placement vs. pain relief:

Placement	Successful (50-100% relief)		Unsuccessful (0-49% pain relief)		Total
	N	(%)	N	(%)	
Sciatic	25	(71)	10	(29)	35
Ulnar	4	(44)	5	(56)	9
Occipital	4	(100)	0	(0)	4
Femoral	1	(34)	2	(66)	3
Brachial Plexus	3	(75)	1	(25)	4
Pudendal	1	(100)	0	(0)	1
Peroneal	1	(100)	0	(0)	1
Total	39	(52)	18	(24)	57[a]

[a] 18 patients (24%) have either had their PNS device removed or have discontinued its use.

Brain Stimulation

In Table 6, one finds a resumé of 28 patients who are the total population of this one-year-average implant study. Under the column "Implant site", one also sees a listing of the pain etiologies treated by each particular implant technique. In general, this technique shows the highest degree of efficacy for relief of chronic pain of the techniques reported in this paper. The majority of these patients were treated by ADAMS and HOSOBUCHI (12)(both of San Francisco) and RICHARDSON (of New Orleans). This technique, while the most complex of those reported here, appears to affect far more directly the pathways of pain, and therefore the smallest electrical field has the greatest overall initial and lasting results.

Table 6. Brain stimulation for relief of chronic pain. 28 patients: 1 year average implant

Implant site	N	Successful % (50-100% relief)		Unsuccessful % (0-49% relief)	
Internal Capsule					
CNS lesions	11	9	82%	2	18%
PNS lesions	2	2	100%		
Sensory thalamic (VPM)					
Facial pain	4	3	75%	1	25%
Medial Thalamus (PVG)					
CNS lesions	1	1	100%		
PNS lesions	1	1	100%		
Cancer head	1			1	100%
Cancer trunk	4	4	100%		
LB syndrome	3	3	100%		
Brain stem					
Facial pain	1	1	100%		
Total	28	24	86%	4	14%

At 75-100% relief: 6 successes, CNS lesion, internal capsule stimulation; 2 successes, facial pain, VPM stimulation.

Discussion and Summary

Presented here are clinical results and follow-ups of cases comprising patients in the series of 25 neurosurgeons in North America. Reported are four modalities of therapy using electrical stimulation to control chronic pain. In general, the long term results using transcutaneous nerve stimulation for chronic pain were favorable in 63% and 55% of patients whose results were reported at the end of 7 and 12 months of therapy, respectively. Due to the rather selective nature of these cases, it is felt that these results compare favorably with those now being reported elsewhere which indicate that transcutaneous nerve stimulation may have an overall efficacy of about 25% of cases for *chronic* pain control. Approximately 80% of the cases with acute, traumatic or postoperative pain may be successfully managed with little or no additional medication while employing skin surface stimulation. Overall results for dorsal column and peripheral nerve stimulation indicate that about 50% of the patients will be helped by removing 50% or more of their pain for periods of time ranging up to more than 18 months. Recent reports indicate that where the good results of dorsal column stimulation may show a decline in many cases, a number of these patients may be returned to good pain control if the electrode is moved to another site along the spinal cord. This appears to be often related to the development of fibrosis around the surface of the electrode with long term stimulation. A few cases similarly have been reported with peripheral nerve stimulation. These conclusions indicate that in all stimulation techniques, the relocation of electrodes should be considered before discontinuing the therapy entirely. Deep brain stimulation has the highest overall rate of success, although this method is applied in what are probably the most severe pain cases. In summary, this report, as well as others which are now appearing regarding the use of electrical stimulation for the control of acute and chronic pain, indicates that this is a viable therapy in selected cases that compares favorably with existing methods of treatment in the management of intractable chronic pain, particularly in relation to certain pain etiologies.

Acknowledgements. The author wishes to acknowledge the considerable effort given the preparation of this material and gathering of the data by his colleagues and members of the department: Constance CARTIER, Rollin DENNISTON, and Rita HIRSCH, Neuro/Rehab Division, Medical Programs Department, Medtronic, Incorporated.

Appreciation is also given for members of the study group who made their patients and clinical data available for this report.

The clinical study status reports containing the above information are available from Medtronic, Inc., as:

"Follow-Up Survey on Peripheral Nerve Stimulation Implants," NR503, July 12, 1974.

"Follow-Up Survey on Dorsal Cord Stimulator Implants," NR510, February 27, 1975.

"3583 Electrode Clinical Study Status Report," NR511, April 15, 1975.

Patient Use and Acceptance of the Neuromod™ Transcutaneous Nerve Stimulator, NR512, March 31, 1975.

REFERENCES

1. MELZACK, R., WALL, P.D.: Pain mechanism: a new theory. Science 150, 971 (1965).

2. SHEALY, C.N., MORTIMER, J.T., RESWICK, J.B.: Electrical inhibition of pain stimulation of the dorsal column: preliminary clinical reports. Anesth. Analg. 46, 489 (1967).

3. SHEALY, C.N., TASLITZ, N., MORTIMER, J.T., BECKER, D.P.: Electrical inhibition of pain: experimental evaluation. Anesth. Analg. 46, 299 (1967).

4. PICAZA, J.A., CANNAN, B.W. et al.: Pain suppression by peripheral nerve stimulation. Surg. Neurol., Minneapolis Pain Seminar (ed. C.D. RAY) (in press).

5. SHEALY, C.N., MAURER, D.: Transcutaneous nerve stimulation for control of pain. Surg. Neurol. 2, 45 (1974).

6. SHEALY, C.N.: Transcutaneous electroanalyzing. Surg. Forum 23, 419 (1972).

7. LONG, D.M.: External electrical stimulation as a treatment of chronic pain. Minn. Med. 57, 195 (1974).

8. HORWITZ, N.: New uses found for electrical skin stimulation. Med. Trib. 45, 1 (1974).

9. SHEALY, C.N.: Transcutaneous electrical stimulation for control of pain. Clin. Neurosurg. 21, 269 (1974).

10. BURTON, C.V.: Dorsal column stimulation: optimization of application. Surg. Neurol., Minneapolis Pain Seminar (ed. C.D. RAY) (in press).

11. LONG, D.M., ERICKSON, D.E.: Stimulation of the posterior columns of the spinal cord for relief of intractable pain. Surg. Neurol., Minneapolis Pain Seminar (ed. C.D. RAY) (in press).

12. HOSOBUCHI, Y., ADAMS, J.E., RUTKIN, B.: Chronic thalamic and internal capsule stimulation for the control of central pain. Surg. Neurol., Minneapolis Pain Seminar (ed. C.D. RAY) (in press).

The Clinical Value of Dorsal Column Stimulation (DCS)

W. WINKELMÜLLER, H. DIETZ, and D. STOLKE

Since SHEALY (2, 3) and NASHOLD (1) reported about good results in the treatment of intractable pain by DCS, an increase in clinical and experimental work about pain pathophysiology could be observed. There are different views on the value and effectivity of DCS as a method of pain surgery: some tend to an optimistic judgment, others are skeptical and regard DCS implantation as a passing trend.

With this discussion in mind we made a follow-up study of 40 patients who have undergone implantation of a dorsal column stimulator during the last 2 1/2 years in our clinic. The analysis of these cases was made in order to clarify failures, complications, the qualification of selection procedures and the value of technical improvements.

DCS implantation was performed to control various types of pain, caused by malignant tumors with infiltration of a nerve plexus, traumatic lesions of peripheral nerves and spinal cord, arachnoiditis, peridural scar compressions following disc operations, as well as stump and phantom limb pain.

Patients with obvious signs of hysteria, depression and hypochondria were excluded from implantation. Special psychological tests were not used. Implantation was carried out when a repeated pain relieving effect was achieved by transcutaneous or percutaneous stimulation. In the beginning we did not eliminate drug addicted patients.

Unipolar electrodes were implanted in 34 patients, bipolar in 6 cases, all were fixed endodurally. The electrodes were placed at an upper thoracic level, the cable was led over the shoulder and the receiver was buried subcutaneously in the infraclavicular region. Stimulation started on the first postoperative day.

According to pain etiology we differentiated four groups of patients (Table 1):

1. Malignant tumors with infiltration of a nerve plexus.

2. Stump and phantom limb pain.

3. Chronic low back pain following multiple lumbar disc operations.

4. In this group we summarize all other intractable pain syndromes.

Our follow-up study covers up to 30 months after operation. At this time we can overlook 15 good to very good results and 19 failures out of 40 patients. 6 patients with only fair pain relief needed analgetic substitution. We have to point out that there are up to 70% long-term failures in malignant tumor patients. These data, however, include those cases in which pain could be relieved temporarily, at least for several months.

Table 1. Follow-up study after DCS-implantation (up to 30 months)

Primary disease	Cases	Pain relief in %			
		0-25	25-50	50-75	75-100
Malignant tumor	14	10	-	1	3
Stump and phantom limb	16	5	-	3	8
Low back syndrome	6	2	-	1	3
Miscellaneous	4	2	1	-	1
Total	40	19	1	5	15

Therefore we classified the results into groups of early failures, pain relief up to 6 months and pain relief of more than 6 months (Fig. 1). The malignant tumor group shows the least success rate, especially when tumor expansion led to reduced survival time. The judgment of survival time, however, is difficult, because in 6 patients who died during the following 6 months no signs of tumor metastasis were present at the time of implantation, neither by x-ray screening nor scintigraphically.

31% primary failures in the group of stump and phantom limb pain is a rather high percentage. A long-term pain relief could be achieved in 50% and 60% of benign pain syndromes. These patients had complete pain relief and did not need additional analgetic medication.

Furthermore we examined postoperative complications and side effects of DCS (Table 2).

4 patients experienced unpleasant radicular sensations and compressing dysesthesias at the implantation level, probably induced by direct irritation of neighboring dorsal roots. Even by increasing the voltage, stimulation-induced paresthesia did not spread into distant parts of the body. Pain relief occurred only if the paresthesia produced by DCS was referred into the painful area. By changing the transmitter and setting the pulse width to a maximum of 1 msec, we succeeded in abolishing the unpleasant radicular sensation and obtained analgesia by a more diffuse current propagation. In two patients we failed in taking this range of stimulation parameters, so that we plan to replace the monopolar electrode by a bipolar one.

Table 2. Postoperative complications

		Cases
1. Side effects of DCS	a) unpleasant sensation at implantation level	4
	b) loss of gait control	4
2. Technical failure	defect of cable isolation	3
3. Infection	local decubital ulcer 6 months following implantation	1
4. Epidural bleeding	transient motor and sensory loss	1

4 patients complained of being unsteady in the upright position and of loss of motor control during stimulation. They performed stimulation in a lying position and thus obtained a sufficient analgetic effect. We suppose that this impairment of motor control is due to current spread in the cord involving the dorso-lateral spino-cerebellar tracts.

3 patients, who previously obtained excellent relief from pain, reported on irregular stimulus impulses until transmission had completely stopped. Twice we reoperated and found an insulation defect in the monopolar device which led to a short circuit between defferent and indifferent cable. The third patient was satisfied by additional application of a transcutaneous set, so that we desisted from reoperation.

The quota of operative complications was low. One dorsal column stimulator had to be removed 6 months after implantation because of an infected decubital ulcer along the cable at the level of collarbone. More serious was a postoperative subfascial bleeding, which caused an incomplete paraplegia by cord compression. After immediate reoperation it took more than 4 months to recover completely.

In three cases no pain relief was achieved in spite of good function of the DCS implant. But even stereotactic thalamotomy and bilateral open as well as percutaneous cordotomy could bring sufficient lasting pain relief. All patients experienced pain recurrence within 6 months after the interruption of the spinothalamic pathway.

If we look upon our follow-up study critically, a modification of selection criteria and an adequate correction of technical complications is indicated:

(1) Our figures show that pain due to carcinoma is not worthwhile being treated by DCS. A better result would be obtained by cordotomy and thalamotomy.

(2) The treatment of benign pain syndromes by DCS is considered more promising, because a lasting pain relief is achieved at least in 50%. The rather high percentage of primary failures may be diminished by a better selection of patients and by technical improvements. We would, for example, exclude drug addicted and so-called career patients who have undergone multiple operative procedures. Further improvement is expected by the application of bipolar electrodes together with more effective transmitters. The concentration of electrical current in bipolar electrodes has the advantage of avoiding unpleasant radicular sensations and of better covering the painful area by stimulation-induced paresthesia.

Comparing destructive operations like cordotomy and thalamotomy with DCS, the first method is incriminated by defect symptoms and a rather high rate of complications. The latter achieves pain relief by a more physiological neuronal modulation.

The confrontation of both methods in respect to their results in the treatment of cancer favors cordotomy: the published cases of WHITE and SWEET (4) show that a total of 54% have good relief of pain by cordotomy opposed to 25% early failures. In benign pain syndromes, too, the early successes of open cordotomy (70%) are better than our results of DCS. But, regarding long-term results, the failure rate of cordotomy (64%) - due to the dropping level of analgesia - is higher than the failure rate of DCS. But much longer follow-ups are necessary in order to evaluate the efficiency of this system.

As to the clinical value of DCS at present, this method offers the possibility of long lasting pain relief in most forms of benign pain syndromes, if a careful selection of patients was made.

REFERENCES

1. NASHOLD, B.S., FRIEDMAN, H.: Dorsal column stimulation for control of pain. Preliminary report of 30 patients. J. Neurosurg. 36, 590-597 (1972).

2. SHEALY, C.N., MORTIMER, J.T., RESWICK, J.B.: Electrical inhibition of pain stimulation of the dorsal columns: Preliminary clinical report. Anesth. Analg. Curr. Res. 46, 489 (1967).

3. SHEALY, C.N., MORTIMER, J.T., HAGFORS, N.R.: Dorsal column electroanalgesia. J. Neurosurg. 32, 560-564 (1970).

4. WHITE, J.C., SWEET, W.H.: Pain and the Neurosurgeon, p. 699. Springfield/Ill.: Charles C. Thomas 1969.

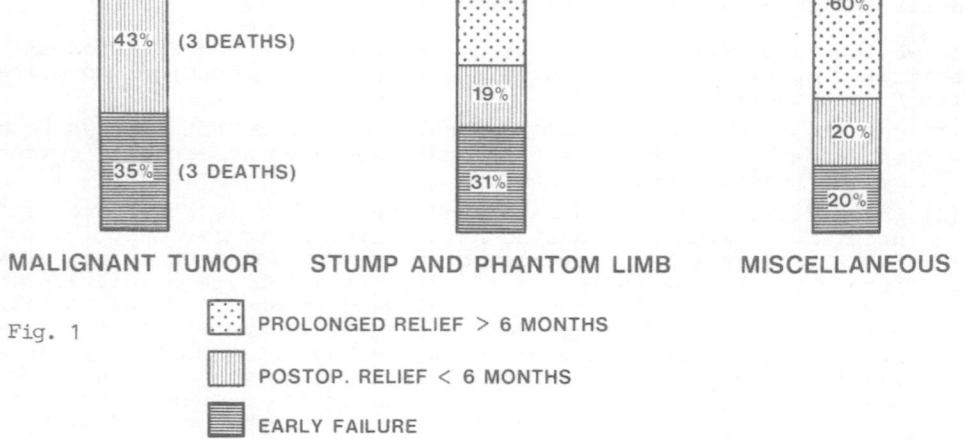

MALIGNANT TUMOR   STUMP AND PHANTOM LIMB   MISCELLANEOUS

Fig. 1   PROLONGED RELIEF > 6 MONTHS

                  POSTOP. RELIEF < 6 MONTHS

                  EARLY FAILURE

Central Stereotactic Interventions for Intractable Pain

G. Dieckmann

Stereotactic procedures were first performed by KIRSCHNER (15). In his original publication the term "gezielte Operationen" was already used. KIRSCHNER's apparatus and the method of denaturation of the trigeminal ganglion had already fulfilled all criteria of operations later performed under the term "stereotactic operations". Modern stereotactic procedures against pain started with SPIEGEL and WYCIS, whose first stereotactic papers were concerned with interventions in the mesencephalon and the thalamus against pain (33). TALAIRACH and co-workers (13) first correlated stereotactic lesions in chronic pain patients with the clinical result. They were followed-up by HASSLER and RIECHERT (11). First long-term results were then reported by HAS-SLER and RIECHERT (12), MARK et al. (19, 20) and SPIEGEL and WYCIS (33).

Today, the indications for central stereotactic procedures are all pain states not to be influenced by direct or pharmacological means or by the usual neurosurgical interventions. These indications are: essential neuralgias, post-herpetic neuralgias, anaesthesia dolorosa, causalgias, phantom limb pain, thalamic syndrome and pain in the course of a neoplastic disease.

Nucleotomy of the Tractus Spinalis Nervi Trigemini

This intervention is the same as the open operation of SJÖQUIST (32). The procedure was made possible after the introduction of spinal stereotactic interventions by CRUE et al. (4) and HITCHCOCK (14). An approach is made to the caudal nucleus, i.e. the lower part of the trigeminal nucleus. Electrical stimulation of this nucleus causes pain responses in the face in the area of the classical onion-skin arrangement. Deep recordings show evoked potentials after nocioceptive stimulation in the ipsilateral periphery. At the present time the method of SCHVARCZ (31) seems to be the therapy of choice for destroying the caudal part of the trigeminal nucleus. A tungsten electrode with a tip diameter of 50 μ is introduced through the atlanto-occipital interspace by means of a HITCHCOCK device. Impedance changes indicate cord contact and penetration. Control of exact electrode placement is indicated by the results of electrical stimulation. Lesions of 2,5 to 3,5 mm are produced fractionally by radiofrequency. After each coagulation quality and extent of sensory changes are checked.

The indication for stereotactic nucleotomy are all chronic pain states of the trigeminal nerve, mainly essential neuralgias in which surgical pretreatment was unsuccessful. Furthermore, anaesthesia dolorosa, post-herpetic neuralgias and malignant tumors of the head. SCHVARCZ's method is a new one and various postoperative follow-up studies are available showing very good results in patients with malignant tumors as well as those with non-malignant diseases (4, 14, 31). Postoperatively an analgesia occurs. The aesthesia of the skin is preserved thus enabling a bilateral intervention. Persisting complications were not observed.

Mesencephalotomy

Stereotactic mesencephalotomy was introduced by SPIEGEL and WYCIS (33). Principally, it corresponds to the open operation of DOGLIOTTI (5) and of WALKER (38). These operations interrupt spinothalamic and quintothalamic pathways at the level of or rostral to the colliculus superior. Later reports on this topic were given by TORVIK (37), MAZARS et al. (23) and ROEDER and ORTHNER (30). Recently NASHOLD and WILSON (25, 26) reported on mesencephalic stimulation and destruction by means of chronic implanted electrodes. The stimulation of this region produced pain in the trigeminally supplied skin. Inversely spontaneous pain was removed by radiofrequency lesions in this region. As did SPIEGEL and WYCIS, NASHOLD and WILSON recommended the combination of mesencephalotomy with the destruction of the thalamic dorsomedial nucleus in patients with pronounced psychological reactions to their pain.

The authors recorded epileptic discharges from the mesencephalic region during spontaneous pain attacks. After radiofrequency lesions, these attacks no longer appeared. Because of the possibility of producing pain by electrical stimulation in this mesencephalic area and the disappearance of pain after radiofrequency lesions, NASHOLD and WILSON presumed that central pain was possibly caused by an irritation at the midbrain level (25).

Pain, particularly of the head and neck, can disappear by this intervention. Postoperatively, about 72% of the patients are immediately and totally free of pain according to SPIEGEL and WYCIS (33). The long-term results are essentially unfavorable, i.e. only 31% of the patients are free of pain. The mortality in the cases reported by SPIEGEL and WYCIS was 7,4%. This is remarkably more than the usual stereotactic mortality which is commonly about 1%. Today this procedure is hardly used, the target point itself being dangerous, and long-term results are more unsatisfactory than those of stereotactic thalamotomy.

Thalamotomy

The thalamic interventions occur in three neuronal systems concerned with pain experience as specifically described by HASSLER (see page 1). Accordingly there are three different target points which are attacked. The interruption of the specific or cortical pain conducting system is at the relay point between the 2nd and 3rd neuron, i.e. the end point of part of the fibres from the spinothalamic tract (the basal part of the sensory relay nucleus of the thalamus). In the awake patient, low frequency electrical stimulation of this nucleus causes a prickling or feeling of heat; higher frequency stimulation is followed by pain sensation in circumscribed contralateral parts of the body (12). The interruption of the specific pain conducting system always results in an analgesia and thermalgesia. In cases of lesions within the specific sensory relay nucleus alone, only temporary relief of pain is obtained.

This is explained by the so-called "dichotomy" of the pain pathways (10). From the spinothalamic tract, fibres merge into nuclei (such as nucleus limitans, parafascicular complex, centre median, intralaminar nuclei) of the unspecific thalamic projecting system. All of these nuclei belong to the so-called subthalamic pain-conducting system. Electrical stimulation of these nuclei causes in awake patients - according to the site of the stimulation - disagreeable sensations which are difficult to define and localize. Electrical high-frequency stimulation in the nucleus limitans evokes strong pain feeling in the contralateral part of the body without local differentiation. Lesion of these nuclei augment the analgesia and make it more lasting as BETTAG and YOSHIDA (3) have already reported. Also, the selective lesion in the subcortical pain conducting system is often followed by complete relief of pain without any sensory deficits (13, 20). The interruption of this system diminishes attention to the pain and the subjective "feeling" of pain.

The interruption of thalamo-frontal pathways takes place at one thalamic level by lesions in the dorso-medial nucleus and the adjacent internal lamella. Thereby, the anxious fixation of the patient on his pain as well as the estimation of the pain still present can be diminished or removed.

In general, the thalamic interventions show immediate postoperative good to very good pain relief in 70-100% of the patients (3, 19, 12, 27, 28). This good immediate effect is due less to a selective lesion in the cortical pain conducting system, but rather brought about by a combined lesion in both the cortical and subcortical pain-conducting systems or at times in the subcortical system alone (3, 13, 27, 34, 35). But what brings this good result about is still a matter of discussion. More recently a single lesion in the subcortical system seems to be preferred by certain authors, although from the anatomical point of view, combined lesions in both systems seem to be necessary. About 1 year after the intervention the relapse rate increases greatly. For the non-malignant pain patients then only about 50% of them were free of pain, another 20% showed partial amelioration. On the other hand, 70-90% of the patients with malignant tumors remained free of pain until their death because of the short survival time. In these latter cases, the lesion can be limited to the subcortical pain conducting system.

Remaining side-effects consisting of analgesia, thermanaesthesia, ataxia, sometimes also hypaesthesia, occur after a lesion in the cortical pain-conducting system. After destruction in the subcortical system sometimes only paraesthesia or dysaesthesia is seen. Lesions in the dorso-medial nucleus and the adjacent internal lamella, even if only performed unilaterally, can be followed by apathy and loss of initiative. Such thalamic procedures are definitely ineffectual in drug addicted patients. The mortality is generally 0-7% (29).

In recent years, good results were sometimes reported after interventions in the pulvinar, the great integrative nucleus of the thalamus (27, 28, 41). The mode of action of this intervention is not yet clear. Clinically, the effect of operation is similar to that obtained after a lesion in the central median nucleus, although the neurophysiology of both nuclei is different. Postoperatively one can find pain improvement without sensory deficits. The immediate results are not only postoperatively good, but also often last a longer period of time (27, 41).

Sharply delineated lesions are not only produced by high frequency, electrolytic or cryolesions by means of intracerebral electrodes, but more recently also by radiosurgical procedures, the so-called γ-thalamotomy of LEKSELL (17). This is a cross-radiation with γ-beams from 169 Co-sources, i.e. a closed, unbloody technique in the course of which a burr hole need not be performed. The procedure is still expensive; probably it points to a future method of stereotactic lesioning.

Chronic Thalamic Stimulation

Aside from the previous methods mentioned to obtain pain relief by the interruption of neuronal systems, more recently the possibility of avoiding central pain by chronic stimulation of cerebral structures, analogous to DC-stimulation of the spinal cord, has been introduced. It is known from animal experiments that electricl stimulation of periventricular and periaquaeductal grey matter causes a general analgesia. Neurophysiologically this analgesia is explained by activation of a pain inhibiting system which modulates pain inputs (1, 24). Clinical application of this finding was carried out by RICHARDSON (27, 28). Chronic intermittent stimulation with 50 and 75 Hz produced good pain relief, outlasting stimulation by up to 20 minutes. Similar good results with intermittent electrical stimulation of the sensory thalamic relay nucleus by means of chronic implanted electrodes were reported by MAZARS (22).

Psychosurgical Procedures

In the beginnings of psychosurgery, it was found that in patients with unbearable pain, the suffering was diminished by frontal leucotomy, although the operation had no specific effect on the pain threshold itself (39). Searching for possibilities to replace the relatively rough method of frontal leucotomy by more selective lesions led to the method of resection of the cingulate gyrus (16) and later to radiofrequency lesioning of the cingulum bundle in the rostral cingulate gyrus (2, 6, 7).

Stereotactically, the cingulum interruption was performed bilaterally in the rostral third. The electrodes were situated just above the corpus callosum, not too far rostrally to avoid fronto-thalamic projecting fibres. Rostral cingulotomy does not cause analgesia, it reduces or removes the suffering in a way so that the patient no longer suffers from his pain. Postoperatively, there is little or no preoccupation with the pain. At the same time, the need for medication is diminished. However, the problem is, as usual, the indication as to intervention. Probably this decision is best made in conjunction with a psychiatrist. Appropriate patients are those with psychogenic pains or with pain of non-malignant origin or of a non-recognisable probably organic nature respectively, and when a strong emotional factor dominates. These patients show good pain relief for a longer period of time. In judging the operative effect, not the verbal complaints of the patients, but the actual behavior should be considered. Recently GUTIERREZ-LARA (9) reported complete pain relief in 10 of 14 patients. The remaining 4 patients at times needed some medication against pain. 6 of the patients were addicted to drugs; postoperatively they showed no withdrawal symptoms.

Another possibility of a selective leucotomy consists of a circumscribed destruction of fronto-thalamic fibres in the rostral part of the internal capsule. MARTINEZ et al. (21) reported such a stereo-tactic interruption of the fronto-thalamic fibres in the anterior capsule. During this procedure, it is possible to define the cranial and basal borders of the internal capsule by means of microelectrode recordings in order to delimit the lesions as exactly as possible.

Hypophysectomy

Surgical ablation of the hypophysis has a good effect on bone meta-stases as well as on pain. The pituitary can be destroyed by simple surgical means, semistereotactically with radioactive isotopes, or stereotactically by high frequency or cryolesions respectively as well as by implantation of radioactive isotopes. The method of pref-erence is usually personally determined. The stereotactic approach avoids all risks of open cranial surgery. By a simple transnasal, transphenoidal approach, radioactive isotopes can be implanted to de-stroy the pituitary as first reported by TALAIRACH et al. (36).

Final Remarks

Stereotactic interventions are performed for a symptomatic relief of unbearable pain:

(1) At the caudal nucleus of the spinal tract of the trigeminal nerve for pain relief in the trigeminal region.

(2) At the mesencephalic level, mostly against pain in the head and neck region.

(3) In the basal thalamus with an interruption of the specific as well as the subcortical pain conducting system to interrupt the systems of pain sensation and pain "feeling".

(4) In the pulvinar, where the mode of action is not yet known.

(5) In the thalamic dorso-medial nucleus to interrupt thalamo-frontal systems because of psychiatric indications. All thalamic target points are effective against all the pain states mentioned above.

(6) Above the thalamic level the interruptions are performed in the cingulate gyrus or,

(7) In the fronto-thalamic projecting systems, in the rostral part of the internal capsule for psychosurgical reasons.

(8) A special indication for pain relief is hypophysectomy in hormone-dependent malignant tumors.

There are basic reasons for being very careful with regard to the in-dications for stereotactic procedures in central pain of non-malignant origin because of the unfavorable long-term results. However, thera-peutic alternatives are lacking in such cases, so that the possibili-ty of a stereotactic operation should be discussed from time to time. On the other hand, the indication is given in cases of unbearable pain caused by malignant tumors because of the good immediate results. Indeed, such an indication should be considered more often than is now the case.

REFERENCES

1. AKIL, H., MAYER, D.J.: Antagonismus of stimulation-produced analgesia by p-CPA, a serotonin synthesis inhibitor. Brain Res. 44,
   692-697 (1972).

2. BALLANTINE, H.Ph., Jr., CASSIDY, W.L., FLANAGAN, N.B., MARINO,
   R., Jr.: Stereotaxic anterior cingulotomy for neuropsychiatric
   illness and intractable pain. J. Neurosurg. 26, 488-495 (1967).

3. BETTAG, W., YOSHIDA, T.: Über stereotaktische Schmerzoperationen.
   Acta Neurochir. (Wien) 8, 299-317 (1960).

4. CRUE, B.L., TODD, E.M., CARREGAL, E.J.A.: Posterior approach for
   high cervical percutaneous radio frequency cordotomy. Confin.
   neurol. 30, 41-52 (1968).

5. DOGLIOTTI, M.: First surgical sections in man of the lemniscus
   lateralis (pain-temperature path) at the brain stem for the treatment of diffused rebellious pain. Anesth. Analg. 17, 143-145
   (1938).

6. FOLTZ, E.L., WHITE, L.E., Jr.: Pain "relief" by frontal cingulumotomy. J. Neurosurg. 19, 89-100 (1962).

7. FOLTZ, E.L., WHITE, L.E., Jr.: The role of rostral cingulumotomy
   in "pain" relief. Int. J. Neurol. 6, 353-373 (1967).

8. FORSTER, D.M.C., LESELL, L., MEYERSON, B.A., STEINER, L.: Gamma-
   thalamotomie bei therapieresistenten Schmerzen. In: Schmerz
   (Hrsg. R. JANZEN, W.D. KEIDEL, A. HERZ, C. STEICHELE), s. 207-
   212. Stuttgart: Georg Thieme 1972.

9. GUTIERREZ-LARA, F.: Stereotactic cingulotomy: A rational and effective approach for causalgia (report of 14 cases). Exc. Med.
   293, 38 (1973).

10. HASSLER, R.: Die zentralen Systeme des Schmerzes. Acta Neurochir.
    pp. 1-10, 1. Europ. Neurochir. Kongr. Zürich 1959.

11. HASSLER, R., RIECHERT, T.: Indikationen und Lokalisationsmethode
    der gezielten Hirnoperationen. Nervenarzt 25, 441-447 (1954).

12. HASSLER, R., RIECHERT, T.: Klinische und anatomische Befunde bei
    stereotaktischen Schmerzoperationen im Thalamus. Arch. Psychiat.
    Neurol. 200, 93-122 (1959).

13. HÉCAEN, H., TALAIRACH, J., DAVID, M., DELL, M.B.: Coagulations
    limitées du thalamus dans les algies du syndrome thalamique.
    Résultats thérapeutiques et physiologiques. Rev. neurol. 81, 917-
    931 (1949).

14. HITCHCOCK, E.: Stereotaxic spinal surgery. J. Neurosurg. 31, 386-
    392 (1969).

15. KIRSCHNER: Die Punktionstechnik und die Elektrokoagulation des
    Ganglion Gasseri. Über "gezielte" Operationen. Arch. klin. Chir.
    176, 581-620 (1933).

16. LeBEAU, J.: La résection bilatérale de certaines aires corticales
    préfrontales. La Sem. des Hôp. de Paris 24, 1937-1942 (1948).

17. LEKSELL, L.: Stereotaxis and radiosurgery. An operative system.
    Springfield/Ill.: Ch. C. Thomas 1970.

18. MARK, V.H., ERVIN, E.R.: Stereotactic surgery for the relief of
    pain. In: Pain and the Neurosurgeon: A forty-Year Experience
    (eds. J.C. WHITE, W. H. SWEET), pp. 843-887. Springfield/Ill.:
    Ch.C. Thomas 1969.

19. MARK, V.H., ERVIN, F.R., HACKET, T.P.: Clinical aspects of stereotactic thalamotomy in the human. I. The treatment of chronic severe pain. Arch. Neurol. 3, 351-367 (1960).

20. MARK, V.H., ERVIN, F.R., YAKOVLEV, P.: Stereotactic thalamotomy. III. The verification of anatomical lesion sites in the human thalamus. Arch. Neurol. 8, 528-538 (1963).

21. MARTINEZ, S.N., BERTRAND, C., MOLINA NEGRO, P.: Alteration of pain perception by stereotactic lesions of the fronto-thalamic pathways. Abstr. 6th Symp. Inter. Soc. Res. Stereoencephalotomy, p. 26. Tokyo 1973.

22. MAZARS, G., MERIENNE, L., CIOLOCA, C.: Intermittent thalamic stimulations in the management of intractable pain. 25. Jahrestagung Dtsch. Ges. Neurochir., Heidelberg 1975.

23. MAZARS, G., PANSINI, A., CHIARELLI, J.: Coagulation du faisceau spinothalamique et du faisceau quintothalamique par stéréotaxie. Indication-resultats. Acta Neurochir. (Wien) 8, 324-326 (1960).

24. MAYER, D.J., WOLFE, T.L., AKIL, H., CARDER, B., LIEBESKIND, C.J.: Analgesia from electrical stimulation in the brainstem of the rat. Science 174, 1351-1354 (1971).

25. NASHOLD, B.S., Jr., WILSON, W.P.: Central pain and the irritable midbrain. In: Pain and Suffering (ed. B.L. CRUE), pp. 95-118. Springfield/Ill.: Ch.C. Thomas 1970.

26. NASHOLD, B.S., Jr., WILSON, W.P.: Central pain: an epileptic phenomenon. In: Special Topics in Stereotaxis (ed. W. UMBACH), pp. 112-120. Stuttgart: Hippocrates 1972.

27. RICHARDSON, D.E.: Thalamotomy for intractable pain. Confin. Neurol. 29, 139-145 (1967).

28. RICHARDSON, D.E., AKIL, H.: Pain relief by electrical stimulation of the brain in human patients. Exc. Med. 293, (1973).

29. RIECHERT, T.: Relief of certain types of intractable pain. In: Pain (eds. R.S. Knighton, P.R. Dumke), Henry Ford Hospital International Symposium. pp. 519-529. Boston: Little, Brown & Co. 1966.

30. ROEDER, F., ORTHNER, H.: Erfahrungen mit stereotaktischen Eingriffen. III. Über zerebrale Schmerzoperationen, insbesondere mediale Mesencephalotomie bei thalamischer Hyperpathie und bei Anaesthesia dolorosa. Conf. Neurol. 21, 51-97 (1961).

31. SCHVARCZ, J.R.: Spinal cord stereotactic surgery. Exc. Med. 320, 234-241 (1973).

32. SJÖQUIST, O.: Eine neue Operationsmethode bei Trigeminusneuralgie: Durchschneidung des Tractus spinalis trigemini. Zbl. Neurochir. 2, 274-281 (1937).

33. SPIEGEL, E.A., WYCIS, H.T.: Stereoencephalotomy. Part II: Clinical and physiological applications, pp. 206, 210-221. New York: Grune and Stratton 1962.

34. SPIEGEL, E.A., WYCIS, H.T., SZEKELY, E.G., GILDENBERG, P.L.: Medial and basal thalamotomy in so-called intractable pain. In: Pain (eds. R.S. Knighton, P.R. Dumke), Henry Ford Hospital International Symposium, pp. 503-517. Boston: Little, Brown & Co. 1966.

35. SUGITA, K., MUTSUGA, N., TAKAOKA, Y., DOI, T.: Results of Stereotaxic Thalamotomy for Pain. Confin. Neurol. 34, 265-274 (1972).

36. TALAIRACH, J., SZIKLA, G., TOURNOUX, P.B., BANCAUD, J.: La chirurgie stéréotaxique hypophysaire. Confin. Neurol. 22, 204-213 (1962).

37. TORVIK, A.: Sensory, motor and reflex changes in two cases of intractable pain after stereotactic mesencephalic tractotomy. J. Neurol. Neurosurg. & Psychiat. 22, 299-305 (1959).

38. WALKER, A.E.: Relief of pain by mesencephalic tractotomy. Arch. Neurol. Psychiat. 48, 865-883 (1942).

39. WATTS, J.W., FREEMAN, W.: Psychosurgery for relief of unbearable pain. J. Int. Coll. Surg. 9, 679-683 (1946).

40. WYCIS, H.T., SPIEGEL, E.A.: Long-range results in the treatment of intractable pain by stereotaxic midbrain surgery. J. Neurosurg. 19, 101-107 (1962).

41. YOSHII, N., TATSUYUKI, K.: Clinical and experimental studies of thalamic pulvinotomy. 6th Symp. Inter. Soc. for Res. Stereoencephalotomy, p. 203. Tokyo 1973.

Long-Term Results of Central Stereotactic Interventions for Pain

F. MUNDINGER and P. BECKER

The treatment of chronic pain and pain due to malignant tumours is one of the problems dealt with by functional neurosurgery. The traditional use of the cordotomy and tractotomy performed either with the percutaneous or the stereotactic puncture technique has been supplemented in recent years by direct, permanent radio-stimulation of interneuronal connections on the dorsal surface of the spinal medulla (so-called dorsal column stimulation). Apart from these procedures performed at the periphery, we have been carrying out stereotactic interventions on the structures of the central nervous system itself since 1952 in Freiburg. Beginning in April 1952 one of the authors (MUNDINGER) operated 137 patients with intractable pain (Fig. 1), by stereotaxy. The first such operation was performed on the primary sensory nuclei together with RIECHERT following a suggestion by HASSLER (5, 6, 7, 9). The proportion of operations for pain is small in relation to the total number of stereotactic operations: 5,112 of these were performed up till February 28, 1975 (1, 2, 10, 12, 13). The reason for this is that from the outset we have severely restricted the indications for central pain operations.

Essentially we differentiate three pain-conducting systems (5) (Fig. 2):

1) the spinothalamic system which terminates in the parvocellular ventro-caudal nucleus (V.c.pc) of the posterior thalamus and in the nucleus limitans (Li). After coagulation at these points, pain impulses can neither be transmitted further nor processed.

2) the lemniscus-medialis system or the thalamic reticular system which terminates in the caudal ventral nuclei (v.c.) and the lamella medialis (la.m.) and transmits unpleasant sensations in a cortico-pedal direction. The cortical representations are, however, of little significance for the experience of pain, as the cortectomies show (10).

3) the trunco-thalamic system (Ce.Pf) which is a non-specific system of secondary subcortical pathways for pain impulses to the reticular activating system, to the central grey matter and to the dynamogenous zone of HESS in the caudal hypothalamus. This system is important for the affective reaction to pain stimuli.

The pulvinar (PU) contains multisensorial impulses from both cortical regions (8). It is the structure responsible for integrating sensory perception and is activated by sensory stimuli. For the most part these stimuli pass via the dorsal column or, alternatively, via the antero-lateral tract and the mesencephalic formatio reticularis to the lateral pulvinar (11). Finally, the connection between the prefrontal cortex and the medial fascicular nucleus (M.fa.p.) is of therapeutic significance since it produces a change in the auto-representation of pain as well as in the emotional components of the pain experience. Interruptions are performed on these structures (9, 10) (see Fig. 2).

Assessment

We performed 63 operations on 35 patients whom we were able to observe post-operatively for a period of up to 14 1/2 years. Excluded here are the stereotactic interventions with coagulation of the ganglion Gasseri.

Fig. 3 gives a survey of the various diagnoses, the number of patients in each category and the number of stereotactic operations performed.

Phantom pain with or without causalgia is numerically the largest category, followed by trigeminal neuralgia - for the most part postherpetic with anaesthesia dolorosa - and by the thalamus syndroms. The other groups are composed of patients with chronic pain syndromes of other origins, such as the intercostal neuralgia caused by tabes dorsalis, etc. With the exception of the thalamic pain syndrome, one or more neurosurgical operations on the pain-conducting systems have usually been performed previously. The average age of the patients at the time of the first stereotactic operation was 59 years.

For our assessment we made use of the patients' health records with the results of post-operative examinations and catamnestic investigations. After more than 2 decades 20 of the 35 patients had died of causes not related to the operation.

The results are broken down in categories according to the positions of the lesions (Table 1). In the first column we find the cases in which lesions have been performed in the primary (specific) senso-motor nuclei, the small-cell ventro-caudal nuclei (V.c.pc) and the nucleus limitans (ncl.li); the second colums shows the cases of lesions in the secondary (nonspecific) senso-motor nuclei (the lemniscus medialis and trunco-thalamic system); and in the third column we have the break-down of the cases in which a combination of these loci was used.

We differentiate, moreover, between post-operative and long-term results.

The best results can be obtained for treating phantom pain without causalgia (Table 1) by making lesions in the non-specific pain nuclei as well as by combined lesions in the specific thalamic pain nuclei. In comparison, the patients who underwent coagulations in the primary senso-motor nuclei alone did not show as good post-operative improvement and in the course of further observation only registered moderate improvement.

For the patients suffering from phantom pain combined with causalgia, good results were achieved post-operatively with the combined coagulation, while long-term results showed only modest improvement for one patient following the combined coagulation. The patients with causalgias that had not responded to other methods of treatment reported good long-term improvement.

Thus, out of a total of 22 patients with phantom pain and causalgia, 17 or nearly 4/5 improved, 6 of them (approx. 1/3) showing good or very good results.

Table 1. Postoperative and late results depending on targets

Diagnosis		prim. sens.-mot. ncl		sec. sens.-mot. ncl		combined target	
		postop.	long-term	postop.	long-term	postop.	long-term
a) phantom pains and causalgia	a	3	–	4	1	6	–
	b	3	1	2	1	3	3
	c	–	4	1	3	–	4
	d	–	–	–	1	–	1
	e	–	1	–	1	–	1
b) trigeminal neuralgia	a	2	–	1	–	5	–
	b	1	1	–	–	3	4
	c	2	1	2	–	2	4
	d	–	2	–	3	–	2
	e	–	1	–	–	–	–
c) thalamic pain	a	1	–	3	1	1	–
	b	2	2	3	3	4	3
	c	–	–	3	4	–	1
	d	–	1	–	1	–	1
	e	–	–	–	–	–	–
d) other intractable pains	a	1	–	1	–	3	–
	b	–	–	2	1	–	1
	c	–	1	–	2	1	–
	d	–	–	–	–	–	1

a = painfree, b = good improved, c = improved, d = unimproved or worse, e = unknown.

For the most part, the patients with trigeminal neuralgia accompanied by anaesthesia dolorosa (Table 1b) showed good to very good improvement immediately following the intervention - which was a coagulation of the primary pain-conducting system or especially the combined coagulation of all 3 pain-conducting systems. However, here again, long-term results revealed that only the combination produced satisfactory results. Following coagulation in the primary senso-motor nuclei alone just half of the patients reported moderate to good improvement as compared to 80% of those treated with the combined procedure. Coagulation of the secondary senso-motor nuclei alone did not bring any long-term improvement.

Best late results in the thalamic pain syndrome were observed after combined lesions including the dorsomedial nucleus (4/5 remained improved). But after lesions of the secondary senso-motor nuclei 8/9 also remained improved, the dorsomedial nucleus being lesioned in 5/9 of the patients.

For the other conditions of chronic intractable pain (Table 1c), the post-operative results of 5 interventions (on 4 patients) where secondary and combined coagulations in the pain-conducting systems had been performed were very satisfactory. On a long-term basis, even the group with lesions in the non-specific system showed lasting improvement; however, the small number of cases in this group prevents an adequate assessment.

Summary

Long-term evaluation (up to 14,5 years) of 56 patients with intractable pain demonstrates that:

a) Combined coagulation of the primary and secondary senso-motor nuclei (in 2/5 additionally combined with coagulation of the medial nucleus) gives the best results with an over-all improvement rate in 4/5 of the patients; 2/5 of these show improvement ranging from good to pain-free.

b) Bearing in mind that these operations were performed as an *ultima ratio* after all other operative measures had failed, we may conclude that central stereotactic interventions for pain performed at the level of the thalamus and capable of extension to other systems such as the posterior hypothalamus (14) and the cingulum (10) represent a method which can even produce an effect on these patients.

REFERENCES

1. BIRG, W., MUNDINGER, F.: Computer Calculations of Target Parameters for a Stereotactic Apparatus. Acta Neurochir. 29, 123 - 129 (1973).

2. BIRG, W., MUNDINGER, F.: Computer Programmes for Stereotactic Neurosurgery. Confin. Neurol. 36, 326 - 333 (1974).

3. GUTIERREZ-MAHONEY, C.G. de: The treatment of painful phantom limb by removal of postcentral cortex. J. Neurosurg. 1, 156 - 162 (1944).

4. HASSLER, R.: Die zentralen Systeme des Schmerzes. Acta neurochir. (Wien) 8, 353 - 423 (1960).

5. HASSLER, R., RIECHERT, T.: Die Beeinflussung des Phantomerlebnisses durch gezielte Hirnoperationen. W. Internationaler Neurologenkongreß, Lissabon, 1953.

6. HASSLER, R., RIECHERT, T.: Indikationen und Lokalisationsmethode der gezielten Hirnoperationen. Nervenarzt 25, 441 - 447 (1954).

7. HASSLER, R., RIECHERT, T.: Klinische und anatomische Befunde bei stereotaktischen Schmerzoperationen im Thalamus. Arch. Psychiatr. 200, 93 - 122 (1959).

8. KREINDLER, A., CRIGHEL, E., MARINCHESCU, C.: Integrative activity of the thalamic pulvinar lateralis posterior complex and interrelations with the neocortex. Exp. Neurol. 22, 423 - 435 (1968).

9. MUNDINGER, F.: Die stereotaktische Unterbrechung der Schmerzbahn im Thalamus. I. Neurochirurg. Diskussionstag, Salzburg/Österr. 26. 10. 1968.

10. MUNDINGER, F.: Stereotaktische Operationen am Gehirn. Stuttgart: Hippokrates 1975.

11. RICHARDSON, D.E., ZORUB, D.S.: Sensory Function of the Pulvinar. 4th Symp. Int. Cos. Res. Stereoencephalotomy, New York, 1969. Confin. Neurol. 32, 165 - 173 (1970).

12. RIECHERT, T., MUNDINGER, F.: Beschreibung und Anwendung eines Zielgerätes für stereotaktische Hirnoperationen (II. Modell). Acta Neurochir. (Wien) 3, 308 - 337 (1956).

13. RIECHERT, T., MUNDINGER, F.: Stereotaktische Geräte. In: Einführung in die stereotaktischen Operationen mit einem Atlas des menschlichen Gehirns. (Hrsg. G. SCHALTENBRAND, P. BAILEY). Stuttgart: GEORG THIEME 1959.

14. SANO, K., MAYANAGI, Y., ISHIJIMA, B.: Results of stimulation and destruction of the posterior hypothalamus in man. J. Neurosurg. <u>33</u>, 689 - 707 (1970).

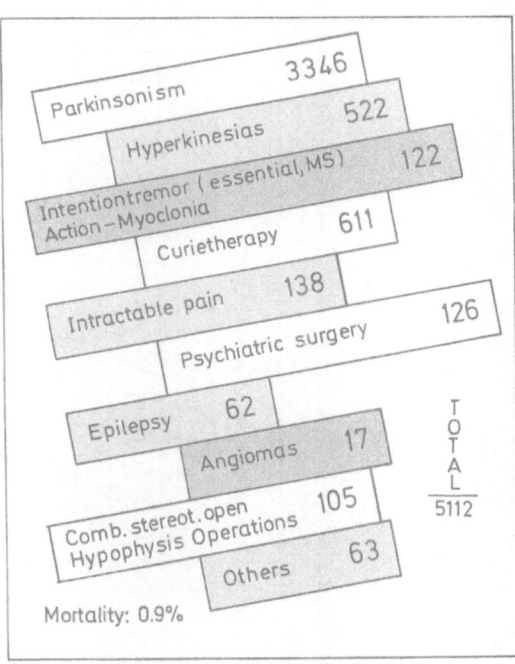

Fig. 1.
Number of stereotactic operations
1950 - February 28, 1975

241

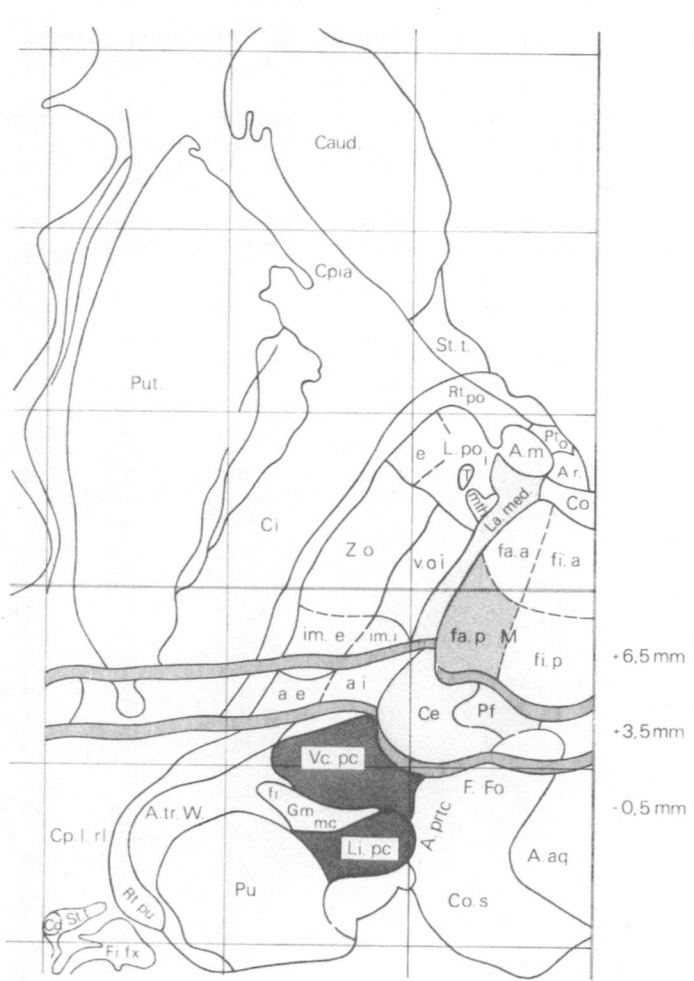

Caud.

Cpia

St. t.

Put.

Rt po

e L. po   A. m   Pt o

A. r

Co

Ci

Z o   v o i   fa. a   fi. a

im. e   im. i   fa. p M   fi. p   +6.5 mm

a e   a i

Ce   Pf   +3.5 mm

Vc. pc   F. Fo   -0.5 mm

fi

A. tr. W.   Gm mc   A. prc

Cp. l. rl.   Li. pc   A. aq

Rt pu   Pu   Co. s

Cd St.

Fi fx

Fig. 2.
Anatomic substrate
of pain thalamotomy.
Horizontal section
to the Ca-CP-level

Diagnosis	n patients	n operations
phantom pains	16	17
phantom p. + causalgia	3	3
causalgia	2	2
trigeminal neuralgia (anaesthesia dolorosa)	16	18
thalamic pain	13	17
other	6	7
Σ	56	64

Fig. 3.
Stereotactic central
operations of
patients with intrac-
table pain

Intermittent Thalamic Stimulation in the Management of Intractable Pain

G. Mazars, L. Merienne, C. Cioloca, and M. Prendeville

Prior to 1961, an extensive study of stimulation of the sensory pathways and sensory nuclei in man suggested the use of intermittent stimulation of the nucleus ventralis posterolateralis (VPL) in the management of some types of pain (1).

Since 1962, we have been investigating thalamic stimulation, in order to select the best parameters of stimulation and the criteria for selecting the patients.

In a first period, stereotactically implanted electrodes were connected through the scalp to an external stimulator for periods of several weeks, but, since 1972, implanted stimulators with built in batteries and a magnetic switch are connected to the electrodes. Bipolar electrodes with 4 mm between poles are placed in the VPL in a frontal plane 3 to 6 mm in front of the posterior white commissure. The distance from the midline depends on the localization of pain since the target is the somatotopic representation of the painful area; in most instances it ranges between 8 mm for the head and face to 10 mm for the shoulder and arm, and 14 to 16 mm for the leg.

The best criteria for a correct placement are obtained through electrical stimulation with 3 volts, 2 msec pulses, 20 Hertz: this should produce a sensation of light shocks, vibration or throbbing in the area affected with pain and nowhere else. Recording of action potentials, though interesting, cannot be used when the long sensory pathways are impaired.

At lower voltages, viz. between 0,6 volts and 2,2 volts, electrical stimulation is not perceived or produces just a feeling of light throbbing; yet, at these low intensities, stimulation during one to three minutes is able to result in "fading out" of pain. The most surprising fact is that pain does not recur when stimulation is discontinued; the relief of pain lasts for one hour to several days, and stimulation with the same parameters affords for a new and often longer period of pain relief. Implanted stimulators built to our specifications by BIOMEDIX deliver 1 or 2 volts impulses of 2 msec at a duration at a rate of 10 per second; a switch can activate the stimulator by holding a magnet in front it. The batteries can last for several years, owing to the low amount of energy used during the short periods of stimulation.

Electrodes are made of fine silicon coated gold wires, and the connections are made through miniature plugs.

Selection of Patients

Our experience concerns 44 patients studied over a period of 13 years; it enables us to draw some criteria for future selection of patients: *Thalamic lesions*, as might well be guessed, do not respond to posterior thalamic stimulation: an intact thalamus is a must to be pain free.

Tic douloureux or idiopathic trigeminal neuralgia has never been relieved, in our experience, with thalamic stimulation.

Compression of peripheral nerves or nerve roots and most forms of pain due to cancer are unaffected by VPL stimulation.

Amputation stumps are responsible for several types of pain:

(1) acute, sharp and non lasting pain produced by manipulation of the stump: this type of pain is best stopped by chordotomies and is not affected by thalamic stimulation.
(2) chronic, diffuse pain in the stump or in the phantom limb, not improved by section of the spino-thalamic tract, is relieved by thalamic stimulation and, in our opinion, by no other methods.

One of our patients had received an implanted dorsal column stimulator a year before: even high intensity stimulations producing unpleasant sensations in most of the body failed to reduce pain in the missing arm. From the very first thalamic stimulation, complete relief of pain was obtained for three hours and, since operation, the frequency of stimulations has dropped to 4 or 5 daily.

Altogether, 4 patients with diffuse chronic pain in the stump and/or phantom limb pain can be recorded as fully successful, although we had to remove the stimulator after 3 weeks in a case of severe acute osteomyelitis.

Post herpetic pain seems to be one of the most frequent indications although 2 of 7 of our cases were failures. However, 5 of our patients (including 2 aged 81 and 82!) have been fully successful: one needs only one daily stimulation and the others, two to four stimulations. These patients consider that a stimulation in time is able to prevent the recurrence of pain.

Peripheral nerve lesions include a caustic lesion of the sciatic nerve, an avulsion of several intercostal nerves and a "crushed foot"; all may be classified as successful, although arthralgias persist at manipulations of the foot in one case and will need a complementary chordotomy. *Traumatic avulsions of the brachial plexus*, responsible for causalgic pain and hyperesthesia or anesthesia dolorosa gave excellent results in three cases, although, in one, trouble with an earlier type of stimulator occurred after one month. *Postradiotherapeutic lesions* of the brachial plexus seem to respond well to posterior thalamic stimulation: 2 cases are fully successful, although an earlier case did not experience a noticeable relief of pain after a single stimulation of over 10 minutes; an uncorrect electrode placement is questionable.

Analgesia dolorosa following alcohol blocks (2 cases) and MONBRUN BENISTY syndromes (orbital pain following enucleation of eyeball) (2 cases) are pain free after 1 to 4 years, and one of them has discontinued stimulations for two years. One case of atypic trigeminal neuralgia also had an excellent result although the electrodes had to be replaced twice.

Paraplegias with diffuse pain in both legs and the lower part of the body are not uncommon; simultaneous bilateral implantations with one single stimulator has been performed twice with excellent result.

Vascular lesions at the pontine and penduncular levels are sometimes responsible for pain, often described as "thalamic". In these cases posterior thalamic stimulation works very well, and has provided an excellent recovery of motor function as well in one case.

It is noteworthy that posterior thalamic stimulations can stop pain only when it is related to a lack of proprioceptive informations, and have no effect on pain due to an excess of nociception as show the following examples:

- causalgia of pontine origin has been successfully relieved by thalamic stimulation, but an attack of gout required administration of colchicine to stop this new type of pain;

- scapular periarthritis required injections of corticoids in patients who had been relieved of their chronic causalgic pain from avulsion of the brachial plexus.

- radicular pain (S1) persists in one case of painful paraplegia successfully improved by thalamic stimulation;

- in a few instances, combined operations associating spinothalamic coagulation to intermittent stimulation of the VPL seems to be an almost perfect answer to cancer pain.

These facts apparently prove that electrical stimulation delivered to the VPL works as a substitute to physiological proprioceptive stimuli and fit well with the theory of HEAD and HOLMES. The need for an intact thalamus is an additional proof that MELZACK's gate theory is inadequate and that the integration level of pain is thalamic while "protection reflexes" are integrated at spinal and medullary levels.

Summary

Intermittent stimulation of the nucleus ventralis posterolateralis proved to be a worthy method of treatment of pain due to a lack of proprioceptive informations, such as pain following herpetic lesions, peripheral nerve lesions, avulsions of the brachial plexus, amputations or anesthesia dolorosa. It can be combined with interruption of the spinothalamic tract in cases where the two types of pain are associated, as happens in some cases of cancer pain. The implanted stimulators are reliable and can work several years without needing replacement.

REFERENCES

1. MAZARS, G., ROGĖ, R., MAZARS, Y.: Résultats de la stimulation du faisceau spinothalamique sur la physiopathologie de la douleur. Revue neurologique, 103, 136-138 (1960).

2. MAZARS, G., MÉRIENNE, L., CIOLOCA, C.: Stimulations thalamiques intermittentes antalgiques. Revue neurol. 128, 273-279 (1973).

3. MAZARS, G., MÉRIENNE, L., CIOLOCA, C.: Traitement de certains types de douleurs par des stimulateurs thalamiques implantables. Neuro-Chirurg. 20, 117-124 (1974).

Results of Stereotaxic Operations in Patients With Intractable Pain

A. STRUPPLER, C. H. LÜCKING, W. REISS, and W. HUBERLE

15 patients suffering from chronic, medically not controllable pain were operated on; in all patients stereotactic lesions were made in the area of the c.m., V.c.pc. and the medial lemniscus.

Lesions were made not only in the unspecific but also in the specific pain-conducting cortical systems.

Table 1

N° of patients	Cause of pain
2	pancoast tumor
6	metastasis of various carcinomas
2	intractable zoster neuralgia
2	plexus damage by X-rays
2	thalamic syndromes
3	traumatic spinal cord damage

The exact area of the stereotactic lesion was determined in 3 ways:
(1) by ventriculography,
(2) by recording of evoked potentials produced by cutaneous stimulation and
(3) by observations following intracerebral electric stimulation.

The sites of the stereotactic lesions in various planes are shown Figs. 1 and 2.
They were calculated from X-rays films made following the coagulation while the electrodes where still in place.
It has been shown in animal experiments that the average size of the lesion is between 2 and 3 mm.

Results

Complete pain relief lasting longer than 3 months was obtained only in 6 patients. In another 6 patients pain relief lasted 4 weeks and in 3 patients it was even shorter.

The etiology of the pain as well as its duration did not seem to influence the duration of pain relief in our 15 patients.

Discussion

In a previously reported series of 13 patients (1972), unilateral
lesions in the area of the c.m. and V.c.pc. produced pain relief of
shorter duration as compared to the last group of patients with more
extensive lesions.

The fairly short duration of pain relief may be explained by the
small size of the lesion and the by fact that they are unilateral.
We did not observe hypersensitivity to sensory stimulation following
lesions in the cortical pain systems, even in patients with thalamic
syndromes. This may have been prevented by the lesions in the c.m..

Summary

In patients with intractable pain in whom other surgical methods
such as percutaneous cordotomy cannot be performed, stereotactic lesions in thesspecific and unspecific pain systems are quite effective in obtaining a temporary pain relief.

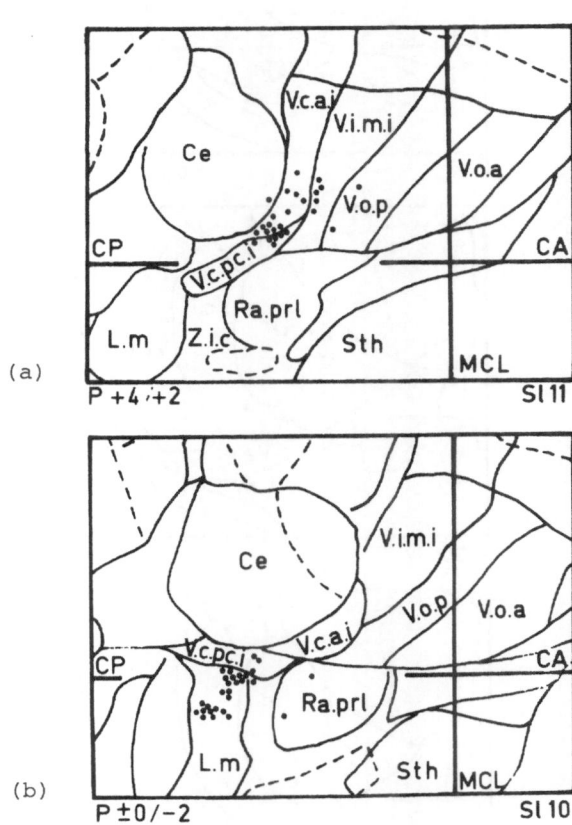

(a)

(b)

Fig. 1. a,b. Lesions in the lateral plane (according to Schaltenbrand
and Bailey, 1957). Positions of electrodes: P +4, +2, ±0, -2

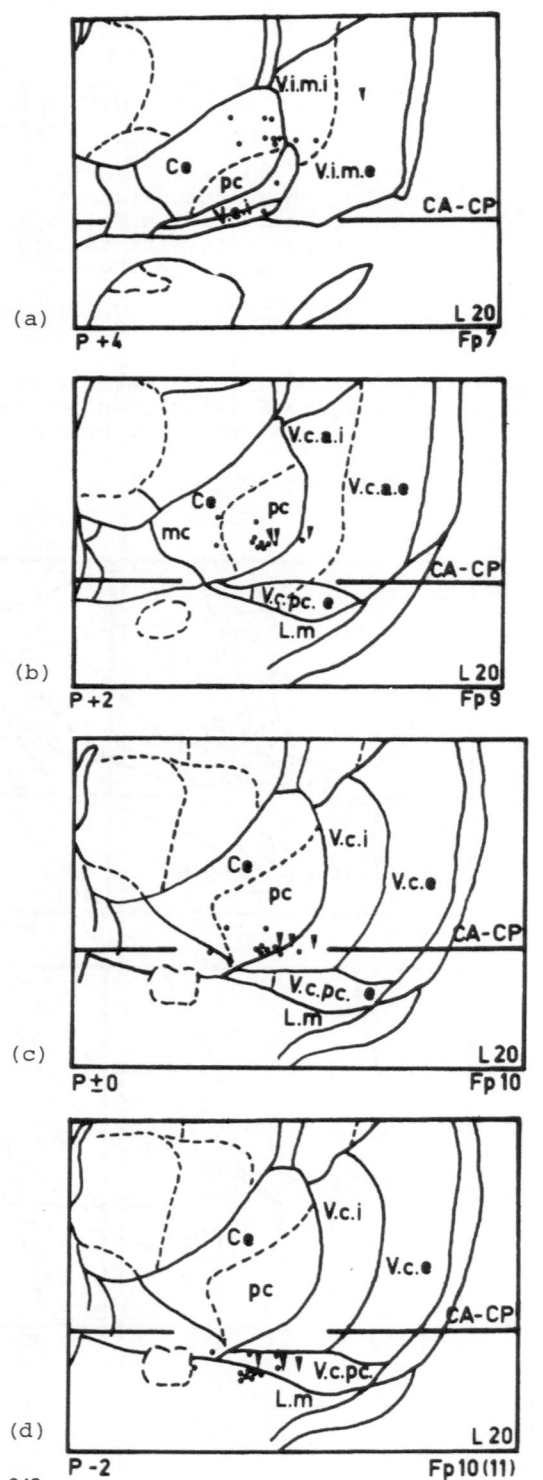

Fig. 2. a, b, c, d.
Lesions in the sagittal plane
(according to Schaltenbrand
Bailey, 1957). Positions of
electrodes: P +4, +2, ± O, -2
head and arm •, leg ▼

Cerebral Stereotaxic Operations for Pain

G. Bouchard, T. Fukushima, and L. F. Martins

For years we have given preference to cerebral stereotaxic operations for the treatment of pain, particularly in malignant diseases, not only because of their limited life expectancy, but also because of their good risks and short recovery period, especially when cachexia is present.

Our patients are divided in four groups:
(1) Malignant tumors of the head and neck.
(2) Malignant tumors of the upper half of the body (Fig.1).
(3) Malignant tumors of the lower half of the body (Fig.2).
(4) Severe anesthesia dolorosa, vascular thalamic pain syndromes (Dèjérine-Roussy syndromes) and phantom pain (Fig. 3).

In the figures, the four degrees of shading of the horizontal columns indicate the relief of pain. Interruption in the columns indicate a second contralateral operation. This was seldom necessary in cases of malignancy of the head and neck. The coagulated areas are given at the right margin of the diagrams. Three schematic drawings (Fig. 4-6) represent the different operative techniques, with steeper insertion of the elctrodes and the tendency to coagulate the median thalamic nucleus more medially and occipitally, to perform additional pulvinar lesions, and to restrict the coagulations in the median center and the subthalamic region. Only in the group of malignancies of the upper part of the body are better results not obvious in late cases. Perhaps this is due to a sudden stress from multilocular skeletal metastases. This also occurs even after an additional bilateral chordotomy. Spontaneous thalamic pain and anesthesia dolorosa can apparently be treated with success as shown by our limited number of cases. One patient was not operated on at our typical targets because of progredient vascular disease, and was, consequently, unsuccessful. Phantom pain did not respond.

The phenomenon of decreased emotional response to pain due to destractions in the median thalamic nucleus is also desirable in cases of pain due to non-malignant disease. There is , however, no obvious alteration even of differentiated personalities. Transitory acute organic brain syndromes occur seldom now, even after bilateral operations at an interval of about three weeks. They last no longer than the healing period of one week the patients usually spend in the hospital.

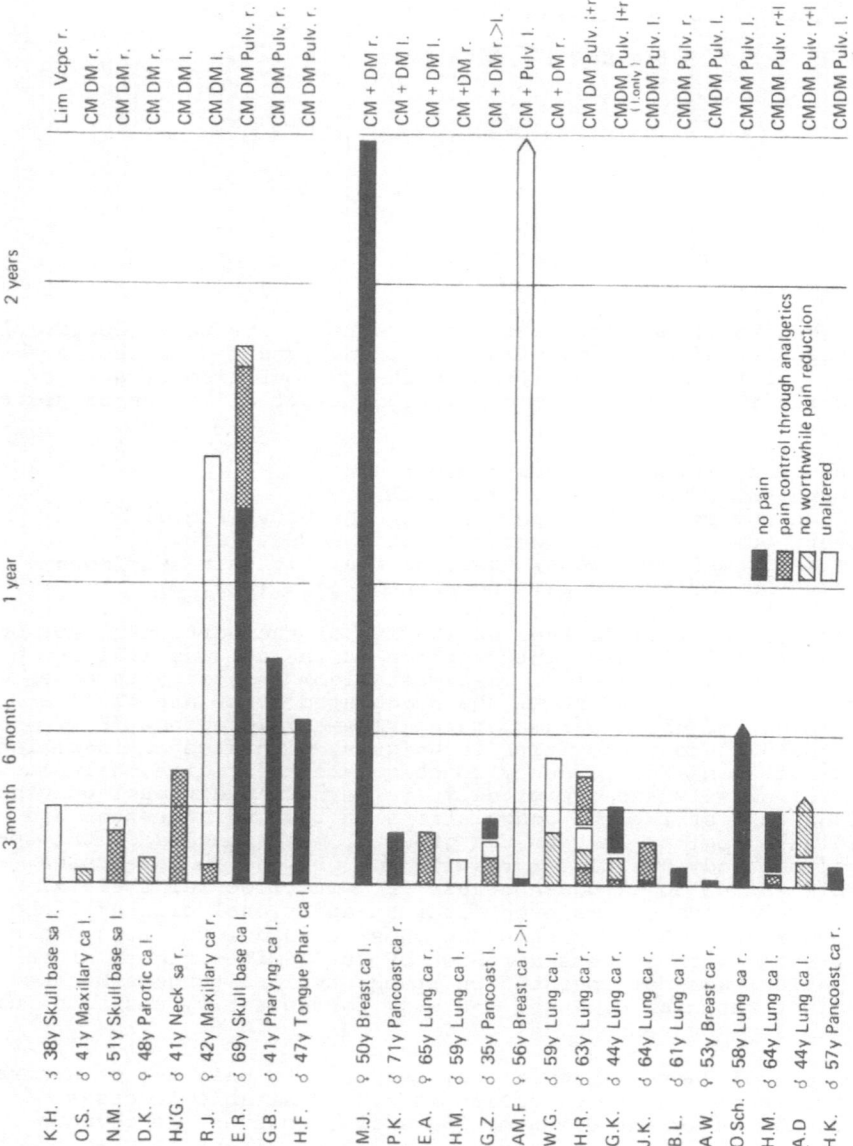

Fig. 1. Groups of malignancies in the head and neck and in the upper half of the body

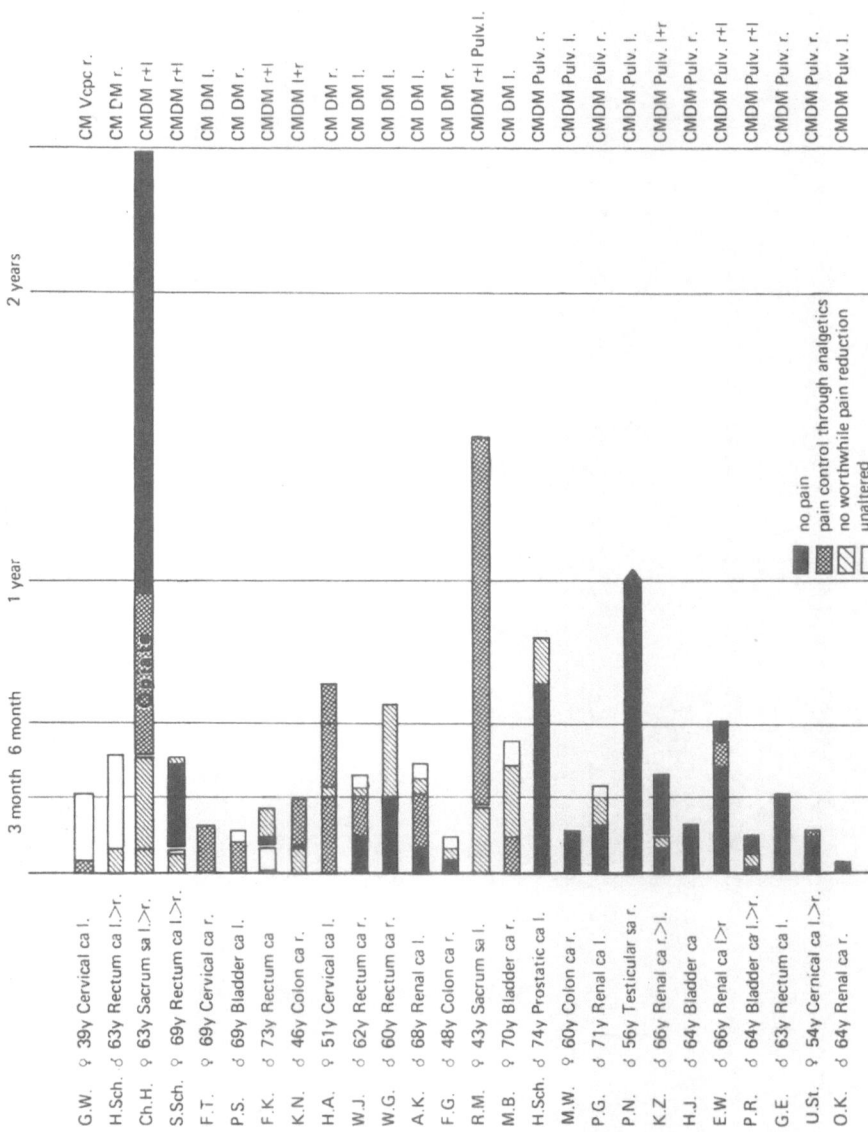

Fig. 2. Group of malignancies in the lower half of the body

251

252

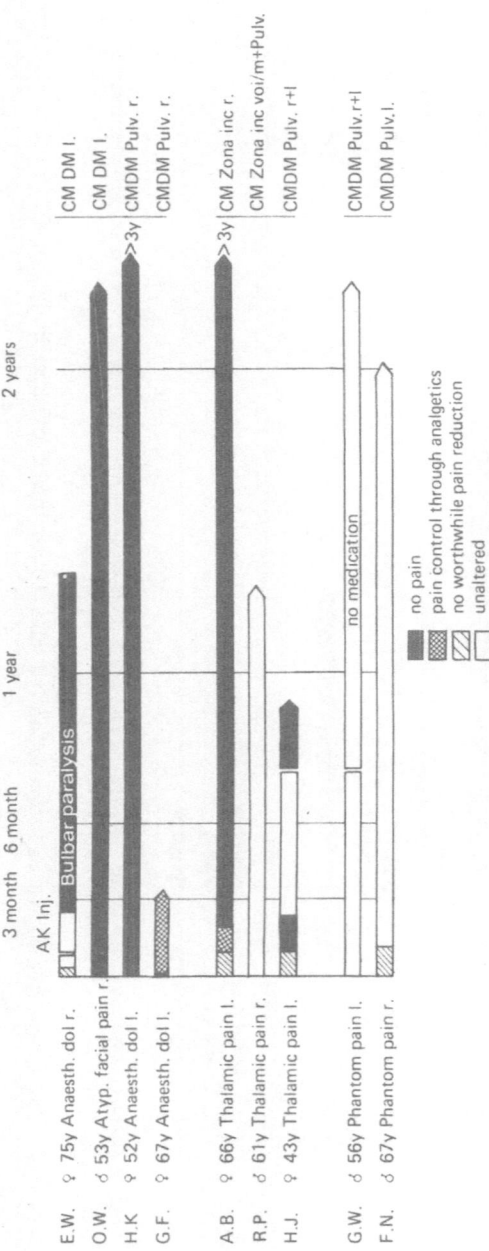

Fig. 3. Group of anesthesia dolorosa, thalamic pain and phantom pain

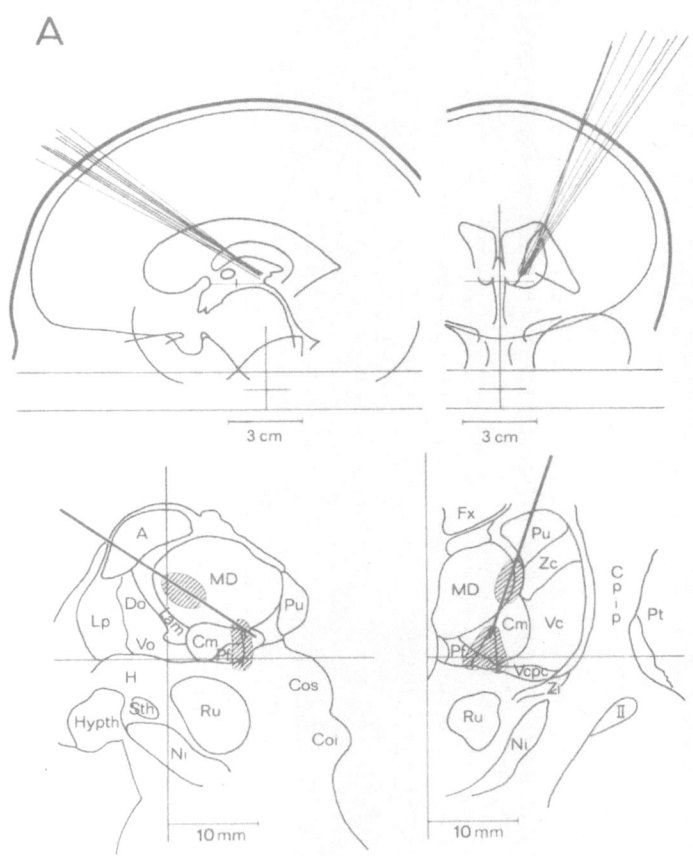

Fig. 4. Schematic drawings of the angle of insertion of the electrode on intraoperative X-ray pictures, and of the coagulations in corresponding atlas sections (Schaltenbrand-Bailey and Van Buren-Borke) in the former group of patients

B

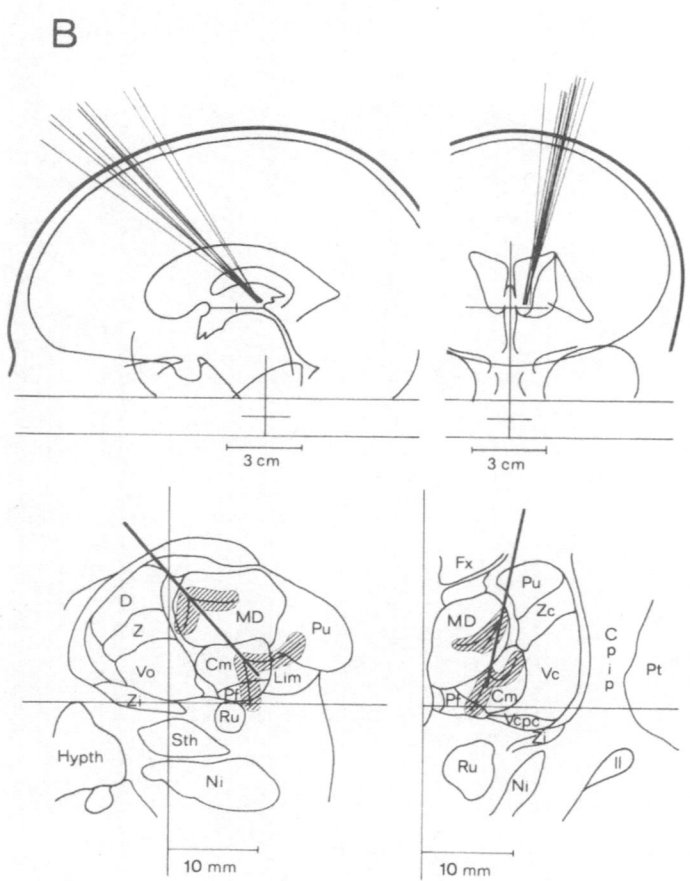

Fig. 5. Same as Fig. 4 in the following patients

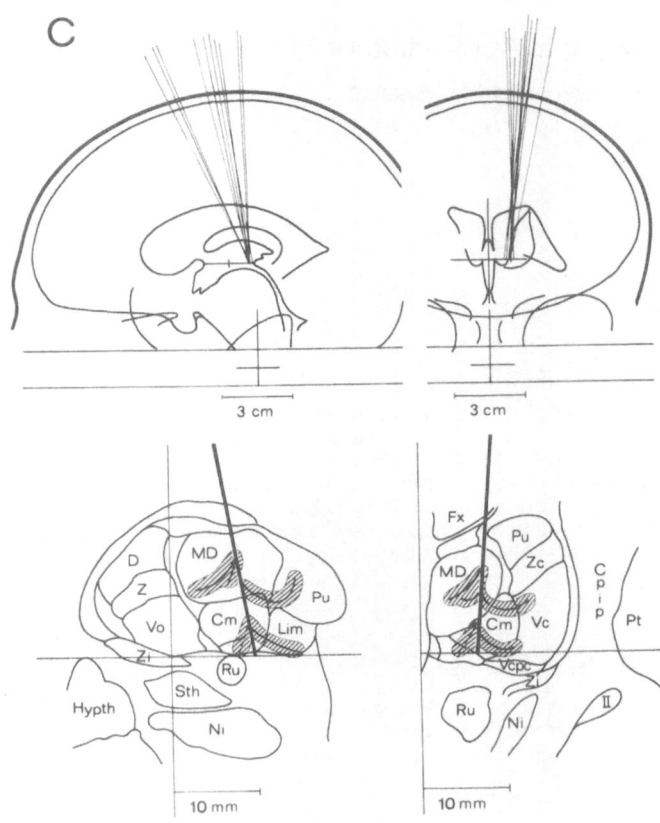

Fig. 6. Same as Fig. 4 in the late patients since 1974

Intrathecal Application of Phenol in the Treatment of Intractable Pain

A. KÜHNER and H. ASSMUS

Introduction

Nerve blocks for relief of intractable pain were first performed by DOGLIOTTI in 1931 by means of intrathecal injeciton of absolute alcohol. MAHER (1955) was the first to make use hypertonic solutions of phenol in glycerine and Pantopaque. Encouraged by the results of operative rhizotomy in symptomatic coccygodynia due to pelvic cancers (26), chemical rhizotomy seemed to us to be worth a trial in such cases, which, otherwise, give rise to important therapeutical problems.

Mode of Action of Phenol

Phenol in a watery solution of only 0,5% is a strong sclerosing agent producing severe nerve fiber damage (10, 23). Due to their rapid diffusion into the CSF, aqueous solutions cannot be employed for selective rhizotomy. Suspended in hypertonic agents such as glycerine or Pantopaque, the hygroscopic phenol cristals diffuse slowly into the CSF, creating a relatively high concentration near the hypertonic "vehicle" and, therefore, near the root to be destroyed. The diffusion rate of the agent out of glycerine is somewhat faster than from Pantopaque, so that phenol-glycerine is more effective at equal concentrations (4, 11, 20, 32). The usual concentration is 5,0%, that of phenol-Pantopaque 7,5%. However, higher concentrations up to 20% have also been used (9, 11, 12, 14, 21, 22). The diffusion rate of phenol was studied by NATHAN (21), who stated that immediately after injection the phenol concentration in CSF is very high and falls considerably within the first hour. This author also stated that the effects on nervous conduction begin 2 minutes after injection and are over within 10 minutes.

Clinically, phenol acts in two phases (16): there is an initial complete sensorymotor paresis by anaesthetic block lasting for about 15 minutes, followed by a definitive or chronic effect with pain relief without major neurologic disturbances. These facts as well as electrophysiologic studies (10, 20, 23) suggested the hypothesis that phenol may produce selective destruction of C-fibers. Histological investigations (2, 3, 4, 8, 9, 20, 27, 28), however, clearly showed that there is a non-selective destruction of all fibers. Superficial fibers are more affected than those within the root (3, 28). The histological findings generally consist demyelination, axon degeneration, and proliferation of Schwann cells.

Techniques

The puncture of the spinal canal is performed in lateral position at the level of the involved segment, with the affected side lowermost. Before injection into the cervical and thoracic areas the patient has to be turned about 45° backwards to ensure that the neurolytic agent will be in contact with only the posterior roots. In the lumbar region there is no spatial separation of anterior and posterior roots, so that the patient has to be turned about 45° ventrally to ensure filling of the radicular pockets. This is easy to perform when Pantopaque solution is used (Fig. 1).

Chemical rhizotomy of the sacral roots is done in the sitting position with the patient bent about 30° to the affected side. If bilateral rhizotomy is wanted the patient will be bent to the other side 5 minutes later and a second injection performed. The usual dose varies from 0,5 ml to 2,0 ml.

Indications

Phenol is mainly employed in cases of intractable pain due to cancer. An analysis of 596 published cases (Table 1) shows that pelvic cancers represent the most frequent indication. These lesions also have the most favorable results, while the results in cases of thoracic cancers or those of the upper extremities are less favorable. Chemical rhizotomies have also been performed in cases of chronic pain due to benign lesions. Pain syndromes of radicular, arthritic or spondylotic origin gave poor results, while pain associated with spasticity, and spasticity itself, offered good results in about 90% of the reported cases. Two cases of successfully treated phantom limb pain (4) which could not be influenced by previous cordotomy deserve to be mentioned here. A global analysis of 1365 published cases (Table 2) shows that pain relief by intrathecal phenol can be obtained in about 57%. Success rates in pelvic cancer are even higher (Table 1).

Table 1. Results of chemical rhizotomy in cancer pain

Localisation	Total nb	Complete relief %	Partial relief	No relief
Urogenital	291	66,6	22,5	10,9
Rectum	108	78,7	12,9	8,4
Pelvis + lower extr.	39	51,3	38,5	10,2
Abdominal	49	34,7	20,4	44,9
Lungs	88	57,9	20,5	21,6
Chest	16	62,5	12,5	25,0
Upper extr.	5	0	40,0	60,0
Total	596	50,3	23,9	25,8

Table 2. Global results of phenol blocks as reported in literature

Author	number	complete relief	partial relief	no relief
MAHER	253	178		75
PAPO	213	83	54	76
CIACOTTO	207	162	19	26
STOVNER	151	116		35
TANK	100	48	18	34
SWERDLOW	100	44	30	26
MARK	87	24	26	37
WHITE	63	31		32
BALL	51	21	17	13
LOURIE	47	6	14	27
BROWN	38	30		8
GORDON	37	19	13	5
KENNEDY	15	10		5
BERRY	3	0	0	3
Total	1365	772	191	402
%	100	56,5	13,9	29,6

The duration of pain relief is a very important point to consider.
The analysis of 156 reported cases shows that the effect of chemical
rhizotomy lasts up to 3 months in 60%. However, among these 60%, 25%
were pain-free for less than one week. Thus, a longlasting effect from
1 to 3 months could be observed in 35%. Another 20% had complete relief for more than 3 months, the longest follow-up being 2 1/2 years.
20% were pain-free until death.

Complications

It has been demonstrated that there are no toxic side effects on CSF
except a slight increase in albumin and cells within the first day
(21).

Important neurologic complications are rare. One case of lethal meningitis (27), Brown-Sequard-Syndrome (5) and 2 cases of paraplegia
(5, 21) have been reported.

Other side effects like incontinence, sensory loss, or paresis were
more frequent, especially within the first days. Thus, transient incontinence occurred in 12%, motor paresis in 11%, and sensory loss in
26%. Permanent neurologic lesions were seen in about 18%. Sensory
losses were the most frequent (15%), bladder dysfunction occurring in
2% and permanent motor paresis in 1%.

Material

We limited indications of intrathecal phenol to cancers of the pelvis except in one case. Thus, chemical rhizotomy was performed in 7 cases. Five of them had rectal cancer, another a collum cancer. The last case exhibited spastic pain in the left thigh. In most cases (Table 3), pain was situated in the sacrum and the perineum. Sometimes there was pain also in the dermatome S 1. Complete relief could be obtained in 2 cases with a follow-up of 2 and 3 months respectively. In 5 cases a partial but good result was obtained, but in 2, there were recurrences which did not respond to a second block.

Both these cases were successfully treated by percutaneous chordotomy. The complications observed were mostly transient (Table 4). In one case definitive incontinentia occurred. There were no motor losses but permanent sensory loss to pinprick occurred in 3 cases. Touch perception was never disturbed permanently. The typical two-phase action was seen in most cases: a large zone of complete sensory loss from (L 5) S 1 to S 5 with recovery of touch perception within 3 to 5 hours and recovery of pain perception within 4 to 6 hours. In 3 cases there was a permanent sensory loss to pinprick in the dermatomes S 4 and S 5 (Fig. 2).

Table 3. Own experience: etiology and results

Case	etiology	site of pain	dosis		complete relief	partial relief	no relief
1	rectum cancer	perianal	0,8 ml 1,4 ml	5,0% 5,0%	1 month 2 months		
2	rectum cancer	sacral	1,4 ml	5,0%		4 months	
3	rectum cancer	sacral S 1	1,0 ml	7,5%	3 months		
4	rectum cancer	sacral	1,4 ml	5,0%		6 months	
5	rectum cancer	sacral S 1	1,5 ml	7,0%		1 month	
6	collum cancer	L 5 + S 1	1,5 ml 1,5 ml	7,5% 25,0%		0,5 month	+
7	spasticity	L 2 - L 4	1,0 ml 1,8 ml	7,5% 7,0%		1,5 months	+

Conclusion

Intrathecal phenol is a valuable method for the treatment of intractable pain in selected cases. According to literature, however, its indications should be restricted to well-defined cases such as local and/or radicular pain in pelvic cancers. Thus, chemical rhizotomy may be an alternative to percutaneous chordotomy. On the other hand, we think that phenol may be used also as a supplement to chordotomy so as to avoid the high bilateral cervical approach for pain syndromes of the midline.

Table 4. Own experience: dosis and neurologic changes observed

Case	dosis		Disturbance of pain perception	touch perception	bladder
1	0,8 ml	5,0%	definitive	–	–
	1,4 ml	7,5%			
2	1,4 ml	5,0%	4 hrs	3 hrs	–
3	1,0 ml	7,5%	definitive	5 hrs	+
4	1,4 ml	5,0%	4 hrs	3 hrs	–
5	1,5 ml	7,0%	6 hrs	4 hrs	–
6	1,5 ml	7,5%	definitive	–	–
	1,5 ml	25,0%	–	–	–
7	1,0 ml	7,5%	–	–	–
	1,8 ml	7,0%	–	–	–

Summary

Indications, technique and results of chemical rhizotomy in cases of intractable pain are discussed. The authors conclude that intrathecal block with phenol is worthwhile in the treatment of pain due to pelvic cancers. It may be an alternative or sometimes even a supplement to chordotomy. The rate of side-effects is not higher than that of other methods.

REFERENCES

1. BALL, H. C. G., PEARCE, D. J., DAVIES, J. A. M.: Experiences with therapeutic nerve blocks. Anaesthesia 19, 250 - 264 (1964).

2. BAXTER, D. W., SCHACHERL, U.: Experimental studies on the morphological changes produced by intrathecal phenol. Canad. Med. Ass. J. 86, 1200 - 1205 (1962).

3. BERRY, K., OLSZEWSKI, J.: Pathology of intrathecal phenol injection in man. Neurology (Minn.) 13, 152 - 154 (1963).

4. BROWN, A. S.: Treatment of intractable pain by subarachnoid injection of carbolic acid. Lancet 2, 975 - 978 (1958).

5. CIOCATTO, E., MORICCA, G., CAVALIERE, R.: L'infiltration sous-arachnoidenne antalgique. Cah. Anaest. 15, 748-757 (1967).

6. DOGLIOTTI, A.M.: Traitement des syndromes douloureux de la périphérie par l'alcoholisation sous-arachnoidiennes des racines postérieures à leur émergence de la moelle épinière. Presse Méd. 39, 1249-1252 (1931).

7. EVANS, R.J., MACKAY, I.M.: Subarachnoid phenol nerve blocks for relief of pain in advanced malignancy. Can. J. Surg. 15, 50-53 (1972).

8. GORDON, R.A.: Intrathecal phenol block in treatment of intractable pain of malignant disease. Can. Anaesth. Soc. J. 4, 357-363 (1963).

9. HANSEBOUT, R., COSGROVE, J.R.B.: Effects of intrathecal phenol in man. Neurology 16, 277-282 (1966).

10. IGGO, A., WALSH, E.G.: Selective block of small fibers in the spinal roots by phenol. Brain 83, 701-708 (1960).

11. KHALILI, A.A.: Pathophysiology, Clinical picture and management of spasticity. In: Clinical anaesthesia, pp. 126-136. Oxford: Blackwell 1967.

12. KELLY, R.E., GAUTHIER-SMITH, P.C.: Intrathecal phenol in the treatment of reflex spasms and spasticity. Lancet 12, 1102-1105 (1959).

13. KENNEDY, W.F., AKAMATSU, T.: Subarachnoid block with phenol-glycerine for the relief of intractable pain. Anaesthesiology 24, 584-585 (1963).

14. LOURIE, H., VANASUPA, P.: Comments on the use of intraspinal phenol-pantopaque for relief of pain and spasticity. J. Neurosurg. 20, 60-63 (1963).

15. LUND, P.L.: Principles and practice of spinal anaesthesia, pp. 818-823. Springfield, Ill.: Charles C. Thomas 1971.

16. MAHER, R.M.: Relief of pain in incurable cancer. Lancet 1, 18-20 (1955).

17. MAHER, R.M.: Neurone selection in relief of pain. Lancet 1, 16-19 (1957).

18. MAHER, R.M.: Further experiences with intrathecal and subdural phenol. Lancet 1, 895-899 (1960).

19. MAHER, R.M.: Intrathecal chlorocresol in the treatment of pain in cancer. Lancet 1, 965-967 (1963).

20. MARK, V.H., WHITE, J.C., ZERVAS, N.T., ERVIN, F.R., RICHARDSON, E.P.: Intrathecal use of phenol for the relief of chronic severe pain. New Engl. J. Med. 267, 589-593 (1962).

21. NATHAN, P.W.: Intrathecal phenol for intractable pain. Lancet 1, 76-80 (1958).

22. NATHAN, P.W.: Intrathecal phenol to relief spasticity in para-plegia. Lancet 12, 1099-1102 (1959).

23. NATHAN, P.W., SEARS, T.A.: Effects of phenol on nervous conduction. J. Physiol. 150, 565-580 (1960).

24. PAPO, I., VISCA, A.: Intrathecal phenol in the treatment of cancer pain. J. Neurosurg. Sci. 12, 146-156 (1973).

25. PEDERSEN, E., JUUL-JENSEN, P.: Treatment of spasticity by sub-arachnoid phenol-glycerin. Neurology 15, 256 (1965).

26. PENZHOLZ, H.: Neurochirurgische Behandlung der Coccygodynie. Arch. Psych. Z. Ges. Neurol. 204, 163-171 (1963).

27. SMITH, M.C.: Histological findings following intrathecal injections of phenol solutions for relief pain. Brit. J. Anaesth. 36, 387-405 (1964).

28. STEWART, W.A., LOURIE, H.: An experimental evaluation of the effects of subarachnoid injection of phenol-pantopaque in cats. J. Neurosurg. 20, 64-72 (1963).

29. STOVNER, J., ENDERSEN, R.: Intrathecal phenol for cancer pain. Act. Anaesth. Scand. 16, 17-21 (1972).

30. SWERDLOW, M.: Relief of intractable pain, pp. 148-175. Amsterdam: Excerpta Medica 1974.

31. TANK, T.M., DOHN, D.F., GARDNER, W.J.: Intrathecal injections of alcohol or phenol for relief of intractable pain. Cleveland Clin. Quart. 30, 111 (1963).

32. WHITE, J.C., SWEET, W.H.: Pain and neurosurgeon, pp. 524-513. Springfield, Ill.: Charles C. Thomas 1969.

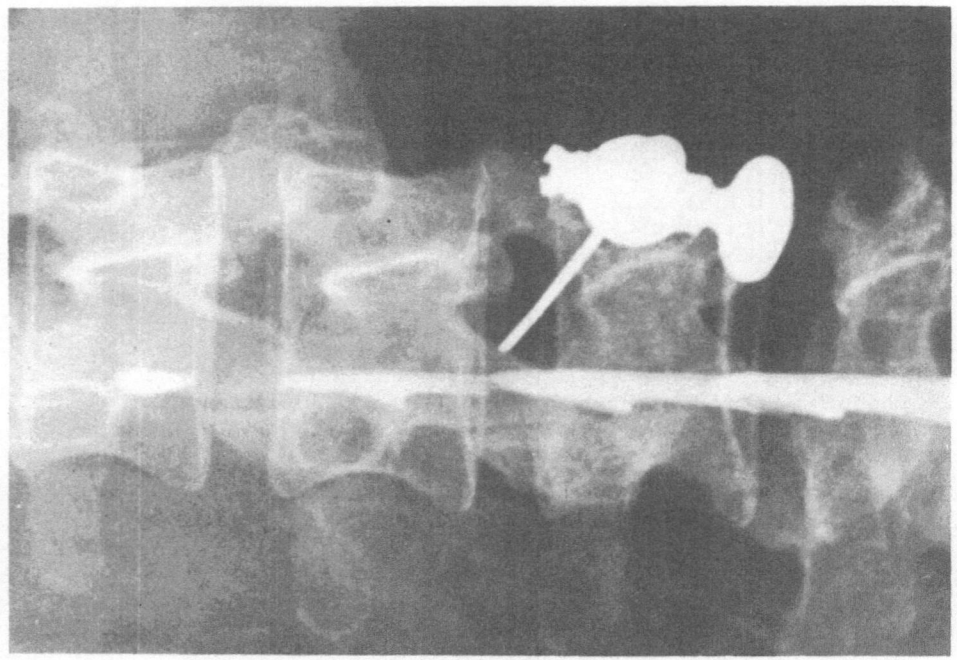

Fig. 1. Radioscopically controlled phenol-Pantopaque injection for pain at the dermatomes L 4, L 5 and S 1 (case N^O 6)

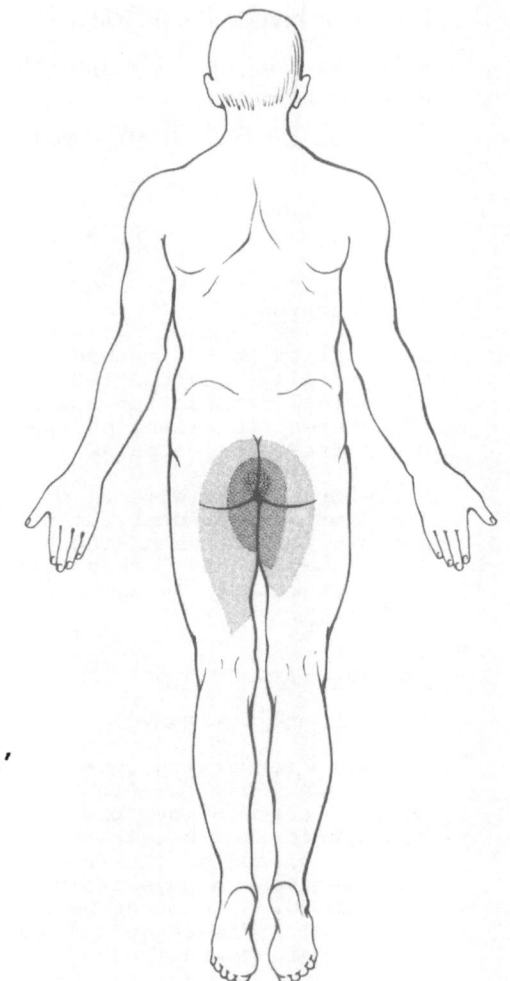

Fig. 2. Typical two-phase action on sensibility (case N° 3) 10 min ('), four hours (▮) and 48 hours (✿) after injection

Place of Hypophysectomy in the Neurosurgical Treatment of Pain

A Comparative Study of Surgical Hypophysectomy and Radio-Isotope Implants: Report of 124 Cases

CL. GROS, PH. FREREBEAU, J. M. PRIVAT, and J. BENEZECH

Introduction

In addition to the methods acting directly on pain pathways, either mechanically (destruction neurotomy, radicotomy, cordotomy) or by electrical stimulation according to WALL and MELZACK's theory, it is of interest to establish the place of hypophysectomy in the neurosurgical treatment of pain.

We report on the effects of hypophysectomy on pain due to metastases from hormonodependent tumours: breast and prostate. Our experience amounts to 128 cases since 1954. The effect of hypophysectomy on pain in acromegaly and Cushing syndrome due to pituitary adenomas will not be dealt with in detail, since their interest lies in their physiopathology.

Material and Methods

Methods and Their Evolution

Our experience with total hypophysectomy, for carcinoma metastases starts in 1954. The first 14 cases reported - MARTELLI thesis (20) - were of surgical hypophysectomy by frontal approach. 8 cases were metastasis from breast cancer. Since 1958, following the works of BAUER (14) and of TALAIRACH (29), surgical treatment gave way to radioactive hypophysectomy by means of intra-sellar implants of Yttrium 90. A comparative study of both methods was published in 1960 (10). Efficiency and uneventful postoperative course of the 2nd method were emphasized.

From 1958 to 1970 a series of 100 cases of radioactive hypophysectomy for the treatment of tumoral metastases has been carried out. We applied a simplified stereotactic transsphenoidal technique according to the GUIOT et al. (13) technique, modified by HARDY (14). 14 cases have since been operated upon by this procedure.

Results

Table 2 summarizes the first series of transfrontal surgical (group A) and radioactive hypophysectomies (group B) already published in 1960 (10) as well as those published in 1966 (11) (group C).

Table 3 contains details of the 20 cases of transsphenoidal surgical hypophysectomy carried out since 1971 (group C).

Table 4 gives the complications noted with the different techniques in the 3 series (groups A-B-C).

Table 1. Technical evolution and material

Technique	Cases	Period
S.H. (frontal approach) (Group A)	8	1954-1959
R.A.H. (Group B)	100	1958-1970
S.H. (transsphenoidal) (Group C)	20	1971-1974

S.H.   : surgical hypophysectomy
R.A.H.: radioactive hypophysectomy

Table 2. Results

	Group A S.H. (frontal) Breast: 8	Group B R.A.H.: 100 cases Breast: 92 Prostate:8		Group C S.H. (transsphenoidal) 20 cases Breast: 19 Prostate: 1	
Mortality (< 1 month)	3 (38%)	11 (11%)		2 (10%)	
Good results					
. on pain	5 (60%)	65 (65%)		15 (75%)	
. objective improvement	2 (25%)	9 (9%)		3 (15%)	
Delayed improvement	0	11 (11%)		2 (10%)	
Metastatic localization		solitary metas- tasis	multiple metas- tases	solitary metas- tasis	multiple metas- tases
Breast { Bone	7	12	55	3	15
Skin	0	12	22		2
Viscera	1	1	21	1	1
Brain	0	2	6		
Prostrate → Bone	0	8		1	

S.H.   : surgical hypophysectomy
R.A.H.: radioactive hypophysectomy

Table 3. Cases of transsphenoidal surgical hypophysectomy for pain due to metastases of breast cancer and prostatic cancer.

Case N°	Age-Sex	Cancer Primary	Metastatic	Pain	Previous Treatment	Associated Treatment	Improvement Survival	of pain	objective
1	26 F	Breast	Bone	Lumbar Dorsal	X-ray Therapy		8 months	+++	-
2	38 F	Breast	Bone	Inferior limbs	Halstedt +ovariec- tomy		6 months	+++	-
3	62 F	Breast	Bone Skin	Sternum	Mammectomy +Cobalt (Co) therapy		3 months	+	0
4	58 F	Breast	Bone	Hips++	Mammectomy +Co		4 months	+	0
5	48 F	Breast	Bone	Dorsal	Mammectomy Ovariectomy Co		> 3 months	+++	+ ↓skin infiltr.
6	44 F	Breast	Bone	Lumbar	0		> 3 months	+++	0
7	70 F	Breast	Bone	Lumbar sciatic	Tumorectomy +X raythera- py		15 days	+++	0
8	63 F	Breast	Bone	dorsal++	Tumorectomy + Xray	decompres- sive laminectomy fication (metal plate)	15 months	+++	+ ossific.
9	51 F	Breast	Bone	Lumbar	Halstedt +Co		4 months	+++	0
10	47 F	Breast	Bone	Lumbar sacral	Halstedt +ovariec- tomy		> 3 months	+++	0
11	48 F	Breast	Bone	pelvis++	Mammectomy + Xray therapy		3 weeks	0	0

12	49 F	Breast	Bone	fronto-orbital	Mammectomy ovariectomy + Xray ther.		2 months	+++	0
13	45 F	Breast	Bone +pleura	Diffuse to bones	Mammectomy + Xray ther.		> 3 months	++ (4th day)	
14	72 F	Breast	Lymphatic nodes	pruritus	0		10 months	++ (12th day)	0
15	69 F	Breast	Bone	Thoracic lumbar	Mammectomy + Xray ther.		> 8 months	+++	0
16	59 F	Breast	Bone	Diffuse to bones	Mammectomy + Xray ther.		> 7 months	+++	0
17	60 F	Breast	Bone	Lumbar sciatic	Mammectomy + Xray ther.		> 3 months	0	0
18	47 F	Breast	Bone	Neck	Halstedt + Xray ther. chemother.	Arthrodesis occipito-C2 (plate)	9 months	+++	+ ossific.
19	46 F	Breast	Bone	Neck	Halstedt Ovariectomy Xray ther.	Arthrodesis C2-C5 (plate)	1 year	+++	0
20	41 M	pros-tate	Bone	Pelvis	Prostatecto-my hormono-ther. chemo-ther.		>20 months	± transient improv.	0

Improvement of pain is evaluated by:
+++ : immediate good result.
++ : good but delayed result.
+ : incomplete or transient improvement.
0 : no result

Table 4. Complications

	S.H. (frontal) (Group A) 8 cases	R.A.H. (Group B) 100 cases	S.H. (trans- sphenoidal) (Group C) 20 cases
Exitus (< 1 month)	3 (38%)	11 (11%)	2 (10%)
Diabetes insipidus	8 (100%)	47 (47%)	16 (80%)
C.S.F. Temp	O	14((14%)	2 (10%)
Leak Perm	O	9 (9%)	1 (5%)

S.H. : surgical hypophysectomy
R.A.H.: radioactive hypophysectomy

Discussion

Several points must be discussed in regard to the results of hypophysectomy in cases of cancer.

Analgetic effects

a) *Subjective results are noted early postoperatively*. With pain relief comes a sensation of good feeling. This is observed in a complete and permanent way in 60 to 65% of the cases belonging to group
A and B. The percentage reaches 75% in group C. Most frequently,
favorable results on pain are obtained immediately, as soon as patient awakes from anesthesia. However, in 10% of our series, relief
was recorded between the 24th hour and 14th day (case N° 14 Table 3).

In 15% of these cases, a transitory improvement of pain without complete relief is obtained. This, however, allows an adjustment to the
major analgetic drugs administered, over a variable period, shorter
than in cases of complete relief.

The apparently better results of group C seem to be related to a better selection of cases, bone metastases alone, without visceral involvement, being more numerous in this group than in group B.

b) *Delay of action: Physiopathology*. It is surprising that the same
immediate results (10 times more frequent than in late improvement)
are obtained with radioactive or surgical hypophysectomy. If one considers the post-mortem data of TALAIRACH, SEDAN, SZIKLA et al. (29).
These authors, found a 90% pituitary destruction in 5 or 6 days, following Yttrium implants. One must, therefore, admit a "sideration" in
pituitary activity which is caused by the trauma of radioactive implants. We do not, however, possess sufficient biological proof
(early postoperative hormonal check) to support this hypothesis. A
very previous report (11) has shown the correlation between good clinical results and the degree of hormonal pituitary deficit as evaluated by hormonal tests one week after surgery. The same is confirmed
by many authors, namely LINQUETTE and LAINE (18), POMMATEAU et al.
(23), FORREST (9), JADRESIC et al. (15), BONIS et COVELLO (5). From
the physiopathological point of view, a relation must be established

to the results obtained by surgical or interstitial radioactive hypophysectomy (implant of Au 198) for pain in acromegaly and Cushing
syndrome provoked by secretory adenomas. Acromegalic arthralgia and
pain of the extremities (acromegalic rheumatism), as well as headache,
are relieved almost constantly and immediately. At the same time, objective improvement is noted; infiltration of teguments especially of
the hands, diminishes. In our series, this result is constant and supports similar results of other authors (6, 16).

In the Cushing syndrome (24, 16, 27), relief of osseous pain, due to
osteoporosis and myalgia, is less constant, incomplete and delayed.
Analysis of our series shows complete relief of pain in 15%, incomplete in 60% and none in 25%. Immediate postoperative pain improvement has never been registered.

These data lend support to the role of the growth hormone (GH) and of
Prolactine (LTH), both of close chemical structure, for the course of
pain in bone metastases from hormono-dependent tumours.

c) *Time of action*. Analgetic effects of hypophysectomy are variable
in duration, lasting from a few days to 4 years in the extreme cases
of our series. This surgical treatment does not prevent pain recurrence due to other metastatic localizations.

d) *Associated objective results* are appreciated on the basis of periods of survival, recalcification of lytic lesions, improvement of
cutaneous signs (regression or resorption of nodules), and of local
or regional signs (peritumoral and periganglionic edematous infiltration).

According to the technique used, roetgenographic improvement of bone
lesions and cutaneous signs occur in 9 to 25%. However, the objective
results seem essentially related to the group with longer period of
survival. In group A the 2 patients objectively improved have survived over a one-year period. In group B and C the same survival period has been noted in 15% of the cases. The mean survival period is,
however, longer in group C, especially for the range covering 3 to
12 months.

A case reported by DUFY (7), where hypophysectomy alone without de-
compressive laminectomy led to subtotal recovery of a metastatic paraplegia, demonstrates the objective effect of hypophysectomy.

One can conclude, in view of these reports, that in each group there
is a statistic relation between survival period and objective signs
of relief. In individual cases this correlation is not so marked. One
must also stress the fact that frequently efficient results in pain
relief are noted without alteration of objective signs. However, improvement of objective signs has never been recorded without relief
of pain. We do not want to discuss here the remission of the disease
as caused by hypophysectomy. This is difficult to establish on series
that do not allow comparison in their evolutive course. In our cases,
however, periods of remission of over 3 months are recorded in 50 to
60%, similar findings have been stated in literature, and in LUFT and
OLIVECRONA's report (19).

e) *Localization of the metastases*. Comparison of the 3 series (Table 2) shows a more marked subjective improvement in cases of bone
metastases alone. If viscera are also involved, the percentage of
subjective relief falls, as also shown. BONIS and COVELLO (5) reported 164 cases of metastatic mammary cancer treated by radioactive

hypophysectomy. The authors stated that incidence of subjective improvement was not higher than in any other secondary localization. However, subjective response to pain, mainly originated from bone localizations, is practically constant. However, this must not be the rule, as our case 14 (Table 3) reported an important subjective, though delayed, relief, although lymphatic node metastases were noted without bone involvement.

In our experience, and in other series (5), failures were predominantly observed in older women, post-menopausic forms and generalized visceral involvement. Prognosis in cases of isolated bone metastasis can not be based on localization and on radiological aspects.

f) *Nature of primary tumor*. Despite our small experience (9 cases), subjective signs of improvement are more pronounced in breast rather than in prostatic cancer. If comparison of immediate postoperative results is possible, improvement is frequently transitory: a few days to a few weeks, as also noted by SEDAN and HARTER (26) and by FERGUSON (8). The latter finds a lasting relief of metastatic pain in 45% of his cases. However, according to these authors, to STAUBITZ et al. (28), and to our own experience, subjective improvement (regression of perineal oedema, survival period) is more constant than in breast cancer.

Complications

A review of our results as related to the different techniques reveals a lower rate of postoperative mortality in groups B and C. It also indicates that surgical transsphenoidal hypophysectomy in cases of tumor and metastases is not more hazardous than radioactive hypophysectomy .

The incidence of diabetes insipidus is twice as frequent in cases surgically treated, while rhinorrhea is produced with the same frequency in radioactive hypophysectomy. Reoperation through a tranfrontal approach has been undertaken 7 times in group B and once in group C. Two other patients belonging to group B, who underwent surgery for obturation of a rhinorrhea, died of meningitis. Finally, radioactive hypophysectomy may provoke late rhinorrhea all the more serious since the patients are out of hospital control and care.

Indications

Pain due to isolated bone metastases alone of hormonodependent tumors (breast, prostate) presents the ideal indication for hypophysectomy by transsphenoidal approach. However, an associated visceral metastasis must not outrule surgery radically, all the more if it does not threaten short-term survival. Absolute contraindications are cases of hepatic involvement, multiple intracranial metastases with intracranial hypertension and pleuropulmonary impairment with latent cardio-circulatory disbalance.

In our opinion the ideal technique is the transsphenoidal approach. Results are slightly better and complications less frequent (late rhinorrhea) by this route. Radioisotope irradiation is conducted when the general condition is mediocre or metastatic diffusion is advanced.

This is the attitude we have adopted after reviewing our cases and the progress of our experience.

Associated surgical treatment

We shall not discuss the moment and indications for hypophysectomy as related to other endocrine-suppressive surgery (ovariectomy, adrenalectomy, orchidectomy), since this has already been done by others for cases of breast cancer (1, 2, 3, 21, 22) and prostatic cancer (17). Nevertheless, in accordance with ROY-CAMILLE (25), we want to emphasize the importance of decompression-fixation procedures, using a metal plate screwed to pedicles bridging the metastatic vertebral lesion and providing stability in special cases of vertebral metastases. We have applied this treatment in association with hypophysectomy in 3 cases (NOS 8, 18, 19, Table 3) and we have published elsewhere (12) the good results obtained thereby.

Conclusion

According to our experience, hypophysectomy has its place in the neurosurgical treatment of pain.

The ideal indication remains the metastases from breast cancer involving bones only, although visceral localization does not outrule this surgery radically, under specific conditions.

In prostatic cancer, relief of pain is obtained in a lower rate, but objective improvement is more frequent.

From the physiopathological point of view, comparison can be made with the results obtained by hypophysectomy for the treatment of pain in cases of acromegaly and Cushing syndrome. As compared to the subfrontal procedure and to the radioactive implants, the best approach remains the transsphenoidal route. Thus, the best results are achieved, and complications are less frequent. Moreover, material is obtained for pathological examination whereby some pituitary metastases have been diagnosed.

Finally, the association of surgical treatment with fixation of vertebral metastases by means of metal plates is reported as a complement to hypophysectomy in the relief of pain.

Summary

The authors report on 128 cases of hypophysectomy for treatment of pain in hormonodependent cancers. Three different techniques were employed: surgical hypophysectomy by subfrontal (8 cases) or transsphenoidal (20 cases) approach and radioactive hypophysectomy (100 cases). Breast cancer had better results as concerns pain relief than prostate cancer, but bone metastases of the latter showed better objective improvement. Pain relief was obtained in 60% to 75%. Transsphenoidal approach gave the best results and less complications and this is proposed as the treatment of choice. Despite the higher risk of rhinorrhea, radioactive hypophysectomy is considered as a valuable method in cases which otherwise present a high surgical risk.

REFERENCES

1. ATKINS, H. J. B.: Comparison and results of adrenalectomy and hypophysectomy for advanced cancer of the breast. LANCET 1, 1148-1157 (1960).

2. BARON, D.N.: Endocrine factors in the treatment of human cancer. West Africa M.J. 8, 125-126 (19).

3. BARON, D.N., GURLING, K.J., RADLEY-SMITH, E.J.: The effect of hypophysectomy in advanced carcinoma of the breast. Brit. J. Surg. 45, 593-606 (1958).

4. BAUER, K.H.: Über die Hypophysenausschaltung bei inkurablen Krebsfällen mit Hilfe perkutaner, intrasellärer Implantation von radioaktivem Gold. Langenbecks Arch. u. Dtsch. Z. Chir. 284, 439-446 (1956).

5. BONIS, A., COVELLO, L.: Hypophysectomie dans les cancers du sein. XVIème Congrès annuel de la Société de Neurochirurgie de Langue Française. Neurochirurgie 12, 169-186 (1966).

6. BONIS, A.: L'irradiation intersticielle hypophysaire dans l'acromégalie. Neurochirurgie 12, 274-290 (1966).

7. DUFY, G.P.: Hypophysectomy in the treatment of certain cases of paraplegia due to secondary deposits from carcinoma of the breast. J. Neurosurg. 30, 602-610 (1969).

8. FERGUSON, J.D., PHILLIPIS, D.E.: A clinical evaluation of radio-active pituitary implantation in the treatment of advanced carci-noma of the prostate. Brit. J. Urol. 34, 485-492 (1962).

9. FORREST, A.P.M., SIM, A.W., STEWART, H.T.: Pituitary function tests after radioactive implantation of the pituitary. Proc. Roy. Soc. Méd. 53, 84-88 (1959).

10. GROS, C., ROILGEN, A., VLAHOVITCH, B.: Hypophysectomie pour can-cer. Voie chirurgicale, voie stéréotaxique. Etude comparative de 28 cas. Ann. Chir. 14, 253-260 (1960).

11. GROS, C., VLAHOVITCH, B., FREREBEAU, Ph.: Considérations sur une série de 87 cas d'hypophysectomie radioactive. Neurochirurgie 12, 663-670 (1966).

12. GROS, C., FREREBEAU, Ph., PRIVAT, J.M., et al.: Les possibilités neurochirurgicales dans le traitement des métastases du rachis. Montpellier Chir. 20, 255-274 (1974).

13. GUIOT, G., THIBAUT, B.: L'extirpation des adénomes hypophysaires par voie trans-sphénoïdale. Neurochirurgie 1, 133-150 (1959).

14. HARDY, J.: Trans-sphenoïdal microsurgery of the normal and patho-logical pituitary. Clin. Neurosurg. 16, 185-217 (1969).

15. JADRESSIC, A.V., POBLETTE, P., REID, A., et al.: Therapeutic hypo-pituitarism induced by stereotaxic trans-frontal implantation of Ytrium 90 in patients with breast cancer. J. Clin. Endocrinol. Metab. 25, 686-697 (1965).

16. JOPLIN, G.F., FRASER, R., STETNER, R.: Partial putuitary ablation by needle implantation of gold 198 seeds for acromegaly and Cushing's disease. Lancet 12, 1277-1280 (1961).

17. JURET, P.: Traitement des cancers humains par les interventions endocriniennes. Paris: Flammariou 1962.

18. LINQUETTE, M., LAINE, E., FASSATI, G.: Conséquences hormonales et métaboliques des hypophysectomies chirurgicales pour cancer du sein. Actual. Endocrinol. 12, 209-225 (1963).

19. LUFT, R., OLIVECRONA, H.: Hypophysectomy in management of neo-plastic disease. Bull. New York Acad. Méd. 33, 5-16 (1957).

20. MARTELLI, F.: Premier bilan de l'hypophysectomie totale d'indica-tion tumorale. Thèse Montpellier 1960.

21. NETTER, A., GORINS, A.: Une observation de cancer du sein avec hypercalcémie; étude des effects de la castration et de l'hypophysiolyse. Sem. des Hôp. 38, 1712-1719 (1962).

22. PEARSON, O.H., RAY, B.S.: Hypophysectomy in the treatment of metastatic mammary cancer. Am. J. Surg. 99, 544-552 (1960).

23. POMMATEAU, E., POULAIN, S., COLON, J.: Le test à la Métopirone dans le cancer du sein en phase avancée, avant et après implantation hypophysaire è l'Ytrium. Lyon Médical 210, 1005-1117 (1963).

24. ROVIT, R.L., BERRY, R.: Cushing's syndrome and the hypophysis. J. Neurosurg. 3, 270-295 (1965).

25. ROY-CAMILLE, R., ROY-CAMILLE, M., DEMEULENAERE, C.: Fixation par plaques des métastases vertébrales dorso-lombaires. Nouv. Press. Méd. 1, 2463-2466 (1972).

26. SEDAN, R., HARTER, M.: Hypophysectomie dans les cancers de la prostate. Neurochirurgie 12, 202-208 (1966).

27. SCHAUB, C.: L'irradiation interstitielle hypophysaire dans la maladie de Cushing. Neurochirurgie 12, 241-273 (1966).

28. STAUBITZ, W.J., OBERKIRCHER, O.J., LENT, M.H.: Prostatic carcinoma - Ten year results. J. Urol. 939-944 (1954).

29. TALAIRACH, J., SEDAN, R., SZIKLA, G.: La chirurgie stéréotaxique de l'hypophyse non tumorale par les radio-isotopes. Neurochirurgie 12, 141-302 (1966).

30. TALAIRACH, J., BONIS, A., SZIKLA, G., et al.: Resultats de la radiothérapie interstitielle (Au 198 - In 122) dans 30 cas d'acromégalie. Presse Méd. 73, 473-477 (1965).

Percutaneous Differential Thermal Trigeminal Rhizotomy for the Management of Facial Pain

W. H. SWEET

Introduction

To discuss electrothermal destruction of the trigeminal pathways before the German Neurosurgical Society is truly to bring coals to Newcastle or owls to Athena. In particular one acknowledges the pioneering work of the Heidelberg Professor KIRSCHNER (4). More important for us today are the excellent studies of Professor SCHÜRMANN and colleagues (10), of STÖWSAND'S group (12) and the recent paper of our hosts MENZEL and your President Professor PENZHOLZ (5).

My hope that it might be feasible differentially to destroy the poorly myelinated fibers for pain, in the trigger zones in trigeminal neuralgia and in the painful facial areas in other intractable neuralgias, has led me to continue work begun in 1955 with the heat generated by a radiofrequency current. This is transmitted to a cannula-electrode whose tip lies preferably among the trigeminal rootlets in cerebrospinal fluid and behind the ganglion. This I first reported in my monograph on pain with Dr. WHITE in 1969 (22). The selective production of analgesia has usually been achieved as a consequence of the following aids: (1) Electrical generators of a precisely controllable heat source; (2) small thermistors measuring the heat developed; (3) neurolept anasthetics to keep the patient calm and cooperative for sensory testing; (4) ultra-short-acting Methohexital (Brevital) to produce brief unconsciousness during the painful parts of the procedure; and (5) patient application on only 5 - 10° C. increments of heating each lasting 1 minute or less. Even when Dilantin and Tegretol are giving not quite adequate relief at tolerated doses, many patients are unwilling to take the 1+% mortality risk and the larger risk of extratrigeminal morbidity entailed by open operation in the middle or posterior fossa. The fact that we can not offer a procedure with a mortality and extratrigeminal morbidity close to zero has led to an increasing influx of patients to clinics where this operation is done. In the last 23 months, for example, I have personally done 177 of these procedures.

I propose in this paper to describe what to some may appear to be excessively elaborate safeguards not only to keep the extratrigeminal morbidity near zero, but also to reduce the undesired intratrigeminal morbidity.

Clinical Material

My conclusion are based mainly on the 669 procedures on 570 patients which have been done at the Massachusetts General Hospital since I initiated the method in October 1965. The diagnostic categories and the number of procedures in each are shown in Table 1. I use the term

atypical trigeminal neuralgia, much as does TAARNHØJ (13), to describe
those patients whose paroxysmal pains occur on a background of continous aching or burning, or have other atypical features such as incon-
sistent provokability of the pain or spontaneous hypesthesia.

Table 1. Differential thermal rhizotomy

Diagnosis	# of patients	# of procedures
Typical V neuralgia	430	505
Atypical V neuralgia	54	58
Multiple sclerosis	16	22
Cancer	20	23
Post-herpetic neuralgia	3	3
Periodic migrainous neuralgia	8	9
Trigeminal neuropathy	3	3
Central pain	2	2
Post-traumatic neuralgia	16	17
Atypical facial neuralgia	18	27
Total	570	669

I shall depart from the usual policy in presenting a scientific paper
by first summarizing the results we and others have obtained with differential thermal rhizotomy in trigeminal neuralgia, and then indicating how we are trying to improve these results in all types of facial
pain. Table 2 shows the late recurrence rate. The longer the followup
the higher this is. THIRY'S figures (15) refer fo his entire series
from 1950 thru 1970. My 28% figure refers only to the 125 patients
followed for more than 4 1/2 years and up to 9 years. In the unusual
series of our host Professor PENZHOLZ (5) 315 cases were followed for
an average of 12.7 years with a relapse rate of 80%. 46.6% of these
occured during the first two post-operative years. Those operations
were done before the present refinement became available. Table 2 also
depicts the encouraging lack of significant morbidity and almost no
mortality which has been the feature of all reports. The only 2 deaths
in the series of NUGENT (6) and STÖWSAND (12) (not cited in the table)
occured in debilitated patients aged 87 and 91 years respectively from
pneumonia. To avoid this we use much less neurolept anesthesia and
prophylactic broad spectrum antibiotics in the ultra-frail patients.

Technique and its Rationale

I shall discuss only the features relevant to increasing the safety
and precision of HÄRTEL's anterior approach to the foramen ovale. It
is usually so easy by the free hand approach to enter this foramen,
that I use neither fluoroscopy nor special aiming apparatus. If this
tactic fails the oblique position of the head for fluoroscopy and a
film as suggested by WHISLER (21) and by ONOFRIO (7) are helpful. The
head is hyperextended if necessary and rotated 15 - 20° away from the
side of the pain. At times the foramen ovale is hard to make out in
any projection. A useful guide to it is the foramen spinosum. This
smaller opening in the denser sphenoid spine, is more readily identi-

fied by virtue of the contrast. In only one patient in the past 2
years has it been impossible for me to enter the foramen ovale. In
patients with either cancer, PAGET's disease or basilar impression in
whom the landmarks were destroyed, I have nevertheless been able to
make lesions in the ganglion or rootlets.

Table 2. Differential thermal rhizotomy

	# of pa-tients	# of proce-dures	Late recur-rence	Permanent extra V loss	Death	Corneal anes-thesia	Severe dyses-thesias
NUGENT	65	72		O	1	8%	4,6%
ONOFRIO	135	142	12%	O	O	7,4%	1,5%
SCHÜRMANN	285	351	5%	O	O		0,4%
SIEGFRIED	34	35		O	O		
SWEET	484	563	28%	O	O	5,1%	1,2%
TEW	205		12%	O	O	12 %	0,5%
THIRY	365	441	18,8%	1 hemi-plegia 1 XII	O	4,2%	< 3,5%
TURNBULL	41	44	12%	O	O	20%	2,4%

From the approach 2,5 - 3,0 cm lateral to the labial commissure there
may be 3 basal cranial openings other than the foramen ovale which
can enter. Fig. 1 shows a spurious oval foramen which may be formed
by failure of ossification of part of the wall of the intrapetrous
canal for the carotid artery. I have traversed this vessel and entered the intracranial cavity in a cadaver; thus far I have avoided
this in vivo. I have also entered the intracranial cavity in the posterior fossa on one occasion at which my initial cannula-electrode
placement yielded slightly pink spinal fluid. Stimulation at 0,6 V
with our usual 60 cycle square wave pulse of 1 duration caused a
sensation in the ipsilateral throat alongside the pharynx. Fig. 2 a
and b reveals that I had wandered into the antero-medial component of
the jugular foramen which represents its pars nervosa. In the 1 subsequent patient I have had with intractable vago-glossopharyngeal neuralgia I could enter only the pars venosa, the jugular bulb, despite
rereated attempts with the assistance of my neuroradiologic colleague
Dr. New. I mention this because one of you, knowing about this percutaneous route to the roots of cranial nerves IX and X, may be able to
do better. I also unintentionally entered on 5 occasions a small foramen anterior to the foramen ovale lateral to the base of the lateral
pterygoid plate not present in many skulls. DE ROUGEMONT (9) had described to me a similar experience, referring to the opening as a
"trou inominé". In the first patient in whom I did this, virtually
clear spinal fluid appeared after my tentative electrode placement.
Gradually increasing the electrical stimulation, I was in the 4,5 volt
range when a brief convulsive seizure occured with turning of head and
eyes to the opposite side. I then took a lateral radiograph which
showed the electrode tip athwart the profile of the anterior wall of
the sella. It had to be lying medial to the temporal lobe and lateral
to the cavernous sinus. This experience has led me not to use a stimulus above 1,5 volts since then. Intracranial entry thru this anterior
foramen led to no sequel in 3 patients. Fig. 3 a shows the position in
one of them. However, in the fifth patient treated only 1 month ago

there occurred the first neurologic deficit outside the trigeminal zone in the Massachusetts General Hospital series. I had just taken the film shown in Fig. 3 b when I noted proptosis of the ipsilateral eye. The eye was blind and the IIIrd, IVth and VIth cranial nerve functions were impaired. There was no change in any aspect of trigeminal sensation. The electrode was removed and within a few minutes vision began to return. To my great relief the entire deficit cleared within 2 days and I made the appropriate trigeminal lesion on the third day. It was a graphic demonstration of the way in which abrupt increase in pressure from bleeding near a nerve can cause immediate gross, though temporary, impairment of function.

On one other occasion, that time the electrode tip shown by the radiographs in a position usually excellent for a lesion, an arterial puncture was revealed by my withdrawal of the stilet. Prompt removal of the needle was followed by an uneventful lack of clinical change in the patient and no blood in her lumbar CSF. However, I elected to treat her by open operation.

The hazards of *vascular* injury from inserting a sharp electrode tip for a heat lesion are of course much greater than from using a needle to inject a chemical. For example, HARRIS (2) by 1940 had treated over 2500 cases of trigeminal neuralgia by intracranial alcohol injection and THUREL's (16, 17, 18, 19) series of such treatments for facial pain had reached 3000 cases by 1961 - with only modest numbers of extratrigeminal complications. Contrariwise KIRSCHNER's electrocoagulation methods yielded so many complications that the method fell into disrepute in some quarters. To decrease the chance of vascular injury - hemorrhage or thrombosis - I have always introduced a device of the smallest feasible diameter, a 20 gauge needle (outside diameter 0,89 mm). An 18 gauge needle has the much larger diameter of 1,23 mm. I am exploring the use of a more rigid shaft of 0,7 mm diameter. I think it may be important also not to insert a small sharp lesion-making electrode beyond the outer sheath needle, as is done by a number of neurosurgeons. One has no warning that the point may have penetrated a vessel wall e. g. the cavernous sinus, which would not bleed until after the heat lesion is made. APFELBAUM (1) has kindly given me a detailed account of a major sequel involving this tactic. Lesion making was underway following satisfactory reference of sensation on stimulation with a solid electrode extending 5 mm beyond the cannula when the patient became progressively less cooperative. He drifted into coma with a contralateral hemiplegia and ipsilateral dilated fixed pupil before the neurosurgeon could remove a large apparently intratemporal hematoma. The hemiplegia persists. THIRY (15) has also reported one permanent and one temporary hemiplegia in patients in whom an arterial puncture was done during the course of introducing the needle electrode. I have stopped the procedure when I have punctured an artery, returning to complete it another day. Thus far there has been no sequel. This totally elective procedure can be stopped at any second and we should not hesitate to use this advantage.

One patient with a unilateral hearing loss on the side of his provokable paroxysms of pain refused diagnostic studies until after his pain was relieved by a heat lesion. Vertebral angiogram disclosed a fusiform dilation of the basilar artery 5 cm long and 2 cm in diameter. The electrode tip had been about 5 mm from this huge vessel. I tell patients with probable *symptomatic* trigeminal neuralgia about this experience when they demand treatment without full diagnosis. Table 3 lists these and other intraoperative complications. The second patient with a seizure, severely ill with a collagen disease,

Table 3. Intraoperative complications

Seizure	2
Cardiac episode	3
Brief paralysis II, III, IV, VI	1
III (lidocaine)	1
Arterial blood (intracranial in 1)	7
Venous blood	16
Hematoma cheek	2

had it merely upon hyperextension of her head. The 3 cardiac episodes provoked no sequel. They include 2 with precordial pain and gave us a valuable warning to stop the procedure. When we encountered venous blood intracranially, presumably from puncture of the cavernous sinus, we replaced the electrode and continued the operation. One patient developed such massive hematomas in the cheek on 2 successive occasions that the procedure was terminated. There were many other minor hematomas in the cheek.

To increase our precision we do thorough sensory and electrical stimulation testing after each increasement to the lesion. The threshold sensory reponses to square wave pulses and to radiofrequency heating are checked each time since the reference of sensation may change. Prior to the first lesion we of course seek to have the sensation referred at each type of stimulus only to the division to be partially destroyed. As the lesion is increased stepwise most of that division's fibers may become unresponsive and the sensation be referred to a neighboring division. Especially when this is the first division we withdraw the electrode slightly or heat it again with greater caution. The crucial datum is the sensory testing after each episode of heating. In my last 158 procedures the sensory loss appeared in a division to which stimulus sensation was *not* referred in 9 patients when the stimulus was heat and in 8 patients when the stimulus was a square wave pulse.

The principal problem in avoiding *corneal anesthesia* has been the abrupt tendency for all sensation in the first division to disappear as one is seeking to complete a second division lesion or produce some higher analgesia because of a first division trigger zone or pain. To decrease the incidence of corneal anesthesia I have used the index of facial flushing, a change which may be striking, and gradually appears during the heating in over half of the cases while the patient is unconscious. Analgesia may not develop in the zone of vivid flushing so the sign may be a false alarm. However, it proved a true warning of evolving first division loss after much less than the usual one minute of heating in at least 5 patients in whom corneal anesthesia was averted. An even more reliable way to avoid major first division loss is to carry out the last lesion or two with the patient conscoius enough to moan, wince or describe sharpness upon pinprick. When vigorous jabs in the forehead no longer cause this reponse the heating is stopped. This is the most certain way I know to avoid corneal sensory loss. Table 4 compares our earlier and most recent results with respect to first division analgesia and corneal anesthesia. In the later group a higher percentage had some other syndrome than trigeminal neuralgia requiring the achievement of first division sensory loss. I am, however, disappointed that 5,7% of these later patients still had corneal anesthesia. The response to sensa-

Table 4. Corneal sensation

Operations	V1 analgesia intended	V1 analgesia unintended	Corneal anesthesia
First 353	8.0%	4.5%	8.0% (29)
Next 177	10.7%	5.7%	5.7% (10)

Other Postoperative Complications

Aseptic meningeal reaction	1
Dysphagia (preexistent hemiplegia on side opposite pain)	1
Anesthesia dolorosa	7
Analgesia dolorosa	6
Late temporal lobe abscess[a]	1

[a]A much more serious complication has just been reported to me. In this patient I had required 3 procedures within 5 days to secure adequate analgesia. Five weeks later there began lethargy, difficulty in concentration, and a contralateral hemiparesis including the face. Dr. Robert KNIGHTON removed a well encapsulated temporal lobe abscess 1 week later from which the patient made a good recovery.

tion of the cornea is so predominantly one of pain that there is a very fine line between an analgesic and an anesthetic cornea. At present I am trying to decrease the incidence of anesthesia here by settling for hypalgesia in the first division. This will of course increase our number of prompt failures. These occurred 37 times (5,5%) after our 669 procedures to date. The sensory loss was inadequate or receded in a few days and the pain recurred.

Other Post-Operative Complications

Table 4. The aseptic meningeal reaction with 712 white cells/cmm in the lumbar CSF, severe headache and nuchal rigidity lasted less than 24 hours. The dysphagia in 1 patient, with a pre-existent R. hemiplegia and hemi sensory loss and a global aphasia, was apparently related to bilaterally inadequate sensory cues for swallowing. He could always take liquids and the symptom gradually improved. Incidentally, it was possible to make a differential analgesia confined to the second and third divisions in this speechless man by observing his facial motor response to pin prick. I do not include *masticator weakness or paralysis* as a complication; this gradually or promptly recovers and causes no significant disability. I make no special effort to preserve the motor fibers except in persons with multiple sclerosis, in young individuals (who may have V neuralgia as the first symptom of multiple sclerosis), and those with bilateral attacks. A convenient way to check proximity to the motor fibers is to use single shocks which cause an obvious muscle twitch. A more lateral placement of the electrode is then necessary. I have always been able to avoid masticator paralysis given the above indications for taking the trouble to do so.

The principal complications in addition to the corneal anesthesia are *the disagreeable sensations related to sensory loss*. The severest form of this problem is of course anesthesia dolorosa, the denervation state in which the patient finds the constant sensations accompanying total numbness of an area intensely distressing or even intolerable. It was the hope that preservation of some touch sensation would eliminate this sequel to trigeminal rhizotomy which has led me to concentrate on the procedure described. As we study these patients postoperatively, however, it is apparent that there may be not only an *anesthesia* dolorosa, there is also *analgesia* dolorosa, a constantly painful state - even though some touch sensation is conserved. I have even had one patient whose trigeminal neuralgia was converted to a hypalgesia dolorosa. He could distinguish both touch and pin prick at high threshold in an upper gum but was grossly hampered in practicing law by a new, relentlessly constant, profoundly distressing feeling in that area unrelated to local stimuli.

Direct questioning of the patients after operation reveals a continuous spectrum of abnormal sensations from none through mildly and moderately to severely annoying. I have classified them as severe when they interfere with the patient's productivity or lead him repeatedly to seek help for them. There was severe anesthesia dolorosa in 7 patients, 4 of whom had trigeminal neuralgia, and a severe analgesia (or in 1 patient hypalgesia) dolorosa in 6 patients, 2 of whom had trigeminal neuralgia.

In a detailed analysis of postoperative sensation in 132 consecutive patients with at least some analgesia after this operation 60% were aware of some change in sensation; 12% were somewhat bothered by numbness and 25% were unhappy about other sensations. These were variously described as little electric shocks, stinging, windburn, soreness, cramps, pinching, itching, painful vibrations, scorched feeling, "a bug with wiry feet crawling in the lips" - etc. Eight had sensations referred to the ear - a blocked or queer feeling or a "film over the ear canal" related to the expected analgesia of the anterior wall of the external auditory canal as part of the third division loss. One of the 8 had a major roaring in the ear. Eight more had problems referred to the nearly normal sentient eye; in 4 it watered too much; in 1 it was too dry; in 2 it burned; in 1 it itched.[1]

SCHÜRMANN has also pointed out the high incidence of minor side effects from the procedure in patients *with trigeminal neuralgia*. 45% of his patients disliked the sensations in the analgesic tongue and 2% *bit their tongues*. In general 10% of his patients disliked their paresthesias and in 6% cold and wind irritated the face. Similar figures for incidence of paresthesias are reported by others: TEW (15%) (14), THIRY (10.9%) (15), TURNBULL (10%) (20).

I have sought to deal with this problem by 2 tactics. 1) Retrogasserian differential lidocaine block and 2) appraisal of the patient's subjective reaction to his sensory loss after each increment to the lesion during operation.

---

[1]RIFKINSON (8) has described to me a trigeminal neuralgia patient of his with a retrogasserian rhizotomy on one side about 6 years before, producing analgesia and anesthesia. A recent radiofrequency (RF) heat lesion for tic pains on the other side yielded analgesia without anesthesia in all 3 divisions here. The RF lesion on the second side has been followed by continuing profuse bilateral lacrimation persisting for several months. The tic pains remain relieved.

The incidence of dysesthesias in patients who do not have trigeminal neuralgia is much higher. In them, I now do initially a differential lidocaine block to give the patient a temporary sample of the facial sensations associated in him with the analgesic but non-anesthetic state. With the electrode cannula tip among the trigeminal rootlets as determined by the same technique as that for making a lesion, I have found that as little as 0.1 cc to 6 cc of 1% lidocaine were required to produce this analgesic state. Even if the sensory loss progresses to full anesthesia to touch it will usually recede through a state of analgesia to pin prick for 5-15 minutes so that the patient and doctor have a chance to determine if the constant or the paroxysmal provokable pains are relieved and the new sensations of numbness or paresthesias are acceptable. If as the analgesia clears, the patient is uncertain, the analgesic state can be restored with a few more drops of lidocaine and the patient can resume his introspection. The electrode cannula is inserted under Methohexital anesthesia but with no Innovar in order to decrease confusion from this latter chemical cause. Table 5 summarizes the results after such tests in the 8 disorders mentioned. No lesion was made in any patient unless he was satisfied with the relief of pain and the new sensations which replaced it after a block producing analgesia.

Table 5. Lidocaine block V rootlets

Pain diagnosis	# of cases	Acceptable relief with block	Needed no lesion	Relief with lesion
Atypical trigeminal	3	2	2	
Post-traumatic	4	3	1	2 of 2
Periodic migrainous	7	3	2	0 of 1
Acromegaly	1	1		1 of 1
Post-herpetic	4	1		V2 lesion not achieved
Atypical facial	19	6	No lesion yet in 2	1 of 4
Trigeminal neuropathy	3	0		
Hyp- or analgesia dolorosa	2	0		

The atypical facial neuralgias have remained our major bête noir. In our first series of 274 patients not one of the 14 patients in this intransigent group was relieved. We have submitted another 19 to preliminary lidocaine block. Only 6 of them were clearcut in describing relief; we made lesions in 4 of these. Only one of the four is a success. However, my hope that preservation of touch fibers in these patients would not only decrease denervation dysesthesias but preserve some pain suppressor mechanisms hypothesized by WALL and me to travelling in the large myelinated fibers has *not* been realized.

The second tactic I now use in all of the patients during the procedure is to ask their subjective appraisal of the annoyance of the sensations accompanying sensory loss after each increment to the lesion. Many are emphatic about preferring much more numbness in the hope of permanent elimination of their agonizing paroxysms. Others, though, are wary about the new sensations ans especially if one cannot provoke a bout of pain they prefer to settle for hypalgesia. Asking the patient to participate in the decision re the extent of his lesion leads to less dissatisfaction when the pain returns and less grumbling about dysesthesias. Of course the sensations during either a differential block or a lesion do not cover the gamut of those probably occurring later. We can assure patients that subsequent operations are no more difficult to complete than the original one. This makes them less uneasy about stopping with hypalgesia.

The degree of preservation of touch varies greatly — in some areas the threshold for a calibrated hair is in the 30 to 90 gram range and is more appropriately described as a sense of painless pressure. In skin analgesic to pin jabs, many patients, however, have touch thresholds only moderately elevated such that they localize most calibrated hairs of 1.2 to 5 g corresponding roughly to touch with cotton or gauze. The thresholds on the homologous normal side run from 200 mg to 1.5 g. The complaints of paresthesias tend to be worse in those with the severe loss of touch.

Results Re Pain

Trigeminal neuralgia. In the patients both in the typical and atypical categories with or without multiple sclerosis, the production of analgesia in the trigger zone relieves virtually all of them. I have seen only one exception to this — a man in whom I made over a 6 year period 6 radiofrequency lesions with only a year or less of relief each time, finally producing dense sustained trigeminal analgesia everywhere but the corner of the mouth. From trigger areas in the markedly hypesthetic upper lip, tongue and chin severe paroxysms could still be provoked. In addition he now had constant pain. At my operative exposure of the trigeminal nerve at the pons a convincing posterior indentation into all the trigeminal rootlets, but mainly the motor ones, by 2 branches of the superior cerebellar artery was seen. These branches could be displaced above and parallel to the trigeminal rootlets as described by JANETTA (3). I cut all but the most medial presumably motor rootlets, and the patient has been completely free of pain for the last 3 years.

The results in the 7 other types of facial pain deserve a more detailed analysis and will be described elsewhere.

Table 6. Preservation of some touch

	First 274 operations	My last 165 operations
Some touch throughout analgesic skin	68%	72%
Touch partially in analgesic skin	23%	25%
Analgesia and anesthesia coincided	9%	3%

Conclusions

The encouraging results of differential thermal rhizotomy in the treatment of trigeminal neuralgia can be improved and the technique applied to selected patients in other categories of facial pain by (1) diagnosis of and prophylaxis for potential medical problems especially in the very frail; (2) the use of an electrode of minimal diameter with a lumen extending to its tip; (3) careful attention to the initial trajectory of the electrode shaft; (4) repeated monitoring by radiographs of electrode placement, and of lesion evolution by thermistor readings, 2 forms of the areas of facial flushing, and the patient's own report of his sensory loss and dysesthesias; (5) completion of the lesion in critical areas with the patient semiconscious and undergoing continuous testing with pin pricks; (6) acceptance of severe hypalgesia as the therapeutic goal in those patients who agree; (7) a preliminary trial of differential lidocaine block in the trigeminal rootlets in those patients with facial pain who do not have trigeminal neuralgia.

REFERENCES

1. APFELBAUM, R.I.: personal communication 1974.

2. HARRIS, W.: An analysis of 1433 cases of paroxysmal trigeminal neuralgia (trigeminal-tic) and the end-results of Gasserian alcohol injection. Brain 63, 209 - 224 (1940).

3. JANETTA, P.: Personal communication 1974.

4. KIRSCHNER, M.: Zur Elektrochirurgie. Arch. Klin. Chir. 167, 761 - 768 (1931).

5. MENZEL, J., PIOTROWSKI, W., PENZHOLZ, H.: Long-term results of Gasserian ganglion electrocoagulation. J. Neurosurg. 42, 40 - 143 (1975).

6. NUGENT, G.R., BERRY, B.: Trigeminal neuralgia treated with percutaneous radiofrequency lesions. J. Neurosurg. 40, 517 - 523 (1974).

7. ONOFRIO, B.M.: Radiofrequency percutaneous Gasserian ganglion lesions. Results in 140 patients with trigeminal pain. J. Neurosurg. 42, 132 - 139 (1975).

8. RIFKINSON, N.: Personal communication 1974.

9. DE ROUGEMONT, J.: Personal communication 1973.

10. SCHÜRMANN, K., BUTZ, M., BROCK, M.: Temporal retrogasserian resection of trigeminal root versus controlled elective persutaneous electrocoagulation of the ganglion of Gasser in the treatment of trigeminal neuralgia. Report on a series of 531 cases. Acta Neurochir. (Wien) 26, 33 - 35 (1972).

11. SIEGFRIED, J.: Un nouveau traitement neurochirurgical de la névralgie du trijumeau: analgésie sans anesthésie. Neuro-Chirurgie 19, 585 - 587 (1973).

12. STÖWSAND, D., MARKAKIS, E., LAUBNER, P.: Zur Elektrokoagulation des Ganglion Gasseri bei der idiopathischen Trigeminus-Neuralgie. Nervenarzt 44, 44 - 47 (1973).

13. TAARNHØJ, P.: Decompression of the trigeminal root. J. Neurosurg. 11, 299 - 305 (1954).

14. TEW, J., MAYFIELD, F.: Trigeminal neuralgia: A new surgical approach. (Percutaneous electrocoagulation of the trigeminal nerve.) Laryngoscope 83, 1096 - 1101 (1973).

15. THIRY, S., HOTERMANS, J.M.: Traitement de la névralgie essentielle du trijumeau per stéreotaxie et electrocoagulation partielle sélective du ganglion de Gasser. Expérience portant sur 365 cas traités entre 1950 et 1970. Neuro-Chirurgie 20, 55 - 60 (1974).

16. THUREL, R.: Névralgie faciale et alcoolisation du ganglion de Gasser. Sem. Ther. 37, 608 - 610 (1961a) also Reve. Neurol. 104, 75 - 77 (1961a).

17. THUREL, R.: Alcoolisation du ganglion de Gasser et diffusion de l'alcool aux formations nerveuses du voisinage. Rev. Neurol. 104, 78 - 79 (1961b).

18. THUREL, R.: Névralgie faciale et sclérose en plaques. Rev. Neurol. 105, 346 - 347 (1961e).

19. THUREL, R.: Névralgie faciale et névrite du trijumeau. Rev. Neurol. 105, 347 - 349 (1961f).

20. TURNBULL, I.: Percuntaneous rhizotomy for trigeminal neuralgia. Surg. Neurol. 2, 385 - 392 (1974).

21. WHISLER, W., HILL, B.J.: A simplified technique for injection of the Gasserian ganglion, using the fluoroscope for localization. Neurochirurgie 15, 167-172 (1972).

22. WHITE, J.C., SWEET, W.H.: Pain and the Neurosurgeon. A Forty Year Experience. Springfield I11.: Charles C. Thomas 1969.

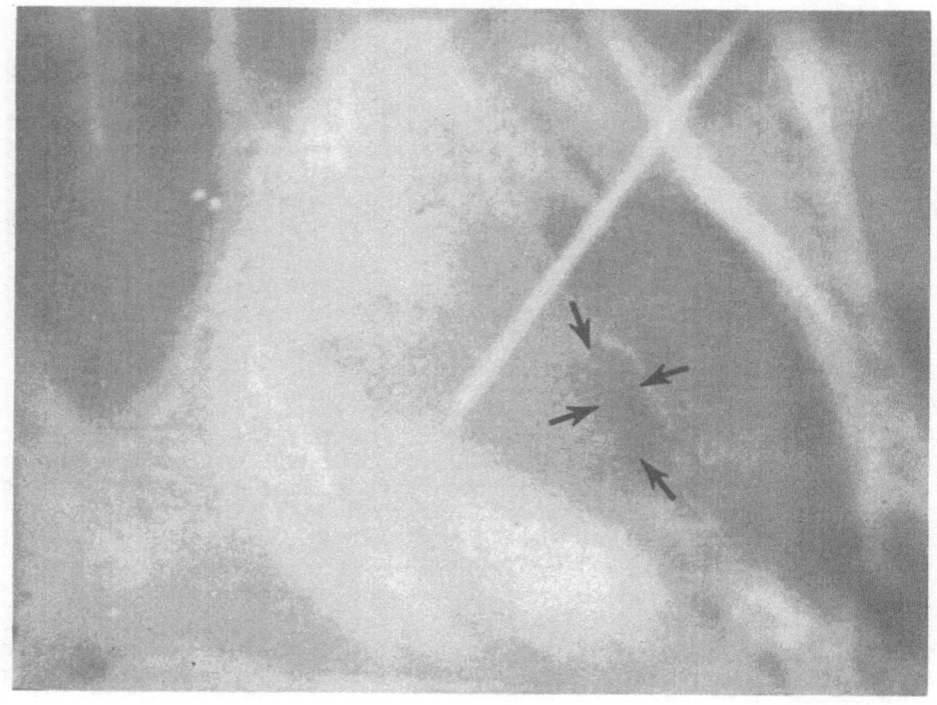

Fig. 1. Electrode traverses foramen ovale. Posterior to this is a larger oval foramen (arrows) due to incomplete ossification of the canal for the intrapetrous internal carotid artery. This is an inconstant but dangerous route to the intracranial cavity. (Courtesy J. Neurosurg. 39: 146, 1974)

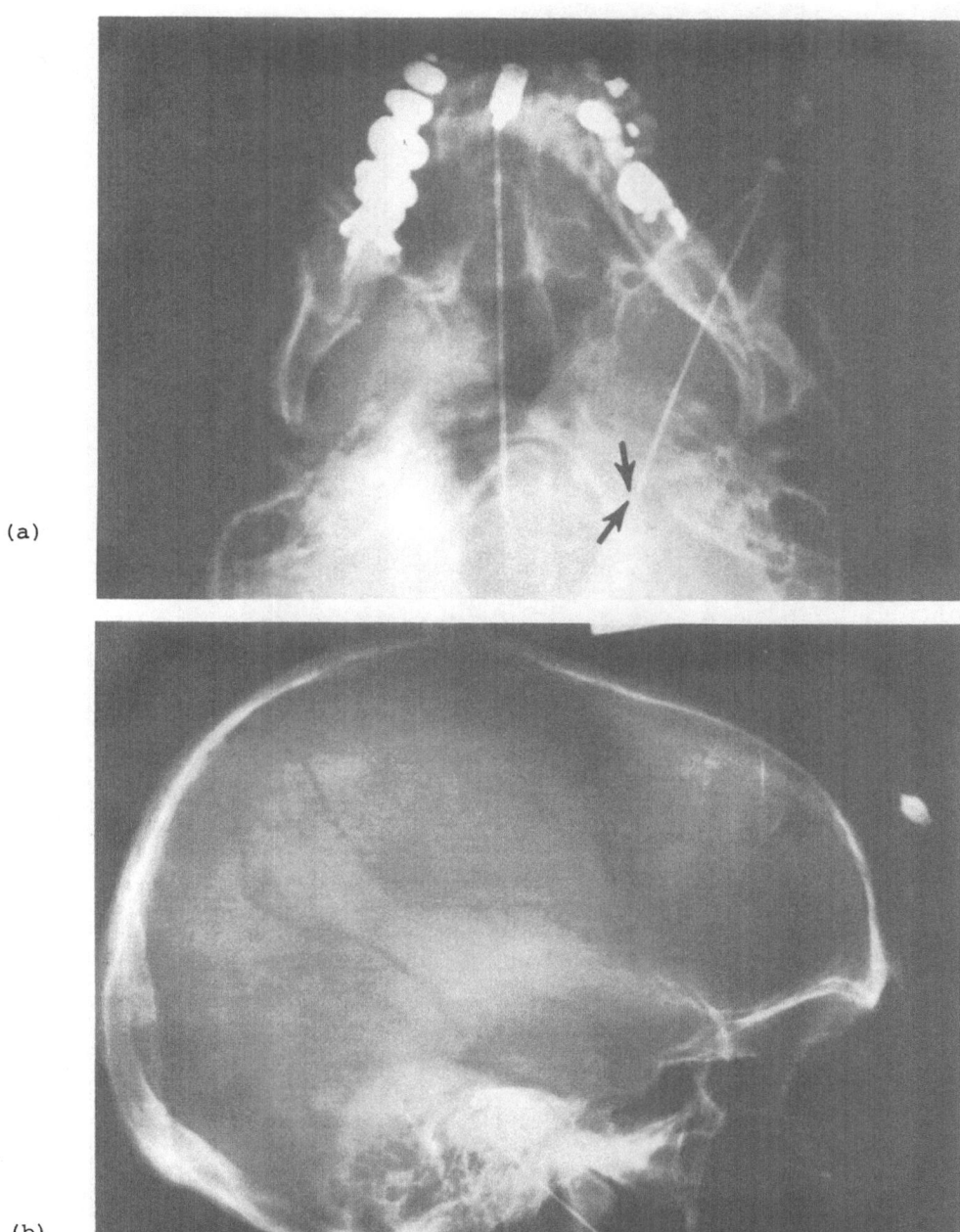

(a)

(b)

Fig. 2 a, b. Electrode tip has passed below the base of the skull lateral to the foramen ovale and medial to the internal carotid artery and the spinous process of the sphenoid bone to penetrate into CSF in the antero-medial component of the jugular foramen, its pars nervosa. (Arrows) In this position it might have been feasible to make a differential lesion in the vago-glossopharyngeal rootlets

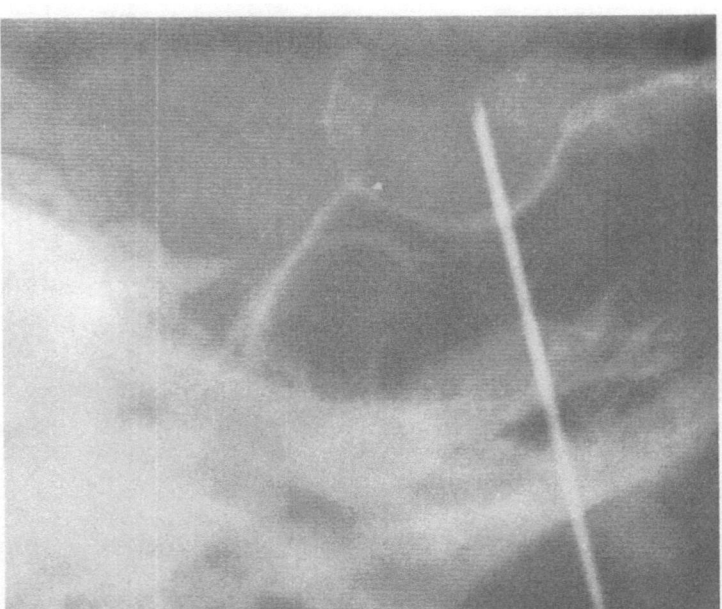

(a)

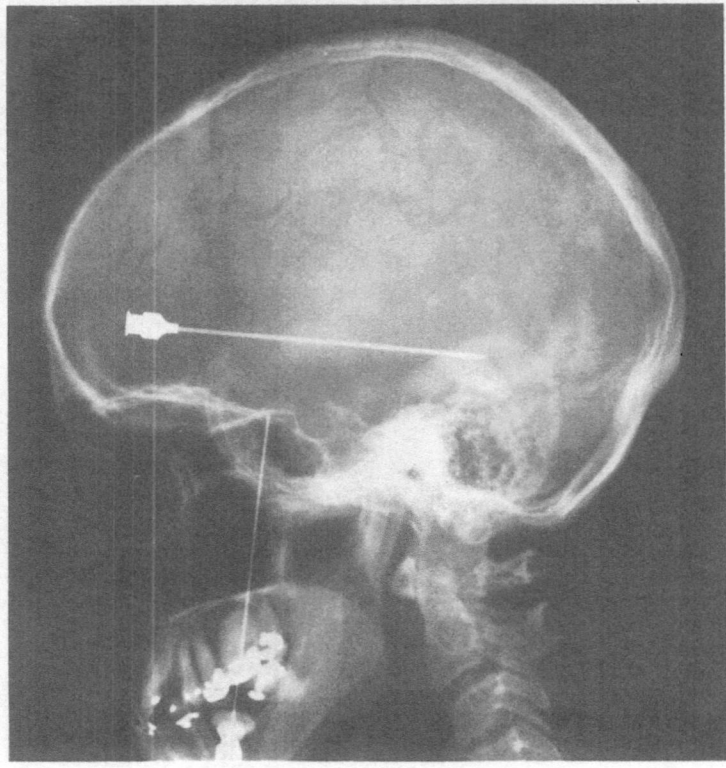

(b)

Fig. 3.a,b.
The electrode
placement in one
pateint depicted
in 3.a caused no
clinical sign or
symptom; the
placement in an-
other patient
shown in 3.b was
followed at once
by a temporary
ipsilateral
proptosis and a
temporary deficit
in cranial nerves
II, III, IV and VI.
(The horizontal
electrode is the
ground electrode
beneath the tem-
poral sclap)

Results of Percutaneous Controlled Thermocoagulation of the Gasserian Ganglion in 300 Cases of Trigeminal Pain

J. SIEGFRIED

Introduction

Every year some 5.000 to 10.000 new patients suffer from trigeminal neuralgia in the United States (20), as compared to 2.500 in West Germany and 250 in Switzerland. Three drugs can be recommended in the treatment of this disease: Diphenylhydantoin (Dilantin), Carbamazepine (Tegretol) and Clonazepam (Rivotril). The results of medical treatment are good, but still controversial. In a double blind study of Tegretol, (the drug which is probably the most commonly used) KILLIAN and FROMM (4) showed that only 70% of the patients had continuous relief for periods up to 36 months. Over the years, more and more patients have recurrence of pain, despite the increased dosage of the drug. However, the incidence of serious side-effects requiring withdrawal of the drug (rash, leukopenia, thrombocytopenia, aplastic anemia, abnormal liver function tests, etc.) varies from 5% to 19% (4,8). The best indicator of successful treatment of trigeminal neuralgia is not a decrease in intensity and frequency of the pain attacks, but a definitive disappearance of the neuralgia. This can not be achieved by conservative therapy in all cases. The surgical treatment of trigeminal neuralgia has a long story and a large number of procedures were proposed: alcohol injection and avulsion or section of the sensory root of the nerve distal or proximal to the ganglion. However, lesions peripheral to the gasserian ganglion are usually effective for only a limited period of time, whether induced by injection of caustic agent, thermally or by direct surgery. The classical division of the preganglion generally relieves the patient of his neuralgia permanently, but it is a major neurosurgical procedure, with possible severe complications, particularly in the elderly, which constitute the majority of the patients suffering from trigeminal neuralgia. Besides, it produces facial anesthesia, a condition poorly tolerated by as much as 20% of those who undergo the procedure and intolerable in a smaller but not negligible percentage (19). Postoperative anesthesia dolorosa is one of the worst complications in 4,8% (5), besides corneal keratitis, extraocular palsy, hemiparesis and aphasia. The percutaneous approach to the gasserian ganglion introduced by HÄRTEL avoids the complications of a major neurosurgical operation and its use for more than 60 years has confirmed its effectiveness. The technique of coagulation of the trigeminal ganglion, introduced by KIRSCHNER, has been largely used in the last 40 years, particularly in Europe, but was abandoned in many places because of complications resulting from the uncontrollable spread of heat to adjacent cranial nerves and arteries. Since 1950, THIRY (17, 18) using the relatively crude surgical diathermy for electrocoagulation, had already been able to produce no objective sensory loss or only an hypesthesia in many cases by applying less current to the electrode. SCHÜRMANN et al. also used partial electrocuagulation, checking the sensory deficit each time after a repeated

short period of electrocoagulation (10). In 1965 W.H. SWEET (14) introduced the particularly valuable technique of controlled thermocoagulation of the trigeminal ganglion. Assuming that the less myelinated small pain fibers (A-delta and C) are more sensitive to the
heat transmitted through and electrode than the heavily myelinated
A-beta touch fibers, graduated controlled thermocoagulation could
produce differential destruction of pain fibers (15). We were able
to confirm this assumption recently in experimental neurophysiological studies (1). The large experience obtained by SWEET in 353 such
procedures up to 1974 (16), including our own (6, 11, 12), confirm
clinically all most valuable advantages of the SWEET's modification
of KIRSCHNER's percutaneous electrocoagulation of the preganglion
rootlets and we will present here our 3-years experience with 300
cases (1972 - 1974).

Method

The technique of the percutaneous controlled thermocoagulation of
gasserian ganglion as described in detail by SWEET (16) and by us
(13) will be only mentioned briefly.

The anterior approach to the foramen ovale by percutaneous puncture
technique as described by HÄRTEL (2) is used. Improper placement of
the electrode is very unusual. On 3 occasions we penetrated the carotid artery through the foramen lacerum. We have, nevertheless, in each
case, performed the operation as planned. The electrode is a hollow
20-gauge insulated with an exposed tip of 5 - 10 mm. Submentovertex
and lateral skull films are made to confirm the needle placement
radiologically. Low voltage stimulation is performed until paresthesias are reported in the trigeminal division responsible for pain.
Under an ultra-short-acting barbiturate, a radiofrequency current is
generated to produce a temperature of 65°C for 60 sec as measured by
a thermistor at the needle tip. A sensory testing is than performed.
If a dense hypalgesia or analgesia to pinprick in the division mediating the pain is not obtained, successive lesions are made until
the result is achieved.

Material

From February 1972 to December 1974, 300 patients suffering from trigeminal pain underwent percutaneous controlled thermocoagulation of
gasserian ganglion. 245 patients were suffering from the classical so-
called essential (idiopathic) trigeminal neuralgia (tic-douloureux),
38 from atypical facial pain, and 17 from symptomatic trigeminal neuralgia (10 cases of disseminated sclerosis and 7 cases of miscellaneous ethiology, mainly tumors) (Table 1).

Table 1.

"Idiopathic trigeminal neuralgia" (Tic douloureux)	245
Atypical trigeminal neuralgia	38
Symptomatic trigeminal neuralgia	17

The youngest patient was 20 years old at the time of the procedure
(atypical facial pain), the oldest 89 years old (tic douloureux).

Fig. 1 indicates the age distribution of these patients, with a mean age of 62 years. The sex-ratio is not remarkable: 148 males and 152 females. The operation was performed 172 times on the right and 128 times on the left side. The projection of pain in the second root was most commonly observed. Figure 2 shows the pain distribution when only one root was affected (left figure) and when two or ocasionally three roots were involved (right figure). The number of coagulations necessary to obtain a sufficient analgesia varies from 1 to 9 but in 103 cases, only 1 coagulation of 60 seconds and in 84 cases 2 coagulations were made. The average number of coagulations performed in our series is two. The duration of the trigeminal pain extended from 1 month to 30 years prior to operation.

Results

1. "Idiopathic" Trigeminal Neuralgia (Tic Douloureux)

All 245 patients suffering from tic douloureux underwent the operation after transient success or partial amelioration or unsuccessful treatment with drugs. Alcohol injections into the gasserian ganglion had been previously performed in 92 patients once or more times. A retrogasserian rhizotomy of the Spiller-Frazier type had been previously performed in 23 cases and one patient had been operated on according to the technique of Dandy. Acupuncture was tried in a large number of cases without any improvement.

Percutaneous controlled thermocoagulation was repeated 3 times within 2 days because analgesia or hypalgesia was not obtained following the first procedure and pain attacks recurred on the first postoperative day. All patients were painfree following the procedure but recurrence of pain took place between 6 months and 2 1/2 years in 15 patients (5.8%) (Table 2). In these 15 cases, mild or strong analgesia was not achieved by thermocoagulation, and when the patient was discharged from the hospital we already had the feeling that the success would be only transitory. The majority of these patients was rather old and the neurological examination following thermocoagulation and short anesthesia was not satisfactory since the patient did not give convincing answers.

Analgesia or marked hypesthesia was obtained in 215 cases (87.7%). Immediately postoperatively, an impairment in touch sensation (moderate hypesthesia) was seen in 199 cases (81%), but this number decreased in the following weeks so that after a few months a normal touch sensation was present in 98 cases (40%). In 26 cases (10.6%) postoperative anesthesia remained unchanged during the follow-up time, but anesthesia became dolorosa in only 1 case (Table 3). In 15 cases anesthesia involved the territory supplied by the first and second roots and, as a complication, keratitis had to be treated in 4 patients. In one case, following a corneal scarring an important diminuition of sight was observed. It is generally admitted that the cornea has no tactible sensation. We do not want to discuss this problem here, but we have observed, in many patients operated on for the first and the second root pain, that analgesia and slight anesthesia are not enough to suppress all corneal sensation.

Other compliations are also listed in Table 3. Transitory troubles of ocular motor function from 2 days to 6 months, including double vision, were seen in 6 cases. Numbness or parethesia was a real problem in 10 patients for a period of 4 weeks to 6 months. In 1 case only, after 2 years, the patient still complains of this complication, although neurological examination reveals a very moderate hypesthesia. Two patients were operated on both sides, the second operation having taken place 6 months after the first one. Later both of them complained of difficulty in chewing and swallowing.

Table 2. Short-term and long-term success (at least 4 months and up to 38 months) of the percutaneous controlled thermocoagulation of the gasserian ganglion for tic douloureux, atypical trigeminal neuralgia and symptomatic trigeminal neuralgia.

	Short-term success	Long-term success
Tic douloureux (245 cases)	245 (100%)	231 (94.2%)
Atypical neuralgia (38 cases)	9 (23.6%)	9 (23.6%)
Disseminated sclerosis (10 cases)	10 (100%)	10 (100%)
Other symptomytic (7 cases)	5 (71.4%)	4 (57.1%)

2. Atypical Trigeminal Neuralgia _

In this series of 38 patients no diagnosis has been made which could explain pain projected into one, two or into all three trigeminal divisions. All patients were treated by many specialists without any improvement during many years. This group of patients will be mentioned only briefly and will be published in detail later. Curiously, we do not see a difference between short-term and long-term success in this group. Only 9 patients became pain-free postoperatively (Table 3). Six of these patients were suffering from continous pain at the time of surgery, but the diagnosis of tic douloureux was also suggested, since they had reported that at the beginning of the disease, some years previously, they were suffering from pain attacks of relative short duration. The 23.6% of success in this series is, unfortunately, not an argument to propose the operation in cases of atypical trigeminal neuralgia. Indeed, 6 patients complained of more pain after surgery, probably due to the fact that troublesome numbness was experienced in addition to the original pain which remained uninfluenced. However, neurotic components are very often seen in cases of atypical trigeminal neuralgia. This makes interpretation rather difficult. Hypesthesia became dolorosa in 3 cases and an anesthesia in one. We do not know why this complication was about 10 times more frequent in cases of atypical neuralgia than in cases of tic douloureux. One case of keratitis followed an anesthetic cornea (Table 4).

3. Symptomatic Trigeminal Neuralgia

a) *Disseminated Sclerosis*. 10 patients (3% of the total series) suffering from trigeminal neuralgia due to disseminated sclerosis underwent percutaneous controlled thermogoagulation of the gasserian ganglion. The average age of these patients was 51 years (ranging from 43 to 60 years). The disease had been known from 9 to 20 years (mean:

15 years and trigeminal pain had existed from 1 month to 7 years prior to surgery (mean: 4 years). 3 patients were suffering from bilateral trigeminal pain: 2 had successfully been operated on unilaterally by the technique of Spiller-Frazier. In one case, thermocoagulation of the gasserian ganglion was performed on both sides with an interval of one month. No complications followed these bilateral operations. The follow-up of this series is short, from 7 to 16 months. All patients are painfree so far, with the desired analgesia. Total anesthesia never occurred, and in only one case the corneal reflex was diminished postoperatively. There is, therefore, a very good indication for percutaneous controlled thermocoagulation of gasserian ganglion in trigeminal neuralgia due to disseminated sclerosis (Tables 2 and 5).

Table 3. Short- and long-term complications following percutaneous controlled thermocoagulation of the gasserian ganglion for tic douloureux (245 cases)

Tic douloureux 245 cases	Short-term	Long-term
VI palsy	2 (0.8%)	O
IV palsy	2 (0.8%)	O
III palsy	2 (0.8%)	O
Keratitis	4 (1.6%)	4 (1.6%)
Anesthesia/hypesthesia dolorosa	1 (0.4%)	1 (0.4%)
Parethesias	10 (4%)	1 (0.4%)

Table 4. Short-term and long-term complications after percutaneous controlled thermocoagulation of gasserian ganglion for atypical trigeminal neuralgia (38 cases)

Atypical neuralgia 38 cases	Short-term	Long-term
Ocular palsy	O	O
Keratitis	1 (2.6%)	1 (2.6%)
Anesthesia/hypesthesia dolorosa	4 (10.5%)	3 (7.9%)
Paresthesias	6 (15.7%)	6 (15.7%)

b) *Other Forms of Symptomatic Trigeminal Neuralgia*. The 7 patients in this group had the following diagnoses: 1) one case of Paget, with significant bone thickening at the base of the skull and narrowing of the foramen ovale compressing the third trigeminal root; 2) one case of giant aneurysm of the internal carotid siphon which had thrombosed following carotid ligature; 3) one case of basal meningitis; 4) one case of postherpetic neuralgia who already had hypesthesia dolorosa; 5) three cases of metastatic or direct invasion of the middle fossa by carcinomas.

The patient with postherpetic neuralgia and the tumor patients were not improved by thermocoagulation of gasserian ganglion. The trigeminal pain as sequel of a basal meningitis initially improved, but recurred after a few weeks. All other cases have so far remained pain-free, and no postoperative complications have been observed (Tables 2 and 6).

Table 5. Short-term and long-term complications after percutaneous controlled thermocoagulation of gasserian ganglion for disseminated sclerosis (10 cases)

MS 10 cases	Short-term	Long-term
	no complications	

Table 6. Short-term and long-term complications after percutaneous controlled thermocoagulation of gasserian ganglion for symptomatic trigeminal neuralgia (except disseminated sclerosis) (7 cases)

Symptomatic neuralgia (no MS) 7 cases	Short-term	Long-term
	no complications	

Table 7. Recurrence and complication rate of trigeminal neuralgia following different surgical approaches (completed apud MARGUTH (7) 1972)

	N.$^{\circ}$	Recurrence	Complication
Peripheral surgical procedures	~ 3.500	~ 50 - 80%	~ 5%
Alcohol injection	~ 9.000	~ 25 - 40%	~ 10 - 15%
Division of preganglionic rootlets	~ 10.000	~ 5 - 10%	~ 5 - 10%
Parapontine neurotomy	670	15%	5 - 10%
Percutaneous controlled thermocoagulation of gasserian ganglion	8 800	5 - 22%	5 - 10%

completed apud MARGUTH, 1972

Discussion

A new surgical procedure must have definite advantages against older techniques, and should proven to be satisfactory for a long period of time. Percutaneous controlled thermocoagulation of the gasserian ganglion for trigeminal neuralgia provides a very good relief of trigeminal pain while avoiding many objectionable side-effects associated with other surgical methods. Since the majority of patients suffering of typical trigeminal neuralgia are elderly people, the surgical procedure must be devoid of stress. Percutaneous puncture of the gasserian ganglion through the foramen ovale enables the patient to remain substantially ambulatory. The comfortable position of the patient on the table and the general anesthesia of 2 to 3 minutes with an ultra-short-acting barbiturate is always well tolerated by the patient, and no mortality occurred in the 800 patients reported in literature. Some complications of the surgery of the trigeminal nerve or trigeminal ganglion are also encountered following percutaneous controlled thermocoagulation of the gasserian ganglion: keratitis, cranial nerve palsies, troublesome numbness and masseter weakness. Hemiparesis, facial paresis and retrotympanic hemorrhage, which have been reported following different surgical approaches, has never occurred following percutaneous thermocoagulation of the gasserian ganglion, white cranial nerve palsies and masseter weakness were always transitory. Troublesome numbness usually regressed and disappeared following a few months, in the majority of patients, but sometimes only after a very long period of time. The recurrence rate and that of troublesome numbness with anesthesia depends on the patients cooperation. To attain the goal of analgesia without anesthesia or with a slight hypesthesia, a very good cooperation of the patient following the first thermocoagulation is necessary. In elderly patients short anesthesia is sometimes followed by a prolonged drowsy state. When the patient is not sufficiently awake to give adequate information about pinprick and touch sensations, thermocoagulation will be repeated or the operation ended if the surgeon is not patient enough. As a consequence, excessive thermocoagulation can lead to an undesirable anesthesia, which can be followed by some troublesome numbness or anesthesia dolorosa. If analgesia or strong hypalgesia is not obtained, a recurrence of trigeminal pain can be observed. This also explains why these problems are more frequent in cases of idiopathic trigeminal neuralgia than in those of symptomatic or of atypical facial pain: patients of the first group are definitely older than those of the other two.

A survey of the literature shows that we have about the same rate of recurrences and of complications as reported by others with other surgical techniques (Table 7). However, the complications are transitory in the majority of cases. Interestingly, also, we have observed only one case of postoperative herpes simplex, a very frequent complication (22.7% in the large series of PETR) following retrogasserian rhizotomy.

The absence of stress for the patient, even for the elderly, less complications, very few of which are permanent, and the same rate of success as other surgical procedures have already made the percutaneous controlled thermocoagulation of the gasserian ganglion the operation of choice for trigeminal neuralgia. Besides, the great advantage of this technique is the possibility to preserve touch sensation.

Summary

From February 1972 to December 1974, 300 patients suffering from
trigeminal neuralgia have been operated on by the technique of percutaneous controlled thermocoagulation of the gasserian ganglion as
described by SWEET. 245 patients were suffering from the classical
so-called idiopathic trigeminal neuralgia, 38 from atypical facial
pain, 10 from disseminated sclerosis and 7 from other symptomytic
trigeminal pain. In cases of classical trigeminal neuralgia (tic
douloureux), the author always succeeded in relieving pain; in cases
of symptomatic facial pain the results are fairly good, but in cases
of atypical facial pain only less than 25% of the patients were improved. The relatively short follow-up period probably gives a false
view of the recurrence rate, which was only 5%. Anesthesia dolorosa
occured in 5 cases as a complication. The simplicity of the method,
the very good results, the low complication rate and the advantages
of this operation as compared with other different procedures make
the percutaneous controlled thermocoagulation of the gasserian ganglion the operation of choice in cases of trigeminal neuralgia.

REFERENCES

1. BROGGI, G., FRIGYESI, T.L., SIEGFRIED, J.: Evoked potentials in
   the trigeminal dorsal root: their selective vulnerability to
   graded thermocoagulation. Exp. Neurol. (in press).

2. HÄRTEL, F.: Die Behandlung der Trigeminusneuralgie mit intrakra-
   niellen Alkoholeinspritzungen. Deutsch. Z. Chir. 126, 429 - 552
   (1914).

3. KILLIAN, J.M.: Tegretol in trigeminal neuralgia with special reference to hematoppietic side effects. Headache 9, 58 - 63 (1969).

4. KILLIAN, J.M., FROMM, G.H.: Carbamazepine in the treatment of
   neuralgia. Use and side-effect. Arch. Neurol. 19, 129 - 136 (1968).

5. KRAYENBÜHL, H.: Die idiopathische Trigeminusneuralgie. Acta Clinica 9, Documenta Geigy (1968).

6. KRAYENBÜHL, H., SIEGFRIED, J.: La termorrizomia en el tratamiento
   de la neuralgia esencial del trigemino. Rev. Esp. Oto-Neuro-Oft-
   alm. 31, 107 - 112 (1973).

7. MARGUTH, F.: Die chirurgische Behandlung der Trigeminusneuralgie.
   In: Schmerz (ed. R. JANZEN et al.) pp. 228 - 229. Stuttgart:
   GEORG THIEME 1972.

8. NICHOL, C.F.: A four year double-blind study of Tegretol in facial
   pain. Headache 9, 54 - 57 (1969).

9. PETR, R.: Results of trigeminal rhizotomy. In: Trigeminal Neuralgia (eds. R. HASSLER, A.E. WALKER), Vol. I pp. 22 - 25. Stuttgart:
   GEORG THIEME 1970.

10. SCHÜRMANN, M., BUTZ, M., BROCK, M.: Temporal retrogasserian re-
    section of trigeminal root versus controlled elective percutane-
    ous electrocoagulation of the ganglion of GASSER in the treatment
    of trigeminal neuralgia. Acta Neurochir. 26, 33 - 53 (1972).

11. SIEGFRIED, J.: Un nouveau traitement de la névralgie du trijumeau:
    analgésie sans anesthésie. Neuro-Chirurgie 19, 585 - 587 (1973).

12. SIEGFRIED, J., KRAYENBÜHL, H.: Die Thermoehizotomie in der Behand-
    lung der idiopathischen Trigeminusneuralgie. Rundschau Med. (Pra-
    xis) 61, 219 - 223 (1973).

13. SIEGFRIED, J., VOSMANSKY, M.: Technique of the controlled thermo-coagulation of trigeminal ganglion and spinal roots. Advances and Technical Standards in Neurosurgery 2, (1975) (in press).

14. SWEET, W.H.: Pain, Vol. I, pp. 167 - 197; 607 - 609. Springfield/Ill.: CHARLES C. THOMAS 1969.

15. SWEET, W.H., WESPIC, J.G.: Relation of fibers size in trigeminal posterior root condition of impulses for pain and touch: production of analgesia without anesthesia in the effective treatment of trigeminal neuralgia. Trans. Am. Neurol. Assoc. 95, 134 - 137 (1970).

16. SWEET, W.H., WESPIC, J.G.: Controlled thermocoagulation of trigeminal ganglion and rootlets for differential destruction of pain fibers. Part 1: Trigeminal neuralgia. J. Neurosurg. 39, 143 - 156 (1974).

17. THIRY, S.: Expérience personnelle basée sur 225 cas de névralgie essentielle du trijumeau traités par électro-coagulation du ganglion de Gasser entre 1950 et 1962. Neuro-Chirurgie 8, 86 - 92 (1962).

18. THIRY, S., HOTERMANS, J.M.: Traitement de la névralgie essentielle du trijumeau par stéréotaxie et électrocoagulation partielle sélective du ganglion de GASSER. Expérience portant sur 365 cas traités entre 1950 et 1970. Neuro-Chirurgie 20, 55 - 60 (1974).

19. WESPIC, J.G.: Tic douloureux: etiology, refined treatment. New Engl. J. Med. 288, 680 - 681 (1973).

20. YOSHIMASU, F., KURLAND, L.T., ELVEBACK, L.R.: Tic douloureux in Rochester, Minnesota, 1945 - 1969. Neurology 22, 952 - 956 (1972).

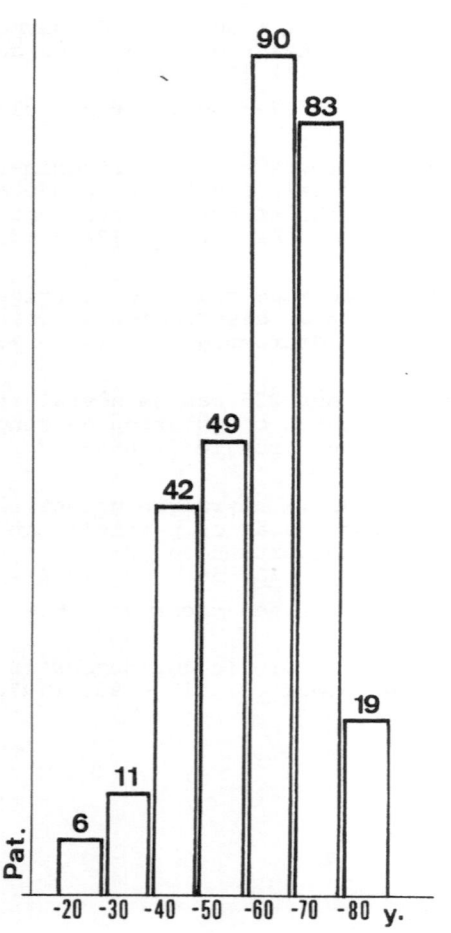

Fig. 1. Age and distribution of 300 patients suffering from trige-minal neuralgia

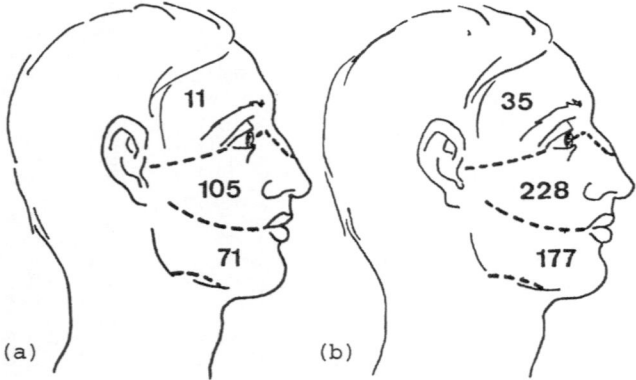

Fig. 2. Pain distribution in the trigeminal roots. On the left (a), repartition of pain projection when one root only was affected and on the right (b) when two or eventually three roots were involved

Thermorhizotomy in Trigeminal Neuralgia: Preliminary Considerations on 46 Cases

G. BROGGI

Introduction

Percutaneous approach to the gasserian ganglion and its rootlets for the treatement of trigeminal neuralgia have proven effective since long (9, 3). However, only after WHITE and SWEET (11) introduced radiofrequency (R.F.) graded thermocoagulation, did trigeminal neuralgia have a more selective treatement, it being possible to achieve facial analgesia without tactile deficit (7, 8, 5, 10, 6). Aim of this paper is to report briefly experience on a group of 46 patients suffering from "essential" trigeminal neuralgia treated by this percutaneous technique, and followed up from 3 to 12 months.

Method

The forty-six patients were operated on at the Istituto Neurologico "C. Besta", Milan between april 1974 and december 1974). All were suffering from "essential" trigeminal neuralgia except two, one of which had multiple sclerosis, while the second had an ipsilateral frontotemporal glioblastoma, operated on in 1973. Age ranged from 27 to 86 years. 21 were males and 25 females. Neuralgia was right-sided in 30 patients. 43 patients had been previously treated with Tegretol (3 to 9 tablets per day) from 1 to 6 years. Only 36 had experienced remission of pain. However, side-effects (leucopenia, drowsiness, dizziness and unsteadiness, cutaneous rash etc.) had led to discontinue the medical treatement and to recommend surgery.

The surgical technique is as described by WHITE and SWEET (11), and by SIEGFRIED (7), but we use fluoroscopic control (Siremobil Siemens) during the entire surgical procedure. Repeated intravenous Penthotal was employed as short-acting anaesthetic. Introduction of the needle into the foramen ovale was achieved under local anaesthesia (Xylocaine 2%) and sedation with intravenous Fentanest (Phentanyl, average dosage 0.10 mg.) plus Sintodian (Dehydrobenzperidol, 2.5 mg.) or Valium (Diazepam, 10 mg.). Under the above circumstances a good cooperation by the patient was usually achieved. The R.F. coagulation of the retrogasserian portion of trigeminal nerve was performed under control of the needle tip temperature, which reflects the temperature in the surrounding tissue. A RFG-5 Radionics Inc. equipement has been used. The procedure included impedance measurement as well as low and high frequency stimulation at different voltages, so as to evoke masseter muscle twitching and paraesthesia on the face. The patients were instructed beforehand to identify the territory of paraesthesia. After obtention of a brief unconsciousness with intravenous Penthotal, repetitive R.F. coagulation was performing checking the face sensitivity with a sharp needle and pinching slightly with a surgical forceps every time the patient awakened. The overall dosage of Penthotal

ranged from 200 to 600 mg. The number of R.F. coagulations ranged
from 3 to 100. Temperature measured at the electrode tip ranged from
56° C to 95° C with different durations (from 10" to 60"), for every
single coagulation. This procedure was repeated untill satisfactory
analgesia was obtained. The foramen ovale was always reached through
the anterior way of HÄRTEL (3); in about 60% of the cases some cerebrospinal fluid dropped out from the needle. In two cases the internal carotid artery was puntured, but no neurological deficit nor
sequelae were present in the postoperative follow up. In both cases
the procedure was continued following a new electrode placement. In
many cases a transient rash of the skin limited to a well defined
territory of one or two trigeminal branches appeared as an expression
of a vasomotor reaction. Only in one case complete hemifacial pallor
appeared following a single R.F. coagulation performed to achieve
second and third branches analgesia.

Table 1

	Mor-tal-ity	Relapse of pain	Unwanted trigeminal nerve morbidity		Topographic selectivity	Other neurological morbidity
			severe	slight		
Number of cases	46	O	5	4	14	32	O
Percent-age	100%	0%	10.9%	8.7%	30.5%	69%	0%

Results

The surgical procedure was succesfull in all (100%) 46 cases, leading
to complete disappearance of lightening trigeminal pain. Operative
mortality has been zero. Pain relapsed in 5 cases (10.9%), in 3 of
which on the day following to the procudure, while in the other two
it returned one and three months later, respectively. All patients
underwent a second procedure which has proven successfull to present.

Neurological morbidity other than related to the trigeminal nerve
has been none, also in the two cases in which the internal carotid
artery had been accidentaly punctured. Analgesia of topographic se-
lectivity as desired has been achieved in 32 (69%) of the cases.

Unwanted severe impairement of trigeminal function appeared in four
cases (8.7%), specifically, corneal complications in one and masticatory weakeness in three. Undesired but slight trigeminal impairement such as excessive analgesia or tactile hypesthesia was present
in 14 cases (30.5%). No tactile anesthesia has been found following
surgery. A slight but not disappointing hitching in the analgesic
territory was reported in 22% of the cases. No "anaesthesia dolorosa"
syndrome has developed to present.

Discussion and Conclusions

Although our follow-up is not very long yet, some preliminary considerations can be made based on these 46 cases.

Controlled thermorhizotomy is a safe, simple and successful treatment of trigeminal neuralgia, being possible without discomfort to the patient even under bad general condition or in late age (our oldest patient was 86 years). It is possible to achieve either qualitative (analgesia vs. tactile deficit) or quantitative (only the desidered branch territory) selective lesion. This is very important because it seems that the more uncomfortable consequence of the SPILLER-FRAZIER or DANDY's operation, anaesthesia dolorosa, requires a heavy tactile deficit. Thermorhizotomy, providing the best possibility of sparing tactile fibers, should free the patient operated on from this potential discomfort.

To achieve the best results good cooperation by the patient and a time consuming electrophysiological procedure are required.

Electrophysiological data supporting the selective action of R.F. heating on trigeminal fibers, come from one *in vitro* study of LETCHER and GOLDRING (4) on the isolated sciatic nerve of the cat, and from one *in vivo* study on the retrogasserian portion of the trigeminal nerve in anesthetized cats (1). Both studies showed that the various components of the compound action potentials of the nerve have different sensitivities. A-delta fiber and C-fiber components are the more sensitive to graded R.F. heating, and disappear well before the large diameter nervous fiber potentials do.

It seems that there is not only a hystological reason for this (smaller diameter and little shielding from myelin sheath), but also a metabolic interference of R.F. heating which affects A-delta and C-fibers at lower temperature. Probably only more sophisticated electrophysiological recordings as well as electromicroscopic studies now in progress (2) will permit more precise conclusions in view of the excellent clinical results (5, 6, 7, 8, 9, 10, 11) of graded thermorhizotomy for the treatment of trigeminal neuralgia.

REFERENCES

1. BROGGI, G., SIEGFRIED, J., FRIGYESI, T.: Evoked potentials in the trigeminal dorsal root: their selective vulnerability to graded thermocoagulation. Expt. Neurol. (in press, 1975).

2. BROGGI, G., SIEGFRIED, J., PELUCHETTI, D.: Unpublished observation, 1975.

3. LECTHER, F.S., GOLDRING, S.: The effect of radiofrequency current and heat on peripheral nerve action potential in the cat. J. Neurosurg. 29, 42-47 (1968).

4. HÄRTEL, F.: Die Behandlung der Trigeminusneuralgie mit intrakarniellen Alkoholeinspritzungen. Deutsch Z. Chir. 126, 429-552 (1914).

5. NUGENT, R.G., BERRY, B.: Trigeminal neuralgia treated by differential percutaneous radiofrequency coagulation of the gasserian ganglion. J. Neurosurg. 40, 517-523 (1974).

6. ONOFRIO, B.M.: Radiofrequency percutaneous Gasserian ganglion lesions. J. Neurosurg. 42, 132-139 (1975).

7. SIEGFRIED, J.: Un nouveau traitement neurochirugical de la nèvralgie du trijumeau: analgesie sans anesthésie. Neuro-Chirugie 19, 585-587 (1973).

8. SWEET, W.H., WEPSIC, J.G.: Controlled thermocoagulation of trigeminal ganglion and rootlets for differential destruction of pain fibers. Part 1: Trigeminal neuralgia. J. Neurosurg. 39, 143-156 (1974).

9. TAPTAS, N.: Les injections d'alcool dans le ganglion de Gasser à travers le trou ovale. Presse Med. 19, 798 (1911).

10. TURNBULL, I.M.: Percutaneous rhizotomy for trigeminal neuralgia. Surg. Neurol. 2, 385-389 (1974).

11. WHITE, J.C., SWEET, W.H.: Pain and the neurosurgeon: A forty-years experience, pp. 184-197. Springfield/Ill.: Charles C. Thomas 1969.

Controlled and Partial Percutaneous Electrocoagulation of the Gasserian Ganglion in Facial Pain

E. Schürmann and K. Schürmann

Each neurosurgeon has his own experience in the treatment of trigeminal neuralgia as well as a good knowledge of the historical aspects of the various surgical procedures. Therefore I can restrict my statements to the own experience with o p e n and c l o s e d operations during a period of about twenty years. However, I would like to start by explaining some of the reasons which have led us to our present technique. I think it was a long and curved yet natural and logical road. It now seems to be an unintended double blind study. Many times in the past 20 years we have changed our mind about the seemingly optimal operative therapy for trigeminal pain attacks (Table 1).

Table 1. Survey of 638 procedures between 1955 and 1973 (201 *open* operations and 437 *closed* procedures)

Neurectomy 1st branch	14
Open cranotomies - 187	
Temporal retrogasserian root section (SPILLER-FRAZIER)	79
Temporal gasserian decompression (TAARNHØJ, extradural modification)	70
Intramedullary tractotomy (SJÖQVIST)	38
Percutaneous procedures - 437	
Gasserian ganglion (alcohol destruction)	24
Gasserian ganglion (electrocoagulation)	413
Total	

Presently we aim at performing the s m a l l e s t procedure and s m a l l e s t lesion with the h i g h e s t possible effect. However, there are certain barriers, as shall be shown below.

Let me point out some steps of the curved way to our present technique. In their recent paper on thermocoagulation, SWEET and WEPSIC (13) stressed that "in North America various forms of open operations have been the preferred definitive treatment for patients with trigeminal neuralgia refractory to medical management". But the authors are somewhat mistaken in stating that "in Europe the feasibility, relative safety, and effectiveness of a percutaneous approach to the Gasserian ganglion and its rootlets have been convincingly demonstrated for over two-thirds of a century".

It is true that *until* World War II trigeminal neuralgia had been preferably treated by using the *uncontrolled* Gasserian ganglion destruction techniques of HÄRTEL (2) (1913, alcohol injection) and KIRSCHNER (3) (1936, electrocoagulation with his ingenious stereotactic apparatus).

The simplicity of these techniques led to their widespread use, particularly in the hands of general surgeons, due to the absence of Neurosurgery at that early time. The radical application of these methods, however, led to many sequelae and complications, such as corneal ulcers, enucleated eyes, blindness, palsies of the sixth, fourth, third and seventh and also twelfth cranial nerves, partial or total deafness, hemiplegia, carotid thrombosis, bulbar syndromes, cardiac and respiratory arrests, meningitis, death and, last but not least, a high incidence of a n e s t h e s i a d o l o r o s a, one of the most unpleasant sequelae. This is why, following World War II, in Germany and other European countries - parallel to the progress in establishing Neurosurgery - a distinct preference for open craniotomies was seen, as vehemently advocated by my teacher TÖNNIS (15) and others.

Nevertheless, while I was still a pupil of TÖNNIS he gave me the task of treating virtually inoperable patients - i.e. very old people and patients with serious heart or pulmonary diseases - by means of alcohol injection into the Gasserian ganglion. Actually no one was permitted to notice this sacrilege. Therefore, I had to hide the patient and myself in a small separated chamber of the radiological department. Alone with the patient and my thoughts, I had my first encounters with a defamed method. In spite of a high rate of recurrences and complications - one sixth cranial nerve palsy in the, nevertheless, thankful wife of a colonel, and three corneal ulcers, as well as three cases of anesthesia dolorosa - among a total of 24 cases, the final results after several very carefully repeated procedures in some patients, was indeed not so bad (12,5% of failures).

Notwithstanding, we continued to prefer o p e n operations during the following years, preferably temporal retrogasserian root section (1) in elderly, and by the technique of SJÖQVIST (11) in younger patients and those with 1st division neuralgia, because of the superficial intramedullary site of the 1st branch fibers and the preservation of touch. However, the advantages of differential loss of pain and of prevention of anesthetic keratitis were outbalanced by several disadvantages, particularly hemiataxia, hemianalgesia, disturbances of equilibrium, as sequelae of lesions to the neighbouring restiform body, spinothalamic tract and vagal fibers. I remember a violinist, who was postoperatively disabled because of hemiataxia. With more precise and restricted indication the results became better, but we gave up in 1957, parallel to the growing experience in other procedures.

Following the report of TAARNHØJ (14) on the operation of decompression, we performed this procedure by an extradural modification in 70 patients. However, about half of this series had recurrences and underwent root section or electrocoagulation, which I had slowly introduced in the meantime.

Then a period of uncertainty in the handling of facial pain patients followed. Temporal retrogasserian root section v e r s u s percutaneous electrocoagulation. Initially we performed electrocoagulation without peroperative sensitivity control. 53 cases were treated under local anesthesia of Gasserian ganglion and 75 cases under general anesthesia, giving a total of 128 more or less uncontrolled procedures. Despite very careful conduct, the surgeon was in the unpleasant and unsafe position of having to perform an uncontrolled destruction of the Gasserian ganglion. The risk was decreased somewhat by using a test in each procedure. The size of the individual lesion was tested on a piece of meat prior to coagulating the ganglion.

Despite the relatively high incidence of recurrences and the insufficient primary effect in cases of a too cautious lesion, the rivalry between open root section and limited percutaneous destruction of the Gasserian ganglion had been decided in favour of the latter, particularly when it became evident that repeated interventions led to the desired positive result in a very large number of cases and had a very low rate of complications.

The most important step, that of control, was introduced with "neurolept-anesthesia" in 1963 (8, 9, 10). This form of anesthesia allows an almost painless puncture of the ganglion of Gasser in the "awake" resp. "semi-awake" patient. That means that, despite the dramatic reduction of pain caused by direct puncture of the ganglion, it is possible to control and check immediately the partial destruction of the ganglion and the resultant sensory deficit. Thus, for the first time, the procedure of electrocoagulation of the Gasserian ganglion came under the control of the surgeon even during its performance. Following each short period of coagulation the surgeon immediately checks the extent of the inflicted damage by performing a sensitivity test. Furthermore, the surgeon can vary the position of the needle tip within the ganglion until the desired effect is obtained. It is possible, for instance, to "hit" only the mandibular territory when the skull films show the needle tip has barely passed two to three millimeters through the foramen ovale. If an additional destruction of the second division is desired or necessary, the needle tip is advanced further into the ganglion so that it comes to lie midway between the base of middle fossa and the upper border of the petrous bone. When the elimination of the first branch is also necessary, the needle tip has to be introduced until it is barely below the upper border of the petrous bone.

Obviously, these are only gross topographical landmarks, the real effect of the procedure being estimated by testing the sensory loss and the corneal reflex. The application of electric current and the correction of the needle position are performed as long as necessary until the desired localization and effect are obtained. This is why we speak of a "controlled, elective, partial electrocoagulation" of the Gasserian ganglion.

Technique of Electrode Introduction and Coagulation

One does not need more than 1) a common but long injection needle of 12 to 14 cm length, with an outer diameter of 1.2 mm, inner diameter of 0.8 mm, and insulated except for 5.0 mm at the needle tip and the opposite end; 2) a common Bovie coagulation apparatus; 3) drugs for neuroleptanesthesia (Thalamonal, Dehydrobenzperidol, Dextromoramid, Fentanyl, and Lorfan); 4) an ordinary x-ray apparatus, perhaps combined with a television monitor for lateral view; 5) a small piece of fresh meat, about 5 to 5 cm in diameter.

The procedure is carried out in the x-ray room under neurolept-anesthesia. Previous to anesthesia the patient is informed of what will happen, and command respiration is trained.

Neurolept-Anesthesia

30 minutes prior to the procedure the patient is given an intramus-
cular injection of 1.0 ml Thalamonal and 0.5 ml Atropine, followed
by intravenous infusion of 10 to 15 mg Dehydrobenzperidol. Five minutes later 2 ml Dextromoramid (1:10 solution) and 13.8 mg Dextromor-
amidbitartrat per ml are administered intravenously. Following placement of the needle tip into the foramen ovale, 2 to 4 ml of the Dex-
tromoramid-solution are injected again.

The mean duration of the coagulation procedure amounted to 40 minutes, and the patient usually needed 11.6 mg Dehydrobenzperidol and
7.8 mg Dextromoramid-Base.

Following the procedure, the patient always receives 1 ml Lorfan i.v.
and 1 ml Lorfan s.c.

Blood gases (ASTRUP method) change only slightly (initially a slight
temporary diminution of pO_2 is common).

During the whole procedure the patient remains in speaking contact
with the surgeon.

Before describing the technique of puncture I would like to demonstrate the procedure in a skull model to show some possible mistakes
(Fig. 1).

In the center of the middle fossa is the foramen ovale, through which
the 3rd division of the trigeminal nerve leaves the skull. The tip
of the insulated needle in the position demonstrated would lie in the
center of the ganglion and close to the rootlets. To the right of the
needle is the foramen spinosum (middle meningeal artery), and dorso-
medially the foramen lacerum (internal carotid artery). Anteriorly
there is the foramen rotundum for the 2nd trigeminal division, and
still more anteriorly and somewhat more cranial the superior orbital
fissure, through which pass the 1st trigeminal division and the motor
nerves to the eye muscles. Since these are to be preserved, x-ray
studies are necessary.

Puncture is performed freehand, that is, without using KIRSCHNER's
(3) or another stereotactic apparatus. HÄRTEL's (2) anterior approach
to the foramen ovale is followed (Fig. 2).

In order to reach the foramen ovale the needle is directed towards a
point placed at the crossing of an imaginary anteroposterior line
through the pupil and a second imaginary transverse line from the superior edge of one ear to a corresponding point on the opposite side.
The needle tip penetrates the skin about 20 mm lateral to the corner
of the mouth, being advanced in the direction of the crossing of the
two described vertical and horizontal lines until the needle tip
passes through the foramen ovale.

At this moment the patient feels sudden pain projected to the skin
area of the mandibular branch. In more than 50% of patients CSF drops
out of the needle. We like it because this means the needle tip lies
behind the ganglion and the lesion will affect mainly rootlets and/or
ganglion.

Correct positioning of the needle is then roentgenologically checked.
If the foramen ovale is not entered at the first puncture, the needle
is usually stopped by the temporal bone at the skull base near to the

304

foramen ovale. In this case the radiographs aid in correcting the position of the needle tip. Care has to be taken not to introduce the needle into the neighbouring foramen lacerum (lesion of internal carotid artery leading to hematoma of pterygopalatine fossa and cheek) or into the ventrally placed superior orbital fissure (danger for ocular and optic nerves).

After passing through the foramen ovale, the needle tip is advanced to the desired depth of about three to twelve mm, depending on whether the 3rd, 2nd or 1st division is to be coagulated.

When radiographic examination in lateral view and base projection has confirmed correct placement of the needle tip, coagulation can be started. Usually we test the size of the lesion on a small piece of meat placed on the plate-electrode. In the patient, following each short period of coagulation (2 to 3 seconds), the resultant sensory deficit is checked. As said, the position of the needle within the Gasserian ganglion can be varied during the procedure until the desired coagulation is obtained. It is very important to obtain a sensory loss or diminution in the trigger zone and to preserve the corneal reflex, as discussed below. In the whole series of 285 patients with 351 controlled coagulations, the average time of the procedure was about 39 minutes (9, 10).

Results

Table 2 summarizes the results of the various procedures during a twenty years period. It is obvious that only in the group of percutaneous procedures immediate repeated interventions (usually a few days after the first operation) were necessary because of deficient primary effect. This occurs more frequently in u n c o n t r o l l e d (16.6% to 24%) than in c o n t r o l l e d procedures (only 8%), what is not difficult to explain, since we were too cautious in handling uncontrolled interventions. Furthermore, when a sensory loss is obtained in the trigger zone the results are, in total, better.

In some patients we observed the unintended effect of loss of painful sensation with simultaneous preservation of touch. In such patients - in whom the effect is comparable to that of differential destruction of pain fibers with sparing of fibers for touch by means of thermocoagulation (12, 13) - recurrences were distinctly less intense and protracted in time (late recurrence) but more frequent than in patients with total sensory loss in trigger zone.

We treated patients with recurrences following temporal retrogasserian root section by means of coagulation of the Gasserian ganglion. Patients with recurrences following temporal Gasserian decompression were treated by root section or electrocoagulation until the definitive result was obtained (Table 3).

Finally, we would like to comment briefly on the last series of 285 patients, treated by 351 c o n t r o l l e d procedures, which doubtlessly led to the best results. Table 3 shows the well known fact that the highest incidence of trigger zones was found in the territory of the 2nd division, followed by the combined 2nd/3rd division, and by 3rd division. By relating the trigger zone to the rate or recurrences and failures it becomes evident that the best results are obtained in patients with 3rd division neuralgia, in which group all patients (100%) eventually had definitive pain relief. More than one recurrence we found particularly in 2nd division and in combined 2nd/

Table 2. Results obtained with the various procedures

Kind of Surgery	No.	Immediate repeated procedure	Early recurrence before 6 months	Late recurrence after 6 months	Negative effect after several OPs	Complications Meningitis, Keratitis, Cheek hematoma	Anesthesia dolorosa	Mortality
Neurectomy 1st Branch	14	–	2 (14%)	4 (28%)	3 (21%)	–	–	–
Temporal Retrogasserian Root Section (SPILLER-FRAZIER)	79	–	5 (5,5%)	11 (13,6%)	6 (7,5%)	6 (7,5%)	3 (3,7%)	2 (1,8%)
Temporal Gasserian Decompression (TAARNHOJ, extradural modified)	70	–	12 (16%)	25 (35%)	5 (7%)	4 (5,8%)	–	–
Intramedullary Tractotomy	38	–	3 (8%)	7 (18%)	?	4 (10,5%)	–	1 (2,6%)
Gasserian Ganglion (*alcohol* destruction)	24	4 (16,6%)	6 (25%)	4 (16,6%)	3 (12,5%)	4 (16,6%)	3 (12,5%)	–
Gasserian Ganglion (electrocoagul., *uncontrolled*)	128	31 (24%)	9 (7%)	8 (6,3%)	7 (5%)	5 (4%)	2 (1,5%)	–
Gasserian Ganglion (electrocoagul., *controlled*)	285	23 (8%)	11 (4%)	14 (5%)	18 (6%)	7 (2,5%)	1 (0,4%)	–
Total	638							

Table 3. The highest frequency trigger zones was found in the second
division of trigeminal nerve (45%), followed by the combined second
and third division and by third division. A trigger zone in the territory of the first division was very rare. The best results are obtained in patients with third branch neuralgia (100% definitively
painless). More than one recurrence was found particularly in second
division and in combined second/third division neuralgia. Repeated
procedures increased the rate of definitive cure (about 94%), although
the relatively highest number of not-cured patients (about 6%) was
also found in this group.

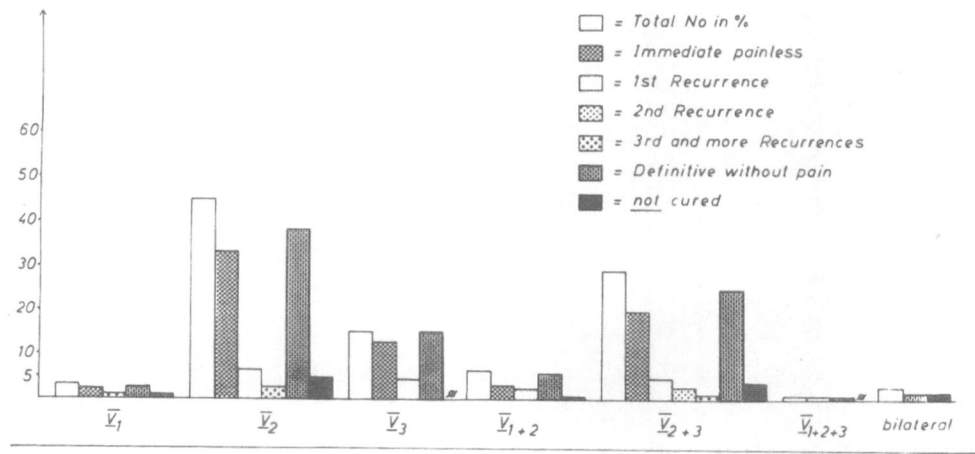

3rd branch neuralgia. In this group we found the highest percentage
of failure to obtain definitive cure, amounting to about 6% (Tables
2 and 3).

The incidence of unpleasant side effects is relatively high. Although
they are actually slight, they may be particularly of subjective importance. Half the patients considered hemianesthesia of the tongue
as a very unpleasant sequela, although it was present in about 80%
(Table 4).

Subjectively unpleasant paresthesias (10%) and locked mandibular
opening (22%) takes the 2nd place among unpleasant subjective sequelae (Table 4). Although weakness of masticator muscles was observed
with a relatively high incidence (12%), patients were subjectively
not very troubled by it. Slight hearing disturbances (7%) are probably caused by injured Eustachian tube during surgery (pterygopalatine
fossa hematoma).

Complications

The complication rate in the recent series of controlled procedures
has been minimal. No neurological deficit outside the territory of
the ipsilateral trigeminal nerve, no paralysis of cranial nerves,
no mortality (Table 5).

Extra- and intracranial morbidity has been temporary, without any
permanent sequelae, with the only exception of slight hearing disturbances, probably due to extracranial hematomas upon unintentional
puncture of the carotid artery and to lesion of the Eustachian tube
(Table 5).

Table 4. The incidence of unpleasant side-effects is relatively high, but of preponderantly subjective importance

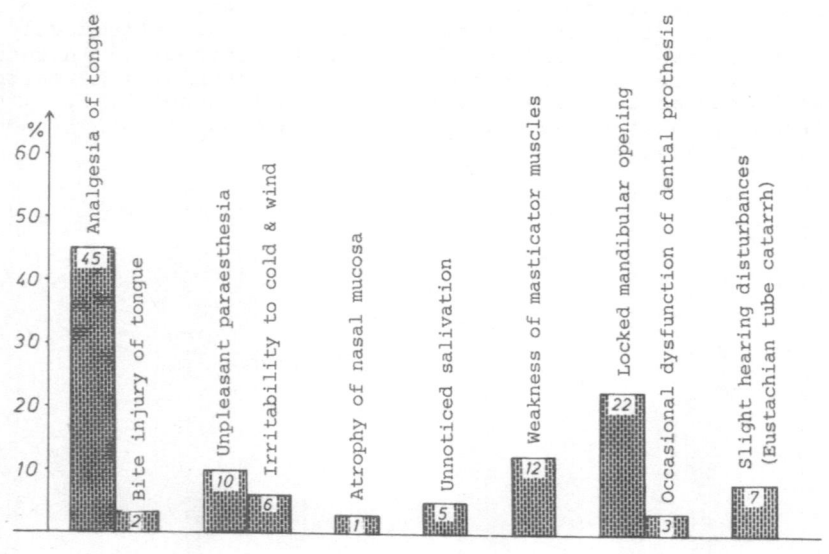

Table 5. Complications were very rare. With the exception of one slight meningitis of three days duration there was   n o   i n t r a - c r a n i a l   complication, particularly no cranial nerve paralysis and no mortality. The most frequent   e x t r a c r a n i a l   compli- cation was a temporary cheek hematoma. Two cases had temporary kera- titis

		Complications		
Intracranial		**Extracranial**		
Blindness (optic nerve lesion)	- 0	Blindness (following Keratitis)	- 0	
Oculomotor n. lesion	- 0	Keratitis, temporary (without corneal ulcer)	- 2	(0,7%)
Abducens n. lesion	- 0			
Facial n. lesion	- 0	Hematoma of the cheek (temporary)	-12	(4,2%)
Epileptic seizures	- 0			
Hemiplegia	- 0			
Intracranial hematoma	- 0			
Bulbar symptoms	- 0			
Brain abscess	- 0			
Meningitis (slight, duration) 3 days	- 1			

In *summary*, the advantages of the c o n t r o l l e d technique are:

(1) Minimal operative risk (no mortality).

(2) Time-saving procedure (mean duration: 40 minutes).

(3) No age limit (oldest patient 92 years) (Fig. 3).

(4) Control of sensory deficit with gradual coagulation during the procedure (preserving corneal reflex).

(5) Possibility of repeating procedure as often as necessary (about 23% in total).

(6) Marked reduction of recurrences as final result (about 6% failures).

(7) Short period of hospitalization of 3 to 5 days in average.

(8) Shortened period of postoperative convalescence with earlier return to work.

Summary

Based on his experience with 638 procedures for the treatment of trigeminal neuralgia between 1955 and 1973 (5, 6, 7, 8, 9), the author developed a strong preference for the percutaneous electrocoagulation of the Gasserian ganglion. Although the method was repeatedly modified in the early years, a standardized technique of controlled, selective and fractional coagulation in the semi-awake patient under neurolept-anesthesia has been used since 1963 in 285 of 437 patients, treated in this manner. The advantages of the method, particularly if compared to 149 cases of open intracranial root sections, are: minimal operative risk, control of the coagulation effect during the procedure, small sensitivity deficit, low complication rate, short period of hospitalization, short convalescence and satisfactory end results in a high percentage, only in some instances after a second or third coagulation, if needed. Hypesthesia of the trigger zone is a prerequisite for success.

REFERENCES

1. FRAZIER, C.H.: Radical operations for major trigeminal neuralgia. J. Amer. Med. Ass. 96, 913 (1931).

2. HÄRTEL, F.: Die Leitungsanästhesie und Injektionsbehandlung des Ganglion Gasseri und der Trigeminusstämme. Arch. Klin. Chir. 100, 193-292 (1913).

3. KIRSCHNER, N.: Zur Behandlung der Trigeminusneuralgie. Erfahrungen an 250 Fällen. Arch. Klin. Chir. 186, 225-234 (1936).

4. KIRSCHNER, N.: Die Behandlung der Trigeminusneuralgie (nach Erfahrungen an 1113 Kranken). Münch. med. Wschr. 89, 235-239 (1942).

5. SCHÜRMANN, K.: Die moderne Behandlung der "idiopathischen" Trigeminusneuralgie mit der subtemporalen extraduralen Wurzeldekompression. Therapiewoche Karlsruhe 6, 380-382 (1956).

6. SCHÜRMANN, K.: Die "Rezidive" nach der Taarnhøj-Norlénschen Wurzeldekompression in der Behandlung der Trigeminusneuralgie. Zbl. Neurochir. 16, 292-298 (1956).

7. SCHÜRMANN, K.: Neurochirurgische Therapie bei Schmerzzuständen. Med. Kurse ärztl. Fortbildung 14, 1-10 (1962).

8. SCHÜRMANN, K., BUTZ, M.: Retroganglionäre Trigeminuswurzelresektion durch temporale Schädeleröffnung oder kontrollierte partielle Elektroverödung des Ganglion Gasseri durch gezielte Punktion in der operativen Behandlung der idiopathischen Trigeminusneuralgie? (Bericht über 435 Fälle). Zbl. Neurochir. <u>29</u>, 131-152 (1968).

9. SCHÜRMANN, K., BUTZ, M., BROCK, M.: Temporal Retrogasserian Resection of Trigeminal Root versus Controlled Elective Percutaneous Electrocoagulation of the Ganglion of Gasser in the Treatment of Trigeminal Neuralgia. Report on a series of 531 Cases. Acta Neuro-chir. <u>26</u>, 33-53 (1972).

10. SCHÜRMANN, K.: Controlled and Partial Percutaneous Electrocoagulation of Gasserian Ganglion in Facial Pain. Annual Meeting American Assoc. Neurological Surgeons, St. Louis, April 22-27, 1974.

11. SJÖQVIST, O.: Eine neue Operationsmethode bei Trigeminusneuralgie. Durchschneidung des Tractus spinalis trigemini. Zbl. Neurochir. <u>5</u>, 274-281 (1937).

12. SWEET, W.H., WEPSIC, J.G.: Relation of fiber size in trigeminal root to conduction of impulses for pain and touch. Production of analgesia without anesthesia in the effective treatment of trigeminal neuralgia. 22nd Annual Meeting of the Scandinavian Neurosurgical Society in Stockholm, August 21-22, 1970.

13. SWEET, W.H., WEPSIC, J.G.: Controlled thermocoagulation of trigeminal ganglion and rootlets for differential destruction of pain fibers. Part 1: Trigeminal neuralgia. J. Neurosurg. <u>40</u>, 143-156 (1974).

14. TAARNHØJ, P.: Decompression of the trigeminal root and the posterior part of the ganglion as treatment in trigeminal neuralgia. J. Neurosurg. <u>9</u>, 288-290 (1952).

15. TÖNNIS, W.: Die Bedeutung einer sorgfältigen Differentialdiagnose für die chirurgische Behandlung der Trigeminusneuralgie. Dtsch. Med. Wschr. <u>76</u>, 1202-1205 (1951).

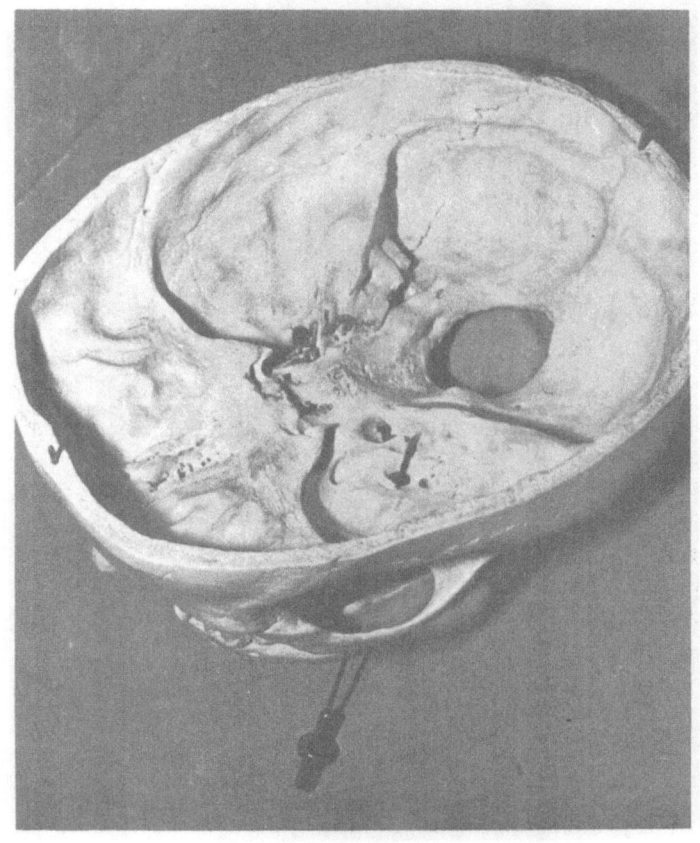

Fig. 1. Model of the base of skull illustrating the free-hand puncture of the Gasserian ganglion. The non-insulated needle tip has been
passed through the foramen ovale. Lateral to it is the foramen spinosum and medial to it the somewhat larger foramen lacerum

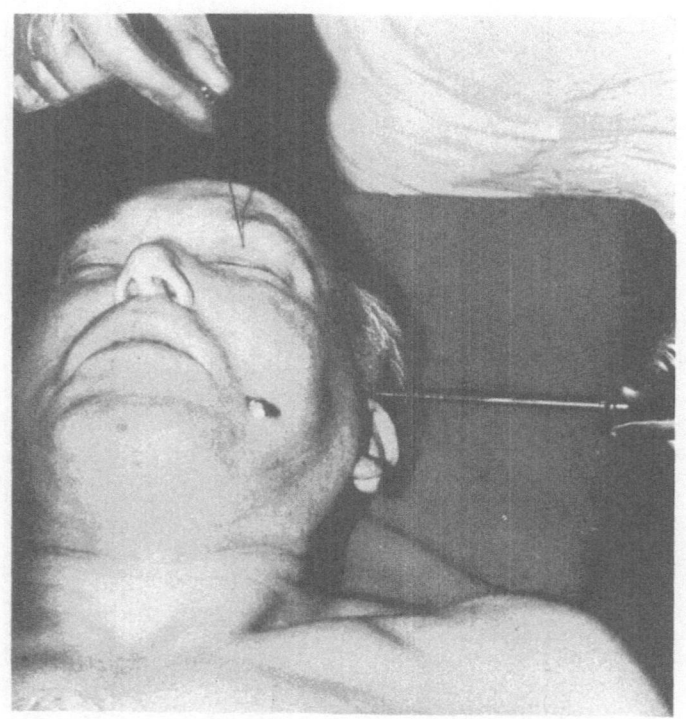

Fig. 2. Reference points for the percutaneous free-hand puncture of the Gasserian ganglion. In order to reach the foramen ovale the needle is directed towards a point placed at the crossing of an imaginary anteroposterior line through the pupil and a second imaginary transverse line from the root of one ear to a corresponding point on the opposite side. The point of entrance of the needle tip through the skin lies about two centimeters lateral to the angle of the mouth. The needle tip is advanced in direction of the crossing of the imaginary anteroposterior and transverse lines until it passes through the foramen ovale. The correct position of the needle tip is then roentgenologically checked

Age   and sex in facial pain patients

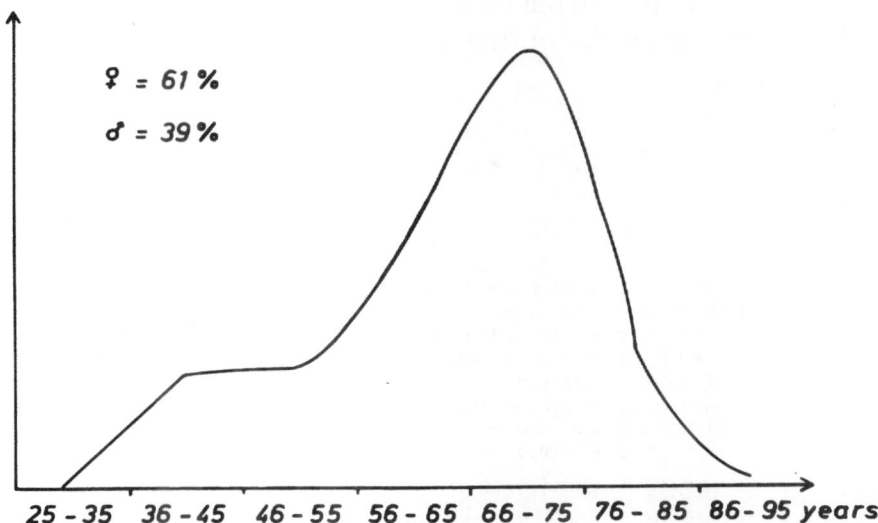

Fig. 3. About two-thirds of the series is female. The youngest patient was aged 23 and the oldest 92 years, while the highest frequency of tic douloureux was found between the ages of 66 and 75 years

Remarks on the Techniques of Electrocoagulation of the Gasserian Ganglion for Trigeminal Neuralgia. Experience With More than 900 Operations Performed in Over 600 Patients from 1952 to 1974

B. HÜBNER

Over the past 22 years we have applied electrocoagulation of the gasserian ganglion according to the method of K.H. BAUER 893 times in 630 patients suffering with trigeminal neuralgia. At the end of my lecture I will provide a short account of the results obtained. The purpose of this lecture is to give some idea of the technical aspects with the aid of which we have been able to obtain reliable results with smallest risk. These techniques have undergone development and improvement in the course of the years.

(1) *Anesthesia*. From 1952 to 1965, the patients were usually submitted to coagulation under hexobarbital anesthesia and later under insufflation anesthesia. For three years now, we have frequently used Ketanest anesthesia, a method which I regard as the most protective and which has certain limitations only in cases of sclerotic patients and persons suffering from hypertension. Premedication is made with Dolantin, Atosil and Atropine.

(2) *The Positioning of the Patient* is best on an operating table capable of being raised and lowered hydraulically. Directly connected to the table is a complete amplifier unit with a television system. This facilitates optimum positioning of the head for puncture of the ganglion as well as for TV-control.

(3) *Puncture* is accomplished with a normal puncture needle (Akufirm) coated with insulating paint, and sterilized in boiling water. Care should be taken not to allow other instruments to come into contact with the varnish coating. The tip of the needle is scraped bright to a length of 5 to 7 mm using a scalpel. The shorter the uncoated surface, the more accurate the obtained coagulation. Coatings consisting of modern plastic insulating material are invariably below our expectations: frequently they burn through even when charged below 600 mA. A needle should be used only once.

(4) *The Method of Puncture* we employ is that described by HÄRTL and K.H. BAUER. Control of the precise position of the needle with the amplifier in an axial position makes it possible to coagulate only the 3rd or 2nd division or all 3 branches, depending on the individual indication. This facility of control avoids inadvertent puncture of the jugular foramen, the foramen lacerum, the Eustachian tube or the pterygopalatine fossa.

(5) *Coagulation of the Ganglion* is performed by means of continuously variable diathermy, employing precision-controlled current up to a maximum of 600 mA. After each circuit closure of a few seconds duration, it can be ascertained, by turning the puncture needle slightly, whether and to what extent coagulation has occurred. Although this

method is an empirical one, it is undoubtedly more accurate than the method of limiting the time of coagulation by using a stop watch, or of precoagulating using a test piece of meat. The complete procedure does not take longer than 5 to 10 minutes.

(6) *Follow-Up Treatment* should definitely include protection of the eye by means of a watch-glass bandage so that a moist chamber safeguards the cornea. Depending on the patient's state of consciousness, we decide, after a period of 6 to 24 hours, whether the protective dressing may be removed in the case of normesthesia of the cornea. To be on the safe side, however, ointment of Bepanthen or a similar agent should always be applied to the conjunctival sac during the first few days. We allow the patients to leave bed after 24 hours and discharge most of them after only two days. For safety, an opthalmological check-up should be made regularly during the first week following the procedure.

Table 1 shows that the relapse rate is relatively high, amounting to 15%, especially since we coagulate only on a selective basis. On the other hand, we have an extremely low rate of complications. Serious late damage to the eye or mucous membranes amounts to less than 2%.

Table 1. Operations on patients suffering from trigeminal neuralgia from 1952 - 1974

Number of patients	630
Number of electrocoagulation operations	893
Relapses included in this number	130
Number of other operations	31
Relapse rate	15%
Postoperative mortality rate (3 cases)	0,33%
Serious early complications (keratitis) (20 cases)	1,31%
Serious late complications (loss of sight, chronic mucosal ulceration) (15 cases)	1,64%
Average age of the patients (924 operations)	63,8 years

Results of Treatment of Trigeminal Neuralgia by the Operation of Dandy

R. WÜLLENWEBER and P. DISTELMAIER

When comparing different surgical methods applied for the treatment
of a disease one has to consider:
(1) the results,
(2) the complications,
(3) the specific indications.
DANDY (1, 2, 3) has described the following advantages of the para-
pontine section of the sensory roots of the trigeminal nerve:
(1) no lesions of the cornea,
(2) no paresis of the masticatory muscles,
(3) no anesthesia of the face,
(4) only one case of transitory facial nerve paresis,
(5) no hemiplegia, aphasia or epileptic seizures as sequelae of the
    operation.
The lethality in a series of 200 patients - operated on by himself -
was 0,5%. He observed recurrences of pain in only 2%, these patients
recovered after reoperation.

Patients

212 patients suffering from a trigeminal neuralgia were operated on
at the Neurosurgical Department of the University of Bonn. The age
distribution corresponds to the morbidity rate of trigeminal neuralgia, with a peak within the 6. and 7. decades (Fig. 1). The relation
of females to males, 3 : 2, confirms the findings of other statistics. The oldest patient was 81 years, the youngest 29 and suffering
from a traumatic lesion of the trigeminal nerve. 64% of the patients
had typical "tic douloureux". This group includes idiopathic as well
as symptomatic neuralgias. 36% were cases with atypical neuralgia,
described in the majority of cases as a continuous pain. From these,
14% were tumors of the base of the skull and 26% sequelae of head
injuries. 60% of the patients had been operated on previously (32%
exeresis of peripheral branches, 58% destruction of the Gasserian
ganglion according to KIRSCHNER or HÄRTL, 10% operations according
to FRAZIER or TAARNHØJ).

Results

145 patients were followed up to 16 years. In the group of typical
tic douloureux 85% recovered to the point that no further medicamen-
tous treatment was necessary. 15% had recurrences, but only 6% had a
typical tic douloureux. The results in cases of atypical pain of the
face without tic douloureux were very poor. 65% of the patients had
recurrences. Most recurrences developed within the first 3 years
following surgery.

Complications

The most common and harmless complication was a herpes labialis in more than 50% (Fig. 2). The symptoms disappeared completely within 2 - 3 weeks after surgery. The rate of transitory facial paresis and of hearing deficits was very high. It may be assumed that these disturbances were caused by traction of the nerves during cerebellar retraction. Persistent facial paresis was observed in only 1 case (0,8%), but persistent hearing deficits occured in 6%. No corneal lesion was recorded. Cerebellar symptoms, observed postoperatively in 6%, persisted in one case. Transitory disturbances of mastication were seen in 4% but persisten in only 2 cases. In these 2 cases lesions of the motor root must be assumed. Anesthesia dolorosa was observed in 5%, 2/3 (4 cases) of which had herpes zoster. The high rate of hearing defects may be caused by vascular lesions, since damage only by traction would probably also have involved the facial nerve. Lethality was 3,7% but only 4 patients died as a consequence of the operation (1 hemorrhage, 2 pontine softenings, 1 purulent meningitis caused by mastoidotomy). In the other 4 cases death was caused by extracerebral complications, 3 patients suffering from arterial hypertension. All patients who died following surgery were in the age group from 60 - 69 years. 2 patients died 2 months following surgery.

Recurrence Operations

As mentioned above, 60% of allpatients operated on by the technique of DANDY had already been operated before. Recurrences following paracerebellar dissection of the trigeminal roots were almost impossible to influence. In 4 cases renewed exposure of the cerebellopontine angle was undertaken to dissect remnants of the sensory roots. In only 2 cases the result of the reoperation was satisfactory. Anesthesia dolorosa, observed in 6 cases, could not be cured by different operations (thalamotomy included). The highest rate of recurrences - besides the zoster-cases- was seen in cases of posttraumatic facid pain. The poor results of reoperations by DANDY's technique suggest that no further operative treatment should be given, particularly since more than 50% of the patients treated with TEGRETAL, recovered and were able to resume their occupation.

Range of Indications

The main indication for DANDY's procedure has been considered to be those patients who did not recover following other more peripheral procedures. Formerly we saw a further indication in cases in which cerebellopontine angle tumor had not been excluded but had also not been proven with the usual diagnostic methods. In fact, we found only 4 tumors - mostly cholesteatomas - affecting the trigeminal roots. As a result of the refinement of diagnostic procedures this specific indication can be considered obsolete nowadays.

Thorough analysis of the operative reports revealed that arachnoidal adhesions were described in more than 30%. Naturally these findings depend on the subjective opinion of the surgeon. It is therefore impossible to answer the question of whether these findings have any importance for the pathogenesis of idiopathic trigeminal neuralgia. Concerning the range of complications, DANDY's comments must be confirmed, except for the hearing disturbances, not metioned by him. No permanent lesions of the cornea, and no focal disturbances attributable to a cerebral hemispheric lesion were observed. The percentage

of permanent facial or masticatory paresis was very low. The high
percentage of permanent hearing deficits in our group of patients
led us to indicate this type of surgery with reserve in all cases
in which uni- or bilateral hearing disturbances already existed.
The excellent results of DANDY's series could not be confirmed.

Summary

212 patients with trigeminal neuralgia were operated on by section
of the sensory root accoring to DANDY. 85% of the cases with typical
tic douloureux recovered, but only 35% of patients suffering from
atypical pain of the face. 60% had previously been operated on by
other methods. 4 patients died as a consequence of surgery. The rate
of transitory disturbances was rather high, but permanent deficits
were only seen in a low percentage. No permanent corneal lesions and
no focal disturbances attributable to a cerebral hemispheric lesion
were observed.

REFERENCES

1. DANDY, W.E.: Section of sensory root of trigeminal nerve at the
   pons. Bull. Hopkins Hosp. 35, 105 (1925).

2. DANDY, W.E.: Operation for cure of tic douloureux; partial section of the sensor root at the pons. Arch. Surg. 18, 687 (1929).

3. DANDY, W.E.: Hirnchirurgie, pp. 201-227 Leipzig: J.A. Barth 1938.

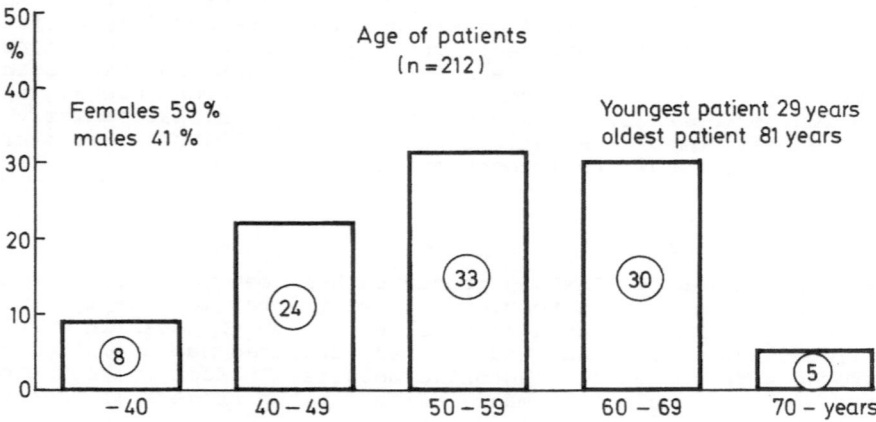

Fig. 1. Age distribution in 212 cases of trigeminal neuralgia treated
by the operation of DANDY

	Transient	Permanent
Herpes labialis	50 %	—
Facial nerve paresis	17 %	1 %
Hearing disturbances	11 %	6 %
Cerebell. symptoms	6 %	1 %
Paresis of masticatory muscles	4 %	2 %
Anesthesia dolorosa	—	5 %
Keratitis	2 %	—

Fig. 2. Complications in 145 cases of trigeminal neuralgia treated by the operation of DANDY

Results of Surgical Treatment of Idiopathic Trigeminal Neuralgia Using Different Operative Techniques

(A Co-Operative Study)*

H. PENZHOLZ, J. MENZEL, and H.-U. HAGENLOCHER

Trigeminal neuralgia is one of the most dreadful pain diseases that is known. Patients suffering from this pain do not die of it, unless they commit suicide; however, their life is a torment. A very effective treatment may be achieved by neurosurgical procedures. The value of different operative techniques is to be judged by (1) the efficiency with which pain relief - transitory or, better permanent - is obtained and by (2) the dangers that accompany surgery.

The aim of this study was to gain better insight into the possibilities, limitations, and risks of the most frequently-used operative methods and to subject them to critical evaluation.

Material and Methodology

For this purpose the co-operation of all German and Austrian neurosurgical units was requested. They were asked to re-examine patients who had been operated in the last 10 years and to list their results in the questionnaire which had been mailed to them and which had been prepared for computer analysis. We intended to gather information on the efficiency and complications of surgical methods used in German-speaking countries.

Seventeen German and Austrian neurosurgical clinics responded to our request, and we would like to express our thanks to all of the collaborators for their co-operation (Table 1). Based on these data, we were able to analyze a total of 1,946 patients who had undergone surgical treatment for idiopathic trigeminal neuralgia.

Results

Table 2 shows age distribution and applied surgical procedures. Analysis showed that 1,051 patients were treated by electrocoagulation or received alcohol injection into the Gasserian ganglion. 477 patients underwent FRAZIER's temporal or DANDY's suboccipital rhizotomy. In 55 cases medullary tractotomy was performed. The discrepancy between the

---

*The following colleagues have collaborated in the present study:

M. Schirmer and H. Schlarb (Berlin-Neukölln), Th. Grumme (Berlin-Westend), V. Hensell, H. Miltz and Roßberg (Düsseldorf), W.-J. Bock (Essen), D. Kirchhoff and H.-W. Pia (Gießen), B. Rama (Göttingen), H. Tritthart (Graz), K. Schmidt and A. Spring (Günzburg), K. Faulhauer (Homburg/Saar), E. Schürmann and K. Schürmann (Mainz), B. Richling (Salzburg), E. Heiß and F. Pampus (Stuttgart), P. Oldenkott and H. Rooschüz (Tübingen), J. Ganglberger and H. Kraus (Wien), P. Gruß and H. Straber (Würzburg), T. Demirel (Wuppertal).

Table 1. Results after different operative procedures for idiopathic trigeminal neuralgia (A cooperative study)

Participating Clinics	Number of Cases
Berlin-Neukölln	13
Berlin-Westend	190
Düsseldorf	281
Essen	50
Giessen	467
Göttingen	106
Graz	57
Günzburg	40
Heidelberg	107
Homburg (Saar)	48
Mainz[a]	102[a]
Salzburg	27
Stuttgart	142
Tübingen	120
Wien	129
Würzburg	30
Wuppertal	37
Total	1 946

[a]Because of a regrettable misunderstanding, only the follow-up of the patients in the time between January 1st 1971 and December 31st 1973 has been taken over in the Computer study. The results of the follow-up of the whole series of 635 cases treated in various procedures by the Neurosurgical Department of the University Clinic in Mainz is compiled and compared in the paper by K. SCHÜRMANN (see Table 3).

Table 2. Frequency of the different surgical procedures in relation to patients age

Age	Electro-coagulation	Alcohol-injection	FRAZIER	DANDY	SJÖQVIST
20	1	0	0	1	0
30	6	4	5	2	1
40	39	2	12	11	1
50	109	18	52	21	8
60	249	22	115	30	10
70	338	19	137	30	23
80	203	14	47	9	12
90	26	1	2	3	0
Total	971	80	370	107	55
	1 051		477		55

total number of patients examined and the sum given in Table 2 is explained by the fact that 300 patients were first subjected to operative techniques, mainly preganglionic procedures, which were not taken into consideration in our questionnaire.

The frequency of pain relief after the first operation and until discharge from clinical care is shown in Table 3. Of the 971 patients who underwent electrocoagulation, 892 (= 91.8%) were free of pain or had at least satisfactory pain relief. 37 patients (= 3.8%) showed no improvement. Of the 80 patients treated by alcohol injection, 58 (= 72.5%) greatly improved or even had no further pain attacks. However, in 14 cases (= 17.5%) this method was ineffective. Of the 370 patients who underwent surgical treatment according to the technique FRAZIER's 349 (= 94.3%) were free of pain or satisfactory pain relief was achieved. This operation was ineffective in 13 cases. According to DANDY's method, which was applied in 107 cases, no improvement was observed in 7 cases (= 6.9%). 96 (= 89.7%) patients, however, were relieved of pain. SJÖQVIST medullary tractotomy led to pain relief in 98.1%. In only one case was the operation unsuccessful.

Table 3. Free of pain after the first operation

	Painless or essentially improved	not improved	n
Electrocoagulation	892 = 91,8%	37 = 3,8%	971
Alcoholinjection	58 = 72,5%	14 = 17,5%	80
FRAZIER	349 = 94,3%	13 = 3,5%	370
DANDY	96 = 89,7%	7 = 6,5%	107
SJÖQVIST	54 = 98,1%		55

The complications resulting from the various procedures are shown in Table 4.

Paralysis of the masseter muscle (masticatory paralysis) after electrocoagulation (6.3%) and alcohol injection (2.5%) is rare, following somewhat more often the FRAZIER procedure (8.9%) and occurring surprisingly frequently in patients who underwent surgical treatment according to DANDY's method (22.4%). But these results must be interpreted with caution, because the assessment of postoperative masticatory paralysis is dependent on very subjective reports both on the part of the patient and clinical investigator.

Facial paralysis resulted in 10.5% and 13.1% following FAZIER's and DANDY's methods respectively. From the 39 patients with facial palsy after FRAZIER's operation 29 could be followed up. Re-examination showed improvement in 14 cases so that in the total of 370 who underwent the FRAZIER procedure there were only 15 cases (= 4.1%) with permanent, complete facial paralysis. In 14 cases of the DANDY group, 13 could be followed up. Here we found improvement in 6 patients so that only 7 were impaired permanently (= 6.5%). In contrast to this the rate of this complication after electrocoagulation was only 0.8% (8 : 971).

Table 4. Surgical procedures and complications

	Masticatory Paralysis	Facial-nerve Paralysis	Oculomotor- N. Paralysis	Impaired Hearing	Hemiparesis	Ataxia	Mental Disturbances	Keratitis Neuroparalytica	Loss of Sight	n
Electrocoagul.	61 6,3%	8 0,8%	5 0,5%	27 2,8%	9 0,9%	6 0,6%	34 3,5%	17 1,7%	1 0,1%	971
Alcoholinject.	2 2,5%	0	2 2,5%	1 1,3%	0	0	9 11,3%	0	0	80
FRAZIER	33 8,9%	39 10,5%	9 2,4%	4 1,1%	7 1,9%	6 1,6%	24 6,5%	8 2,2%	1 0,3%	370
DANDY	24 22,4%	14 13,1%	1 0,9%	19 17,8%	1 0,9%	15 14,0%	9 8,4%	4 3,7%	0	107
SJÖQVIST	0	0	0	0	3 5,5%	1 1,8%	0	0	0	55

Paralysis of the oculomotor nerve, although rare, developed in 9 patients after FRAZIER's operation or 2.4% of the group.

Impaired hearing and cerebellar ataxia occured especially frequently in 17.8% and in 14% respectively after DANDY's operation.

Mental change was most frequently observed after alcohol injection (= 11.3%) and with approximately the same frequency after FRAZIER's temporal (6.5%) and DANDY's suboccipital retroganglionary rhizotomy (8.4%). But these mental changes may also occur after electrocoagulation (3.5%). Here it should be borne in mind that in older patients with arteriosclerosis of the carotid and vertebral arteries and osteochondrosis of the cervical spine, hyperextension of the head, which may be necessary for X-rays of the skull base, may lead to permanent brain damage.

Neuroparalytic keratitis developed in 1.7% of the patients subjected to electrocoagulation, in 2.2% of the FRAZIER group and in 3.7% of the DANDY group. Blindness of the afflicted eye resulted only in one instance each after electrocoagulation and the FRAZIER procedure. It is remarkable that unilateral loss of sight has apparently never occurred in patients who had undergone surgical treatment according to the DANDY technique, in spite of the fact that the frequency of keratitis is much higher in this last group.

The frequency and intensity of postoperative paresthesia as well as of anesthesia dolorosa have been listed separately (see Table 5a and 5b). Severe permanent paresthesia (Table 5a) is most often seen after alcohol injection: 3 patients (3.7%) in a total of 80 cases showed this unpleasant development. Less severe, permanent paresthesia was observed in another 3 patients. Although this complication seems to be rare after electrocoagulation and after temporal rhizotomy, one has to face the possibility. In the group of 971 electrocoagulated patients 5 (= 0.5%) had severe and 40 (= 4.1%) less severe, permanent paresthesia. It is remarkable that no case of severe permanent paresthesia was observed in the 107 patients of the DANDY group and only 3 cases (= 2.8%) developed moderate, permanent paresthesia.

Table 5a. Surgical procedures and paresthesia

| | Transitory | Permanent | | n |
		Slight	Severe	
Electro-coagulation	38 = 3,9%	40 = 4,1%	5 = 0,5%	971
Alcohol-injection	6 = 7,5%	3 = 3,7%	3 = 3,7%	80
FRAZIER	16 = 4,3%	5 = 1,4%	7 = 1,9%	370
DANDY	8 = 7,5%	3 = 2,8%	0	107
SJÖQVIST	0	0	0	55

Anesthesia dolorosa (Table 5b) was most frequent after alcohol injection. After eletrocoagulation, this dreadful complication occurred in 0.8%, after FRAZIER's temporal approach in 2.2% and after the DANDY operation in 1.9% of the cases.

Table 5b. Surgical procedures and anesthesia dolorosa

	Number	n
Electrocoagulation	8 = 0,8%	971
Alcohol injection	4 = 5,0%	80
FRAZIER	8 = 2,2%	370
DANDY	2 = 1,9%	107
SJÖQVIST	O	55

Table 6. Surgical procedures - rate of mortality and causes of death

	Direct causes				Indirect causes				Total	n
	1	2	3	Total %	1	2	3	Total %	† %	
Electro-coagul.	1	O	1	2 = 0,2%	1	1	1	3 = 0,3%	5 = 0,5%	971
Alcohol-inject.	1	1	O	2 = 2,5%	3	O	O	3 = 3,8%	5 = 6,3%	80
FRAZIER	2	2	2	6 = 1,6%	3	1	O	4 = 1,0%	10 = 2,6%	370
DANDY	2	O	O	2 = 1,9%	1	2	2	5 = 4,7%	7 = 6,6%	107
SJÖQVIST	O	O	1	1 = 1,8%	O	1	O	1 = 1,8%	2 = 3,6%	55

1 Postop. Hemor-rhage
2 Meningitis
3 Other causes

1 Infarction
2 Embolism
3 Pneumonia

Table 7. Rate of relapses

	Number	%	n
Electrocoagulation	374	38,5	971
Alcohol injection	61	76,3	80
FRAZIER	61	16,5	370
DANDY	8	7,5	107
SJÖQVIST	16	29,1	55

Table 6 shows the postoperative mortality. The cause of death is related to direct (e.g; hemorrhage, meningitis etc.) and to indirect (pneumonia, embolism etc.) postoperative causes. The lowest rate of mortality was found in the electrocoagulation group (0.5%). In the FRAZIER group, as the second most frequently used method, the mortality rate was 2.6%. Worth mentioning is the high rate of mortality in the group of patients who had undergone the DANDY procedure (6.6%), wheregy 4.7% died from indirect postoperative causes alone.

The frequency of relapse is given in Table 7. Of the 971 patients who were electrocoagulated, 374 (= 38.5%) had to undergo a second operation as a result of a genuine relapse. In another 11 cases a second operation is planned so that the recurrence rate rises to about 40%. 61 patients (= 76.3%) who were treated by alcohol injected into the gasserian ganglion had pain relapse. In the FRAZIER group, recurrence was noted in 61 patients (= 16.5%), whereas in the total of 107 patients who underwent the DANDY operation, 8 cases (= 7.5%) suffered a relapse.

Discussion

The results presented can only give a rough idea about the efficiency of different surgical procedures for trigeminal neuralgia in German-speaking countries. It is probable that the results would have been quite different if the various operations had been performed by only one neurosurgeon who is specialized in this field. This applies equally to the three most frequently used methods, namely electrocoagulation, the FRAZIER temporal operation and the DANDY suboccipital approach. This may also be valid for the at present less frequently used procedures such as HÄRTL's alcohol injection and SJÖQVIST's medullary tractotomy.

Some of the remarkable results in this co-operative study might be explained by different degree of exactness practised by the follow-up investigators in the individual clinics. As an example the diverging data concerning the frequency of masticatory paralysis, neuroparalytic keratitis, and mental changes after the different operative procedures can be mentioned.

Finally the unequal size of the groups could be a factor. This may play a role as to the difference between the frequency of pain recurrence after FRAZIER's procedure (370 cases) and after the DANDY operation (107 cases). The present data seem to favour the suboccipital approach of DANDY as far as the probability of relapse is concerned. However, the significance of the lower rate of recurrences in this latter group was not statistically verified.

Summary

On the basis of the present study involving 1,946 patients from 17 neurosurgical clinics who were operated on for idiopathic trigeminal neuralgia, we can say the following:

(1) Electrocoagulation with 50% of the total test-group was the most frequently used operativ method.

(2) All operative techniques resulted in immediate pain relief or at least satisfactory improvement, in approximately 90% of the cases.

(3) The number of complications was the lowest following electrocoagulation. It was twice as high after the FRAZIER operation and 4 1/2 times higher after the DANDY operation.

(4) Permanent postoperative paresthesia occurred in 4.6% of the cases following electrocoagulation, in 3.3% of the cases after the temporal approach and in 2.8% of the cases after the DANDY operation. Permanent severe paresthesia did not remain in any of the patients who underwent the DANDY procedure.

(5) Anesthesia dolorosa resulted in less than 1% of the cases after electrocoagulation. It occurred after the temporal and suboccipital approaches more than twice as often.

(6) Mortality after electrocoagulation amounted to 0.5%, following FRAZIER's operation 2.6%, and after DANDY's operation 6.6%.

(7) The relapse frequency amounted to 40% after electrocoagulation, 16.5% after the temporal approach and 7.5% after DANDY's approach. The different number of cases in the last two groups permits only a limited comparison.

It seems to be legitimate to state, on the basis of our investigation that electrocoagulation - or its modern variation, thermocoagulation of the ganglion GASSERI - seems at the present time to be the best method for treating idiopathic trigeminal neuralgia surgically the first time.

Free Communications

Complications from Surgery on a Vulnerable Spinal Cord

B. B. WHITCOMB

Certain risks are to be expected in surgery of the spinal cord. There are particular situations, however, where serious complications may occur where there is an obvious vulnerability of the cord. In other situations, the vulnerability may be more obscure due to an abnormal vascular supply. This will be demonstrated in the following cases.

Case I

A 49-year-old female achondroplastic dwarf gave a history of pain in the right upper extremity for several years. On admission, she showed some generalized weakness and long tract signs with ankle clonus, left Babinski and peripheral weakness in the right arm. X-rays showed borderline platybasia with developmental changes at C1-C2. There was some scoliosis of the cervical spine. The myelogram showed an upward course of the cervical roots, suggesting an Arnold-Chiari malformation, but there was no obstruction. An arteriogram showed a *hypoplastic left subclavian artery*. Operation was performed in the *sitting position* under *general anesthesia* with decompression of C1, C2 and the foramen magnum. The spinal cord was not touched or manipulated. Postoperatively, there was a central cervical cord syndrome with flaccid motor paralysis of the hands, which has persisted, plus paralysis of the right shoulder girdle, arm and upper intercostals. She has a bilateral Babinski response but is able to walk.

Here a vulnerable ischemic cord became infarcted because of the procedure, probably from posturing under anesthesia in a patient whose cord circulation was borderline with hypoplastic vessels.

Occurring at about the same time, there were three similar cases in New England of cord or medullary infarctions following rhizotomies for spasmodic torticollis. Dr. William SWEET of Boston described his case as postoperatively having a devastating flaccid paralysis in both upper extremities similar to the case presented above; Dr. Hannibal HAMLIN of Providence reported a similar serious complication with a Left Brown-Sequards Syndrome and Dr. William SCOVILLE had the following case in our clinic in Hartford:

Case II

A 49-year-old male with severe spastic torticollis. Operation was performed in the sitting position with section of the motor roots of C1, 2 and 3 bilaterally plus the spinal accessory nerves. There was transient troublesome bleeding between C1 and 2 roots anteriorly. The immediate postoperative result was satisfactory, but the patient developed sleep apnoea in a few hours. This was immediately recognized, and he was placed on the respirator but found to have a medullary syndrome with inability to swallow, speak or breathe and with a drop in blood pressure, quadriparesis and bladder paralysis. There was slight gradual improvement over a few months. He was ambulatory with assistance and sent to a convalescent hospital for physical therapy and died of sleep respiratory arrest. At autopsy, unfortunately the cervical cord was not removed, but sections of the medulla indicate the infarction that occurred.

In retrospect, we found two other cases at Hartford Hospital which we believe fit into this category although fortunately their neurologic signs were transient.

Discussion

These cases all suggest an unexpected vascular insult to a cord made vulnerable from a preoperative anomaly or pathological vascular change.

Anatomically, from the works of ADAMKIEWICZ, HUGHES and later anatomists and the more recent works of LAZORTHES, PISCOL, TÖNNIS, ZÜLCH, DiCHIRO and others, we know the major anastomotic vessels enter at the cervical and lumbar enlargements producing the so-called "watershed circulation" with its vulnerable areas. We have been warned that the variations in location of the major anastomotic vessels are also a cause for caution.

Pathologically, vulnerability is produced by those conditions reducing the size of the spinal canal and by vascular conditions jeopardizing the circulation of the cord. The bony stenosing lesions may be congenital such as platybasia, achondroplasia, dysraphism, scoliosis, etc. or acquired such as spondylosis, subluxation, fracture, arachnoiditis ossificans, etc. Cases of spondylosis have been made paraplegic simply by manipulation of the neck under general anesthesia for the purpose of intubation; also by chiropractic manipulation when subsequent occlusion of a vertebral artery has been demonstrated. The soft tissue lesions include: tumors, central disc herniations, hematomas, infections (granuloma) etc. There is also vulnerability from vascular lesions and anomalies. The primary vascular lesions include A.V.M. and arteriosclerosis. WILSON et al. reported two cases of A.V.M. in which there was transient paraplegia occurring after eating a large meal. It was assumed these arose from splanchnic steal through enlarged feeding arteries. More important, however, are lesions of the contributing circulation: aortic — as aneurysms, coarctation and trauma; vertebral — as unilateral compression, occlusion or anomalies. We have reason to believe that this latter situation may have been at play from the marked torsion of the neck in the cases of spasmodic torticollis as illustrated by the second case. Of particular interest are lesions affecting the anastomotic feeding vessels to the cord and the consequent ischemia in the watershed areas. Unexpected injury may occur to these vessels because of their variability in location. The great anastomotic artery (Adamkiewicz) is of such importance that the side and level of its entrance into the spinal cord should be established, particularly before surgical attack in the thoracolumbar area. Damage to this vessel in approaching thoracic discs has accounted for some of the complications in these cases. Diagnostic, radiologic agents used intra-arterially by transient blocking of these vessels have produced tragic paralyses. A low systemic blood pressure or a sudden drop during surgery compounds the vulnerability of an already compromised cord circulation.

Surgical factors to be implicated are the posturing and positioning of the patient with a vulnerable cord under general anesthesia. Local or regional block anesthesia may be much safer and is advised her in most cases as well as in tumors of the dominant hemisphere. This is well tolerated particularly by the older people.

The surgical approach must be planned to give no further encroachment to an already compromised cord or vascular supply. A central cervical disc is better approached anteriorly and a thoracic disc through a transthoracic or costotransversectomy approach. However, these are not without accidents. KRIEGER and ROSOMOFF have reported two cases of sleep apnoea which they felt resulted from ischemia of the cord from an anterior surgical approach to C3-4 disc herniation. If operated psoteriorly, the dura must be opened to permit direct visualization of the cord while expressing the disc. The tragedies of the extradural approach are too well known. Manipulation must be avoided, and the preservation of radicular vessels is essential.

In the lumbar canal, cauda equina palsy can occur from severe compression with associated ischemia of these roots or by the resulting arachn oiditis which commonly follows a complete block in the lumbar subarachnoid space. It is curious why some cases of severe arachnoiditis may have neither signs nor symptoms while others may have severe neurologic deficits and pain. It is suggested that, in some of these cases, vascular occlusion of sufficient duration has occurred to produce the deficit.

Summary

(1) Damage to vascular supply of the cord is often more devastating than direct intrinsic cord surgery.
(2) Conditions rendering the cord circulation to be vulnerable must be recognized preoperatively.
(3) Selective arteriography is advisable prior to surgery on some chronic compressive cord lesions.
(4) Bilateral vertebral angiography is a pertinent preoperative test when considering rhizotomy for spasmodic torticollis.
(5) In cord surgery, one must protect all spinal vessels which may appear of secondary importance normally, but which may be of prime importance in a pathological situation.
(6) Arachnoiditis from extradural surgery more commonly arises from a compression lesion of the cauda equina and may become symptomatic when circulation to the cauda equina is involved.

Spinal Cord Injuries

The Immediate Complete Areflexic Tetraplegia Syndrome*,**

R. C. SCHNEIDER

The author (37) and others (11, 21, 22, 41) have stated in the past
that if a spinal cord injury is immediate and complete, without a
block on the jugular vein compression (Queckenstedt) test, for 24
hours or longer, the prognosis for any functional recovery is hope-
less. Spurred on by the developments in basic and clinical research,
this author believes that this view is no longer tenable, for there
has been effective functional recovery in such instances occurring
beyond the 24-hour limit.

Seven years ago, TURNBULL and co-workers (43) reported their important microangiographic study of the spinal cord of the cadaver, describing the intrinsic relationships of the tiny vessels. In order to
study the results of trauma to the spinal cord in the laboratory, the
older techniques of ALLEN (2, 3) of dropping a given weight a specific distance directly on the cord has been revived (1, 13, 30, 31,
46). However, a rather more natural development of a lesion by GOSCH
and co-workers (18, 19), employing the impact track, has been used in
the Michigan Neurosurgical Research Laboratory, with very satisfactory results.

GOODKIN and CAMPBELL (17) presented their preliminary material on the
sequential alterations found in experimental cord trauma. In further
studies, DUCKER and ASSENMACHER (12), studying trauma induced in monkey spinal cords, emphasized the importance of the timing in the microvascular response. They believed that the subacute and delayed
response due to alteration of the vessel wall resulted in a perivascular inflammatory response, vasomotor paralysis, intravascular stasis, and occasional intravascular coagulation, which halted circulation and led to necrosis within the cord. These authors indicated
that such a response was self-destructive and suggested that prevention of this phase was essential. Subsequent studies showed that
the severity of injury was reflected by alterations in the smaller
vessels, and that the failure of their perfusion was responsible for
the irreversible damage (14).

In other important experimental work, WAGNER and co-workers (45) believed that, within four hours following contusion, pathological
changes occurred in the microvasculature of the spinal cord which resulted in depleted circulation through the capillaries and the post-
capillary venules. In further work from that laboratory, DOHRMANN and
others (10) demonstrated by electron microscopy that by one hour after the spinal cord was experimentally contused, the periaxonal

*Partially reprinted from SCHNEIDER, R.C., CROSBY, E.C., RUSSO, R.H.
and GOSCH, H.H.: Clin. Neurosurg. 20: 424-492, 1973 (39).
**(Work supported by the Begole-Brownell Neurosurgical Fund).

spaces of the involved fibers were dilated, and although the myelin
sheaths of the fibers were attenuated, the axonal morphology remained
intact. After four hours, the myelinated nerve fibers had markedly
dilated periaxonal spaces, and the intact but attenuated sheaths contained axons in various stages of degeneration. However, there still
were only partially denuded axons. Since some of their animals only
had a transitory paraplegia, they postulated that the changes in
these less injured fibers were reversible within the first two weeks
after injury. KELLY and co-workers (23) found in studying traumatized
spinal cords in dogs that low tissue pO_2 could be replaced with oxygen under high pressure, and that following the use of hyperbaric
oxygen, recovery of neurological function seemed equal to other
treatment with hypothermia, steroids, etc. (24).

From their observations of monkeys whose spinal cords were submitted
to the weight-dropping technique (2, 3), OSTERHOLM and MATHEWS (30)
discovered the rather rapid accumulation of norepinephrine after injury. The result was first a neural reaction of electrical depression
or paralysis of fiber activity. The second response was a vascular
one which was toxic tissue destruction. Their subsequent studies (31)
demonstrated that α-methyltyrosine blocked the formation of norepinephrine and thus diminished the degree of spinal cord damage. However, α-methyltyrosine is extremely toxic and OSTERHOLM and MATHEWS
(31) have warned against its use in humans. Nevertheless, this
chemical study provides the possibility of an improved outlook for
the spinal cord injury patient of the future. However, recent studies
fail to support their work.

To ALBIN and co-workers (1) and WHITE and ALBIN (46) must go the credit for the current interest in experimental work due to their studies
with local hypothermia. Their work suggested that local cooling of
the traumatized spinal cord, using ALLEN's (2, 3) old techniques,
effected remarkable neurological recovery. However, DUCKER and HAMIT
(13) and BLACK and MARKOWITZ (5) found the administration of steroids in similarly produced experimental trauma to be at least equal
to, and usually superior to, local cooling of the injured cord in
attaining neurological recovery. The report of COLE and co-workers
(8), stemming from the long use of corticosteroids at the University
of Minnesota, suggested that if they are to be effective they should
be administered early, for the effect is probably greatest in three
to six hours.

Although DAWSON studied cerebral responses after electrical peripheral nerve stimulation in 1947 (9) and improved his technique in
1954, the use of evoked responses in studying the prognosis of traumatized peripheral nerves (26) and injured spinal cords in man (15,
16, 20, 32) has only recently received renewed usage. The future application of these techniques may be of aid in estimating the prognosis and the value of various medical and surgical techniques in the
treatment of acute spinal cord injuries in man.

For years, cervical myelography was not used in the cord injury patient for fear of causing increased deficit. However, more recently
the use of percutaneous instillation of contrast medium at the C-2
vertebral level for cervical myelography using the translateral film
in the prone position has eliminated anxiety concerning undue movement at the cervical fracture or dislocation site such as might occur
with tilting of the patient if the radiopaque oil was injected by the
lumbar route. The increasing use of gas myelography (25, 29) with
polytomography in some clinics (28, 33) has demonstrated the presence
of extruded disc or bone fragments anterior to the cervical spinal

cord and reinforced the clinical observation of the "acute anterior cervical spinal cord injury syndrome" (34, 35) with the necessity for urgent operation (35, 37). On the other hand, if there is a smooth gas shadow anterior to the cervical spinal cord, and a fragment is excluded, there may have been destruction or merely vascular insufficiency without compression to the anterior portion of the cervical spinal cord, and surgery may be contraindicated as suggested by ROSSIER to the author (33).

In the light of these old (42) and new developments suggesting the urgency of instituting treatment (6), the following two case reports of immediate complete areflexic tetraplegia are of some interest.

Case 1

This 18-year-old right-handed girl was riding in a car, not wearing a seat belt, when the vehicle went out of control and turned over. She was ejected from the vehicle without sustaining a loss of consciousness on August 29, 1971 at 9:00 p.m. Upon arrival at a local hospital, the x-rays revealed a C-6 on C-7 fracture-dislocation (Fig. 1A) and a comminuted left fractured humerus. She was then sent directly to the University Hospital. The patient had an immediate complete areflexic tetraplegia, with good residual flexion of her biceps, very weak extension of the triceps, and no grip in the hand bilaterally. There was a complete loss of all sensory modalities to the C-7 dermatome on the right and C-8 on the left. Within two hours after injury, by 11:00 p.m., Vinke tongs had been placed and a lumbar puncture demonstrated a complete block on the jugular vein (Queckenstedt) test. At 6:00 a.m. on August 30 a course of dexamethazone was instituted (4 mg every six hours for two weeks). A second lumbar puncture was made at 9:00 p.m. on August 30, 24 hours after injury and 22 hours after the institution of traction and the initiation of steroid therapy. No blockage was noted on this second Queckenstedt test.

By August 31, 1971 at 2:00 p.m., there was recovery of gross touch, vibration and position sense, and deep pain in the toes bilaterally. Both Achilles reflexes were intact and extensor plantar reflexes were noted. On September 5, the sensory level for hypalgesia had dropped to the T-5 dermatome level. At operation on September 16, a disrupted spinous ligament was found at the C-6-C-7 interspace. There was a locked right facette and a free bone fragment compressing the right side of the cord. A complete laminectomy of C-6 and a partial one of C-7 was performed, with removal of the fragment from the posterior aspect of the cord. The dura was opened and the cord appeared normal. The dentate ligaments were cut and no evidence was found of an extruded disc or bone fragment anterior to the cord. Dural closure was performed and posterior fusion was made by wiring the C-5 and C-7 spinous processes and inserting an iliac bone graft (Fig. 1B). Six months after injury the patient was totally independent. She walked well but had slight imbalance. There was good strength in her lower extremities and right arm, but the left leg was weak. There was symmetrical hyperreflexia with bilateral extensor plantar reflexes. Bladder function was controlled by intermittent catheterization. Ten months after injury she was teaching dancing five days a week and spending a sixth day on her ballet lessons. Her only neurological deficit was the hypalgesia to the L-1 dermatome in the right lower extremity, but this appeared to present no handicap in her activities.

Comment

This patient had an immediate complete tetraplegia with a block on the Queckenstedt test demonstrated two hours after injury. The institution of traction immediately thereafter and the administration of dexamethazone six hours later were successful in overcoming the block as shown on lumbar puncture 22 hours later. It is not known which of these factors was responsible for improvement, but her tetraplegia was shown to clear, disappearing 42 hours after injury. Dr. Robert KNIGHTON (27) had first mentioned to the author in 1969 that he had been administering dexamethazone to his spinal cord injury patients with some success for about 1 year.

The advantages of the posterior approach in this case were the ability to reduce the locked right facette and to elevate the depressed laminar fragment, and the opportunity to view the external condition of the cord and cut the dentate ligaments and to check the possible evidence of an anterior ruptured intervertebral disc or bone fragment. The disadvantage was a longer interval on a frame. An anterior approach could have accomplished the anterior exploration of the cord, but reduction of the facettes, elevation of the depressed lamina, visualization of the condition of the cord, and stimulation of it (if it had been desired) above and below the site of the lesion could not have been accomplished.

A second case is presented because this patient and the previous one were hospitalized concurrently with immediate complete tetraplegia, but the timing in the two patients' management varied considerably and is significant in our discussion.

Case 2

An 18-year-old male was riding in the guest-passenger seat of a car without any seat belt when the vehicle struck an abutment at 55 m.p.h. at 1:00 p.m. on August 27, 1971. The car turned end over end and the patient regained consciousness on the ground, having sustained an immediate complete paralysis of the lower extremities; he was barely able to grip with his hands. At the hospital, the immediate complete areflexic tetraplegia was confirmed, with a sensory level to C-8 for hypalgesia. Cervical spine x-rays demonstrated a fracture through the right lateral mass of the C-6 vertebra on the anterior-posterior view (Fig. 2A) with a slight anterior dislocation of the C-6 vertebral body on C-7 on the lateral view (Fig. 2B). The latter film also suggested the presence of a bony fragment either in the spinal canal at the C-6-C-7 interspace or just lateral to it. Because of the anterior-posterior view, the latter condition was suspected. He was placed in halter traction on a frame until 8:00 a.m. on August 28, 1971, at which time a lumbar puncture was performed and a partial block was found on the jugular vein (Queckenstedt) test, with a cerebrospinal fluid protein value of 77 mg per cent. Immediately thereafter, 19 hours after injury, he was placed on a regime of 10 mg of dexamethazone intravenously and continued on a 4-mg dosage every six hours. Skeletal traction was instituted simultaneously, and there was a slight improvement in alignment at the dislocation site. A lumbar puncture was repeated 72 hours after the first one with no evidence of block on the Queckenstedt test and with the protein value recorded at 40 mg per cent. By September 2 his hypalgesia level was at the C-5 dermatome but otherwise there was no neurological change. He was hyperextended slightly. On September 9, 13 days after his injury, he continued to demonstrate his complete areflexic tetraplegia, and a complete laminectomy of C-5, C-6, and C-7 was performed. On the right a fractured C-6 lamina, which had compressed the spinal cord, was removed, the dura opened, and the dentate ligaments were cut. The cord appeared to be normal. Evoked responses were obtained between the C-6 and C-7 posterior nerve roots bilaterally, suggesting posterior continuity of the spinal cord. (It was unfortunate that further attempts to provide similar stimulation to the anterior roots could not be accomplished because of equipment failure.) The dura was then closed and an iliac bone graft made from C-3 to T-1, with care taken to bridge the bony defect and protect the spinal cord from loose fragments.

By March 15, 1972, he had recovered almost completely, being neurologically negative except for weakness in the interossei of both hands; his right showed more involvement than the left. There was minimal weakness in the right hand, with minimal hyperesthesia in the fingers of both hands. There were right hyperactive upper and lower extremity reflexes, with only a right extensor plantar reflex. He had used self-catheterization for his motor paralytic bladder. His lateral cervical spine x-rays showed a solid bony fusion from C-3 through T-1 but he had surprisingly good movement on flexion and extension films, although his extensive fusion was solid. Ten months after injury he returned with only some weakness and atrophy in his interossei muscles. In spite of this neurological pattern his plant physician had let him return to his work as driver of semi-trucks which task he was reported to have performed skillfully.

Comment

There is no doubt that this patient had an immediate complete areflexic tetraplegia, and inasmuch as the block on lumbar puncture and jugular compression was only partial it was thought that surgical decompression could be delayed. This was especially true since the lateral x-ray film suggested the possibility of some encroachment on the spinal canal at the C-6-C-7 interspace. A C-2 percutaneous Pantopaque[1] myelogram might have demonstrated the degree of encroachment on the spinal canal and might have led to earlier operation. However, it was feared that the manipulation necessary to insert an intratracheal tube might further damage an already compromised spinal cord which apparently had had relief of pressure by traction or the relief of spinal cord edema by dexamethazone.

The posterior surgical approach in this case permitted the elevation of the depressed fracture of the lamina and enabled visualization and stimulation of the spinal cord. The posterior cervical spinal fusion was far too extensive and would have been adequate if carried one segment less in both a cephalad and caudad direction. Instead stabilization could have been accomplished by a two-space anterior fusion at another time, perhaps 10 days later. However, in this instance the desired result was accomplished by one operative procedure despite its extent. The recovery from neurological deficit cannot be attributed necessarily to traction, but perhaps dexamethazone administration permitted protection of the spinal cord function by decreasing cord edema. It was administered 19 hours after injury and presumably this is much too late to have prevented the supposed irreversible changes that have been reported in experimental works by so many observers.

---

[1]Pantopaque, ethyl 10-(p-iodophenyl) undecylate, Lafayette Pharmacal, Inc., Fayetteville, Ind.

Discussion

From a discussion of the data above, it is apparent that the goal in
the treatment of acute spinal cord injuries, whether it be on a biochemical or surgical basis, should be the diminution of hypoxia to
the injured spinal cord by the improvement of the microcirculation.
WHITE and ALBIN (46) reported applying their experimental local cooling techniques, which require operative intervention, to 10 patients,
who had "complete or nearly complete" tetraplegia, with some degree
of satisfactory neurological recovery. This paper intimated that such
recovery probably was related to the operation and the hypothermia
technique which was employed. Inasmuch as this work was presented at
a national meeting, and numerous impressionable neurosurgeons may
hasten to provide such therapy, perhaps the author may be permitted
a few constructive critical comments. A lesion is either complete or
incomplete. Since the recognition of the acute central cervical spinal cord injury syndrome (36, 38), the author has discovered that
patients with only a twitch of the quadriceps or minimal movement of
a great toe may progress to complete recovery without operation. If
surgery had been performed, the return of function would have been
attributed to the successful operative procedure. Attention to each
detail in the neurological examination is significant; this is the
reason why large surveys of spinal cord injuries by a multitude of
examiners, some thorough, and others not so compulsive, may produce
evaluations which may be misleading.

Another consideration relative to surgery is the jostling about necessary to introduce an intratracheal tube in a patient who already
has an almost completely compromised respiratory function by a complete lesion at the C-3-C-4 level or higher; this may lead to trag-
edy (37). In the series of the 10 patients which WHITE reported (47),
there were four who were stated to have respiratory and/or cardiac
arrest. It is difficult to understand what effect such occurrences
can have on the microcirculation of the injured spinal cord other
than a deleterious one.

One of the most important factors to be gleaned from recent experimental and clinical work is the fact that the immediate administration of steroids (dexamethazone in the cases reported) at the site of
the accident or shortly thereafter *may be as effective* or perhaps
even better than surgery. However, it is just as dangerous to credit
this type of conservative medical therapy with the neurological improvement (Cases 1 and 2) as it is to state that operation with hypothermia to the cord is responsible for the recovery of some neurological function. In Cases 1 and 2 the presence of a block on the
Queckenstedt test was complete in the former instance and partial in
the latter one. Recovery might well have been attributed to the initiation of skeletal traction.

With regard to the operative approach, the neurosurgeon must use the
anterior or posterior surgical procedure which best fits the patient's
condition. If only cervical bony deformity is present without neurological deficit, locked facettes, the evidence of bone fragments in
the canal, or depressed lamina on laminagraphy and percutaneous myelography (performed at the C-2 level), then the anterior approach may
be desirable (4, 7, 40, 44). Its advantages of the avoidance of a
bony fusion over the dura and the early mobilization and rehabilitation of the patient are very important. However, if there is a neurological deficit, with disc material or a bony fragment seen in the
spinal canal, a locked facette unilaterally or bilaterally, or a depressed lamina on laminagraphy or myelography, then the posterior

approach is perhaps the better. This permits opening the dura, visu-
alizing the cord, cutting the dentate ligaments, and stimulating the
cord, thus evaluating evoked potentials across the site of injury.
The immobilization problem is no longer as great since the development of the halo support permits early ambulation and rehabilitation
even with a posterior cervical fusion.

Summary

The immediate complete areflexic tetraplegic injury syndrome and its
management has been discussed. Two such cases with almost complete
recovery have been reported which were immediate and complete for
over 24 hours. Although the current experimental data suggest that an
irreversible effect may occur in three to six hours after injury,
some of the cases recently treated with steroids after a considerably
longer interval between injury and therapy have shown beneficial results. The dangers of claiming that the steroids were responsible for
achieving the desired effect in these cases, or that results can be
improved by operation and hypothermia, are cited. From the data presented here, the current dictum of speed to perform a decompression
operation within four hours does not seem to be valid. *The importance
of treating each patient with a spinal cord injury as an individual
rather than fitting a single operative approach to the patient is
emphasized.*

REFERENCES

1. ALBIN, M.S., WHITE, R.J., ACOSTA-RUA, G., YASHON, D.: Study of
   functional recovery produced by delayed localized cooling after
   spinal cord injury in primates. J. Neurosurg. 29, 113-120 (1968).

2. ALLEN, A.R.: Surgery of experimental lesion of the spinal cord
   equivalent to crash injury of fracture dislocation of spinal column. A preliminary report. J.A.M.A. 57, 878-890 (1911).

3. ALLEN, A.R.: Remarks on the histopathological changes in the spinal cord due to impact: an experimental study. J. Nerv. Ment. Dis.
   11, 141-147 (1914).

4. BAILEY, R.W., BADGLEY, C.E.: Stabilization of the cervical spine
   by anterior fusion. J. Bone Joint Surg. 42A, 565-594 (1960).

5. BLACK, P., MARKOWITZ, R.S.: Experimental spinal cord injury in
   monkeys: comparison of steroids and local hypothermia. Surg.
   Forum 22, 409-411 (1971).

6. BUCY, P.C.: Acute spinal cord injury. The Fourth Annual Edgar A.
   KAHN Lecture, Ann Arbor/Michigan, October 13, 1972.

7. CLOWARD, R.B.: Treatment of acute fractures and fracture-
   dislocations of the cervical spine by vertebral body fusion. J.
   Neurosurg. 18, 201-209 (1961).

8. COLE, H., LONGBY, D., CHOU, S.: Are corticosteroids effective in
   the treatment of spinal cord lesions. Presented at the 25th Annual
   Meeting of the Neurosurgical Society of America, Pebble Beach/
   Calif., March 22, 1972.

9. DAWSON, G.D.: A summation technique for the detection of small
   evoked potentials. Electroenceph. Clin. Neurophysiol. 6, 65-84
   (1954).

10. DOHRMANN, G.J., WAGNER, F.C., Jr., BUCY, P.C.: Transitory traumatic paraplegia: electron microscopy of early alterations in myelinated nerve fibers. J. Neurosurg. 36, 407-415 (1972).

11. DRAKE, C.G.: Cervical spinal cord injury. J. Neurosurg. 19, 487-494 (1962).

12. DUCKER, T.B., ASSENMACHER, D.R.: Microvascular response to experimental spinal cord trauma. Surg. Forum 20, 428-430 (1969).

13. DUCKER, T.B., HAMIT, H.F.: Experimental treatment of acute spinal cord injury. J. Neurosurg. 30, 693-697 (1969).

14. DUCKER, T.B., KINDT, G.W., KEMPE, L.G.: Pathologic findings in acute experimental cord trauma. J. Neurosurg. 35, 700-708 (1971).

15. DUCKER, T.B., PEROT, P.L., Jr.: Cerebral somatosensory evoked potentials from peripheral nerve stimulation in spinal cord injuries. Presented at the Third Annual Edgar A. KAHN Neurosurgical Meeting, November 19, 1971, Ann Arbor/Michigan.

16. GIBLIN, D.R.: Somatosensory evoked potentials in healthy subjects and in patients with lesions of the nervous system. Ann. N.Y. Acad. Sci. 112, 93-142 (1964).

17. GOODKIN, R., CAMPBELL, J.B.: Sequential pathological changes in spinal cord injury. A preliminary report. Surg. Forum 20, 430-432 (1969).

18. GOSCH, H.H., GOODING, E., SCHNEIDER, R.C.: Mechanism and pathophysiology of experimentally induced cervical spinal cord injuries in adult rhesus monkeys. Surg. Forum 21, 455-457 (1970).

19. GOSCH, H.H., GOODING, E., SCHNEIDER, R.C.: Cervical spinal cord hemorrhages in experimental head injuries. J. Neurosurg. 33, 640-645 (1970).

20. HALLIDAY, A.M., WAKEFIELD, G.S.: Cerebral evoked responses in patients with dissociated sensory loss (Abstract). Electroenceph. Clin. Neurophysiol. 14, 786 (1962).

21. KAHN, E.A.: Spinal cord injuries (Editorial). J. Bone Joint Surg. 41A, 6-11 (1959).

22. KAHN, E.A., ROSSIER, A.B.: Acute injuries of the cervical spine. Postgrad. Med. 39, 37-44 (1966).

23. KELLY, D.L., Jr., LASSITER, K.R.L., CALOGERO, J.A., ALEXANDER, E., Jr.: Effects of local hypothermia and tissue oxygen studies in experimental paraplegia. J. Neurosurg. 33, 554-563 (1970).

24. KELLY, K.L., Jr., LASSITER, K.R.L., VONGSVIVUT, A., SMITH, J.M.: Effects of hyperbaric oxygenation and tissue oxygen studies in experimental paraplegia. J. Neurosurg. 36, 425-429 (1972).

25. KLEFENBERG, G., SALTZMAN, G.F.: Gas myelographic studies in syringomyelia. Acta Radiol. (Stockholm) 52, 129-128 (1959).

26. KLINE, D.G., DeJONGE, B.R.: Evoked potentials to evaluate peripheral nerve injury. Surg. Gynec. Obstet. 127, 1239-1248 (1968).

27. KNIGHTON, R.S.: Personal communication 1969.

28. LARSON, S.J.: Gas myelography in the management of spinal cord injury. Presented at the 25th Annual Meeting of the Neurosurgical Society of America, Pebble Beach/Calif., March 22, 1972.

29. ODEN, S.: Diagnosis of spinal tumours by means of gas myelography. Acta Radiol. (Stockholm) 40, 301-313 (1953).

30. OSTERHOLM, J.L., MATHEWS, G.J.: Altered norepinephrine metabolism following experimental cord injury. Part I: Relationship to hemorrhagic necrosis and post-wounding deficits. J. Neurosurg. 36, 386-394 (1972).

31. OSTERHOLM, J.L., MATHEWS, G.J.: Altered norepinephrine metabolism following experimental spinal cord injury. Part II: Protection against traumatic spinal cord hemorrhagic necrosis by norepinephrine synthesis blockade with alpha methyl tyrosine. J. Neurosurg. 36, 395-401 (1972).

32. PEROT, P.L., Jr.: The use of somato-sensory evoked potentials in the evaluation of brain and spinal cord injuries. A preliminary report. Presented at the 25th Annual Meeting of the Neurosurgical Society of America, Pebble Beach/Calif., March 22, 1972.

33. ROSSIER, A.B.: Personal communication 1971.

34. SCHNEIDER, R.C.: A syndrome in acute cervical injuries for which early operation is indicated. J. Neurosurg. 8, 360-367 (1951).

35. SCHNEIDER, R.C.: The syndrome of acute anterior cervical spinal cord injury. J. Neurosurg. 12, 95-122 (1955).

36. SCHNEIDER, R.C.: Surgical indications and contraindications in spine and spinal cord trauma. Clin. Neurosurg. 8, 157-184 (1962).

37. SCHNEIDER, R.C.: Trauma to the Spine and Spinal Cord. In: Correlative Neurosurgery, Ch. 26 (eds. E.A. KAHN, E.C. CROSBY, R.C. SCHNEIDER, J.A. TAREN). Springfield/Ill.: Charles C. Thomas 1969.

38. SCHNEIDER, R.C., THOMPSON, J.M., BEBIN, J.: The syndrome of acute central cervical spinal cord injury. J. Neurol. Neurosurg. Psychiat. 21, 216-227 (1958).

39. SCHNEIDER, R.C., CROSBY, E.C., RUSSO, R.H., GOSCH, H.H.: Traumatic spinal cord syndromes and their management. Clin. Neurosurg. 20, 424-492 (1973).

40. SMITH, G.W.: Treatment of certain cervical spine disorders by anterior removal of the intervertebral disk and interbody fusion. J. Bone Joint Surg. 40A, 607-624 (1958).

41. SUWANWELA, C., ALEXANDER, E., Jr., DAVIS, C.H., Jr.: Prognosis in spinal cord injury, with special reference to patients with motor paralysis and sensory preservation. J. Neurosurg. 19, 220-227 (1962).

42. TARLOV, I.M., KLINGER, H.: Spinal cord compression studies. II. Time limits for recovery after acute compression in dogs. Arch. Neurol. Psychiat. (Chicago) 71, 271-290 (1954).

43. TURNBULL, I.M., BRIEG, A., HASSLER, O.: Blood supply of cervical spinal cord in man. A microangiographic cadaver study. J. Neurosurg. 24, 951-965 (1966).

44. VERBIEST, H.: Anterior operative approach in cases of spinal cord compression by old irreducible displacement or fresh fracture of cervical spine. J. Neurosurg. 19, 389-400 (1962).

45. WAGNER, F.C., Jr., DOHRMANN, G.J., BUCY, P.C.: Histopathology of transitory traumatic paraplegia in the monkey. J. Neurosurg. 35, 272-276 (1971).

46. WHITE, R.J., ALBIN, M.S.: Spine and spinal cord injury. In: Impact Injury and Crash Protection, Ch. 3 (eds. E.S. GURDJIAN, W.A. LANGE, L.M. PATRICK, L.M. Thomas), pp. 63-85. Springfield/Ill.: Charles C. Thomas 1970.

47. WHITE, R.J., YASHON, D., ALBIN, M.S., DEMIAN, Y.K.: The acute management of cervical cord trauma with quadriplegia. Presented at the meeting of The American Association of Neurological Surgeons, April 16, 1972, Boston/Mass.

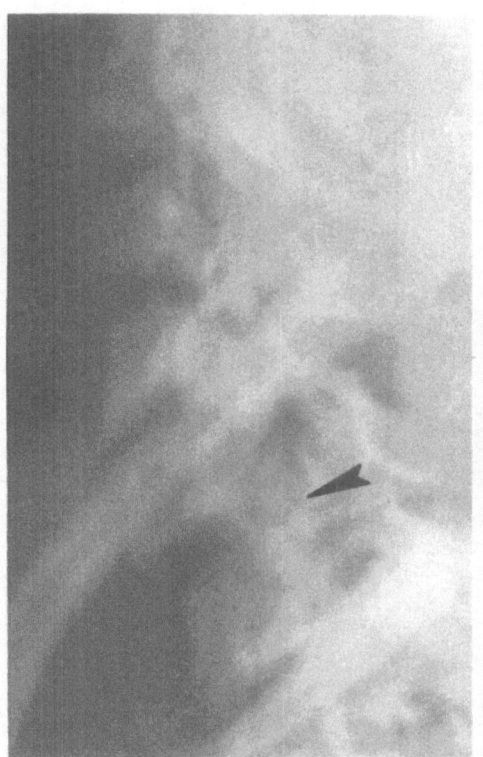
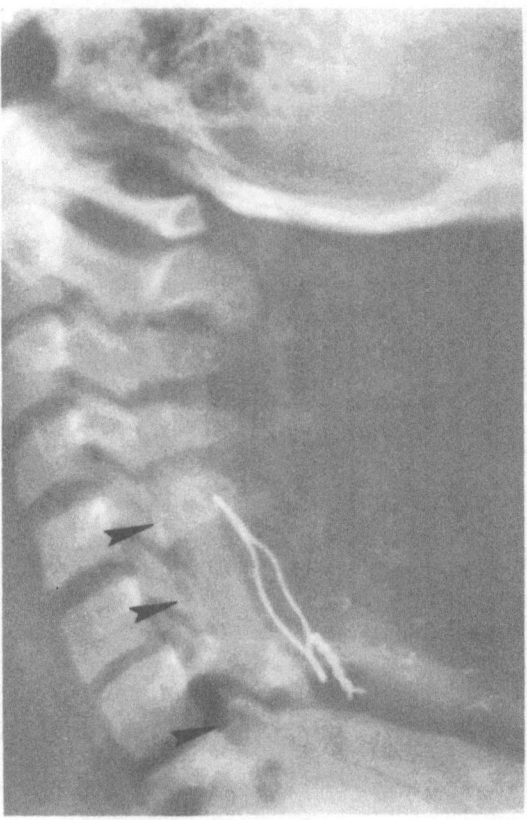

Fig. 1. Case 1. (A) A poor quality film showed the result after 40 lb. of cervical traction. There were locked facettes with a suggestion of bone spicules in the canal (arrow). (B) A film five months after realignment and a posterior spinal fusion, with wiring of the C-5 and C-7 spinous processes and the application of iliac bone, showed solid union (Reprinted courtesy Clin. Neurosurg. 20, 424-492, 1973)

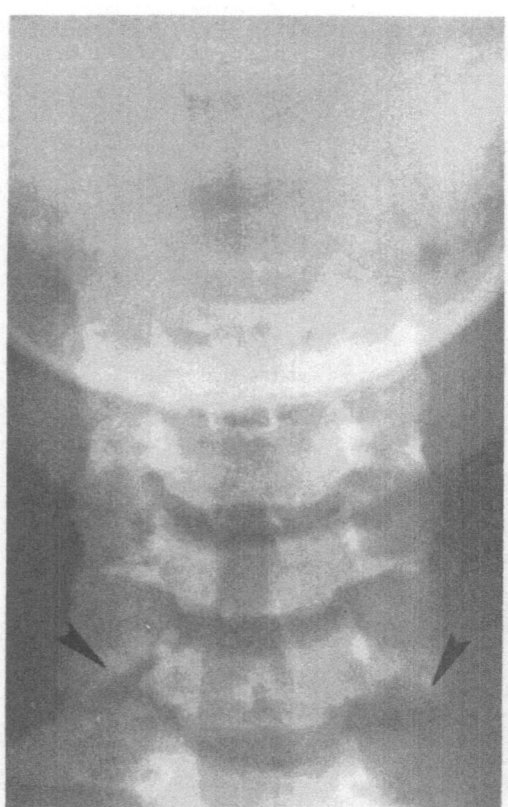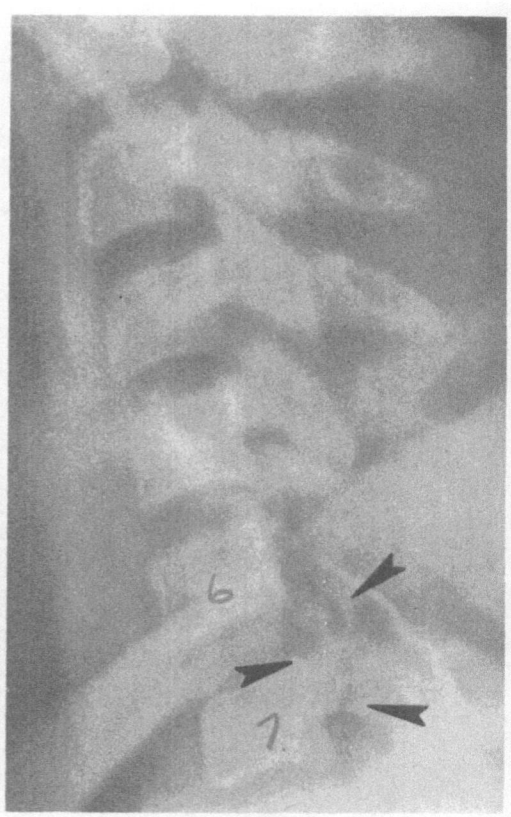

Fig. 2. Case 2. (A) The anterior-posterior view of the x-ray suggested bilateral fractures through the pedicles of the C-6 vertebra with probable joint disruption. (B) The initial lateral x-ray film demonstrated disruption at C-6-C-7 with possible bone fragments in spinal canal (Reprinted courtesy Clin. Neurosurg. 20, 424-492, 1973)

Evoked Potential Studies for the Evaluation of Spinal Function After Experimental Spinal Trauma

D. LINKE and I. VLAJIC

In most experimental studies on spinal trauma dealing with the evaluation of afferent and efferent spinal function by means of neurophysiological techniques, compression was quantified by measures
difficult to correlate to clinical problems (1).

Spinal trauma can be quantified by the following parameters: latitude,
depth, pressure as well as compression time and time course.

In the present study the effects of duration of compression on function of spinal cord are evaluated by neurophysiological methods following sudden spinal cord compression to half its diameter.

Methods

20 adult rabbits were laminectomized at the thoracal level under
Nembutal anesthesia. Compression was performed by means of a device
developed for this purpose, and allowing differentiated variation of
compression parameters. The spinal cord was suddenly compressed to
half its diameter for the following periods of time: less than 1 sec,
for 1 min, 7 min, 15 min, 30 min, 1 h, and 1 h and 15 min.

Cortical potentials were evoked by stimulation of the exposed left
sciatic nerve. Stimulation was performed by means of bipolar electrodes with rectangular pulses of 1 msec duration and an amplitude
of 10 V at rates of one per second. Monopolar recording of evoked
cortical responses was made extradurally on the contralateral hemisphere with the aid of a steel screw electrode in contact with the
dura 1 mm parasagittal. 64 successive responses were amplified by
a Toennies-Physioskop and averaged by a Hewlett Packard 5450A Fourier
Analyzer.

In order to evaluate efferent conduction muscular responses were
evoked by extradural stimulation of the sensorimotor cortex with
amplitudes up to 90 V. Recordings were made in the contralateral
biceps femoris.

Results

In all cases of sudden compression of the spinal cord to half its
diameter for up to 1 h only flat, distorted and delayed cortical
evoked potentials were obtained, demonstrating a severe disturbance
of afferent spinal function, as seen in averaged cortical evoked
responses recorded 1 h to 24 h following the trauma. Controls up to
72 h after compression showed no significant change. No evoked potentials were seen in animals in which the spinal cord was compressed

for 1 h and 15 min. Only in 1 out of 4 cases was there a slight doubt about this finding. Similar results were seen upon cortical stimulation. In intact animals muscular reaction in the biceps femoris was seen about 20 msec after cortical stimulation. Reduction and delay of response was seen in cases of compression lasting up to 1 h. No response appeared after 1 h and 15 min of compression.

Discussion

Following sudden compression of the spinal cord to half its diameter extensive loss of afferent and efferent spinal function is seen. Residual spinal function is significantly dependent of compression time in cases of compression lasting more than 1 h. No function of the longitudinal systems were detected in such cases. There was no significant change of these findings in the course of three postoperative days.

The lack of correlation between residual spinal function and compression time suggests that a circulatory factor may be involved. Further investigations to clarify these problems are planned.

REFERENCE

1. MARTIN, S.H., BLOEDEL, J.R.: Evaluation of experimental spinal cord injury using cortical evoked potentials. J. Neurosurg. 39, 75-81 (1973).

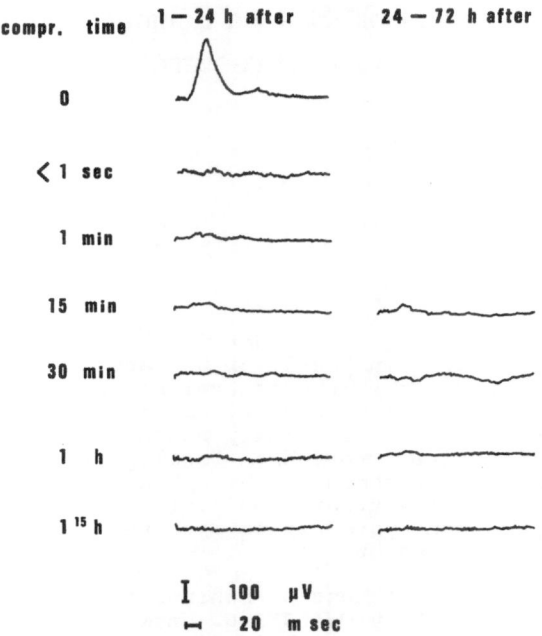

Fig. 1. Evoked potentials following different compression times,
recorded 1 - 24 h after compression (first column) and 24 - 72 h
after compression (second column). No significant responses could
be found upon compression lasting more than 1 h

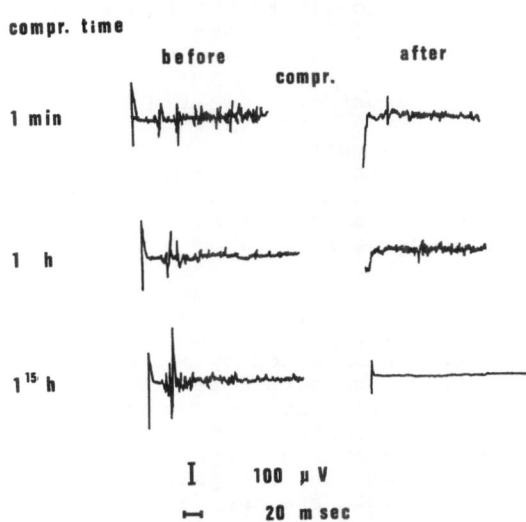

Fig. 2. Muscular responses to cortical stimulation before and after
diffent compression times. No response could be found after compression lasting more than 1 h

"Dumb-Bell"-Shaped Echinococcus in the Spinal Canal

G. Ledinski and L. Negovetić

According to NITTNER (1972) Echinococcus cysts are most frequently
located in the liver 65% and the lungs 10%. Echinococcus cysts localized within the central nervous system (MATTOS PIMENTA; BRANDT, 1960)
are far less common, amounting only to 0.16 to 2%. HENNEBERG noted
that until 1936 only approximately 150 cases of hydatidosis had been
reported. Vertebral localization is particularly frequent. The parasite disseminates by a hematogenous route and reaches the spongiosa
of the vertebral body. In approximately 84% of the cases the Echinococcus cysts extend into the spinal canal resulting in medullary
compression.

The first case of Echinococcus cyst in the spinal canal was described
in 1807 by CHAUSSIER. Until 1950 about 210 cases of this localisation
had been described (ZOLTAN).

For several reasons it is difficult to find a comprehensive survey
of spinal Echinococcosis in literature. First, individual surgeons
have very little personal experience with this problem and do not
always publish their findings. Second, geographic and regional factors influence the extent and percentage of infestation, resulting
in marked statistical variability. Since, however, we believe spinal
Echinococcosis to be of specific importance, we should like to report
on an additional case.

Case Report

B.H., 64 years old married male, father of 8 children, living near to
Banja Luka. Hie was admitted to the Central Institute for Tumors and
Allied Diseases on September 27, 1973. Prior to admission he had been
treated in another hospital, where myelography revealed an exspansive
process at L_1.

The patient's symptoms had begun 8 years previously. First he experienced pain in the back extending along his left leg. The pain was
particularly acute when he coughed or stretched. Temporary pain relief was obtained by means of analgeties. However, pain returned
yearly, becoming more intense. Early 1973 pain had become intolerable
and the patient was sent to a rehabilitation hospital for three
months at which time a lumboishialgic syndrome was diagnosed. There
was a motor and a sensor dysfunction first in the left and then in
the right leg. The patient felt bilateral leg, weakness accompanied
by complete anesthesia in both leg on the following day. From then
on he had difficulties to defecate and urinate. Ten days prior to his
admission complete paraplegia had developed caudal to Th_{12}.

Based on clinical and myelographic findings, a laminectomy from Th$_{12}$ to L$_3$ was performed. Multiple transparent cysts varying from the size of a corn grain to a walnut were found in the dorsal epidural space. Larger cysts were observed ventral to the dural sac, compressing the cauda equina. Some cysts ruptured spontaneously following removal of the vertebral arches (Fig. 1). As soon as the intraspinal cysts had been removed, additional cysts, some of which burst, protruded into the spinal canal through the intervertebral foramina L$_1$-L$_2$ and L$_2$-L$_3$ on the left side. Following enlargement of the foramina, a large cavity was seen underneath the diaphragm, lined by a firm primary membrane and full of smaller cysts (Fig. 2).

The primary membrane and its contents were removed completely. Thereafter another large cavity full of cysts was found extending into the pelvis. There was no primary membrane. All cysts were removed, but some of them burst spontaneously because of the great pressure. The surgical cavity was drained and the wound closed in layers. Hystopathological diagnosis was Echinococcus. The operative wound healed primarily and the patient was transferred to a rehabilitation center, where his symptoms improved during the following 6 months.

Ten months later the patient was readmitted due to recurrence of Echinococcus in the area of the surgical wound, where a large fluctuating soft tumor was found. The repeated antigen test was negative.

Several days later the tumor ruptured spontaneously, giving exit to approximately 200 ml of liquid and to multiple cysts of varying size (Fig. 3). The tumor ruptured several times more: each time the content was the same. The patient was treated for 3 months. During the last month cysts had become more rare but the fistula persisted. The patient was again returned to the rehabilitation center.

Discussion

It is necessary to distinguish primary from secondary spinal hydatidosis. The location of the parasite is either intradural or epidural. Intraparenchimal localization is very rare. POPOW and UMEROW (1935) reported several cases. Intradural localization is likewise very rare (HENNEBERG, 1936). Primary extradural hydatidosis was described by GUSEINOV in 1963. In Yugoslavian literature intradural and extradural Echinococcus were described by HAMERŠAK (1956), POPOV (1935) and FERKOVIC (1966).

One very characteristic aspect of paravertebral hydatidosis is the tendency of the parasite to penetrate through the intervertebral foramina into the spinal canal. The foramina are markedly enlarged, showing that Echinococcus in the spinal canal is secondary. This was so in our case. Sometimes by intense pressure. Parts of the vertebral arches are destroyed, rarely the vertebral body. In our case there were no changes in the roentgenograms, but aimed x-ray studies of the intervertebral foramina had not been made. It is interesting to note that although Echinococcus leaves marked traces on bony structures the dura remains intact and represnets a barrier to further spreading of the parasites.

Paravertebral parasitic cysts can extend to the pleural cavity, to the mediastinum, the kidneys, the peritoneum, to various abdominal organs, to paravertebral muscles and to connective tissue. On the other hand, paravertebral parasites can penetrate into the spinal canal without causing neurological symptoms.

The clinical picture in our case was of radicular nature for a period of 8 years. Sudden sensorimotor paraplegia associated with sphincter disturbances suggested an expansive process which was confirmed by mielography.

Based on the intraoperative findings and on the postoperative X-ray studies, we conclude that our case was of primary paravertebral muscular localization. According to HENNEBERG the most common site for primarily paravertebral muscular Echinococcosis is the lumbosacral region. Prognosis of spinal Echinococcosis is very poor due to the recurrences. Cerebral localization was a better prognosis. Since the cysts are crowded within the spinal canal and often rupture spontaneously, infecting the surroundings, we consider these cases incurable.

Summary

The autors describe a patient who had suffered from a painful left-sided lumboishialgic syndrome for 8 years. Only following the development of paraplegia an intraspinal expansive process was suspected. Suboccipital myelography showed a complete stop at L_1. Surgery revealed secondary Echinococcosis of the spinal canal believed by the authors to be of primary paravertebral muscular location.

REFERENCES

BERKAY, F.: Spinal echinococcosis, J. Internat. Coll. Surgeons, (Chicago) 22, 35-39 (1954).

BRANDT, P.: cit. by Nittner.

DEVE, F.: Echinococcose vertebrale, son processus pathologique et ses lesions. Ann. anat. path. (Paris) 5, 841-865 (1928).

FERKOVIĆ, M.: Povodom slučaja ehinokoka kaude ekvine Liječnički vjesnik 88, 161-165 (1966).

GUSEINOV, A.M.: cit. by Nittner.

HAMERŠAK, B., POPOV, N.: Ehinokok centralnog nervnog sistema Zbornik radova IV. sastanka kirurško ortopedske sekcije Hrvatske i Slovenije (Zagreb) 1956.

HENNEBERG, R.: cit. by Nittner.

MATTOS PIMENTA, A.: cit by Nittner.

NITTNER, K.: Raumbeengende Prozesse im Spinalkanal einschließlich Angiome und Parasiten. In: Handbuch der Neurochirurgie, Vol. 7(2), (eds. H. Olivecrona, W. Tönnis). Berlin-Heidelberg-New York: Springer 1972.

POPOW, N.A., UMEROW, B.T.: Echinococcus der Wirbelsäule und des Rükkenmarks. Deutsche Zeitschrift f. Nervenheilkunde 137, 187-196 (1935).

SAMIY, E.: Kompression des Rückenmarks und der Cauda Equina durch Echinococcuscysten. Acta Neurochirurgica 9, 369-384 (1963).

SILOBRČIĆ, I.: Pokušaj medikamentozne supresije eksperimentalne sekundarne ehinokokoze, Anali Kliničke bolnice "Dr. M. Stojanović" 9, 32, (1972).

ZOLTAN, L.: cit. by Nittner.

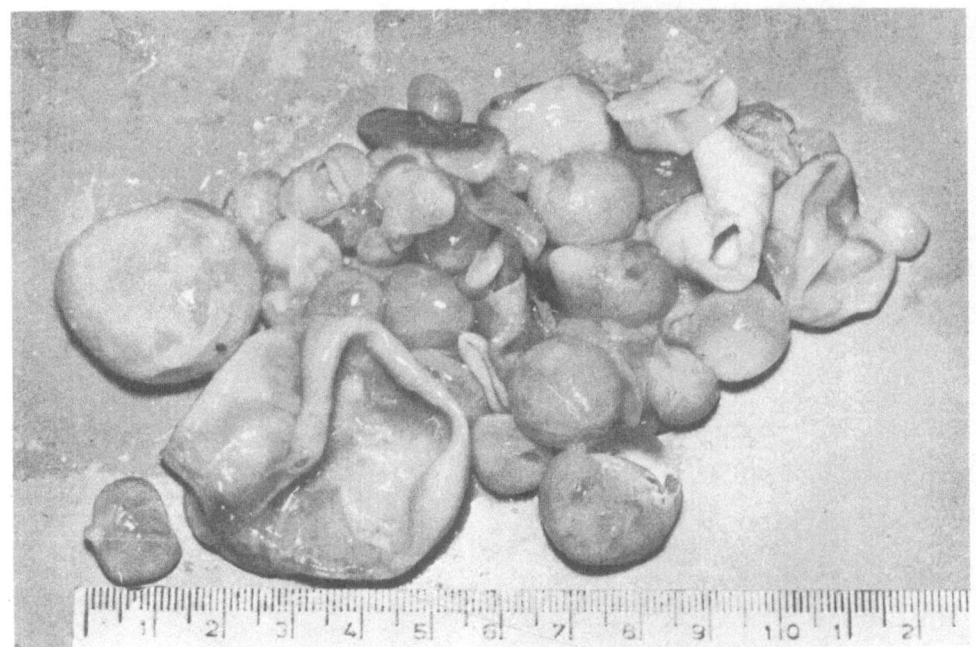

Fig. 1

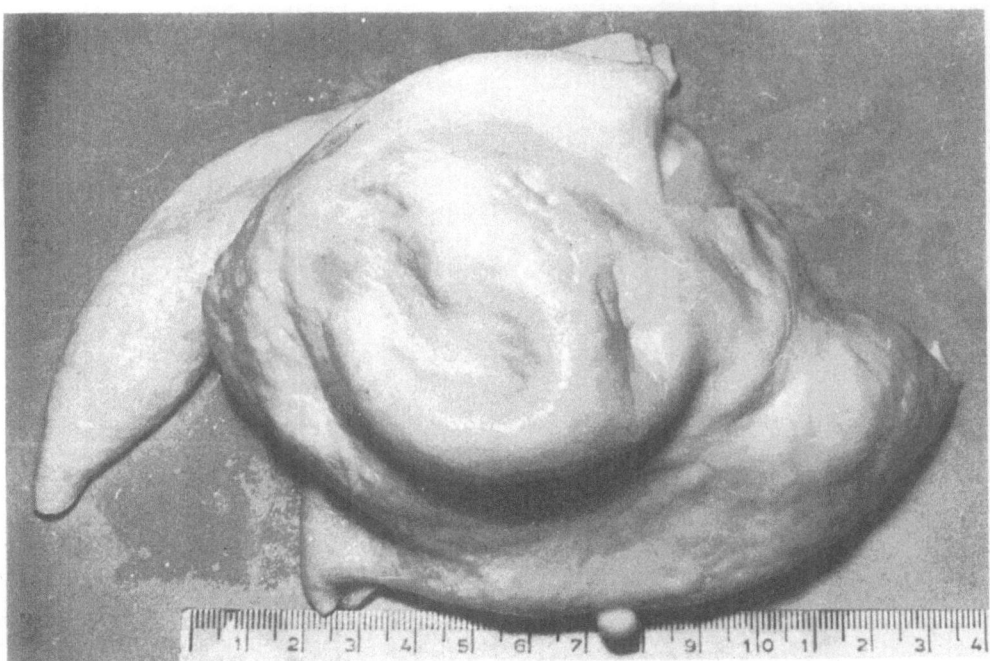

Fig. 2

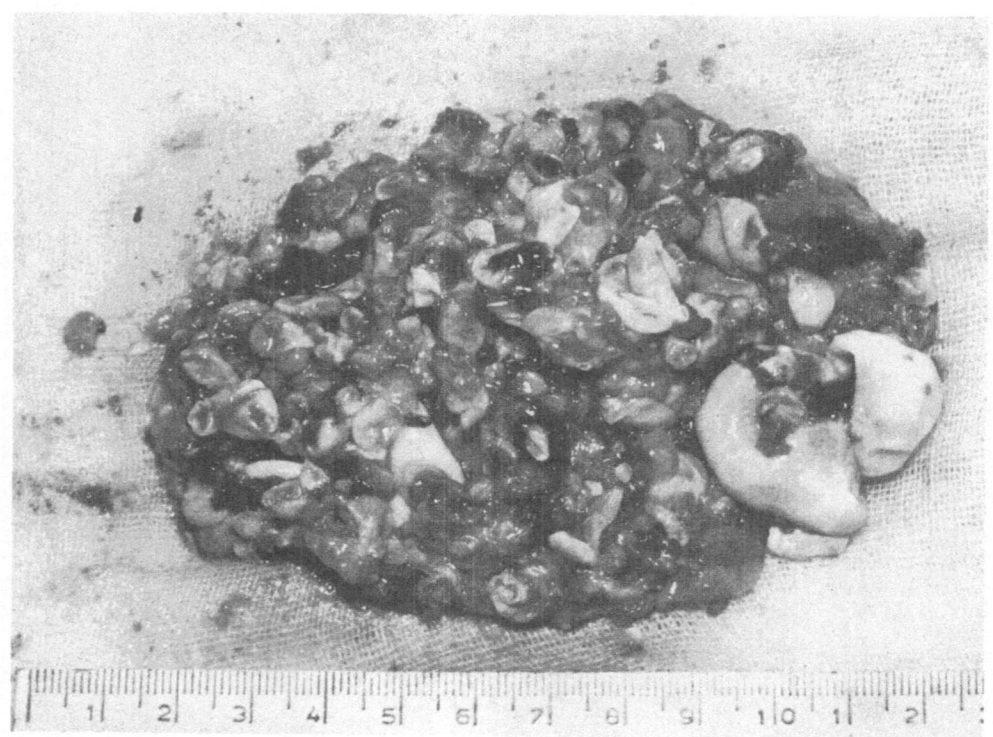

Fig. 3

Atypical Localizations of Pachymeningitis Cervicalis Hypertrophicans

M. Schirmer, G. Kostadinow, and H. Wenker

Pachymeningitis cervicalis hypertrophicans is a rare chronic inflammatory condition of the spinal dura mater. The clinical picture of this disease was first described by CHARCOT (1) in 1872 and is characterised by irritation of the spinal nerve roots and compression of the spinal cord, damaging the long tracts and leading to paraparesis or tetraparesis. JOFFROY (2) described the pathological changes in the dura mater in 1873 and called the disease pachymeningitis cervicalis hypertrophicans, because it was at first known to occur only in the cervical region. Tuberculosis and syphilis are considered as ethiologic factors.

In the past 6 years two patients have been operated on CHARCOT-JOFFROY's disease at the neurosurgical department of the Städtisches Krankenhaus Neukölln in Berlin. In both the typical hypertrophic changes were found outside the cervical region.

The first case was a 63 years old woman with pachymeningitis hypertrophicans in the thoracic region: a spinal cord compression syndrome, already characterised by considerable unsteadiness of gait and pronounced distrubances of sensitivity, could be improved by laminectomy from the 6th to the 9th thoracic vertebrae and removal of the hypertrophic dura mater. After two month of intensive physiotherapy the patient was able to walk slowly without help; the pronounced preoperative disorders of sensitivity were now limited to the dermatomes L5 and S1. Micturition and defaecation were not disturbed, either before or after the operation.

The second patient operated on deserves greater attention. In this case the typical pathological changes were found in the intracranial dura mater. To our knowledge this has been described in only one case so far (3), in contrast to the spinal manifestation of CHARCOT-JOFFROY's disease.

This patient was a 30 years old man who had been in hospital several times over 20 years due to tuberculosis of the lungs and skin, and for tuberculous retinochorioiditis. As long as eight years before the present illness he had been thoroughly examined neurologically and radiologically because of unexplained headaches and bilateral papilledema. No cause was found for the clinical symptoms. Improvement, with regression of the papillary stasis occurred during treatment with tuberculostatics and cortisone. The patient was investigated neurologically once more because of renewed violent headaches, worse on the right side, and incipient bilateral papillary stasis. In the brain-scan[1] a distinct technetium concentration was found in the

[1]We thank Dr.Meisel, head of the radiological department of the Städtisches Wenckebach-Krankenhaus in Berlin for kindly supplying the brain scans.

right occipital region. A less distinct staining in the same region was seen in the cerebral angiograms. Since the erythrocyte sedimentation rate was highly raised, and serum electrophoresis suggested an inflammatory process, we suspected the presence of a tuberculoma. Surgery, however, revealed only a tumor-like thickened tentorium with denser expansion into the supratentorial region. The soft meninges and the cerebral and cerebellar cortices showed distinct inflammatory changes. The affected tentorium was resected.

Histological examination by Prof. K.KÖHN (Pathological Institute of the Städtisches Krankenhaus Neukölln) revealed: fibrous thickening of the tentorial tissue, containing numerous vessels with thickened and extensively hyalinised walls, as well as abundant non-specific chronic infiltrations, partly diffuse, partly focal, interspersed with lymphocytes and particularly histiocytes. Histological diagnosis: pachymeningitis hypertrophicans.

The postoperative course was free of complications. When discharged 4 weeks later, the patient no longer had any headaches and the papilledema had completely regressed. The final neurological examination revealed only an unchanged facial weakness on the right and a mild nystagmus on gaze to the left.

It seems remarkable that in the patient with the intracranial localization of the pachymeningitis hypertrophicans there is an obvious direct relationship with a long existing tuberculosis and that the dura mater changes typical for CHARCOT-JOFFROY's disease were not found exclusively in the cervical region. Therefore we consider it advisable to name this disease simply pachymeningitis hypertrophicans.

REFERENCES

1. CHARCOT, J.M.: Gaz. méd. de Paris, 9 (1872).

2. JOFFROY, A.: De la pachyméningite cervicale hypertrophique curable. Thèsis, Paris 79, 1873.

3. NAFFZIGER, H.C., STERN, W.E.: Chronic pachymeningitis. Arch. Neurol. Psychiat. 62, 383-411 (1949).

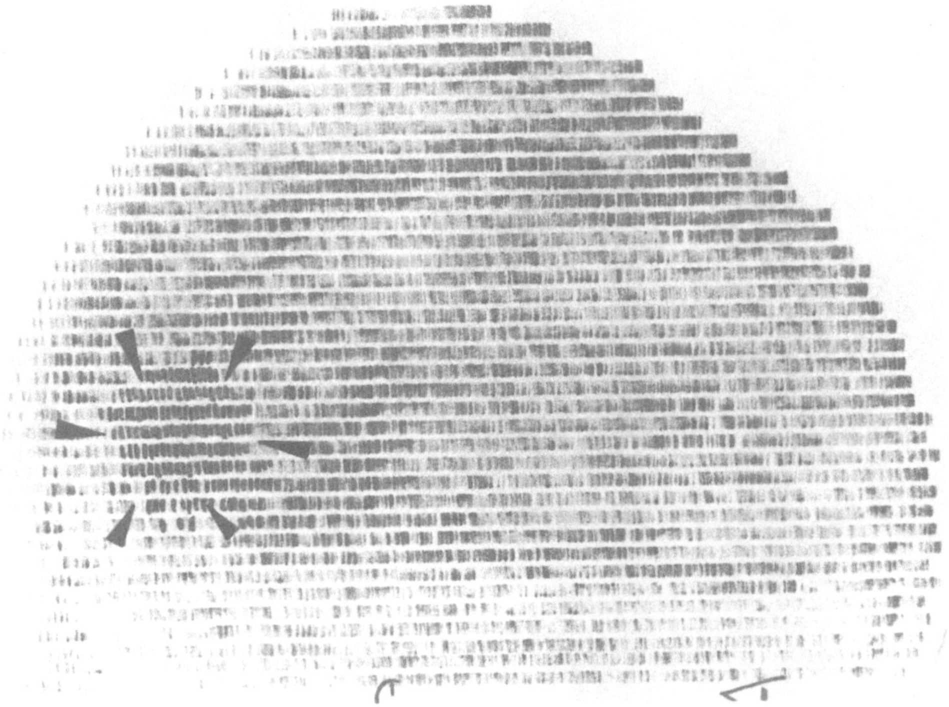

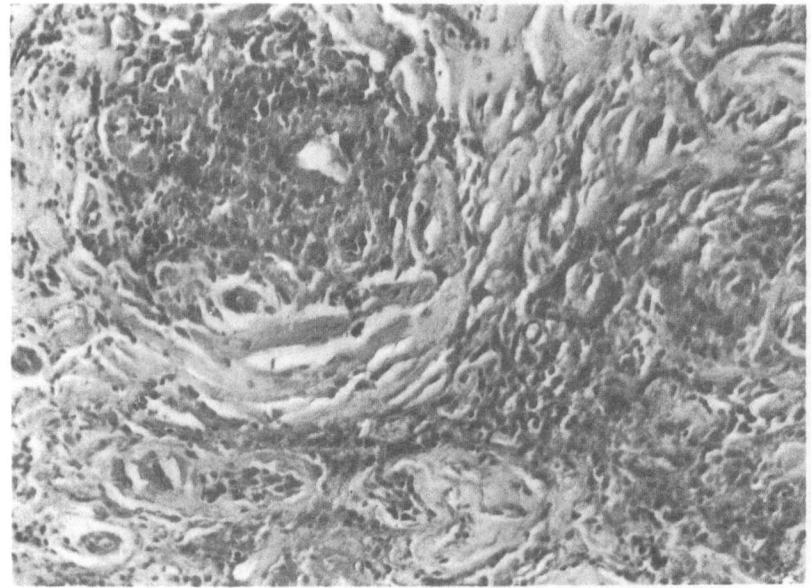

Fig. 1. Brain scan: distinct technetium concentration in the right occipital region (from Dr. MEISEL)

Fig. 2. Pachymeningitis hypertrophicans of the tentorium. Hematoxylin-eosin-staining. Magnification 1:160

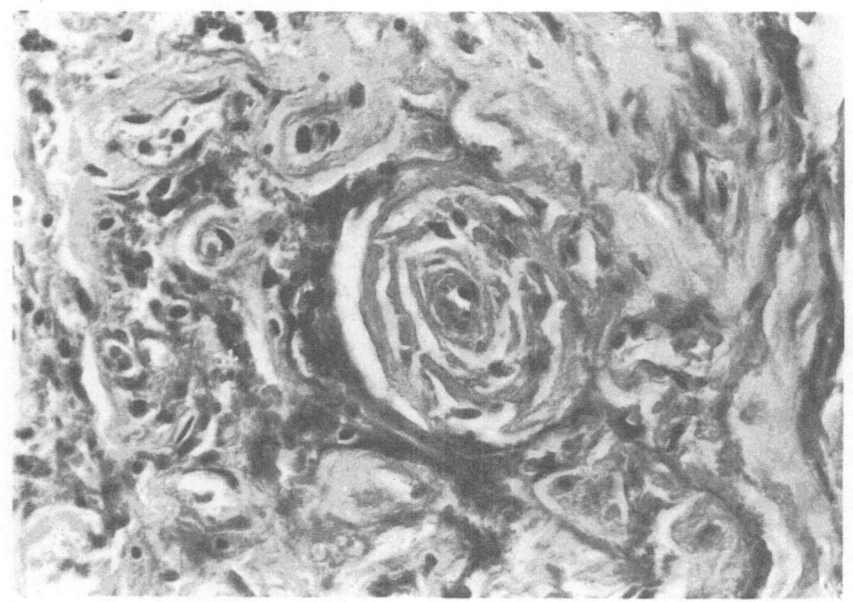

Fig. 3. Hyalinized vessel with thickened wall in pachymeningitis hypertrophicans. Hematoxylin-eosin-staining. Magnification 1:420

First Experiences With the Anterior Discectomy Without Fusion of the Cervical Spine in Cases of Acute Disc Rupture

G. Busch, K. Schürmann, and M. Samii

Since 1967 we have performed the anterior fusion operation in degenerative and traumatic lesions of the cervical spine according to the CLOWARD technique, sometimes with modifications. The results have been reported several times (1, 6, 7). The total amount of operations is 115. Since October 1973 we have performed the anterior discectomy without fusion in 6 patients with acute cervical disc rupture.

The method corresponds to that of MURPHY and GADO 1972 (5), based on publications of HULT (4) and HIRSCH et al. (3). The approach is the same as in the operation of CLOWARD. Following exposure of the ventral surface of the cervical spine, the intervertebral disc is roentgenologically identified by insertion of a cannula. Thereafter the intervertebral space is incised and subtotal removal of the disc performed in a way similar to that of lumbar discs. The posterior longitudinal ligament is not cut, no attempt being made to remove dorsal osteophytes but only to decompress the cervical root laterally by foraminotomy. Finally, a small drainage is inserted and the wound sutured. The cervical spinal column is immobilized by a plastic collar for 2 weeks.

We approached this surgical intervention with skepticism and fear. We knew that, by removing only the anterior part of the segment, we ran the resk of instability. On the other hand, we do not expect postoperative instability for the following anatomic and functional reasons:

(1) The small vertebral joints remain intact.

(2) The uncovertebral processes remain and prevent lateral gliding, resp. dislocation.

Finally, no dislocation has been observed following lumbar disc surgery and following anterior fusion in cases of degenerative disease, particularly during the first postoperative days.

The indication is given only in cases of acute soft herniation of a cervical nucleus pulposus accompanied by neurological deficits. Table 1 gives a short survey of the symptomatology. All patients are male, aged between 32 and 54 years. The involved level was C-5/6 3 times, C-6/7 2 times, and both segments once. In no case did the myelogram show a substantial narrowing or even a stop. CSF protein content was increased in only one case.

The results were very satisfactory. All patients reported relief of pain immediately after surgery, followed by a slow improvement of the neurological deficits. The follow-up is now 18 months. In one patient we observed shoulder and arm pain 9 months after surgery. The preoperative neurological deficits, however, had disappeared.

Table 1. Symptomatology in 6 patients with cervical disc herniation

	Acute Pain Syndrome	Motor Deficit	Reflex Impairment	Sensibility Impairment	Osteo-Chondrosis	Involved Height
CI., B. 42 years	+	+		+	Narrowing	C 5/6
AH., H. 39 years	+	+	+	+	+	C 5/6/7
SÜ., J.P. 32 years	+	+	+	+	+	C 6/7
SI., K. 54 years	+	+	+	+	+	C 5/6
SM., F. 52 years	+	+	+	+	+	C 6/7
HI., C. 35 years	+	+	+	+	Narrowing	C 5/6

The following 3 figures show the course of roentgenological changes. First, x-ray pictures of a patient with a C 6/7 syndrome in retroflexion (left) and anteflexion (right). Obvious narrowing of C 6/7 (Fig. 1). The roentgenograms shown in Fig. 2 were made 8 months following surgery. The intervertebral space is still narrowed, a slight anterior angulation has developed. This angulation has been reported by CLOWARD in 10% of his patients with ventral fusion as due to degenerative changes without an affecting the clinical results, as has been confirmed in our material. It seems, however, that we have to count with a higher percentage in cases of clear discectomy. The x-ray pictures shown in Fig. 3 are from a patient with a disc herniation between C 6/7 before (left) and after (right) surgery. The x-ray films show no marked changes. Fig. 4 shows a lesion at C 5/6, immediately before operation, and 2 months later. Beginning fusion has developed. In no patient was there obvious gliding or dislocation of the vertebral bodies.

Because of the small number of cases, final conclusions should be drawn with care. For a limited number of patients, i.e. with acute soft cervical disc herniation, anterior discectomy seems to be an effective treatment. It would spare the patient the removal of autologous bone as well as the insertion of foreign material.

REFERENCES

1. BUSCH, G., SCHÜRMANN, K.: Anterior fusion in fracture-dislocations and in spontaneous fractures of the cervical spine. In: Proceedings of the German Society of Neurosurgery Vol. 2, Cervical Spine Operations, pp. 340-349. Excerpta Medica Amsterdam 1971.

2. CLOWARD, R.B.: The anterior approach for removal of ruptured cervical disc. J. Neurosurg. 15, 602-617 (1958).

3. HIRSCH, C., WICKBOM, J., LINDSTRÖM, A., ROSENGREN, K.: Cervical-disc resection. A follow-up of myelographic and surgical procedure. J. Bone Jt. Surg. 46A, 1811-1821 (1964).

4. HULT, L.: Antero-lateral diskutrymning vid cervicala diskbrack. Nordisk. Med. 60, 969-970 (1958).

5. MURPHY, M.G., GADO, M.: Anterior cervical discectomy without interbody bone graft. Neurosurg. 37, 71-74 (1972).

6. SCHÜRMANN, K.: The importance for rehabilitation of the interbody fusion and stabilization operation in fracture dislocations of the cervical spine. Scand. J. Rehab. Med. 4, 114-122 (1972).

7. SCHÜRMANN, K., BUSCH, G.: Die Behandlung der cervicalen Luxationsfraktur durch die ventrale Fusion. Chirurg. 41, 225-228 (1970).

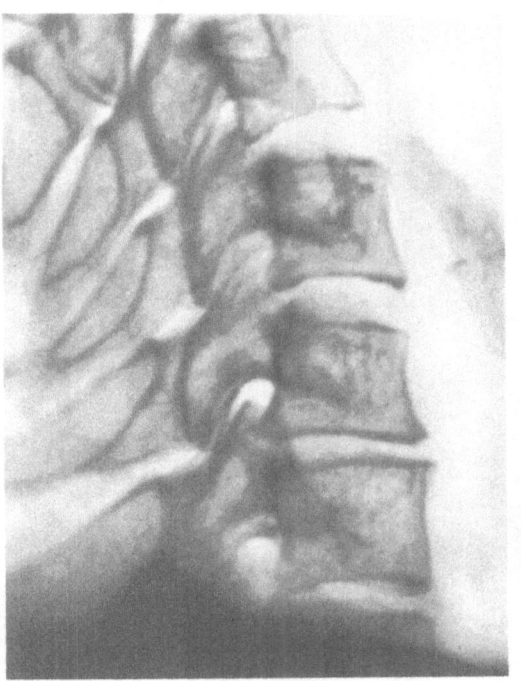 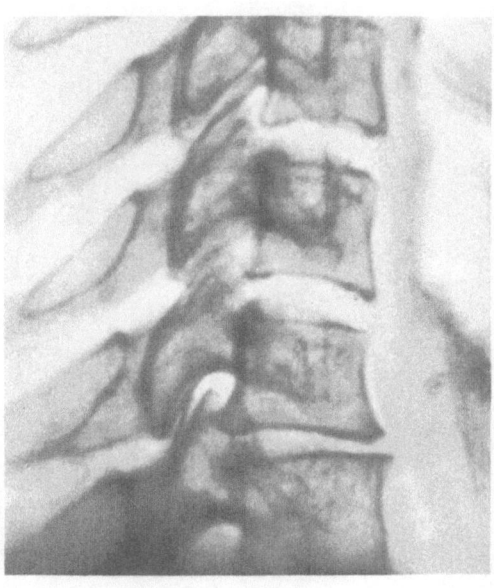

a) Retroflexion   b) Anteflexion

Fig. 1. Osteochondrosis and narrowing of the intervertebral space C 6/7

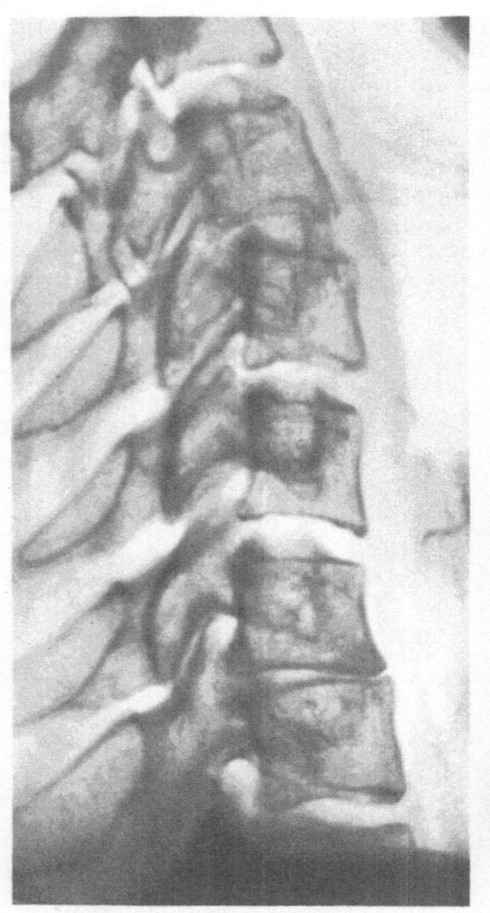 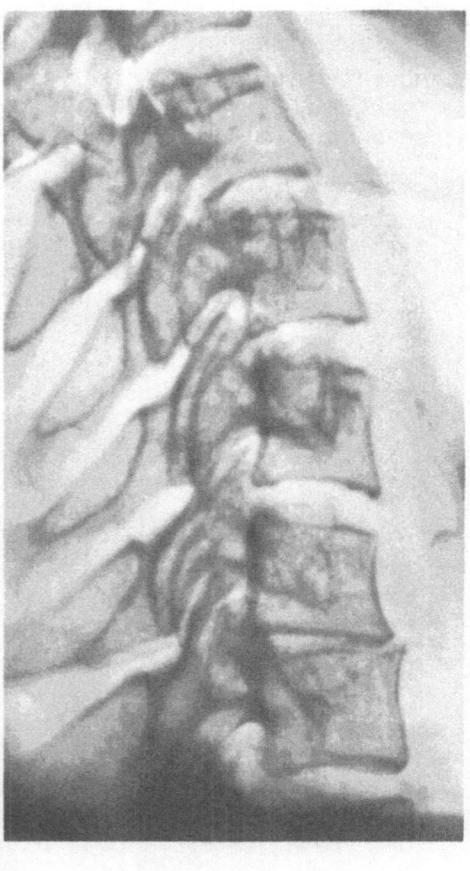

a) Retroflexion　　　　　　　　b) Normal position

Fig. 2. The same patient 8 months after anterior discectomy C 6/7 without fusion

Fig. 2.
c) Anteflexion

Further narrowing and anterior
angulation C 6/7

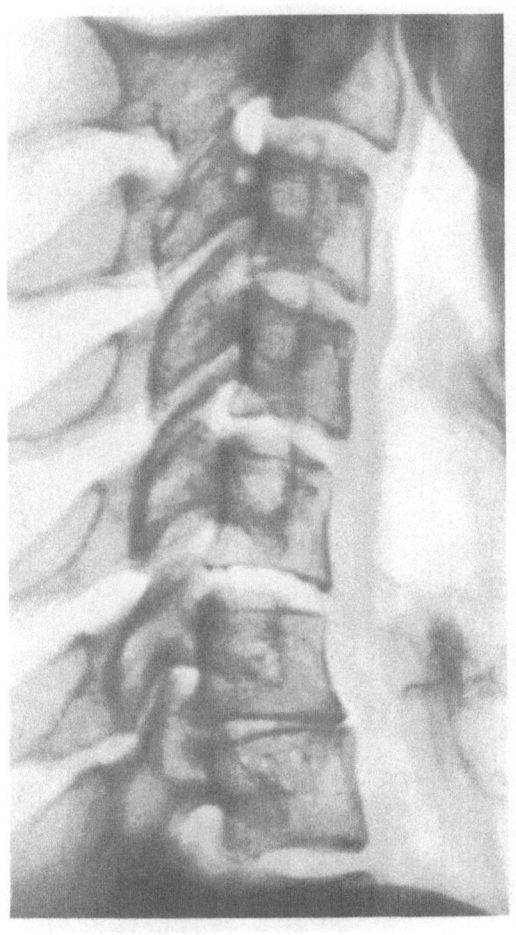

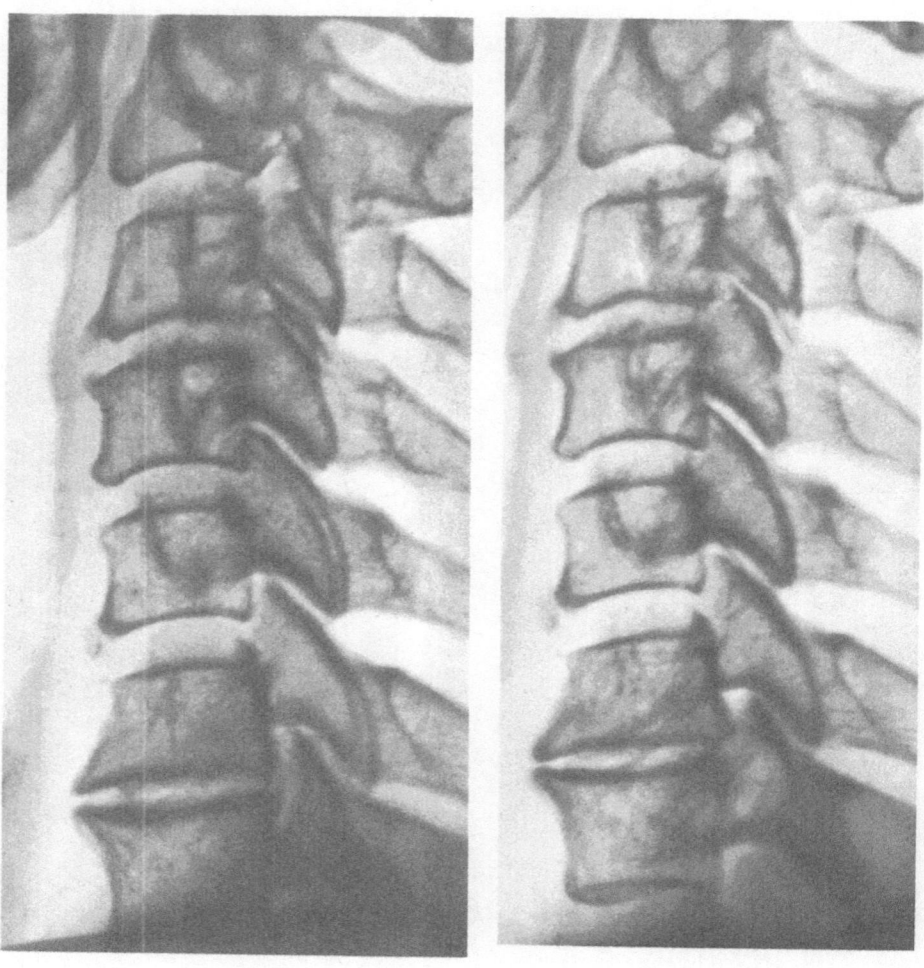

a) before   b) 2 months after the operation

Fig. 3. Nucleus pulposus prolaps C 6/7

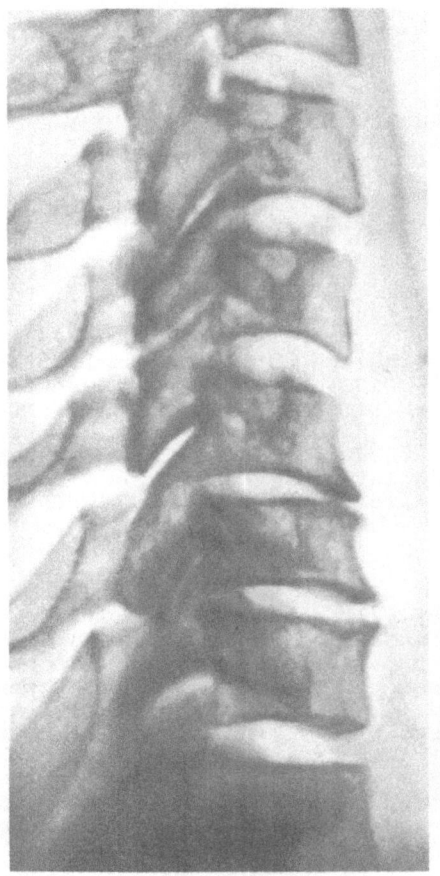 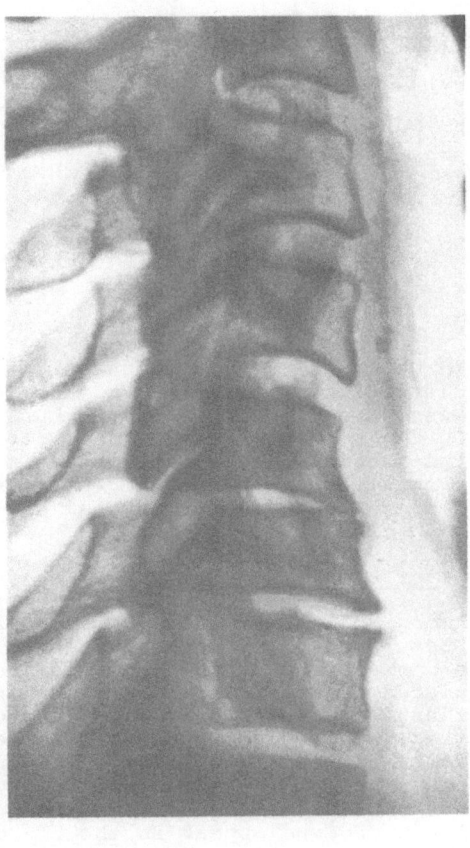

a) 5 days after operation

b) beginning fusion at the anterior part of the vertebral body 2 months later

Fig. 4. Discectomy C 5/6

Computerized Tomography Using the High Definition Matrix (160 x 160) An Early Evaluation*

E. KAZNER, H. STEINHOFF, W. LANKSCH, and F. MARGUTH**

In December 1974, a computerized tomography equipment with the high definition matrix (EMI-Scanner 160 x 160) has been installed at the Neurosurgical Clinic of the Ludwig-Maximilians-University of München. During a 4-months-period 650 patients have been investigated using the standard cross sections as proposed by AMBROSE (1) and a special reconstruction programme (patient's movements correction). The principle of the method has been described in detail by HOUNSFIELD (2).

Material and Results

Among 133 intracranial tumours 129 (97%) could be diagnosed in the plain scan, i.e. without the application of a contrast medium. Two of the four primarily not visible tumours were metastases which appeared in the CT-scan after enhancement. The other two cases were tumours of unknown histology located in the region of the third ventricle and the corpus callosum respectively. The one in the third ventricle became visible after intravenous injection of contrast medium.

Brain tumours appear in the CT-scan partly as areas of *decreased density*, especially low-grade gliomas and metastases. Fig. 1 shows a diffusely growing astrocytoma grade 1 in the left frontal lobe as a dark area. Fig. 2 is an example of a metastasis in the left parietal region. Tumours with generally *increased density* as compared to normal brain tissue are meningiomas (Figs. 3, 8), pituitary adenomas (Fig. 4) and craniopharyngiomas (Fig. 5). With glioblastomas the tomograms show a *variegated picture*, areas of lower, increased and equal density to the brain being found (Fig. 6a). The real tumour size can be delineated exactly only after contrast enhancement (Fig. 6b). The case in Fig. 6b shows the so-called ring-sign of a glioblastoma, caused by central necrosis. Fig. 6c represents the "nodule-sign" of a more solid glioblastoma.

Besides the direct visualization of a tumour, computerized tomography permits recognition of the *histological nature* of neoplasms in many cases. For this purpose, the printouts showing the EMI-numbers are of great advantage. In the case of Fig. 7, the attenuation values of this very large space-occupying lesion represented as a sharply delineated area of markedly reduced density equaled that of CSF with lowest values down to -14 in the basal scan. That means a density be-

*This study was carried out with the EMI-Scanner which was financed by the Stiftung Volkswagenwerk.
**We want to express our appreciation to Dr. WILSKE of the Neuropathological Institute of the University of Munich for the autopsy material containing the cross-sections of the brain.

low that of water. Therefore two types of lesions had to be considered: an epidermoid cyst and a lipoma. Since lipomas usually reach even lower EMI-numbers down to -40 to -50 and considering the location of the lesion, an epidermoid cyst was diagnosed and confirmed at surgery.

The second important criterion for the differential diagnosis of tumours is their *response to intravenous contrast medium injection*. According to our experience with 67 tumours, all meningiomas (Fig. 8), glioblastomas (Fig. 6), acoustic neurinomas (Fig. 12), pituitary adenomas, cerebellar astrocytomas and medulloblastomas show an uptake of contrast medium. The majority of metastases and solid craniopharyngiomas also increases in density. On the other hand, low-grade gliomas remain unchanged. The same is true with tumour calcifications.

A histogram showing the distribution of the EMI-numbers within a tumour before and after contrast enhancement can be printed out by the computer (see Fig. 9). The different types of tumour appearance have been demonstrated already with glioblastomas (see Fig. 6).

The *intensity of contrast medium uptake* followed during a certain period of time after injection permits further conclusions regarding tumour histology. Meningiomas, acoustic neurinomas, metastases and pituitary adenomas show an early peak with the highest density values shortly after the injection and a relatively rapid decrease during the first hour. Glioblastomas have a delayed maximum uptake and a prolonged decrease.

Computerized tomography visualizes *brain edema* of any origin directly for the first time. The hydratation of brain tissue leads to a decreased density which appears as a dark area in the CT-scan (see Figs. 3, 6, 10 and 12). We consider a perifocal edema with a diameter up to 2 cm *edema grade I*, an edema which extends throughout one-half of a cerebral hemisphere as *edema grade II*, and an edema involving nearly a whole hemisphere *edema grade III*. Edema is particularly marked in cases of meningioma. Even tumours of the size of a walnut may cause an edema grade III. Similar observations have been made in the presence of glioblastomas and metastases. The edema follows the white matter and, consequently, shows finger-sized extensions (see Fig. 10). In low-grade gliomas differentiation between the tumour itself and the surrounding edema is not possible with accuracy.

Tumours in the posterior cranial fossa can also be easily diagnosed using CT. Fig. 11 shows an example of a cerebellar astrocytoma of the upper vermis, extending through the aquaeduct into the posterior part of the third ventricle. Acoustic neurinomas may cause diagnostic problems in the plain scan. However, they appear clearly delineated after contrast enhancement (see Fig. 12, a and b).

In *neurosurgical emergencies* CT offers unexpected diagnostic possibilities. Hemorrhages of any location may be accurately differentiated from bran infarction. Coagulated blood appears peak white (see Figs. 13, 15), whereas flowing blood is not visible in the plain scan. The patient of Fig. 14 presented with signs of an acute left-sided hemiplegia. In the CT-scan the whole area supplied by the right middle cerebral artery shows decreased density caused by hypoxemic brain swelling. Angiographically, an occlusion of the right middle cerebral artery was found. In cases of brain infarction the gray matter is also involved in the edematous process.

The high definition matrix shows the extension of a hemorrhage from a *ruptured aneurysm* with great detail as demonstrated in Fig. 15, a to c.

Postoperative complications can be recognized by means of CT with great accuracy. The child of Fig. 16 deteriorated continuously after the removal of a plexus papilloma in the right temporal horn, so that a hematoma was suspected. The CT-scan, however, revealed an edema extending through the whole right cerebral hemisphere and caused by a spasm of the right internal carotid artery and its branches.

In cases of *head injury* a reliable differentiation between brain contusion and intracerebral hematoma is possible. Multiple contusions can be demonstrated (see Fig. 17). All acute posttraumatic intracranial hematomas are easily detected. Examples of intracerebral and acute subdural hematomas are shown in Figs. 18 and 19.

Chronic subdural hematomas may cause diagnostic problems as the density of the hematoma is similar to that of normal brain tissue in certain stages of the illness. However, the most frequent finding in chronic subdural hematomas is a low-density, lens-shaped area between the skull and the brain (see Figs. 20 and 21).

In cases of *infantile hydrocephalus, malformations of the brain* and *subdural effusions*, CT offers a complete diagnosis, so that other neuroradiological investigations can be avoided. Instructive cases are shown in Figs. 22 to 26.

The high resolution of the 160 x 160 matrix is of special advantage in cases of *orbital tumours*. The patient of Fig. 27 presents a dense lesion in the posterior part of the left orbit. A meningioma of the optic nerve sheath was removed at surgery. Orbital scans show very fine details, such as the optic nerve, the lens and the suspension of the eye ball. In cases of orbital lesion computerized tomography will probably replace all the other methods of investigation.

Conclusions

The experience of only a few months already allows the statement that computerized tomography has increased the diagnostic possibilities in cases of brain disorders to an unexpected degree. Many only suspected diagnoses may now be substantiated by a morphological substrate without discomfort to the patient. Without doubt, the genius invention of G.N. HOUNSFIELD will influence thinking and acting of neurosurgeons in a dramatic way.

Summary

The evaluation of 650 patients investigated by means of computerized tomography (CT) reveals a very high detection rate in cases of brain tumour and other intracranial space-occupying lesions. Among 133 brain tumours 129 (97%) could be diagnosed in the plain scan. After contrast enhancement only one false negative case remained. For emergencies and children with brain disease CT is the most informative investigation of all.

The high definition matrix 160 x 160 in connection with the patient's movements correction has led to further improvement of resolution and visibility of details of intracranial anatomy and pathology on CT-scans.

REFERENCES

1. AMBROSE, J.: Computerized transverse axial scanning (tomography):
   Part 2. Clinical application. Brit. J. Radiol. <u>46</u>, 1023-1047
   (1973).

2. HOUNSFIELD, G.N.: Computerized transverse axial scanning (tomography): Part 1. Description of system. Brit. J. Radiol. <u>46</u>, 1016-
   1022 (1973).

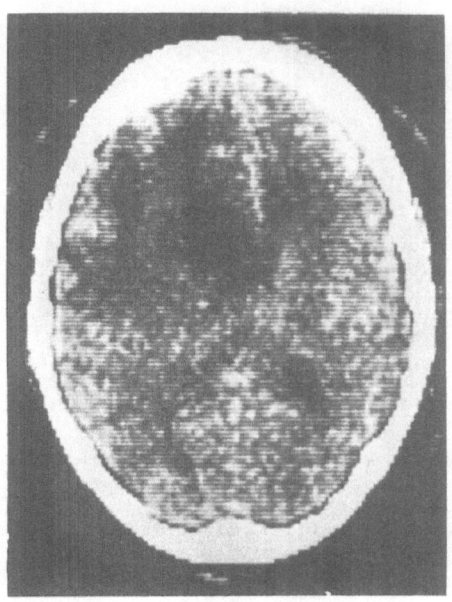 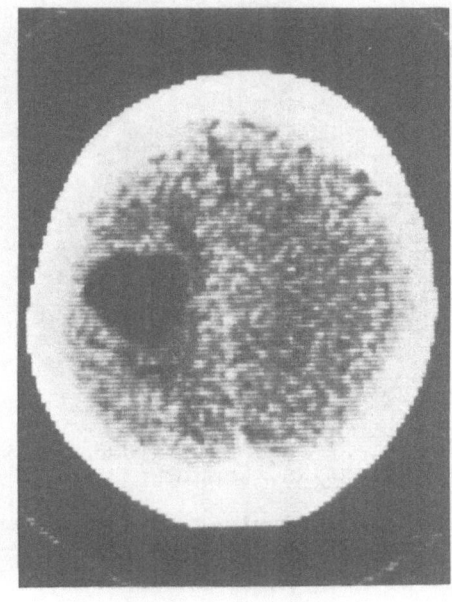

Fig. 1   Fig. 2

Fig. 1. Diffusely growing astrocytoma grade I in the left frontal
lobe, extending into the right frontal lobe in a 25-year-old man (CT
002/75, scan 2A)

Fig. 2. Metastasis of a bronchiogenic carcinoma in the left parietal
region (CT 326/75, scan 3B)

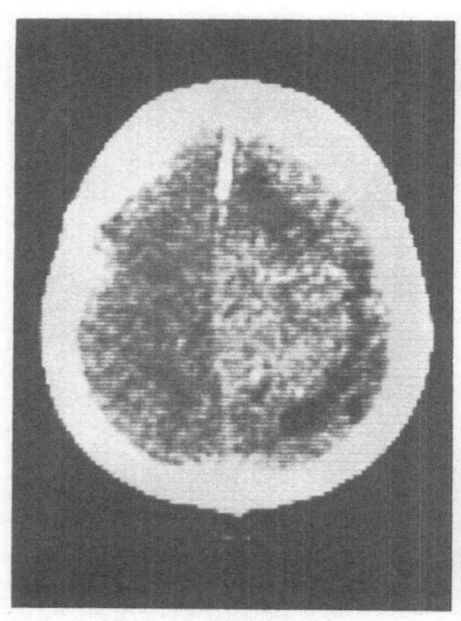 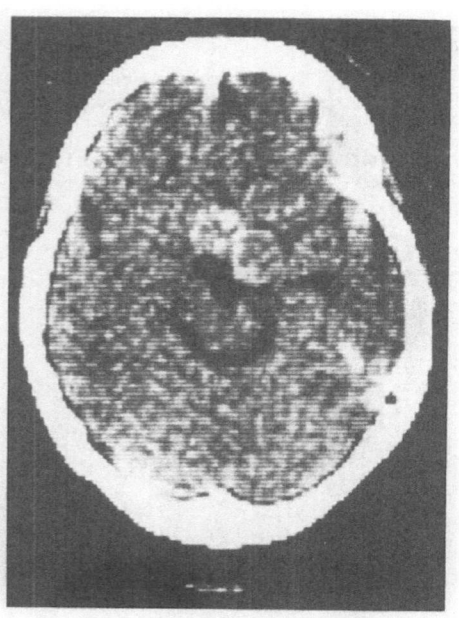

Fig. 3   Fig. 4

Fig. 3. Parasagittal meningioma on the right side. Perifocal edema
(CT 025/75, scan 3B)

Fig. 4. Pituitary adenoma with two tumour nodules of increased density (CT 055/75, scan 1B)

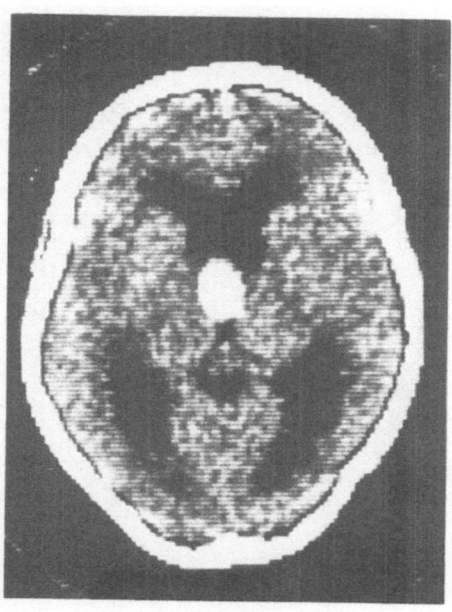

Fig. 5. Predominantly solid cranio-
pharyngioma with markedly increased
density (CT 464/75, scan 2A)

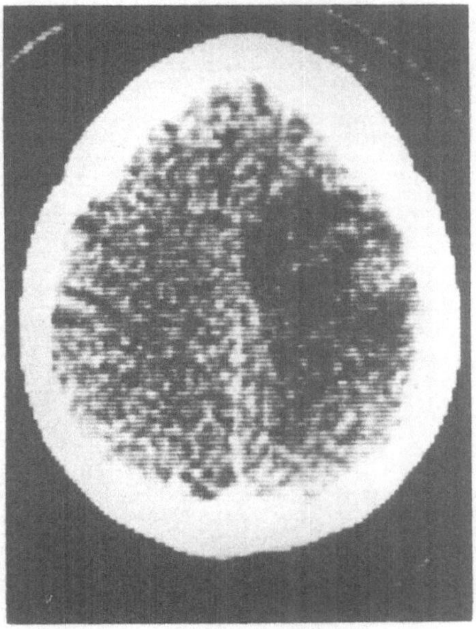

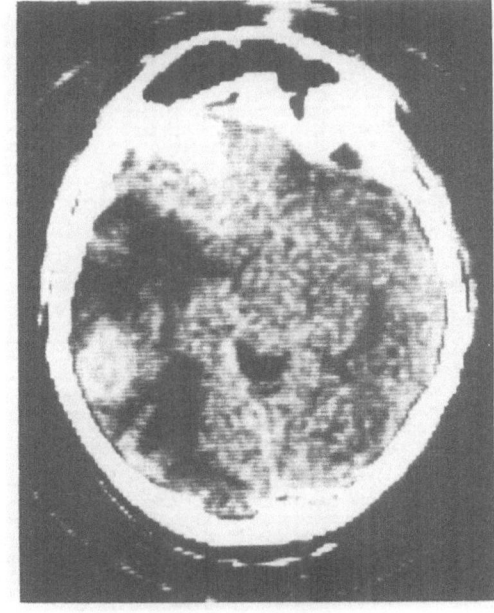

a)

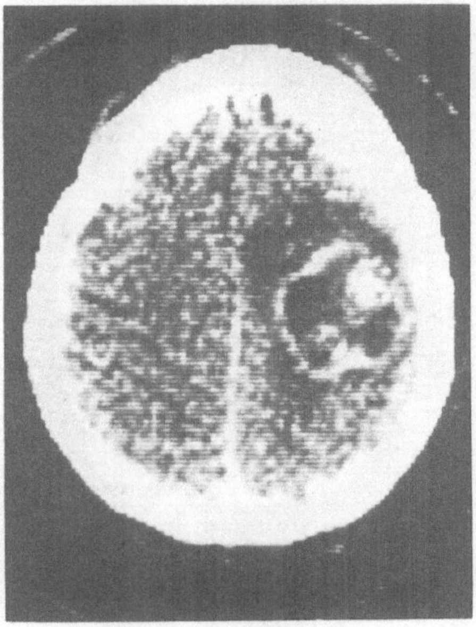

b)

c)

Fig. 6. a) Glioblastoma in the right parietal lobe. Variegated picture of tumour. Exact size of tumour not recognizable (CT 648/75, 3B);
b) After contrast enhancement with Urografin 60R the tumour is clearly delineated. Ring type of glioblastoma with central necrosis. Same
patient as Fig. 6a; c) Glioblastoma in the left cerebral hemisphere
after enhancement. Nodular type of lesion. Note marked edema represented as dark area (CT 473/75, scan 2A)

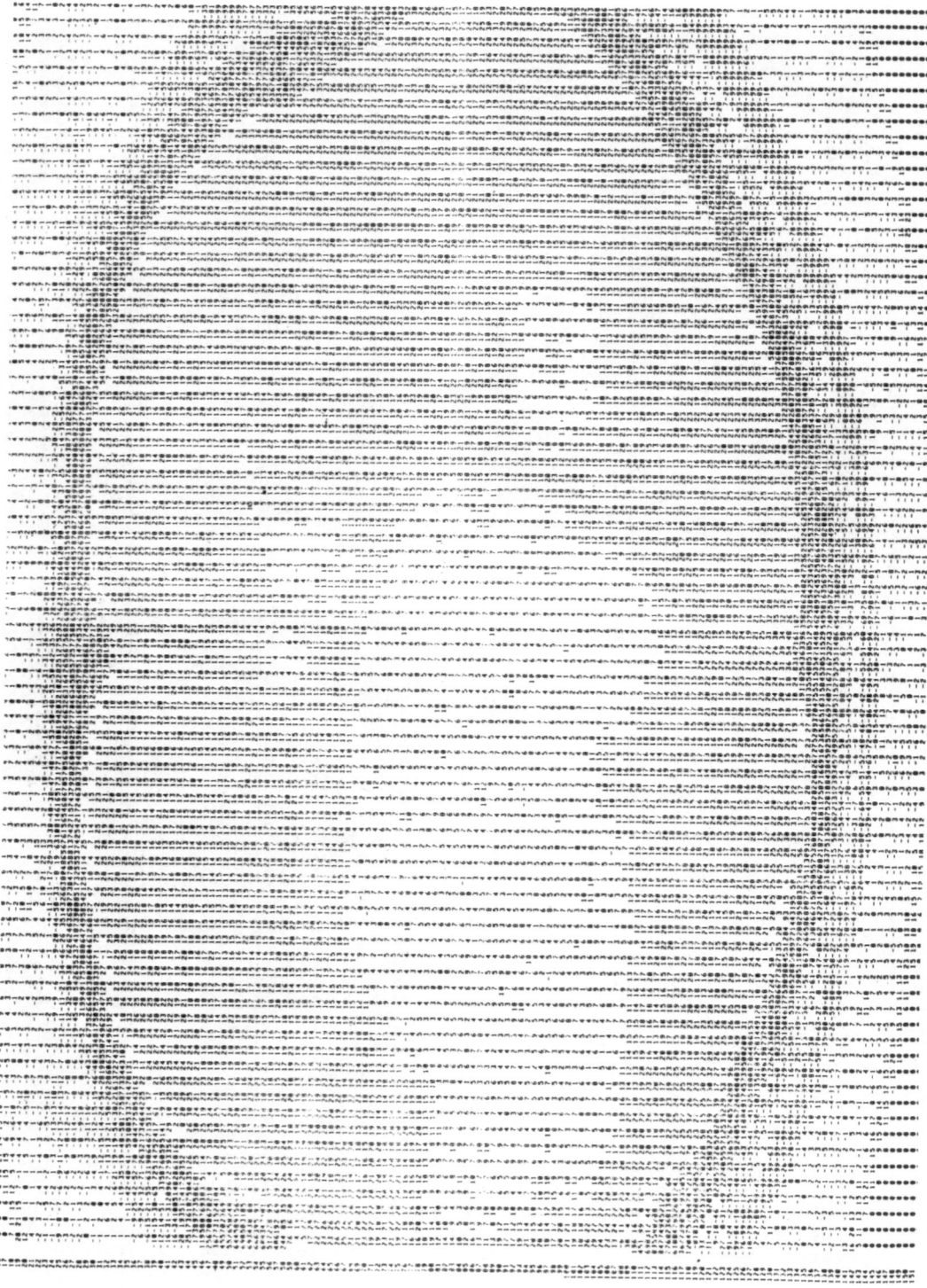

370

Fig. 7.a)

Fig. 7. Epidermoid cyst in the left
cerebral hemisphere
a) (see p.370) print out of scan 2A
with low EMI-numbers in the region
of the lesion.
b) scan 2A showing the lesion as
dark area (CT 476/75)

b)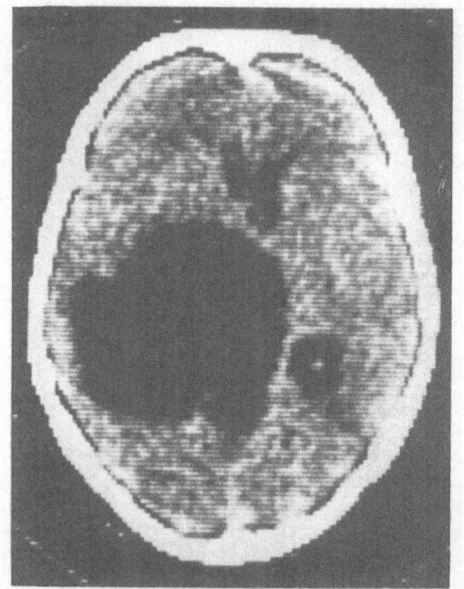

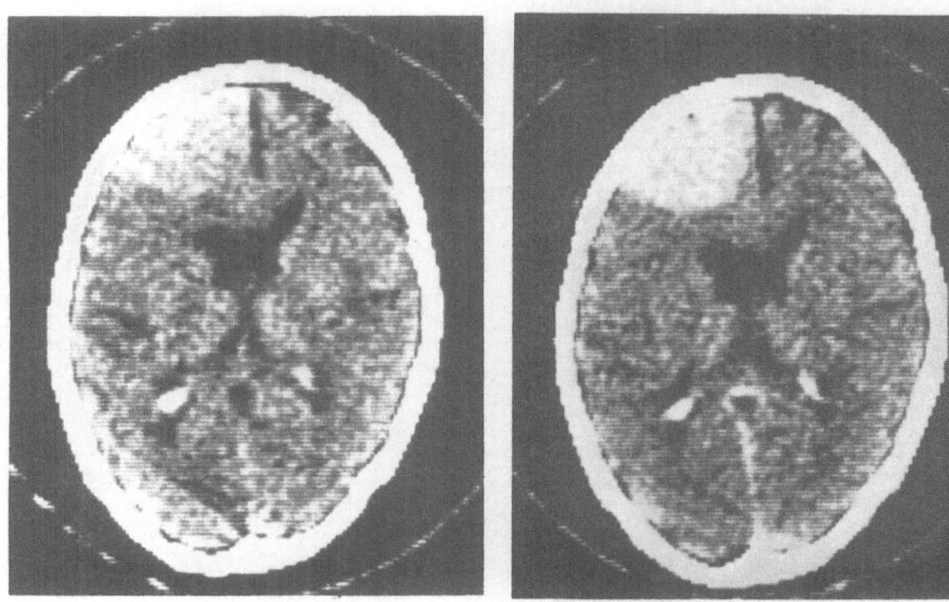

Fig. 8. Effect of contrast enhancement in meningiomas. Marked increase of density following contrast medium injection. Note absence
of edema in this 72-year-old man (CT 568/75, scan 2B)

DISC NAME:- NEUROCHIR. GROSSHADERN 829B
FILE NUMBER:- 35

MEAN= +21.7104
STANDARD DEVIATION= +2.5671

HISTOGRAM

```
15    3   XXX
16    6   XXXXXX
17   10   XXXXXXXXXX
18   21   XXXXXXXXXXXXXXXXXXXXX
19   44   XXXXXXXXXXXXXXXXXXXXXXXXXXXXXXXXXXXXXXXXXXXXXX
20   61   XXXXXXXXXXXXXXXXXXXXXXXXXXXXXXXXXXXXXXXXXXXXXXXXXXXXXXXXXXXXXXX
21   72   XXXXXXXXXXXXXXXXXXXXXXXXXXXXXXXXXXXXXXXXXXXXXXXXXXXXXXXXXXXXXXXXXXXXXXXXXXXX
22   63   XXXXXXXXXXXXXXXXXXXXXXXXXXXXXXXXXXXXXXXXXXXXXXXXXXXXXXXXXXXXXXXXX
23   59   XXXXXXXXXXXXXXXXXXXXXXXXXXXXXXXXXXXXXXXXXXXXXXXXXXXXXXXXXXXXX
24   39   XXXXXXXXXXXXXXXXXXXXXXXXXXXXXXXXXXXXXXXXX
25   28   XXXXXXXXXXXXXXXXXXXXXXXXXXXX
26   21   XXXXXXXXXXXXXXXXXXXXX
27   10   XXXXXXXXXX
28    3   XXX
29    0
30    2   XX
```

DISC NAME:- NEUROCHIR GROSSHADERN 829B
FILE NUMBER.- 37

MEAN= +24.0411
STANDARD DEVIATION= +2.5680

HISTOGRAM

```
18    3   XXX
19   10   XXXXXXXXXX
20   21   XXXXXXXXXXXXXXXXXXXXX
21   49   XXXXXXXXXXXXXXXXXXXXXXXXXXXXXXXXXXXXXXXXXXXXXXXXXXX
22   61   XXXXXXXXXXXXXXXXXXXXXXXXXXXXXXXXXXXXXXXXXXXXXXXXXXXXXXXXXXXXXXX
23   66   XXXXXXXXXXXXXXXXXXXXXXXXXXXXXXXXXXXXXXXXXXXXXXXXXXXXXXXXXXXXXXXXXXXXXX
24   60   XXXXXXXXXXXXXXXXXXXXXXXXXXXXXXXXXXXXXXXXXXXXXXXXXXXXXXXXXXXXXX
25   74   XXXXXXXXXXXXXXXXXXXXXXXXXXXXXXXXXXXXXXXXXXXXXXXXXXXXXXXXXXXXXXXXXXXXXXXXXXXX
26   53   XXXXXXXXXXXXXXXXXXXXXXXXXXXXXXXXXXXXXXXXXXXXXXXXXXXXXXX
27   42   XXXXXXXXXXXXXXXXXXXXXXXXXXXXXXXXXXXXXXXXXX
28   13   XXXXXXXXXXXXX
29   16   XXXXXXXXXXXXXXXX
30    5   XXXXX
31    3   XXX
32    0
33    2   XX
```

Fig. 9. Histograms of an astrocytoma grade II-III before (above) and after enhancement (below). Increase of EMI-numbers from +21,7 to +24,0 (CT 635/75, scan 2B)

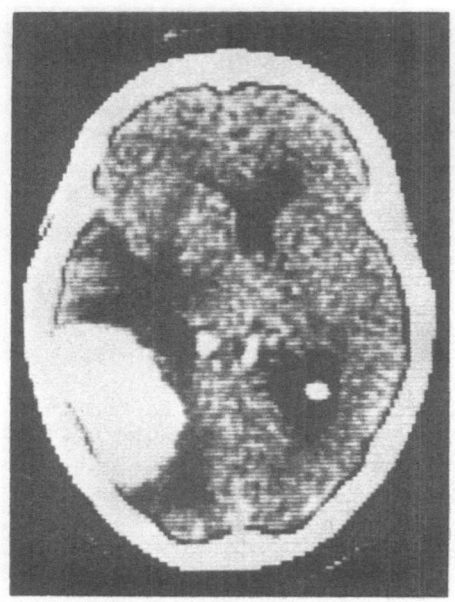

Fig. 10. Edema grade II in a partly calcified meningioma in the left temporo-occipital region. The edema shows finger-sized extensions following the white matter (CT 263/75, scan 2A)

Fig. 12. Acoustic neurinoma before (a) and after enhancement (b). Note perifocal edema (CT 650/75, scan 1B)

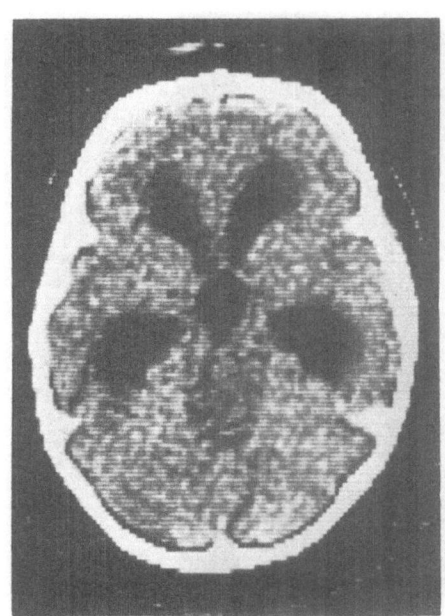 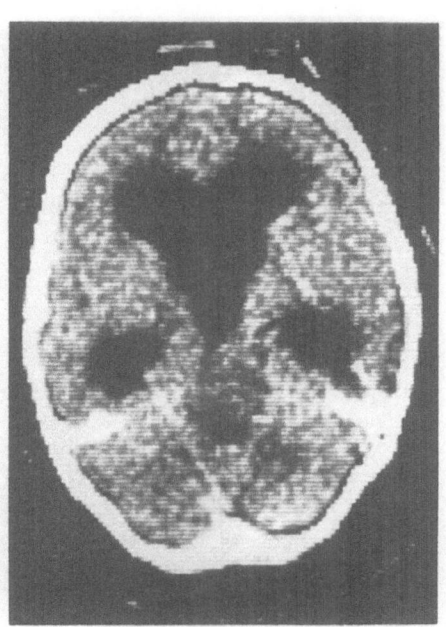

Fig. 11. Cerebellar astrocytoma, demonstrated as low density lesions, extending through the aquaeduct into the posterior part of the third ventricle. Hydrocephalus. (CT 261/75, scans 1B and 2A)

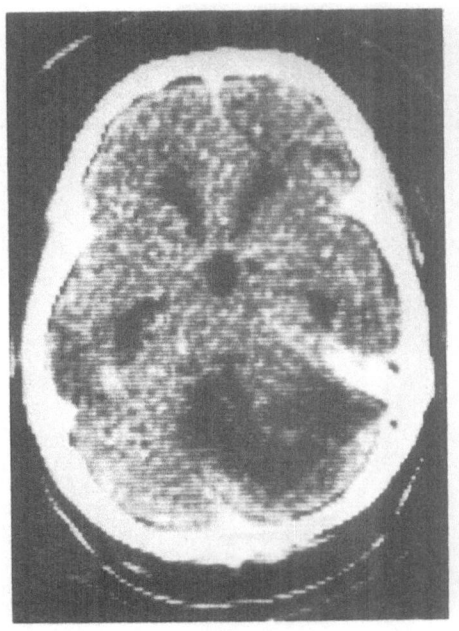 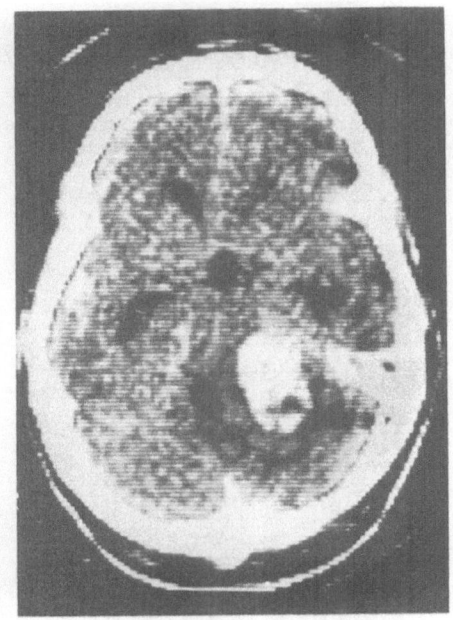

a)   b)

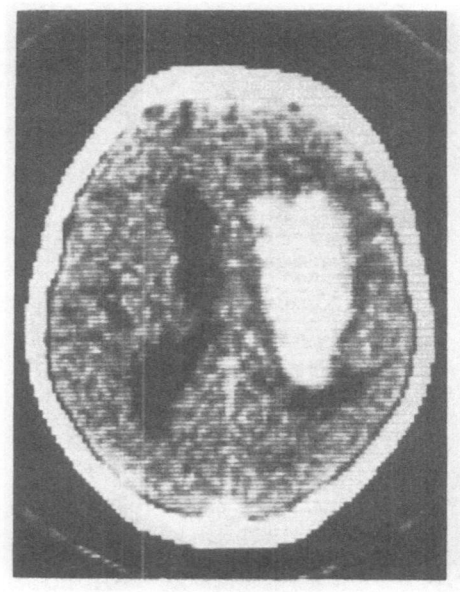 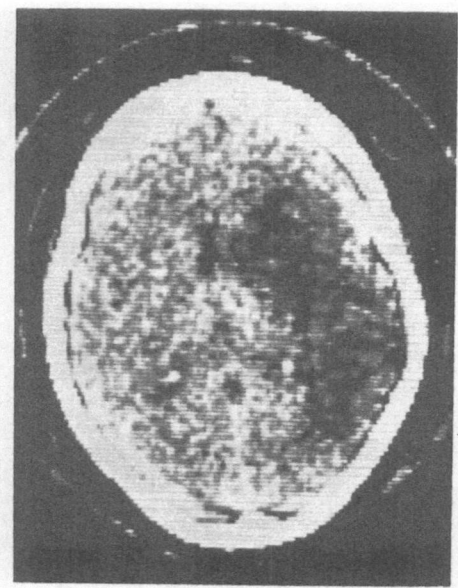

Fig. 13   Fig. 14

Fig. 13. Large intracerebral hematoma in the right cerebral hemisphere due to hypertension (CT 287/75, scan 2B)

Fig. 14. Infarction of the territory supplied by the right middle
cerebral artery. The infarcted area appears as low density zone. Brain
swelling involves gray matter (CT 154/75, scan 2A)

Fig. 15. Computer tomograms and corresponding brain sections in a
case of ruptured aneurysm of the anterior communicating artery (CT
093/75, scans 1B, 2A, 2B)

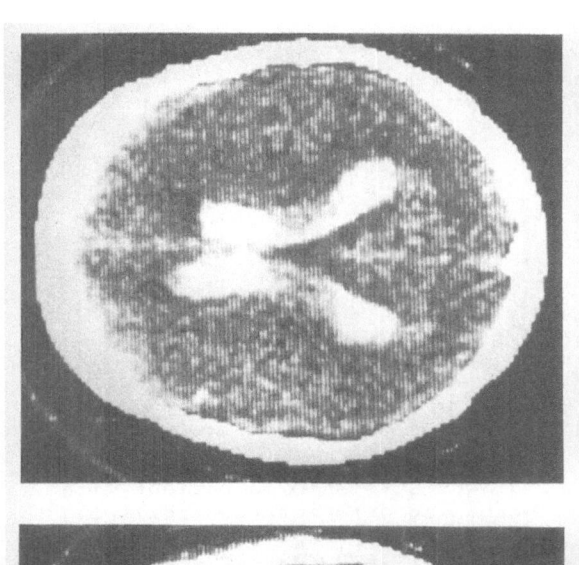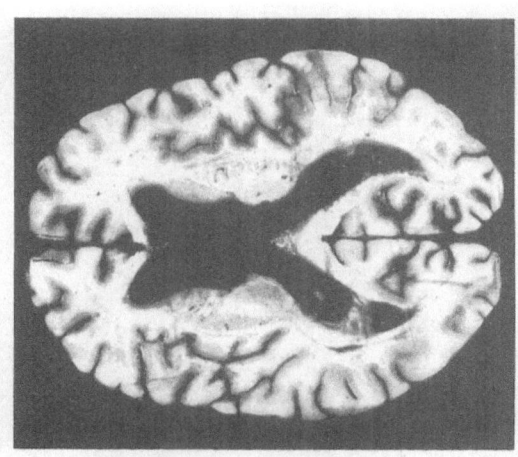

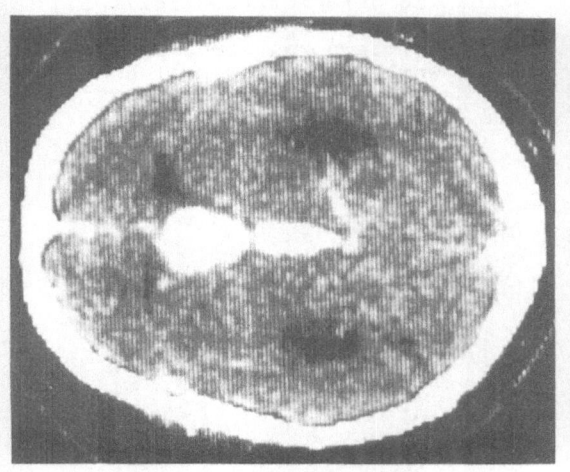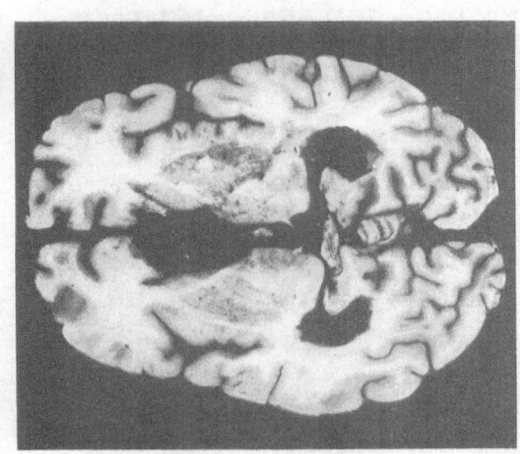

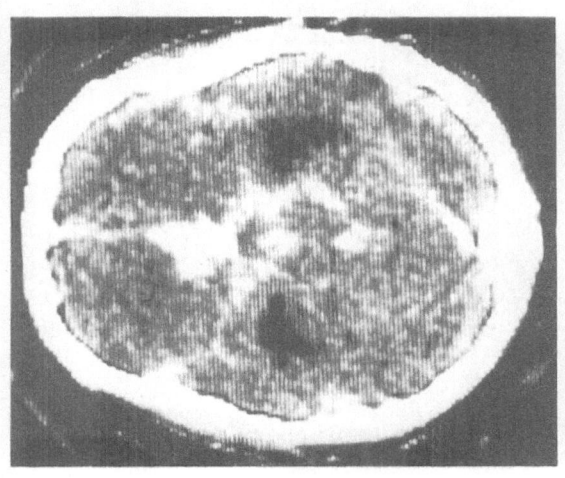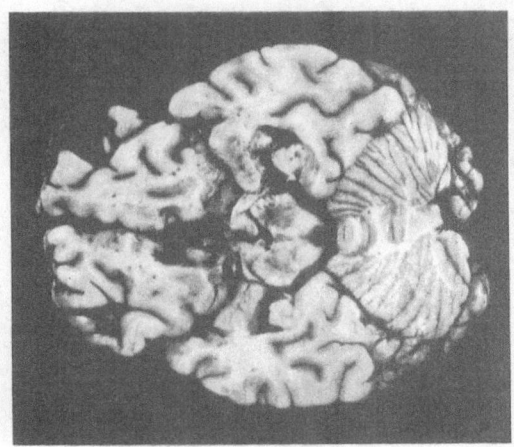

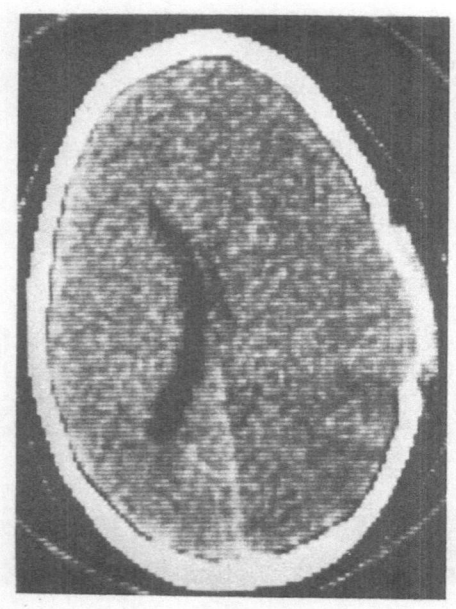

Fig. 16. CT-scan of a patient with increasing deterioration following removal of a plexus papilloma from the right temporal horn. Swelling of the whole right cerebral hemisphere due to vasospasm (CT 376/75, scan 2B)

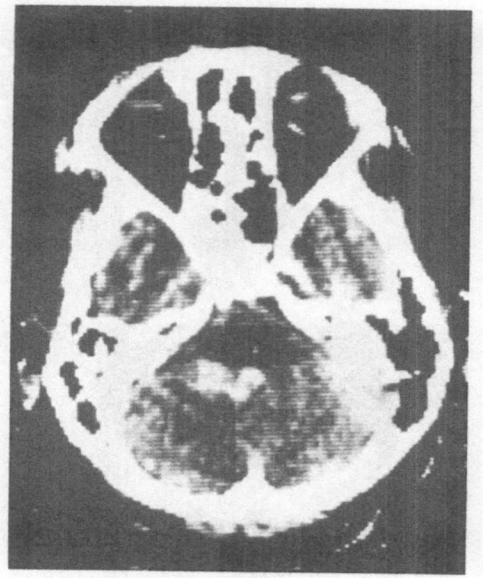

a)

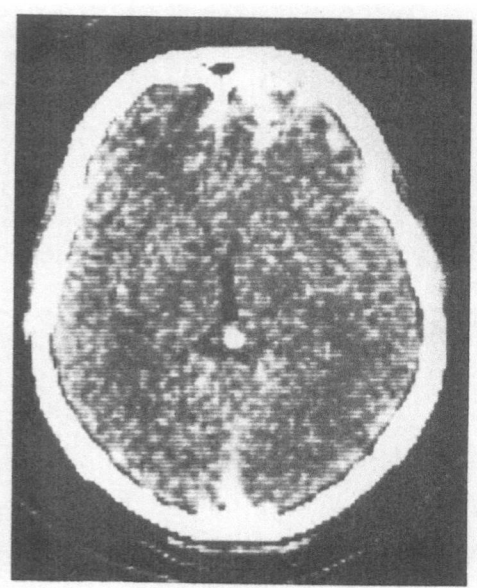

b)

Fig. 17. Multiple contusions in a patient with occipital impact. a) contusion in the depth of the left cerebellar hemisphere in scan 1A. b) contusion of the right frontal lobe in scan 2B. The ventricular system is compressed (CT 460/75)

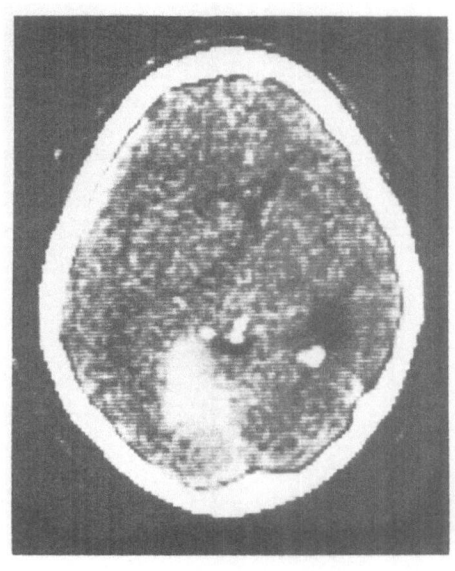 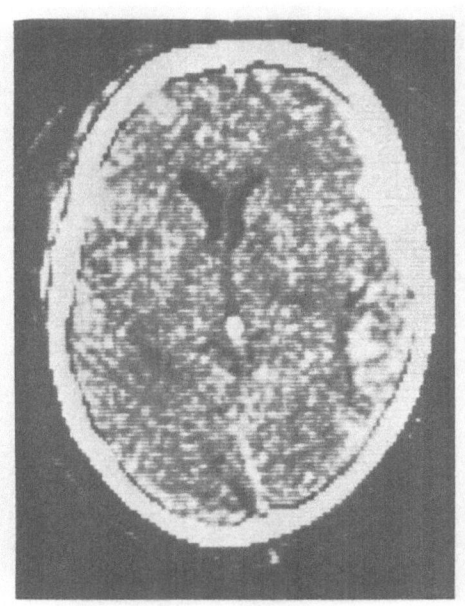

Fig. 18   Fig. 19

Fig. 18. Posttraumatic intracerebral hematoma in the left occipital region (CT 175/75, scan 2A)

Fig. 19. Acute subdural hematoma in the right fronto-temporal region. Note multiple contusions in the right temporal and left fronto-temporal region presented as white-spotted areas (CT 037/75, scan 2A)

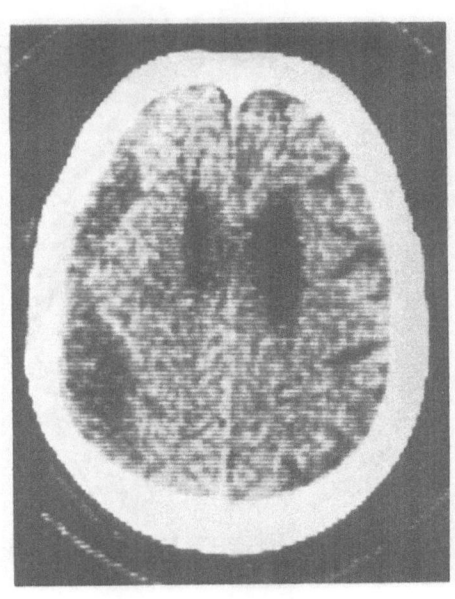

Fig. 20. Chronic subdural hematoma on the left side. Marked cortical atrophy on the right side with broadened sulci (CT 527/75, scan 3B)

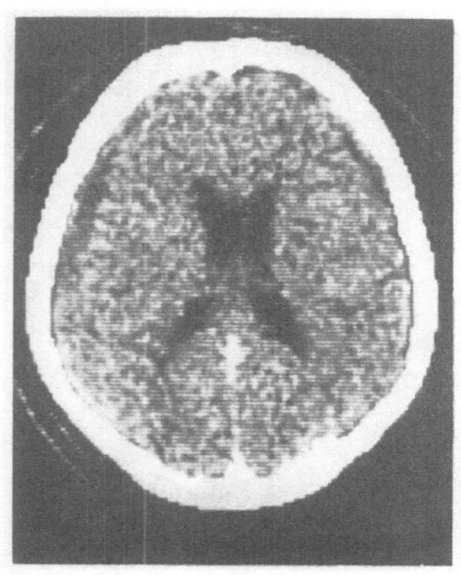

Fig. 21. Small bilateral chronic subdural hematoma (CT 095/75, scan 2B)

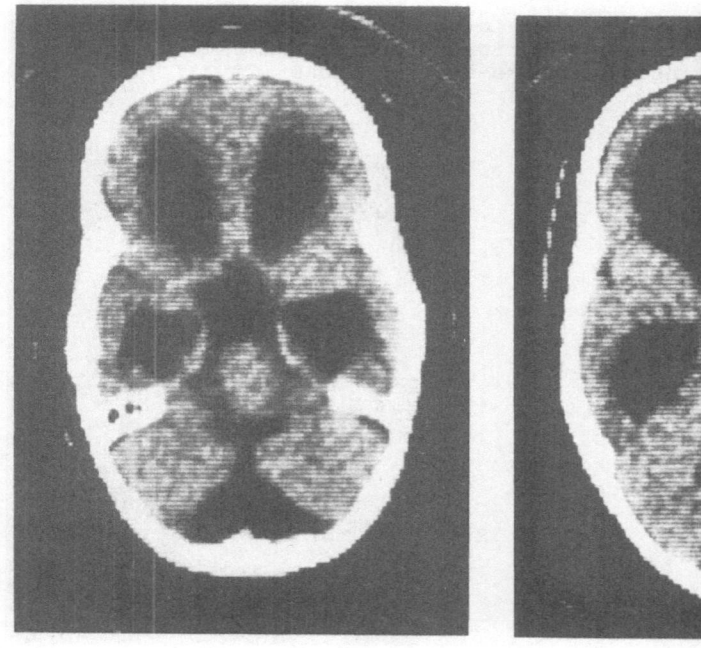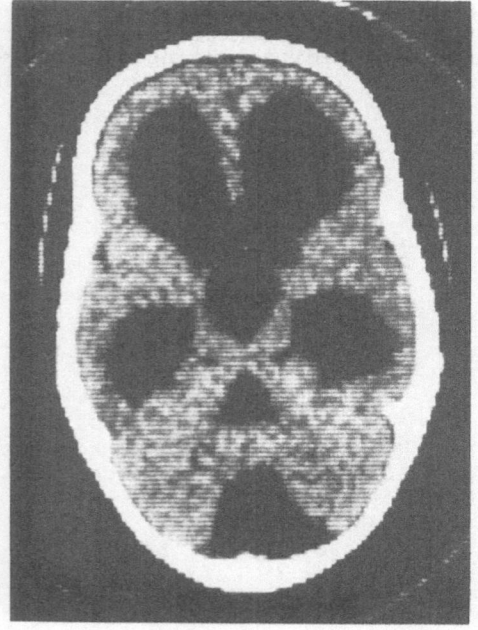

Fig. 22. Diagnosis of communicating hydrocephalus. Wide 4th ventricle, foramen of Magendi and cisterns (CT 489/75, scans 41A and 41B)

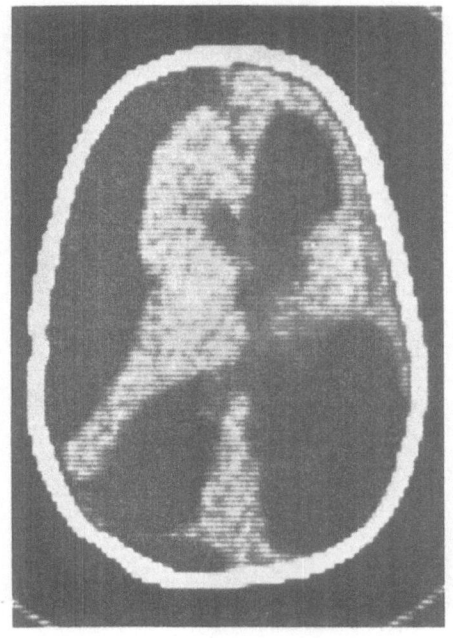

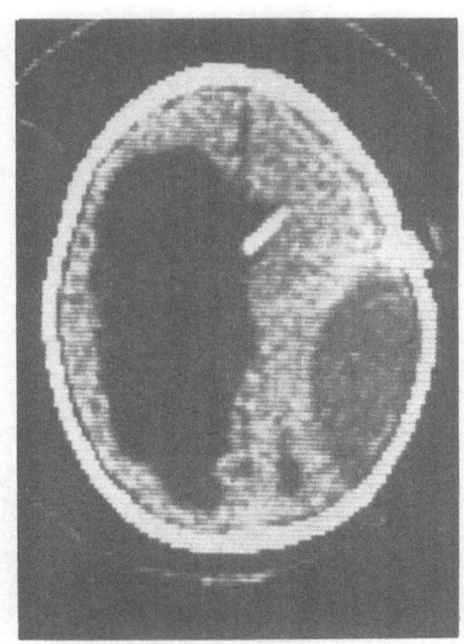

Fig. 23   Fig. 24

Fig. 23. Child with a massive hydrocephalus on the right side and a large subdural effusion covering the left collapsed hemisphere (CT 361/75, scan 2A)

Fig. 24. Chronic subdural hematoma on the right side following a shunt operation. The catheter tip reaches the left dilated porencephalic ventricle (CT 179/75, scan 3A)

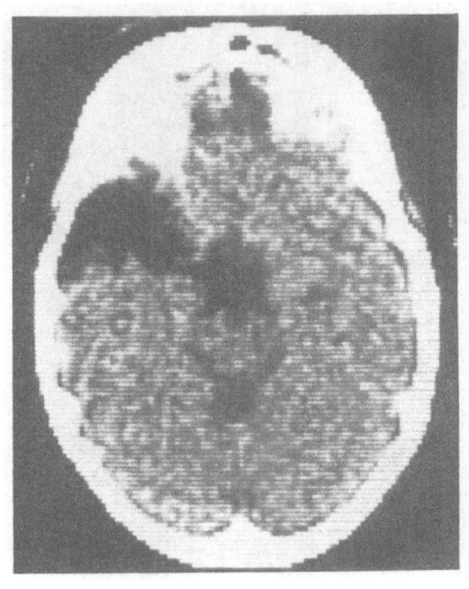

Fig. 25. Arachnoid cyst in the left temporal region (CT 023/75, scan 1B)

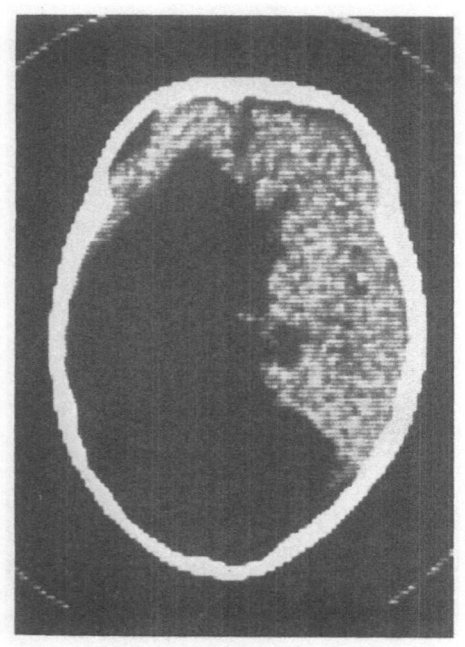

Fig. 26. Aplasia of large parts of the left cerebral hemisphere.
Aplasia of the right occipital lobe in a child with cerebral palsy
(CT 379/75, scan 1B)

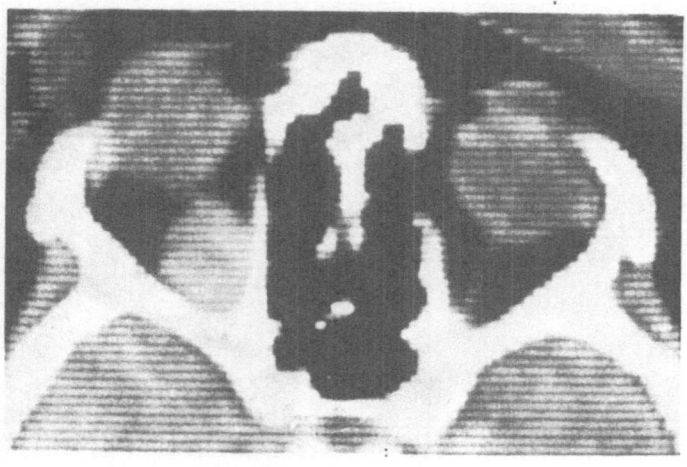

Fig. 27. CT-scans of a patient with a meningioma of the optic nerve
sheath within the left orbit (CT O92/75, scan 71B)

Informational Value and the Therapeutical Application of Selective Angiography

J. WAPPENSCHMIDT and E. LINS

In contrast to a global angiography, selective angiography (S.A.) is performed by introducing a catheter from a principle arterial into certain side branches. By this means it is possible to isolate the region of autochtonous supply of these side branches and to show them without superimposing images of other branches. The following examples demonstrate the informational value and therapeutical possibilities which are offered by S.A. on intracranial tumors fed by external carotid circulation.

The first X-ray displays a paramedian meningioma. Using the trans-femoral method developed by SELDINGER, the catheter was placed at the origin of the middle meningeal artery. We perceived that two strongly meandering branches of the middle meningeal artery were main arterial afflux to the tumor (Fig. 1).

Furthermore, the contrast medium flowed from the middle meningeal artery via a pre-formed anastomose into the anterior meningeal artery which partially fed the tumor.

The following cases also demonstrate both the informational value and the therapeutical use of the method.

The first example is a subtentorial meningioma. In the global brachial angiography of the right side there was no observable deviation of pre-formed arteries.

A hint pointing to a pathological process, however, was provided by a strongly dilated, external occipital artery from which several branches ascended along the occipital region and passed through channels in the bone into the skull.

In the last stage of the arteriogram there was only a discrete homogeneous stain at the falco-tentorial angle which could easily have been overlooked.

However, the selective angiography of the vertebral artery showed a signigicant stain coming from the meningeal branches of the vertebral artery.

During the same session we introduced the catheter into the right external carotid artery and placed its end before the branch-off of the facial artery. The S.A. proved that the supply of blood to the tumor was provided exclusively by the external occipital artery. Again during the last stage of the angiography a homogenous tumor stain could be seen much more distinctly than in the global angiography (Fig. 2). The middle meningeal artery did not participate in feeding the tumor; we tried to block off the blood supply by artificial embolisation. We introduced the catheter into the external occipital artery and injected small pieces of fibrine and tabotamp measuring 1x2x5 mm through it into the vessel in several stages. The control angiography revealed the first effect: the posterior branch of the occipital artery was distally closed; the two anterior branches still remeined open.

In the last phase the tumor stain could be recognized. Therefore we went on injecting small pieces of fibrin and tabotamp. The next control angiography showed that the anterior vessels feeding the tumor were closed and that there was no further stain.

The next case is that of an 56 year old patient. In 1966 an angio-endothelioma underneath the left temporal lobe had been removed surgically and there were the clinical symptoms of a reincidence. The arteriography of the left common carotid artery showed a temporal expansive lesion and also a stain, but it could not be clearly made out if the vessels supplying the tumor were derived from the external carotid artery or from the internal carotid artery circulation.

For the purpose of differentiation a S.A. of the external carotid artery was made and the catheter was placed into the internal maxilary artery. Already in the early stage the selective serial angiography revealed strongly dilatated branches of the middle meningeal artery to be feeding the tumor; during the last stage we saw a homogenous stain of the size of an apple (Fig. 3).

The tumor circulation having consequently been shown to be completely fed by the middle meningeal artery, we tried once again to block this blood supply by artificial embolization, using the same methods as in the first case. The subsequent control X-rays showed the effect: the great supply arteries were closed, only some small branches still remained open.

An additional embolization provided a further reduction of the tumor circulation (Fig. 4). It was necessary, however, to remember that the tumor could find itself new paths of supply from other vascular units. Therefore eight days after the embolization a control angiography was made to establish whether or not this had, in fact, been the case. There was neither a reincidence of the stain to be seen nor any indication of new tumor supplying vessels.

During the subsequent surgery the neurosurgeon noticed that the area in question had remarkably low blood circulation. The histological preparation substantiated the effect of embolization: one could recognize numerous necroses in the tumor region and small balls of fibrine embedded in the tumor.

The following two points demonstrate the significance of the S.A. of the external carotid artery:

(1) By obtaining an isolated image of the discrete branches of the external carotid artery, especially the internal maxillary artery, the occipital artery and the ascending pharyngeal artery, (all arteries involved in supplying the dura), it is possible to identify these vessels feeding the tumor. This in turn provides the information necessary for determining the dimension of the tumor and the diagnosis of the tumor type.

(2) The main advantage of this process is the therapeutical application. It is possible to close intra tumoral sections of vessels directly by embolisation. An occlusion of the main supplying vessels

can always be carried out directly next to the tumor, a process which is impossible in the simple ligature of the carotid external artery. In the latter case the supply of the distal vessel segments comes from the contralateral external carotid artery and ascending branches of the subclavian artery via the callateral vessels. However, it is impossible to estimate the amount of influence that this embolisation method has on the metabolism and the growth of the tumor. An additional possibility is to selectively inject antimetabolic or anti-mitotic substances in high concentrations directly into the tumor in order to influence its metabolism. This method is of special interest in the treatment of malignant tumors. The S.A., with its resulting possibility of blocking the tumor circulation without surgery, un-covers new possibilities in the treatment of certain neoplasms of the central nervous system which do not only justify but almost require its application in appropriate cases.

Summary

In the case of extracerebral tumors which are completely or primarly supplied by the external carotid artery circulation, S.A. provides for the identification of the vessels feeding the tumor. At the same time it is possible to block the blood flow towards the tumor by ar-tificial embolization. At the present time, however, one cannot pre-dict the possibility of the total necrosis of the tumor. In the case of benign tumors, S.A. works as a preoperative measure to provide an area of low blood flow for the surgeon. In the case of malignant tu-mors in the extracerebral part of the head or facial regions, S.A. can be used as an additional measure to allow antimetabolic or anti-mitotic substances to be injected directly into the tumor in high concentrations.

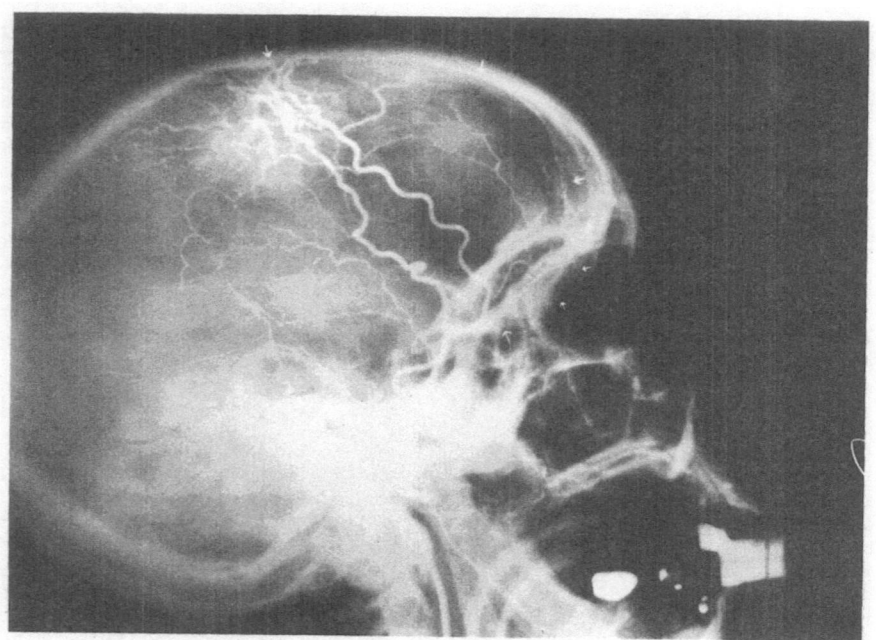

Fig. 1. Feeding meningial artery of paramedian meningioma

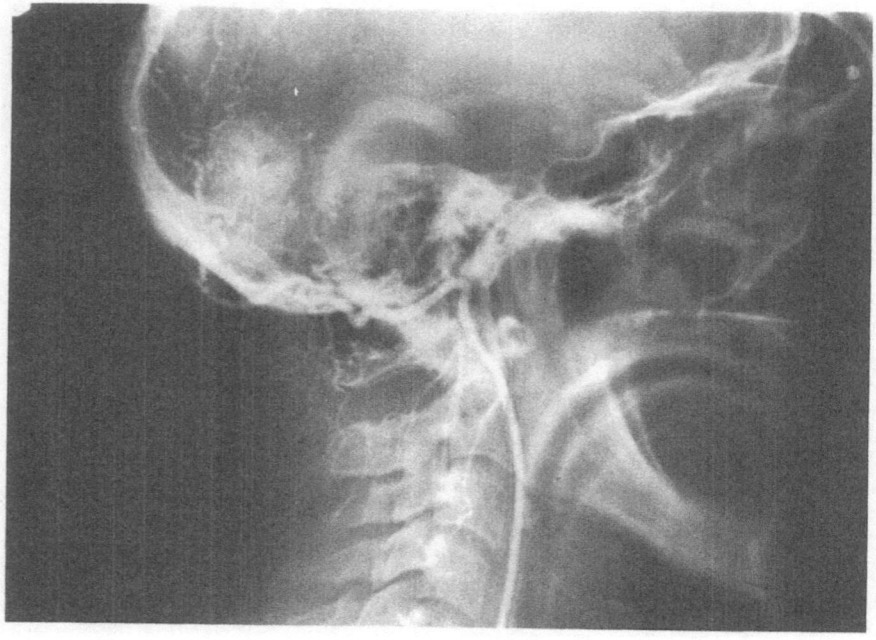

Fig. 2. Meningial branch of occipital artery supplying infratentorial meningioma

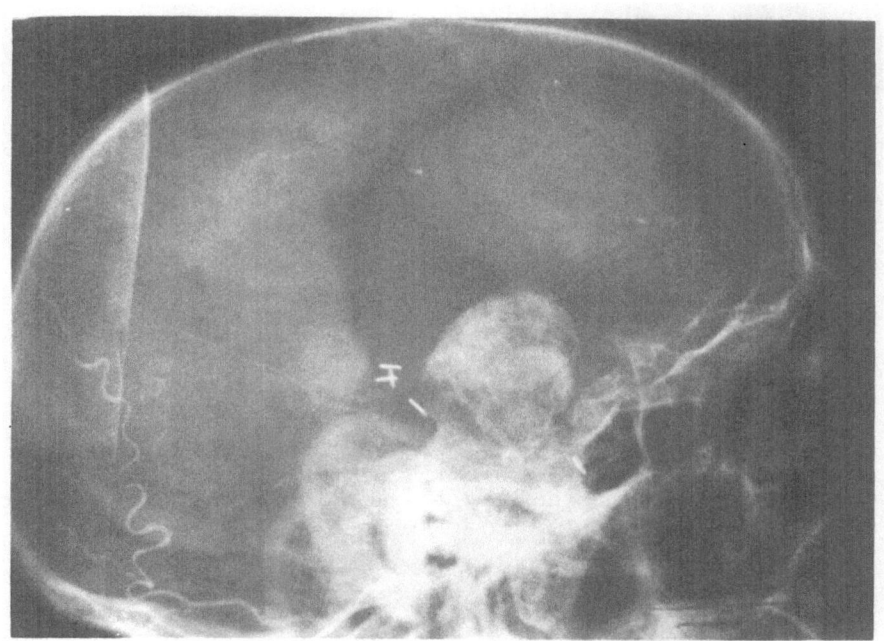

Fig. 3. Temporal angioendothelioma, supplied by middle meningial artery

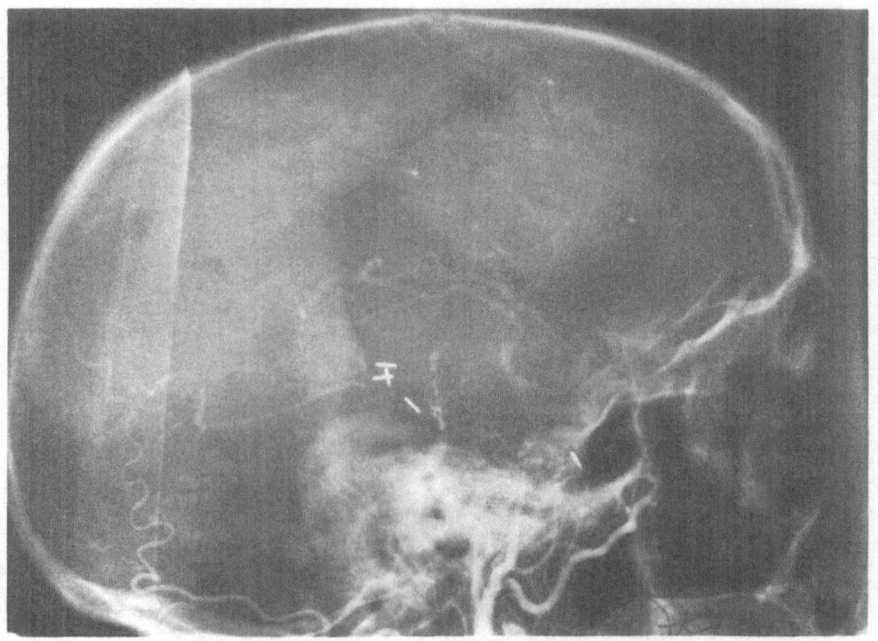

Fig. 4. Reduction of circulation following embolization of feeding arteries

The Meningal Branch of the Occipital Artery

A. Perneczky, S. Salah, and M. Tschabitscher

Introduction

The arterial blood supply of the dura mater in the posterior cranial fossa is often attributed to the pharyngeal artery, whereby the role of the occipital artery is not considered. It is our aim to draw attention to the meningeal ramus of the occipital artery, as this meningeal artery is important in regard to diagnosis as well as to operation.

Material and Method

In 20 cadavers fixed with formalin the occipital artery was injected with Latex and then the meningeal ramus was prepared under the operating microscope. In addition the meningeal ramus of the occipital artery was studied in normal and in pathological angiograms.

Discussion

The meningeal ramus of the occipital artery has its origin exactly at the point where the occipital artery leaves its own sulcus behind the mastoid. The meningeal ramus ascends in the direction of the mastoid foramen (Fig. 1). In the mastoid canal the artery is surrounded by the wide emissary. At the inner mouth of the mastoid canal the meningeal ramus is divided into two big terminal branches (Fig. 2). One terminal branch supplies the dura in the cerebellar fossa of the occipital bone. The second terminal branch leads to the posterior surface of the pyramid, where it supplies the dura, and reaches the inferior surface of the tentorium with its terminal ramification. A small terminal branch leads from the inner mouth of the mastoid canal along the external wall of the sigmoid sinus in the direction of the jugular foramen.

Thus, the meningeal ramus of the occipital artery supplies the dura in the cerebellar fossa, the dura on the posterior surface of the pyramid, and partially the tentorium.

In normal angiograms the relatively slim meningeal ramus of the occipital artery can, for the most part, only be visualized if the vessels are particularly well filled (Fig. 3). In processes in the cerebello-pontine-angle (especially in meningiomas), in dural angiomas of the posterior cranial fossa (Fig. 4), and in tumors of the glomus, the meningeal ramus of the occipital artery is often one of the main supply vessels of the pathological process. This can be verified by angiography.

When planning a neurosurgical operation in the posterior cranial fossa this vessel ought not be excluded from consideration.

Summary

This paper deals with the anatomy and importance of the meningeal ramus of the occipital artery, which, after passing the mastoid foramen, leads to the dura of the posterior cranial fossa, where it supplies the posterior surface of the pyramid and the cerebellar fossa of the occipital bone. We particularly emphasize the clinical importance of the findings.

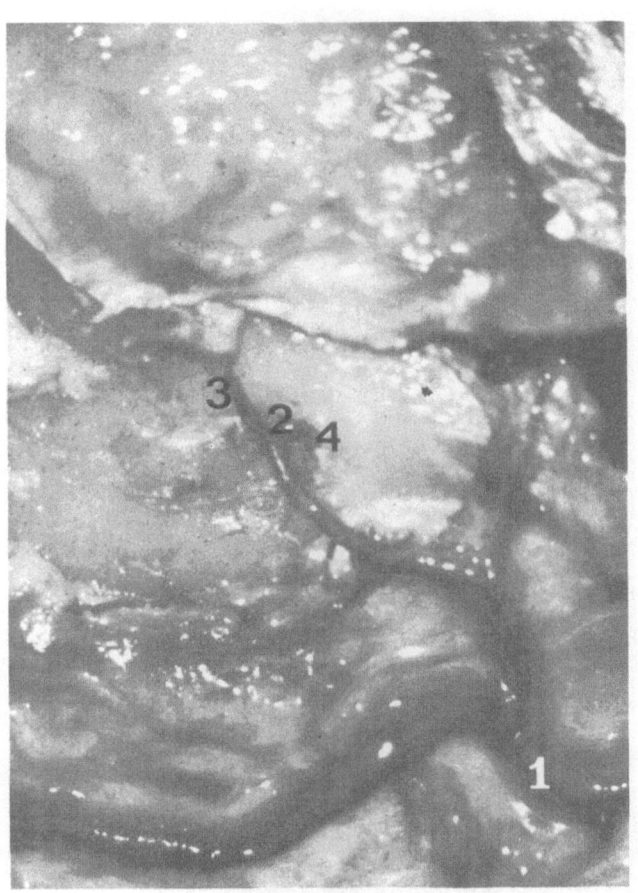

Fig. 1. The extracranial part of the meningeal branch of the occipital artery (right side). 1. occipital artery; 2. meningeal branch; 3. muscular branch; 4. mastoid foramen

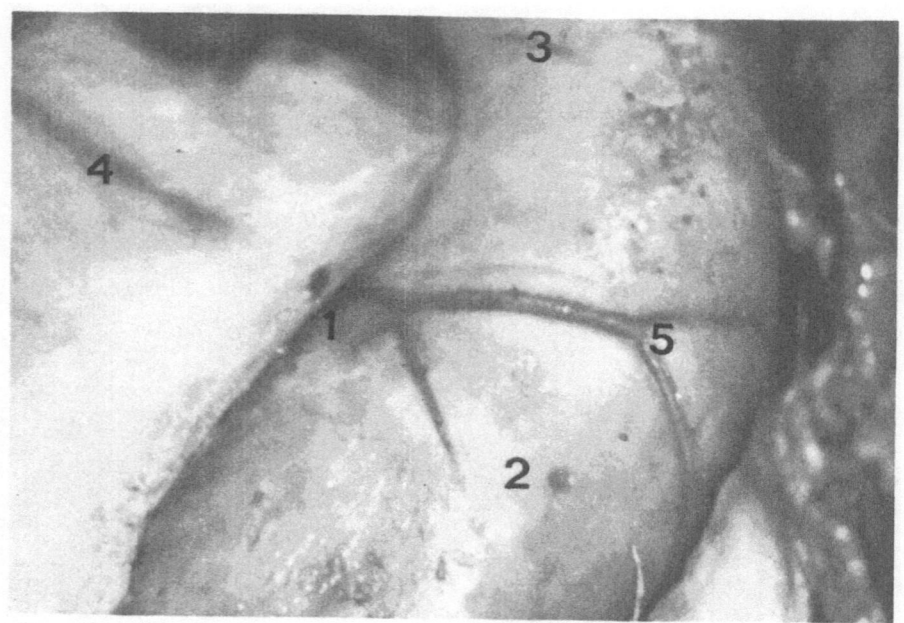

Fig. 2. The mouth of the mastoid emissary into the sigmoid sinus
(left side). 1. mastoid emissary; 2. sigmoid sinus; 3. transversal sinus; 4. branch on the cerebellar fossa; 5. branch on the posterior
surface of the pyramid

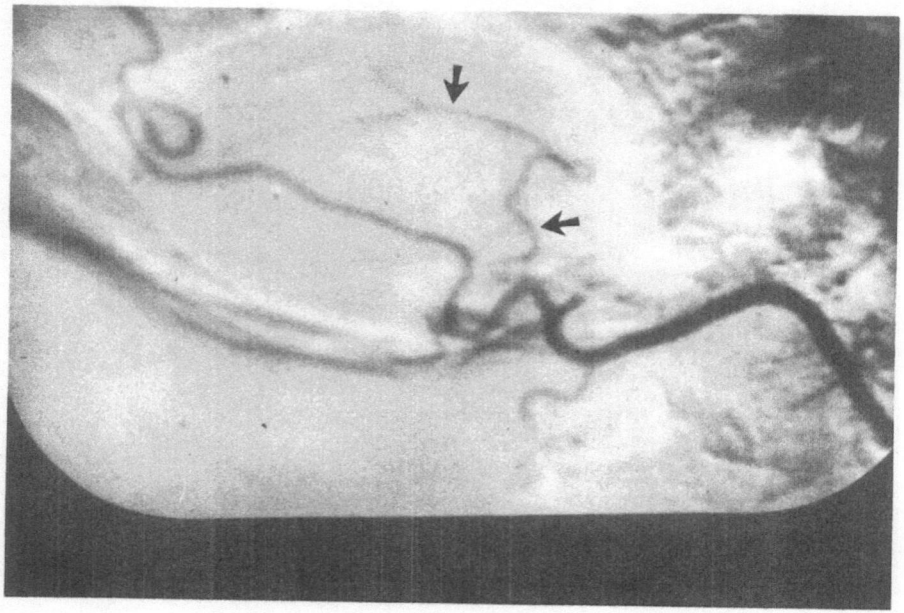

Fig. 3. Normal angiogram of the occipital artery with the meningeal
branch (arrow)

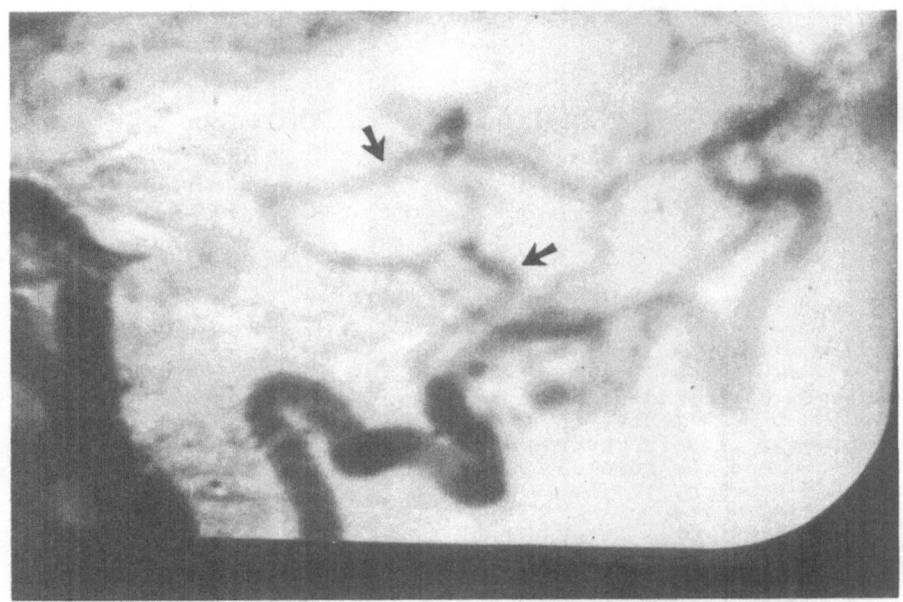

Fig. 4. Angioma of the Dura of the Tentorium with enlarged meningeal
branch (arrow) of the occipital artery

Pediatric Head Injuries

(Follow-Up Study of 625 Cases)

J. P. Chodkiewicz, A. Redondo, L. Merienne, C. Cioloka, and F. Terrazas

Summary

The authors have studied a series of 625 children with head injuries. During the past 7 years, these children have been hospitalized in neurosurgery, closely observed and eventually operated on by the same medical team in the same department. Several observations can be made from these results.

The presence of twice as many boys as girls among the patients has been noted. This masculine predominance remains to be explained.

Traffic accidents are responsible for approximately 50% of the admissions. These are always the most serious accidents involving the greatest number of severe neurological disorders, associated extracranial traumatic lesions and deaths.

The clinical pictures of *benign* and *severe* head traumas are reviewed. The authors emphasize the rarity (4% of the cases) and the bad prognosis of the *epidural hematoma*; the sub-dural hydroma appears to be an uncommon but very interesting lesion.

The diagnostic and therapeutic problems due to associated extracranial traumatic lesions (12% of the cases) have been thoroughly considered.

To evaluate the prognosis as early as possible, several factors have been carefully examined: the *fracture* which plays no part, the *state of consciousness* which is decisive, and the presence or absence of initial hemiplegia seizures or decerebrate rigidity. The sequelae are observed in less than 10% of the cases. In one-third of these cases, complex dyskinesia is present; *post-traumatic epilepsy* does not often appear in the series (3 authentic cases only); prolonged anticonvulsive therapy is of no apparent value.

The results are discussed and compared with those previously published in medical research literature.

Infantile mortality has been stadily diminishing for years in our so-called civilized countries; nevertheless, mortality due to accidents is increasing every year. The greatest percentage of all these accidental deaths is due to head injuries; therefore, many extensive surveys have been devoted to the subject (3, 8, 13, 25, 35, 45).

Material and Methods

In the neurosurgical department of Hôpital SAINTE ANNE in PARIS, we have reviewed 625 cases of children who were admitted in the emergency ward during the past seven years. All these patients were treated and then reexamined many times after hospital discharge by the same neurosurgical team, so that 65% of the cases have been followed up for more than three years.

I. General Data

Table 1 summarizes the age and sex characteristics of the patients studied; they were approximately twice as many boys as girls, but this well known masculine predominance which includes children before 18 months of age, remains to be explained. (18, 25, 30, 31)

18% of the patients studied were of foreign origin (Spain, Portugal, Northern Africa...). This group, which represents statistically less than 10% of the total pediatric population in France, must therefore be considered, in terms of accidental mortality and morbidity, as an underprivileged high risk population. This is of course related to the socio-economic conditions of the people concerned.

Table 1. 625 pediatric head injuries

Girls	226	Boys	399	64%	

Age: 0 - 2.....134 cases
    2 - 5.....127 cases
    5 - 10.....188 cases
    10 - 15.....176 cases

22% total trauma-patients
65% total children admitted
Foreign origin 18%

Table 2. Nature of injury

Traffic Accident	297	48%
Car....... Passenger:	66	
Pedestrian:	134	
2 Wheels... Passenger:	77	
Pedestrian:	20	
Falls	190	30%
Miscellaneous	71	12%
Unknown	67	10%

Nature of Injury (Table 2; excluding birth injuries):

- Traffic accidents were the most common cause of head injuries in children (48%).

- These children were passengers of - or struck by - a two or four wheel vehicle.

- Two wheel accidents represent 13% of the 625 cases and concern *boys* in 88% of the cases.

- Half of these traffic accidents occur when the child is going to or returning from school.

- The severity of these accidents is extreme: 57 children died, representing 73% of the total number of fatalities in our series.

Falls either from a height or at ground level resulted in 30% of the head injuries studied.

There were 24 cases of battered child syndrome with 5 deaths. Finally it must be stressed that these 625 pediatric head injuries represent 65% of the total number of children admitted in our service during the same period of time.

II. Diagnostic Procedures

Clinical experience is of paramount importance to evaluate the neurological condition of a child who sustained a recent head injury. A few diagnostic procedures may contribute to this evaluation.

Skull x-rays are considered a routine procedure: a skull fracture was present in 347 patients (56%). This proportion observed in a neurosurgical ward is much more elevated than the percentage of skull fractures discovered in children coming to a general surgical ward (13, 29).

Lumbar puncture after head injury is, in our opinion, of no help in differentiating surgical and non-surgical cases and may be hazardous.

Echo encephalography and radio-active-brain scanning have not been used routinely in our clinic as an emergency procedure (22, 23).

EEG has been rarely recorded the day of admission except for patients with early seizures and has been, in most of the cases, reserved for secondary problems.

Carotid angiography is from our experience the best diagnostic procedure to identify post-traumatic intracranial lesions such as epidural clots, subdural hematomas, cerebral swelling, multiple contusions etc.; carotid puncture is performed under local or general anesthesia early after admission and biplane films with sometimes cross compression allow a satisfactory investigation of the supratentorial space (19, 34).

The results are very encouraging, sometimes surgically decisive, but the procedure *should not* at all be considered, at least in our hands (8), as totally benign and well-tolerated by a freshly injured infantile brain. In our series carotid angiography was performed in 89 cases (19%); in 17 cases the neurological condition deteriorated immediately and dramatically after angiography; 10 of these severely injured patients died.

III. Benign Head Injuries

249 children in the series (40%) may be classified as benign cases. The patients spent only a few days in our care after injury; all of them were sent back home rapidly and recovered completely. The clinical picture of these cases is very diversified (Table 3).

Table 3. 625 pediatric head injuries

```
- Benign Cases.............................40%
     Minor                             :  97
     Drowsy (transit) ± Fract.         :  81
     Drowsy ± Seizure ± Loc. S.        :  45
- Severe Cases............................52%
     Contusion (Hemisph. or Brain Stem) :136
     Intracranial Hematoma             :  40
     Depressed Fr. + Cranio-CB Wounds  :  97
     CSF Fistula                       :  18
     Moribund at Admission             :  24
- Miscellaneous............................8%
```

Immediate post-traumatic seizures with transitory disorder of consciousness and *no* neurological deficits proved to be always benign, as well as transient post-traumatic drowsiness after impact when strictly isolated with *no* seizures localizing signs or meningeal reaction.

The presence of a skull fracture alone, without any clinical abnormality is, in our experience, of no significance at all. For many authors this type of fracture does not even justify systematic hospitalization (12, 29, 33).

These apparently *benign* cases can pose extremely difficult problems to the physician. The danger is to underestimate the true severity of the situation and the anatomical lesions, and overlook or misinterpret *progressive but subtle evidence* of critical intracranial complication. Four patients in the present group have been initially and erroneously classified as benign cases a few hours after trauma; in fact these four patients who had epidural hematomas did demonstrate discrete but definite early symptoms or signs which were neglected or misunderstood (headaches, diplopia, vomiting...).

This stresses the importance of very careful initial clinical investigation and the necessity of immediate hospitalization of the child to check him with great concern for a few days, each time the clinical picture although apparently benign is equivocal.

IV. Severe Head Injuries

The incidence of *severe* head injuries is 60% (3) in the present series. The classification of these 376 cases is shown in Table 3.

1. Depressed Fractures

Depressed fractures *alone*, with *no* dural tear (54 cases) are seen predominantly in boys (34 cases) and in the frontal region (30 cases). Each time a bone fragment was considered depressed the depth of the skull thickness, or each time there was a neurological deficit (14 cases) or persistent and focalized EEG abnormalities, the fracture was surgically elevated, as a rule 24 hours or more after injury; 90% of the patients recovered completely within 2 weeks or less.

2. Craniocerebral Injuries with Dural Laceration

Include 61 of the cases here studied:

- 18 CSF Fistulas (10 rhynorreas) with basal skull fracture; three cases only had to be surgically treated because of persisting nasal CSF leakage.
- 16 depressed fractures were associated with dural laceration.
- 27 patients had craniocerebral wounds.

The diagnostic problems in these cases are minimal because of evident CSF leakage or patent brain avulsion through the scalp wound; surgical exploration was performed and confirmative in all equivocal cases. With the exception of three children who were moribund at admission, all cases were surgically treated, most of them (63%) 12 hours or more after trauma. In spite of these delays and frequent gross septic contamination of the wound, it must be stressed that post-traumatic brain abcess or meningitis was not seen postoperatively. All patients received large doses of antibiotics (5, 17). The final results in this group of craniocerebral injuries with dural laceration are encouraging: 43 recoveries, 9 sequelae (*no* epilepsy), 9 deaths, among them 6 patients deeply comatose at admission.

3. Post-Traumatic Intracranial Hematomas

Epidural hematoma happens to be in our experience a very rare and murderous lesion, although a considerable amount of literature has been devoted to the subject (6, 13, 19, 20, 21, 25, 34).

- 26 cases only have been identified with 6 deaths and only 20 recoveries.

- 20 of them had a history of typical lucid interval after trauma: this represents less than one-third of the 65 authentic lucid intervals collected among the 625 cases.

- 25 cases out of 26 had a patent skull fracture and 14 of them had unilateral ipsilateral mydriasis.

- 24 patients were comatose at the time of operation.

No case of posterior fossa hematoma was identified angiographically in the operating room or at autopsy.

Acute subdural hydroma is apparently a very rare and not well known intracranial post-traumatic lesion. Twelve cases of this acute collection of clear fluid sometimes mixed with a very small quantity of blood have been seen in our series. The hydroma is often located under a depressed fracture, sometimes associated with minor and superficial brain contusion. The clinical picture is very similar to the epidural hematoma except that severe deterioration of the neurological condition is a matter of days and not hours. A simple burr hole, if not too late, may save the child's life (six recoveries only).

4. Cerebral Contusion

This particular type of severe head injury is neither easily defined nor accurately described in research literature. In our series it represents a very homogenous group of 127 children who sustained very violent cranial impacts due to traffic accidents in 78% of the cases. They were comatose immediately or soon after the accident (87%) and had post-traumatic hemiplegia or hemiparesis (61%) less frequently, general seizures (21%) and skull fractures in only 27% of the cases. EEG was performed in 78 cases and demonstrated very often well limited and focalized abnormalities. Angiography when performed (48 cases) ruled out the presence of patent epidural or subdural collection and demonstrated the classical picture of uni- or bilateral temporo-frontal contusion.

The pathological findings are very similar to those observed in the adult; but in children superficial hemorrhagic cortical contusions seem to be more often located on the side of impact; as shown by COURVILLE (7).

Because of the unpredictable evolution of cerebral post-traumatic edema, especially in children (26, 34), the neurological condition of these patients may deteriorate rapidly, sometimes dramatically with rapid onset of decerebrate rigidity and other brain stem signs of herniation (22, 27, 28).

Subsequently, the prognosis of these brain contusions, thus defined clinically and angiographically, is very severe: only 46 children (36%) recovered completely and 14 died.

It is the authors very firm belief that conservative measures, particularly those designed to control brain edema and to assure a satisfactory airway are of paramount importance in the treatment of cerebral contusion in children. Surgical excision of the contused brain is rarely indicated or justified (25, 26, 34); 7 attempts of that type to resect the swollen and hemorrhagic temporal tip cannot be considered as rewarding from our experience.

V. Traumatic Extracranial Lesions

In the present series of 625 children with head injuries, 77 patients (12%) sustained traumatic associated extracranial lesions; this proportion is very close to those published in other series (4, 13, 24).

Of the fractures, 50% were of the limbs (38 cases): clavicle and femoral shaft were most frequently concerned.

Visceral lesions - either thoracic or abdominal - were uncommon (18 cases).

It is noteworthy to insist upon the fact that among these 77 patients with associated lesions:

- 18 of them sustained very minor head injuries and could, even should have been kept in a general surgical ward and not transferred to a neurosurgical department.

- 59 must be considered as severe or very severe head injuries.

33 of these 77 patients were found in deep state of shock at admission: ten of them died. Hypovolemic shock is said to be uncommon in isolated head injuries (34); in the present series, 3 patients only who were admitted in state of shock were classified as pure head injuries: one suffered a severe blood loss from a scalp laceration not promptly sutured; another one was an infant with a huge epidural hematoma; the third patient bled to death from an enormous craniocerebral wound. As pointed out by HENDRICK and co-workers, it appears evident through our experience as well, that in children sustaining head injuries, if shock is present, the cause is extracranial.

As to the orthopaedic sequelae: 8 patients with their fractures properly treated before admission in neurosurgery recovered completely;
conversely 13 severe sequelae are present in 21 patients with limb
fractures treated lately.

VI. Prognosis

It is of course difficult to evaluate the prognosis of a definite
head injury in the emergency ward when the child is admitted. Nevertheless a few guidelines may be drawn from our experience:

The presence of a skull fracture has no prognostic significance at
all as pointed out by many authors (13, 29, 33).

Table 4 shows that the clinical results in terms of deaths, sequelaes
and recoveries are almost identical in the fracture group and the
patient-group with no evident skull fracture.

Table 4. Prognosis of head injuries in children

Cases	Recovery	Sequelae	Died	Unknown
1. Skull Fracture				
No fracture	60%	10%	8%	22%
Fracture + unknown	60%	11%	12%	17%
2. Consciousness				
Normal or drowsy	72%	4,5%	1,5%	22%
Coma	39%	19%	28%	14%
Coma + fracture	36%	22%	31%	

The level of consciousness noted at admission is the most solid and
faithful element of an early prognosis.

Table 4 demonstrates that the results are far better, even excellent,
when the child is alert or simply drowsy when coming to the neurosurgical ward; initial coma means death or severe sequelae in 47% of
the cases. This is particularly true when initial coma is associated
with decerebrate rigidity: of the 50 patients in the series who were
comatose and decerebrated at admission or within 2 hours, only five
recovered completely; 24 children died and 21 have very severe sequelae making them neurological catastrophies in half of the cases.

Early post-traumatic *hemiplegia or hemiparesis* do not have in our experience any prognostic significance *per se*; of the 129 children with
severe or mild deficit after trauma, 108 survived and 65% of them
recovered completely.

Immediate post-traumatic *epileptic seizures* in children do not necessarily imply a bad prognosis at all: 35 children out of 39 with early
seizures may be classified as full recoveries.

In Conclusion

The careful clinical evaluation of the state of consciousness at admission, and later, is of paramount importance after head trauma in children.

As stressed by HENDRICK and co-workers (24) the decreasing level of consciousness was in their experience, as in ours, the single most important sign of diagnostic and prognostic value.

VII. Neurological Sequelae

Of the 625 children studied: 78 died (12%), 59% recovered completely and 62 cases only had *sequelae* listed in Table 5.

Table 5. 111 sequelae for 65 patients

Psychological problem	51
Hemiparesis, hemiplegia	23
Dyskinesia	18
Visual loss	10
Post-concussional syndrome	6
Epilepsy	3

The rarity of *post-concussional syndrome* in children deserves no comments; (1, 18 bis) post-traumatic neurological deficits are also uncommon.

Our attention has been drawn by 18 cases of post-traumatic *dyskinesia*, sometimes of the cerebellar type, which became evident, as a rule, several months after severe head injuries with initial coma and brain stem symptomatology (2).

The frequency of *post-traumatic epilepsy* has been the subject of many controversial publications (14, 18, 19, 23, 25, 35).

430 patients in the present series have been checked regularly, clinically and by repeated EEG; furthermore, 50% of the families answered a detailed questionnaire; the results of this careful follow-up study are surprising:

- 39 patients had immediate post-traumatic seizures but none of them developed late post-traumatic epilepsy.

- 3 cases only of authentic post-traumatic epilepsy could be found in the 547 survivors of the series studied.

- Out of 215 severe head injuries which could be thoroughly followed, only 29 children have persisting *non*-epileptic EEG abnormalities.

- 134 survivors of head injuries classified as *severe* cases who were admitted in our service between 1967 and 1971 have *not* received any anti-epileptic drug for the past three years and yet have never had a single seizure since.

The present study confirms a well known fact of daily pediatric neurosurgical practice: namely, that in children, even after severe head injuries, systematical and prolonged anti-epileptic treatment and repeated EEG controls are unjustified if not totally useless.

As to the exact frequency of late post-traumatic epilepsy, it is of course necessary to wait a few more years for the cases here reviewed. Nevertheless, as many authors consider that at least 80% of the traumatic epilepsies do appear in the course of the 2 years following trauma, it is fair and logical to assume after others (25, 34) that the frequency of post-traumatic epilepsy in children *is very low*, the risk being apparently well below 2% of the cases.

Conclusion

It seems reasonable and necessary to insist upon two concluding remarks:

- In order to obtain a better knowledge and management of head injuries in children there is still apparently an important need for well coordinated studies on a great number of patients including an extensive follow-up.

- These studies must be focused on *prevention* (30, 31), for accidental mortality and morbidity in children, especially those due to head injuries are at the present time a true challenge if not the most important one to preventive medicine.

REFERENCES

1. ARBUS, L, MORON, P., LAZORTHES, Y., LUXEY, Cl.: Séquelles neuropsychiques des traumatismes crâniens de l'enfant. Neuro-Chir. 15, 27-34 (1969).

2. ARNOULD, G., LEPOIRE, J., TRIDON, P., LAXENAIRE, M., MONTAUT, J., RENARD, M.: Dyskinésies volitionnelles d'attitude. Séquelles de traumatismes graves du tronc cérébral chez l'enfant (à propos de 10 observation Revue Neurologique T 114) 1966.

3. BAUMANN, von W., EMMRICH, P., VOTH, D.: Diagnostische und therapeutische Probleme des schweren kindlichen Schädel-Hirn-Traumas mit Bewusstlosigkeit. Z. Klin. Päd. 70, 60-63 (1973).

4. BERNEY, J.: Head trauma in childhood. Post graduate course in Neurotraumatology, Brussels. September 1974.

5. CHODKIEWICZ, J.P., REDONDO, A., TERRAZAS, F., CIOLOKA, C.: Cranio cerebral wounds in children (follow-up study of 86 cases). Joint Meeting of the German and French Neurosurgical Societies. Agadir, March 1974.

6. CHOUX, M., GRISOLI, F., BAURAND, C., VIGOUROUX, R.P.: Les hématomes extra-duraux traumatiques de l'enfant. Neuro-Chir. 19, 183-197 (1973).

7. COURVILLE, C.G.: Contrecoup injuries of the Brain in Infancy. Arch. Surg. 90, 157-165 (1965).

8. CRAFT, A.W., SHAW, D.A., CARTLIDGE, N.E.D.: Head injuries in children. Brit. Med. J. 4, 200-203 (1972).

9. CREISSARD, P., CHODKIEWICZ, J.P., THEBAULT, A.M.: A propos de cent cas de traumatisme crânio-cérébral chez le nourrisson. Neurochirurgie 14, 759-772 (1968).

10. GROS, G., BALDY-MOLINIER, M., GROS-MASSOUBRE, A., MASQUEFA, C.: L'avenir éloigné des comas traumatiques de l'enfant. Neurochir. 15, 35-50 (1969).

11. HAFFTER, C.: Zur Begutachtung traumatischer Hirnschädigungen im Kindersalter. Ann. Paediat. 199, 134-140 (1962).

12. HARWOOD-NASH, D.C., HENDRICK, E.G., HUDSON, A.R.: The significance of skull fractures in children. Radiology 101, 151-155 (1971).

13. HENDRICK, E.G., HARWOOD-NASH, D.C., HUDSON, A.R.: Head injuries in children: a survey of 4465 consecutive cases at the Hospital for Sick Children (Toronto). Clinical Neuro-Surgery 11-76 (1963).

14. HJERN, B.O., NYLANDER-INGVAR: Acute head injuries in children. Acta Paediatrica 152, 1-37 (1964).

15. JACOBI, von G., KOCH, H., EMRICH, R., RITZ, A.: Neuro-Pädiatrische und Neuro-Radiologische Befunde beim schweren Schädel-Hirn-Trauma des Säuglings und jungen Kleinkindes. Z. Klin. Päd. 70, 63-66 (1973).

16. KASOFF, S.S., ZINGESSER, L.H., SHULMAN, K.: Compartmental abnormalities of regional cerebral blood flow in children with head trauma. J. Neurosurgery 36 (1972).

17. KISELEV, V.P.: Problems concerned with the clinical picture and surgical treatment of open cerebro-cranial injuries in childhood. Surgery (Moscow) 7, 105-110 (1965).

18. KLNOFF, H.: Head injuries in children: predisposing factors, accident conditions, accident proneness and sequelae. Amer. J. Public Health 12, 2405-2417 (1971).

18X. KOUPERNIK, C.: Problèmes posés par l'expertise psychiatrique d'un enfant victime d'un traumatisme crânien. Ann. Med. Leg. 42, 38-46 (1962).

19. LAPRAS, C., DECHAUME, J.P.: Traumatismes crâniens chez le nourrisson et l'enfant. Bull. Med. Leg. et toxicol. 17, 31-42 (1974).

20. LAZORTHES, Y., VANHONG, N., LAZORTHES, G.: Les aggravations secondaires précoces survenant après les traumatismes crânio-cérébraux de l'enfant. A propos de 1193 cas. Neurochirurgie (Paris) 15, 19-26 (1969).

21. LE BEAU, J., CORCOS, A., CHODKIEWICZ, J.P.: Sur la gravité de l'hématome extra-dural traumatique. Bulletin de l'Académie Nationale de Médecine 158, 62-70.

22. LENARD, H.G.: EEG - Veränderungen bei frischen Schädeltraumen im Kindersalter. Münch/med. Wochschr. 107, 1820-1827 (1965).

23. LERIQUE-KOECHLIN, TEYSSONNIERE de GRAMONT: Etude électro-encéphalographique des traumatismes crâniens de l'enfant. Arch. Française de Pédiâtrie 15, 87-93 (1958).

24. PELLERIN, D., RIGAULT, P., N. FETE Cl. et al.: Aspects chirurgicaux des accidents de l'enfant. 13433 cas. Revue de Pédiâtrie 7, 403-416 (1971).

25. MEALEY, J.: Pediatric head injuries. Springfield/Ill.: Charles C. Thomas 1968.

26. PENZHOLZ, H.: Die Schädelhirnverletzung im Kindesalter. Langenbecks Arch. Chir. 332, 651-658 (1972).

27. PHELINE, C.: Les états aigus de souffrance du tronc cérébral chez l'enfant. Etude clinique et thérapeutique. A propos de 12 cas de traumatismes crâniens graves. Pédiâtrie 13 (1958).

28. ROBERTSON, R.C.L., POLLARD, C.J.R.: Decerebrate state in children and adolescents. J. Neurosurg. 12, 13-17 (1955).

29. ROBERTS, F., CHASE-SHOPFNER: Plain skull roentgenograms in children with head trauma. Amer. J. Roentgenology 114 (1972).

30. ROOS, W.: Ursachen und Häufigkeit des Schädelhirntraumas im Kindesalter. Der Nervenarzt 41, 178-181 (1970).

31. SANDELS, S.: Why are children injured in traffic? Can we prevent child accidents in traffic? Skandia Rep. II, June 1974, 1-87, Förlagstjänst, Skandia - S 103-60 Stockholm.

32. SCHIEFER, W.: Das Schädel-Hirntraume beim Kind. Münch.Med.Wschr. 15, 557-561 (1971).

33. SHILLITO, J.: Head Injuries. Ambulatory Pediatrics 837-842 (1968).

34. SHULMAN, K.: Head Injuries in infants and children. In: Injuries of the Brain and Spinal Cord (ed. M. Brock et al.). pp. 503-528. Berlin-Heidelberg-New York: Springer 1974.

35. TISCHER, von W., RICHTER, H., RIEGER, C.: Zur Therapie der Schädelhirnverletzungen im Kindesalter. Zbl. Chr. 98, 156-161 (1973).

Cerebral Artery Occlusion Due to Trauma

I. Schöter

Since inauguration of the "Four-Vessel-Angiography" in 1962 we have observed 207 patients with an occlusion of one of the cerebral arteries and among them 13 patients by whom the occlusion was preceded by a trauma.

The age of the patients ranges from 2 to 73 years.

In 7 cases the arterial occlusion is considered without doubt a consequence of a trauma to the head or to the neck:

5 patients suffered from severe closed head injuries and 2 children tolerated "pencil injuries" (one was injured by a wooden spoon in the region of the right tonsil and the other by a sharp stone in the carotid region of the neck).

One patient tolerated a severe trauma to the whole body with rupture of lien and kidney which probably led to an embolic obstruction.

In 5 other cases a minor trauma preceded the occlusion: 3 children fell on their heads while playing, one girl - and this case is perhaps dubious - while skipping developed a bad headache and lost consciousness, and one patient was hurt by a garage door.

The interval between trauma and the onset of neurological symptoms was less than 24 hours in 7 cases (4 serious and 3 minor injuries), 2 or 3 days in 3 cases (both pencil injuries and the garage door accident), 7 days by one girl who fell while playing, 16 days by one patient who was unconscious for 3 days after a motor car accident, and 7 weeks by the patient who was felt to have had an embolic occlusion.

In 7 cases the internal carotid artery was occluded in its extracranial region; 3 patients suffered from an occlusion of the middle cerebral artery. The supraclinoidal carotid artery was occluded in only one case as were the anterior and posterior cerebral artery.

The mechanism of injury is of great interest. Direct trauma to the vessel wall will probably lead to an intimal tear with following thrombosis or to a subintimal dissection.

Many authors postulate theories concerning other mechanisms. For the most part they presume an overstretching of vessels to be the cause of an intima lesion for instance by hyperextension of the neck (7, 9), especially if the common carotid artery is fixed by bruising the anterior chest wall (4, 5). Others are of the opinion that sudden stretching of the carotid artery over the transverse process of the third cervical vertebra may lead to the lesion (2, 11) or the compression of the internal carotid artery by the transverse process of the first cervical vertebra (1).

FÖDISCH considers an increase of intra-arterial pressure or extra-vasal low pressure to be the cause of intimal damage.

Other authors (4, 8, 10, 12) emphasize the importance of post-traumatic spasm which later can conceivably result in thrombosis.

Genuine vascular anomalies, as for example hypoplasy or pre-existent alterations such as arteriosclerosis may be a contributing factor to this type of arterial occlusion as well as to hypercoagulation.

The intensity of trauma seems to be non-important (3, 10).

Next to the mechanism of injury the modus of obstruction is of great interest.

Two of our patients died; only one autopsy was performed: it revealed a supraclinoidal thrombosis of the carotid artery. In one case the operative revision of the occluded extracranial carotid artery showed an extrvasal and an intramural hematoma.

Once the obstruction had to be considered embolic, as the interval between trauma and onset of neurological symptoms lasted for 7 weeks.

In one patient the occlusion must have been caused by spasm, since the first angiogram showed an extreme stenosis of the supraclinoidal carotid artery and of the proximal anterior and middle cerebral arteries with a blockade of contrast in the Sylvian group. The control angiogram after two weeks was normal.

In all other cases the occlusion persisted angiographically for months and even years.

The prognosis of this disease depends on the collateral blood supply, i.e. on the oxygenation of brain tissue.

Even today we have no possibility to decide whether the lack of blood supply is cellulucidal or whether it simply causes an arrest of cell-function. Visualization of collateral blood flow by contrast is not sufficient, for the angiography seems to be too crude a method to demonstrate the fine terminal vessels (6).

In one of our cases we have angiographically observed a complete collateral circulation very soon after the traumatic occlusion and yet a paresis persists.

In another patient who recovered completely we see no collateral supply.

Thus we have to judge our therapy by its clinical success. Conservative therapy (digitalization, application of pharmaca to improve cerebral oxygenation and glucose metabolism, to combat brain edema and reduce hypercoagulation) has proved to be insufficient in many cases.

For many years the hyperbaric oxygenation therapy has improved the non-surgical treatment.

Four of 11 surviving patients recovered completely. In 7 cases a paresis persisted; one patients had fits.

Desobliteration of obstructed vessels and the performing of extra-intracranial arterial by-passes are the present microsurgical operations to preserve tissue function.

Summary

In 13 cases cerebral artery occlusion was preceded by a trauma: 5 severe closed head injuries, 2 pencil injuries, one trauma to the whole body and 5 minor injuries.

In 7 cases the extracranial carotid artery was obstructed, 6 times other cerebral vessels.

Four patients recovered completely, 2 died, in 7 cases pareses persisted.

Mechanism and intensity of injury and modus of obstruction are discussed. The prognosis depends on the oxygenation of brain tissue trough collateral supply.

Table. Intensity of trauma, localization of occlusion, age and sex of the patients

	DEXTRA				SINISTRA		
EXTRACRAN.	♀ 2 J ⊘	♂ 4 J ○	♂ 35 J ⊗ †	♀ 50 J ⊗	♂ 7 J ⊘	♂ 39 J ⊗	♂ 62 J ○
CAROTIS INT. SUPRACLIN					♂ 73 J ⊗ †		
MEDIA					♀ 7 J ○⊕	♂ 16 J ⊗⊕	♂ 30 J ⊙
ANTERIOR					♀ 11 J ○⊕		
POSTERIOR					♂ 11 J ○⊕		

○ MINOR INJURY ⊙ BODY TRAUMA
⊘ PENCIL INJURY ⊕ RESTITUTION
⊗ SEVERE TRAUMA † EXITUS

REFERENCES

1. BOLDERY, E., MAASS, L., MILLER, E.: The role of atlantoid compression in the etiology of internal carotid thrombosis. J. Neurosurg. 13, 127 (1956).

2. CLARKE, P.R.R., DICKSON, J., SMITH, B.J.: Traumatic thrombosis of the internal carotid artery following a non-penetrating injury and leading to infarction of brain. Brit. J. Surg. 43, 215 (1955).

3. FÖDISCH, H.J.: Hals- und Hirnschlagaderthrombose bei Kindern nach stumpfem Trauma. Pädiat. u. Pädol. 4, 270 (1968).

4. FRANTZEN, E., JACOBSEN, H.H., THERKELSEN, J.: Cerebral artery occlusion in children due to trauma to the head and neck. J.Neurology 11, 695 (1961).

5. GLEAVE, J.R.W.: Thrombosis of the carotid artery in the neck in association with head injury. Proc. Third Int. Congr. Ser. 110, 200, Amsterdam 1966.

6. HIGAZI, I.: Post-traumatic carotid thrombosis. J. Neurosurg. 20, 354 (1963).

7. HOCKADAY, T.D.R.: Traumatic thrombosis of the internal carotid artery. J. Neurol. Neurosurg. Psychiat. 22, 229 (1959).

8. HUBER, P.: Posttraumatische Kaliberschwankungen der Hirngefäße im Angiogramm. Fortschr. Röntgenstr. 98, 292 (1963).

9. MURRAY, D.S.: Post-traumatic thrombosis of the internal carotid artery and vertebral arteries after non-penetrating injuries to the neck. Brit. J. Surg. 44, 425 (1948).

10. OLAFSON, R.A., CHRISTOFERSON, L.A.: The syndrome of carotid occlusion following minor craniocerebral trauma. J. Neurosurg. 33, 636 (1970).

11. RANEY, A.A.: Cerebral embolism following minor wounds of the carotid arteries. Arch. Neurol. u. Psychiat. 60, 425 (1948).

12. YASHON, D., JOHNSON, A.B., JANE, A.J.: Bilateral internal carotid artery occlusion secondary to closed head injuries. J. Neurol. Neurosurg. Psychiat. 27, 547 (1964).

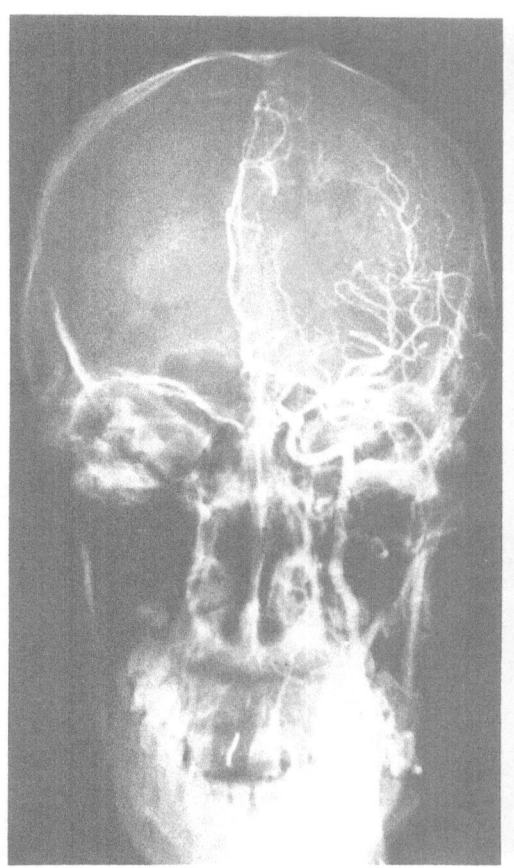 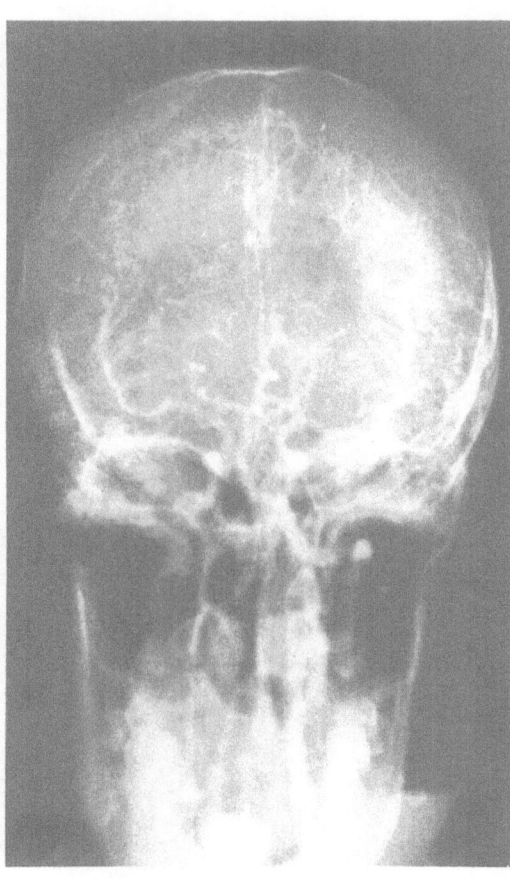

Fig. 1 a. Arterial occlusion
due to spasm

b. The same patient two weeks later

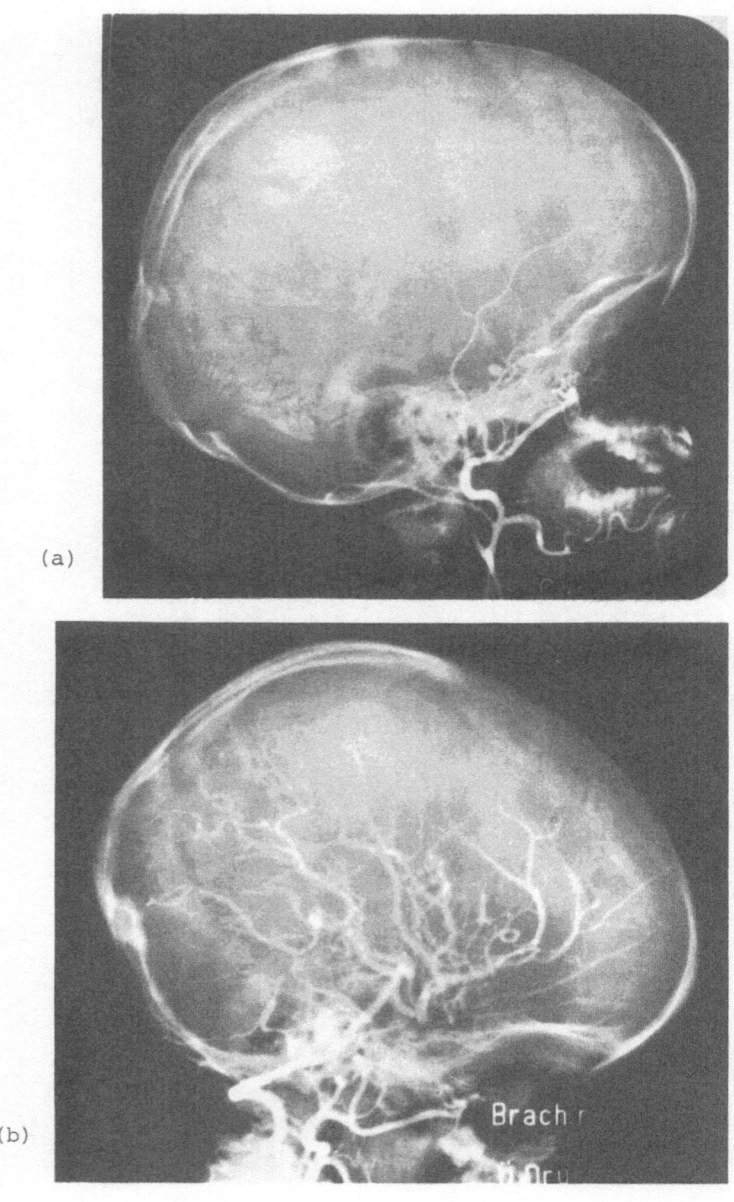

(a)

(b)

Fig. 2 a. Occlusion of the extracranial carotid artery

Fig. 2 b. Complete collateral circulation in the main arteries

Fig. 3. Occlusion of the left posterior cerebral artery, no visible collateral circulation

Right: Left brachial arteriography

Lower: Left carotid arteriography

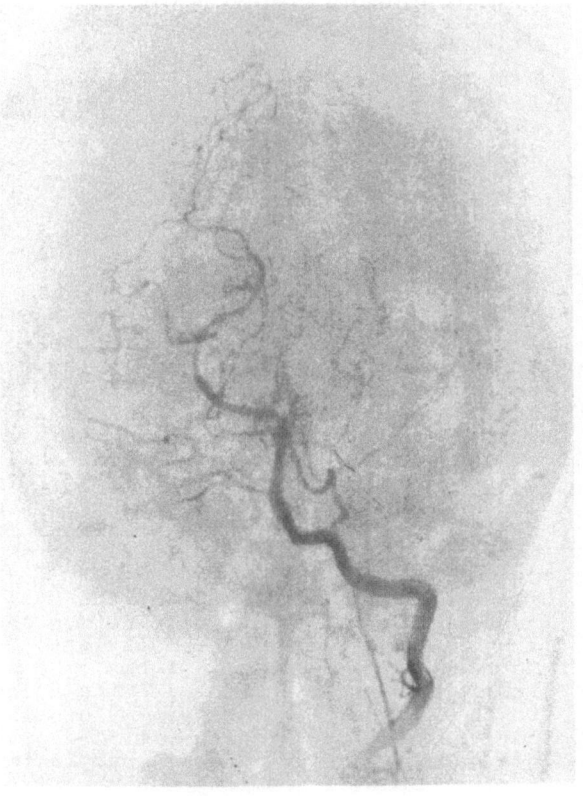

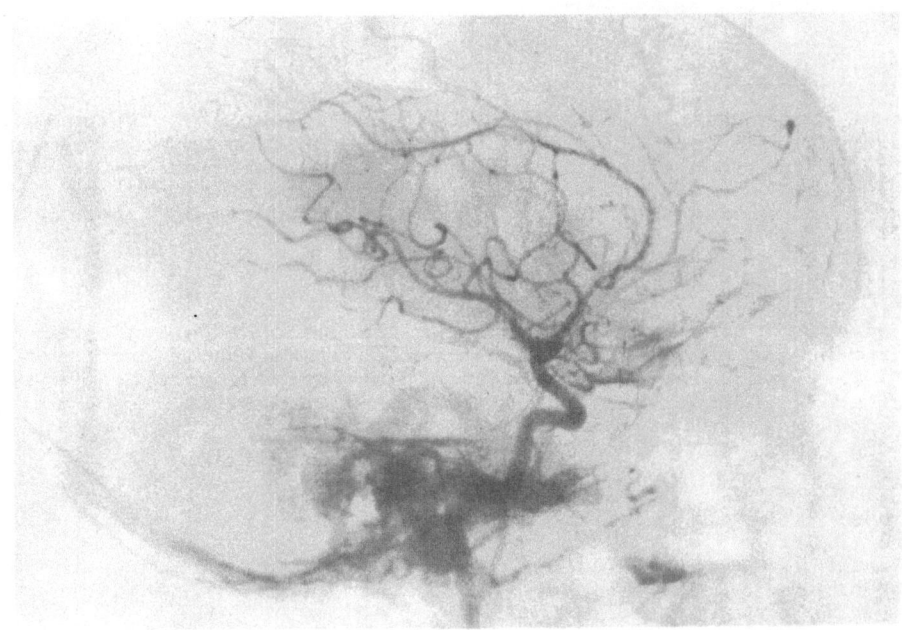

Concentrations of Glycogen, Glucose, Lactate, and Amino Acids in Brain Tumors*

F. WEINHARDT, S. HOYER, H. BERLET, and J. HAMER**

In general, the metabolism of brain tumors has been receiving lesser attention by investigators than that of tumors of non-nervous tissue. Brain tumors were found to display a decreased oxygen consumption and an increased lactate production as BRIERLEY and McILWAIN showed in in-vitro experiments (3). DITTMAN and co-workers found an aerobic glycolysis in both benign and malignant brain tumors and a decrease of the ratio of respiration to aerobic glycolysis in tumors with progressive malignancy (4, 5). Similar findings were reported by KIRSCH and MAHALEY (8, 9). To the contrary, DOHR et al. found that the concentrations of lactate in brain tumors and in normal brain tissue were not significantly different from each other (6).

These findings might support the hypothesis that glycolysis is not necessarily different in cancerous and normal tissue. The prospective aim of this study is to investigate the energy metabolism related to anaerobic glycolysis of benign and malignant tumors and concentrations of free and total amino acids which reflect important metabolic and synthetic activities of tissue. In the following, preliminary results of this study will be presented including values of glycogen, glucose, pyruvate and lactate and of total amino acids in tissue obtained from the central portion of brain tumors and from adjacent perifocal tissue.

Material and Methods

Tissue specimens of 6 meningiomas and 5 malignant tumors including 3 astrocytomas stage II-III and one isomorphic ependymoma and one oligodendroglioma each (2) and, if possible, specimens of adjacent tissue were obtained during brain surgery for the removal of the tumors and frozen at once in liquid N_2 within 2 to 7 s (mean 4 s).

Analytical Methods

Specimens of deep frozen tissue were freed from adhering blood under liquid N_2 and homogenized and extracted with ethanol/perchloric acid (1). The supernatants were analyzed by standard enzyme assays as described (2). The extracted pellets were dissolved in 5N KOH (10) and glycogen was assayed enzymatically following the enzymatic cleavage of the homoglucan polymer (7).

*The studies were supported by grants of the German Research Foundation (DFG).
**We are indebted to Prof. Dr. G. ULE, Institute of Neuropathology of the University, for the neuro-histopathological evaluation.

For the analysis of total amino acids by gas chromatography according to standard methods small pieces of tissue were allowed to thaw, gently washed free of blood in physiological saline and immediately freeze-dried. Thus, average amounts of 12 mg of dry tissue were obtained and hydrolysed in 2 ml 6N HCl in sealed glass vials heated to 150°C for 12 hours. One ml of the hydrolysate was taken to dryness, dissolved in 5 ml of N-butanol-HCl and sonicated for 1 min. The sample was then heated to 150°C for 1 h in an oil bath. N-butanol-HCl was evaporated at 60°C and 0,5 ml of CH_2Cl_2 and 2 drops of TFAA were added. The mixture was briefly sonicated and heated to 150°C for 30 min in sealed glass vials, yielding the amino acid derivatives. Then the samples were ready for the gas chromatographic analysis (Hewlett-Packard gas chromatograph Nr. 7620A).

Results and Comments

The concentrations of some compounds associated with glycolysis are individually represented in Fig. 1. Glucose levels of meningiomas were similar to those of adjacent brain tissue except for one value, which was as high as 16 μmoles/g wet weight. In contrast, malignant tumors, especially three cases of astrocytoma, stage II-III, exhibited lower glucose values. Accordingly, the values of glycogen also tended to be higher in meningiomas (maximum level found 30,6 μmoles/g wet weight) than the malignant tumors. Still, the levels of lactate did not differ in the two groups.

By analyzing perifocal tissue separately an attempt was made to distinguish tumor tissue from tissue which might be considered to be normal or close to normal. In fact, the majority of lactate values of adjacent tissue appears to be definitely lower than in tissue of the tumors proper. There is one exception, however, which was apparently due to marked edema of the specimen. As to glucose and glycogen the differences between focal and perifocal tissue were, if any, less clear-cut.

Values of pyruvate do not reflect a particular pattern due to the small number of analyses available at present for the evaluation.

The concentrations of free and protein-derived amino acids did not vary uniformly in meningiomas, in which low and high concentrations of amino acids were found (Fig. 2). However, in malignant astrocytomas the content of amino acids was markedly lower than in benign gliomas, in which the amino acid concentration was markedly high.

The data including measurements of the concentrations of glycogen, glucose, lactate and pyruvate suggest that in benign brain tumors the energy reserves including glycogen and glucose accumulate, in contrast to gliomas in which the concentrations are diminished.

We found increased concentrations of lactate in both types of brain tumors, that perhaps points to an increased glycolytic flux. Our preliminary data on total AA are considered to indicate a disturbance in nucleic acid metabolism in malignant astrocytomas.

REFERENCES

1. BERLET, H.H.: Comparative study of various methods for the extraction of free creatine and phosphocreatine from mouse skeletal muscle. Anal. Biochem. 60, 347-357 (1974).

2. BERLET, H.H.: Cerebral metabolic rates as determinants of hypoxic survival of adult mice. Advanc. Neurosurg (In Press).

3. BRIERLEY, J.B., McILWAIN: Metabolic properties of cerebral tissues modified by neoplasia and by freezing. J. Neurochem. 1, 109-118 (1956).

4. DITTMAN, J., HERRMANN, H.D., LOEW, F., PALLESKE, H.: Über Atmung und Glukolyse menschlicher Hirntumoren in vitro. Zbl. Neurochir. 30, 119-127 (1969).

5. DITTMANN, J., HERRMANN, H.D., PALLESKE, H.: Normalisierung des Glukosestoffwechsels von Hirntumor-Schnitten durch Hyperosid. Arzneimittel-Forsch. 21, 1999-2003 (1971).

6. DOHR, H., HEUSSEN, B., SCHEITHAUER-HOFFMAN, E., SIMMERT, A.: Lactat in Hirntumoren. Acta Neurochir. 22, 79-84 (1970).

7. KEPPLER, D., DECKER, K.: Glykogen. Bestimmung mit Amyloglucosidase. In: Methoden der enzymatischen Analyse (ed. H.U. BERGMEYER), 3rd ed., p. 1171. Weinheim: Verlag Chemie 1974.

8. KIRSCH, W.M.: Substrates of glycolysis in intracranial tumors during complete ischemia. Cancer Res. 25, 432-439 (1965).

9. MAHALEY, M.S., Jr.: The in vitro respiration of normal brain and brain tumors. Cancer Res. 26, 195-197 (1966).

10. PASSONEAU, J.V., GATFIELD, P.D., SCHULTZ, D.W., LOWRY, O.H.: An enzymic method for measurement of glycogen. Anal. Biochem. 19, 315-326 (1967).

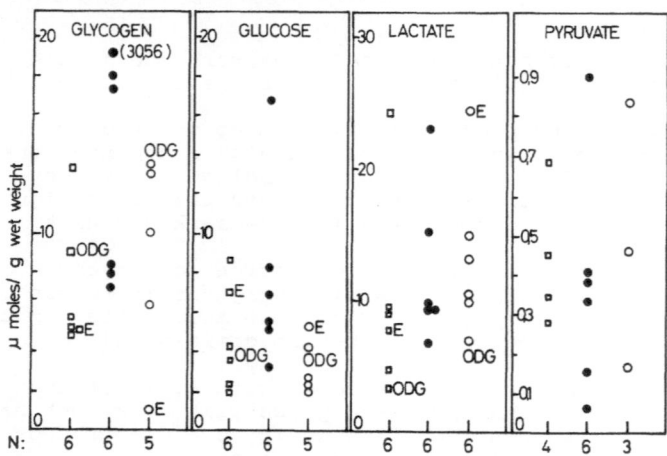

Fig. 1. Concentrations of glycogen, glucose, lactate and pyruvate in brain tumors and adjacent tissue. ODG = oligodendroglioma, E = ependymoma

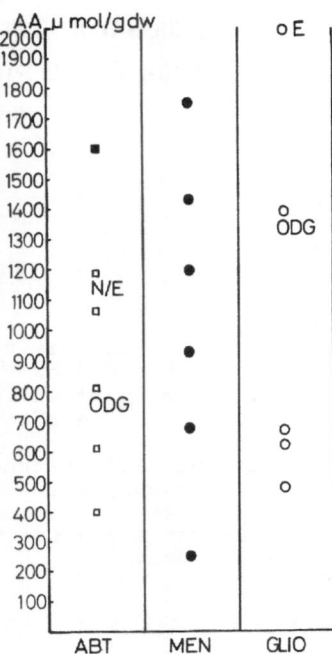

■ EDEMA

Concentrations of total amino acids(AA)
in meningiomas(MEN), gliomas (GLIO)
and adjacent brain tissue (ABT)

Fig. 2. Concentrations of total amino acids in brain tumors and adjacent tissue. ODG = oligodendroglioma, E = ependymoma, N = normal tissue without edema

CBF-Studies from Three Sides in Patients With Intracranial Tumors

A. HARTMANN, E. ALBERTI, D. LANGE, and N. T. MATHEW

The purpose of this study was to evaluate the usefulness of regional cerebral blood flow studies in patients with intracerebral tumours. Brain tumours often form a new blood circulatory system and hence influence the cerebral circulation.

Since the half thickness of the tracer Xenon 133 (Xe 133) is rather small, we suggested that the influence of the tumour tissue on the regional Xe 133 washout curve varies with the localization of the neoplasmatic tissue. Therefore we measured cerebral blood flow from three sides.

Method

21 patients with intracranial tumours form the case material of this study. Diagnosis was achieved by clinical evaluation, angiography, pneumoencephalography, and intravenous 99m-Technetium (99m Tc) scintigraphy. Tables 1 and 2 indicate patients whose diagnosis was proven by biopsy or autopsy.

In 16 patients diagnosis was glioblastoma multiforme, in 4 meningioma and in 1 metastatic adenocarcinoma.

Regional cerebral blood flow (rCBF) was calculated by stochastic method from 12.5 minute washout curve. 4-6 mCi Xe 133 in 1 ml normal saline was injected as a bolus into the internal carotid artery of the involved hemisphere. For that purpose the internal carotid artery was directly punctured after local anesthesia with a 19-gauge Cournaund needle.

Regional cerebral blood transit time (rCBTT) was calculated after injection of 2-4 mCi 99m Tc in a 1 ml bolus into the same artery by taking the full-width-half-maximum of the dilution curve.

16-52 square regions of interest (ROI) were selected from the oscilloscopic display of the hemisphere on the screen of the gamma camera. This camera with a high-sensitivity collimator was connected to a Hewlett-Packard computer for calculation of acquired data.

Size and shape of the tumour was exactly determined by comparing the Xe 133- or 99m Tc-display with the usual intravenous scintigram.

The collimator of the gamma camera was located over the lateral aspect of the skull parallel to the sagittal sinus for $rCBF_{lateral(l)}$ and $rCBTT_1$. For recording the slopes of $rCBF_{vertical(v)}$ and $rCBTT_v$ it was positioned over the vertex parallel to the base of the skull. For estimation of $rCBF_{anterior-posterior(ap)}$ and $rCBTT_{ap}$ it was positioned in ap-direction.

Table 1. Hemispheric CBF from three sides. Except in 5 cases $rCBF_l$ is higher than $rCBF_v$. In 4 out of 15 cases $rCBF_{ap}$ is higher than $rCBF_l$. $rCBF_l$ in patients who were pretreated with Dexamethasone or hyperosmolar solutions hemispheric $rCBF_l$ was often higher than in non-treated patients

rCBF from three sides in patients with intracranial tumours

Patient	Diagnosis	Mean rCBF (ml/100g·min)			
		Lateral	Vertical	A.-P.	
U.B.	metastatic adeno-CA.	38.2 S	30.7 D	37.8 S	
J.W.	G.M.[a]	46.2 D	37.9 S	44.2 D	
F.R.	G.M.[a]	42.3 S	50.2 S	44.1 D	b
E.D.	G.M.[a]	46.7 S	52.8 S	46.5 D	b
A.M.	G.M.	33.6 S	22.0 D	28.9 D	
E.S.	G.M.[a]	36.6 D	37.0 D	37.4 S	
K.F.	G.M.[a]	51.0 D	42.3 S	42.3 S	c
K.P.	G.M.[a]	64.7 S	46.6 D	/	c
A.W.	G.M.[a]	37.8 S	21.2 D	32.6 S	
R.H.	G.M.	48.2 D	44.5 S	41.9 S	
G.G.	G.M.	66.8 S	49.2 D	57.3 S	c
K.S.	G.M.[a]	56.0 S	50.0 D	40.0 S	c
T.J.	G.M.[a]	56.1 D	58.0 S	/	b,c
M.E.	G.M.[a]	40.9 S	43.4 S	42.2 S	b
M.C.	G.M.	70.8 D	79.8 S	79.6 S	b,c
H.S.	G.M.[a]	56.0 S	40.0 D	50.0 D	c
A.S.	G.M.	40.9 D	36.4 D	44.1 D	
mean value		49.0	43.6	44.6	
S.D.		11.3	13.7	11.8	

G.M.: glioblastoma multiforme.
[a]Diagnosis by biopsy/autopsy.
[b]$rCBF_v$ higher than $rCBF_l$.
[c]Patient pretreated with antiedematous substances.
S/D: tumour is *s*uperficially or *d*eeply located.

At least 15 minutes elapsed from the end of one study to the beginning of the next procedure. Serial blood gas check-ups were made from arterial blood with an ASTRUP blood gas analyzer.

Table 2. Mean cerebral blood transit time in 11 patients. Escept in 3 cases mean $rCBTT_l$ was shorter than $rCBTT_v$. The mean value for the whole group is identical for mean $rCBTT_l$ and mean $rCBTT_{ap}$ but not for $rCBTT_v$

rCBTT from three sides in patients with intracranial tumours

Patient	Diagnosis	Mean rCBTT (seconds)			
		Lateral	Vertical	A.-P.	
U.B.	metastatic adeno-CA.	10.9	12.7	9.8	
J.W.	G.M.[a]	7.5	7.1	6.2	b
E.D.	G.M.[a]	8.4	11.3	8.8	
A.M.	G.M.	6.7	10.8	7.2	
E.S.	G.M.[a]	10.1	5.6	12.4	b
K.F.	G.M.[a]	7.8	11.3	8.6	
K.P.	G.M.[a]	7.0	8.2	7.4	
A.W.	G.M.[a]	9.8	11.2	7.2	
G.G.	G.M.	4.0	3.6	4.2	b
M.E.	G.M.[a]	4.8	6.8	5.2	
M.C.	G.M.	4.2	5.4	4.4	
mean value		7.4	8.7	7.4	
S.D.		2.4	3.0	2.4	

G.M.: glioblastoma multiforme.
[a]Diagnosis by biopsy/autopsy.
[b]$rCBTT_l$ longer than $rCBTT_v$.

Results

In the patients with meningiomas there was no abnormal regional pattern of rCBF or rCBTT. However, in 3 out of these cases the hemispheric CBF was decreased. This group is not listed in the tables of this communication.

The results of the rest of the studied patients were as follows: In all but 5 patients mean $rCBF_l$ was higher than mean $rCBF_v$ (Table 1). In 4 out of 17 patients mean $rCBF_{ap}$ was higher than mean $rCBF_l$. In 14 out of 15 cases $rCBF_l$ was closer to $rCBF_{ap}$ than to $rCBF_v$. The mean value of the total group was almost identical for $rCBF_l$ and $rCBF_{ap}$ but not for $rCBF_v$.

Similar results were achieved on testing $rCBTT_{l,v,ap}$ in 11 patients. The mean value for the total group was identical between $rCBTT_l$ and $rCBTT_{ap}$. The mean value for mean $rCBTT_v$ was longer (Table 2). Comparing the localization of the tumour between intravenous scintigraphy and angiography on one hand and the 3-dimensional rCBF-data on the other hand, we got the following impressions: The closer the tumour is to the collimator (i.e. the more superficially it is in the tissue cylinder of the ROI) the better is the correlation between 2 different rCBF-procedures (Pictures 1 and 2). Table 1 contains remarks whether the tumour is localized close to the surface (S = superficial) or away from the surface (D = deep). The flow data of a parasagittal tumour can be reliably measured from vertical, that of a tumour in the frontal lobe with $rCBF_{ap}$ and that of a temporal lobe tumour most reliably with the collimator in lateral position.

Furthermore we found that the distance of the tumour to the surface has less influence on rCBTT-measurement using 99m Tc than on rCBF-measurement with Xe 133.

Patients with decreased hemispheric CBF presented in most of the cases clinical evidence of elevated intracranial pressure (ICP). Even patients without symptoms of increased ICP showed in ROIs close to the tumour depressed rCBF, which was interpreted as a sign of perifocal edema. rCBTT was in these areas prolonged. Some patients with elevated ICP presented in ROIs far away from the neoplasm normal rCBF and rCBTT.

7 patients were treated prior to the circulation study with Dexamethasone or hyperosmolar solutions. These patients are indicated in Table 1. All of them showed normal or supernormal (due to elevated regional tumour-rCBF) hemispheric CBF.

The regional pattern of the glioblastoma multiforme itself showed in 12 out of 16 patients increased rCBF-values and a shortened rCBTT. After injection of 99m Tc, we detected in 8 patients regional peaks in tumour-ROIs, probably due to arterio-venous shunts. 5 cases presented with double peaks (Picture 3). rCBTT in ROIs with peaks or double peaks is moderately short. 4 patients with glioblastoma multiforme have been treated after the first CBF-procedure for 3 to 7 days with intravenous infusion of 10%-glycerol. After that CBF was repeated. In the second CBF-test hemispheric CBF went up, more in non-tumourous than in tumourous areas.

Discussion

Xe 133 and 99m Tc have a rather small half thickness, but that of 99m Tc is better than that of Xe 133. From this fact it has to be concluded that the reliability of achieved data is low if the point of interest is deep under the skull. The deeper a cylinder is over which the washout curve is recorded, the more uncertain are the calculated data. Particularly in areas of decreased flow, the reliability of the values depends heavily on the distance of the lesion from the tissue surface. So far it has not been established numerically how exactly rCBF-data really are if the lesion (infarct, tumour etc.) is located more superficially or more deeply. Patients with ischemic infarction are not ideal subjects for a study about this problem, since the anatomical point of damage to the cerebral tissue can be hardly determined. If cases with cerebral tumours are taken, the shape and size of the neoplasm can be sufficiently established by angiography and intravenous scintigraphy. The use of a gamma camera for measurement of rCBF and rCBTT has the advantage that the filling of the hemisphere with the tracer can be visualized on the display screen. The picture can be compared with that of the scintigram, which is recorded with the same equipment. The correlation between the tumour localization and the significance of calculated data is, by this procedure, much better than data received with a multi-crystal equipment.

So far a number of papers regarding the problem of rCBF in intracranial tumours have been published (1-6, 9-11); however, none of them pay attention to the depth of the tumour in the ROI-cylinder. In our study we detected that the flow data of the whole tumour (taken as one ROI) of at least 2 different aspects correlate better if the tumour is superficially localized. The character of the circulation within the neoplasm is best studied from that aspect in which the lesion is closest to the surface of the tissue. This point should be true for any lesion which is to be detected by rCBF-measurements using Xe 133. There are 2 reasons which account for the fact that there is a better independence of the achieved rCBTT-data from the depth of the tumour: a) the half thickness of 99m Tc is greater than that of Xenon 133; b) the influence of scattered gamma rays from surrounding tissue is less in 99m Tc than in Xe 133.

However, even if a parasagittal tumour might be best characterized by vertical rCBF, this aspect has certain disadvantages. With this aspect the respiratory system is positioned within the field of view of the collimator. The vascular in- and outflow system (the internal carotid artery and the jugular vein) is secondarily within the recorded field. The flow direction is perpendicular to the counting axis and hence does influence the washout slope. The advantage of this and the ap-view is that both hemispheres can be separated. To a certain extent Xe 133, which is injected into one internal carotid artery, crosses via the Circle of Willis into the vascular system of the non-injected hemisphere (7). Lateral rCBF-procedures cannot separate which radioactivity is coming from the injected and which from the non-injected hemisphere. The ap-view should be applied only if the tumour is localized in the frontal area of the brain. With this view it must be remembered that the cylindric segment under the ROI has a rather long axis, so that the posteriorly located tissue does not have a big influence on the washout curve.

Most of the reports regarding the blood flow in cerebral tumours revealed a depressed CBF for the total hemisphere. We separated in our study patients who were treated prior to the test with Dexamethasone or hyperosmolar solutions, from patients who were not treated. The treated group showed a normal to supernormal hemispheric flow but the non-treated group a decreased hemispheric CBF. The supernormal data are based on high regional values, collected from tumour-ROIs. However, even treated patients presented with perifocal depressed rCBF, which we interpret as a sign of perifocal edema. We agree with others who concluded from their experience that an elevated ICP is able to depress rCBF (4). Our opinion is sustained by the fact that longtime treatment of patients with tumours with intravenous infusion of 10%-glycerol does increase cerebral blood flow. This was described before (9). Glycerol is able to decrease ICP (8). We are aware of the fact that for a final interpretation of the effect of glycerol more thoroughly undertaken studies have to be done. Our series presented here is very small.

The character of the circulation system within the neoplasm is better judged if both flow and transit time are studied. Peaks and double peaks due to arteriovenous shunts can be detected with 99m Tc. Apparently, a rather big percentage of glioblastoma do have av-shunts.

rCBF/rCBTT-procedures using Xe 133 and 99m Tc are not helpful in establishing a diagnosis whether a tumour is present or not. But they may contribute to the knowledge about the vascularization of the neoplasm and the presence of brain edema. rCBF-studies in patients with meningiomas are less helpful, since the blood supply is influenced by the external carotid artery.

REFERENCES

1. BROCK, M., HADJIDIMOS, A., DERÜAZ, J.P., SCHÜRMANN, K.: Regional cerebral blood flow and vascular reactivity in cases of brain tumour. In: Brain and blood flow, pp. 281-284. London: Pitman Med. and Scientific 1971.

2. BROCK, M., HADJIDIMOS, A., SCHÜRMANN, K., ELLGER, M., FISCHER, F.: Regional cerebral blood flow and vascular reactivity in cases of brain tumour. In: Brain and blood flow, pp. 281-284. London: Pitman Med. and Scientific 1971. Berlin-Heidelberg-New York: Springer 1969.

3. CRONQVIST, S., AGEE, F.: Regional cerebral blood flow in intracranial tumours. Acta Radiol. Diag. 7, 393-404 (1968).

4. CRONQVIST, A., LUNDBERG, N.: Regional cerebral blood flow in intracranial tumours with special regard to cases with intracranial hypertension. In: Scand. J. Lab & Clin. Invest., Suppl. 102. XV:A (1968).

5. ESPAGNO, J., LAZORTHES, Y.: Cerebral blood flow in tumours. In: Scand. J. Lab & Clin. Invest., Suppl. 102. XV:C (1968).

6. HADJIDIMOS, A., BROCK, M., HAAS, J.P., DIETZ, H., WOLF, R., ELLGER, M., FISCHER, F., SCHÜRMANN, K.: Correlation between rCBF, angiography, EEG and scanning in brain tumours. In: Cerebral blood flow, p. 190-194. Berlin-Heidelberg-New York: Springer 1969.

7. HARTMANN, A., MATHEW, N.T., MEYER, J.S.: Quantitation of collateral crossfilling in internal carotid artery occlusion. In: 7th Salzburg Conference on Cerebral Vascular Disease, held 1974. Stuttgart: Georg Thieme (in press).

8. MATHEW, N.T., MEYER, J.S., RIVERA, V.M., CHARNEY, J.Z., HARTMANN, A.: Double blind evaluation of glycerol therapy in acute cerebral infarction. Lancet, 1327-1329 (1972).

9. MEYER, J.S., FUKUUCHI, Y., SHIMAZU, K., MATHEW, N.T. OHUCHI, T.: Effect on regional cerebral blood flow of compression by a mass lesion. Eur. Neurol. 8, 83-91 (1972).

10. PÅLVÖLGYI, R.: Regional Cerebral blood flow in tumour patients. In: Scand.J.Lab & Clin. Invest., Suppl. 102, XV:B (1968).

11. PÅLVÖLGYI, R.: Paradoxial rCBF reactions in intracranial tumours. In: Cerebral blood flow, pp. 176-177. Berlin-Heidelberg-New York: Springer 1969.

12. ROSENTHALL, L., MARTIN, R.H.: Cerebral transit of pertechnetate given intravenously. Radiology 94, 521-527 (1970).

CORRELATION BETWEEN CBF AND ⁹⁹Tcᵐ SCINTIGRAPHY
IN GLIOBLASTOMA MULTIFORME

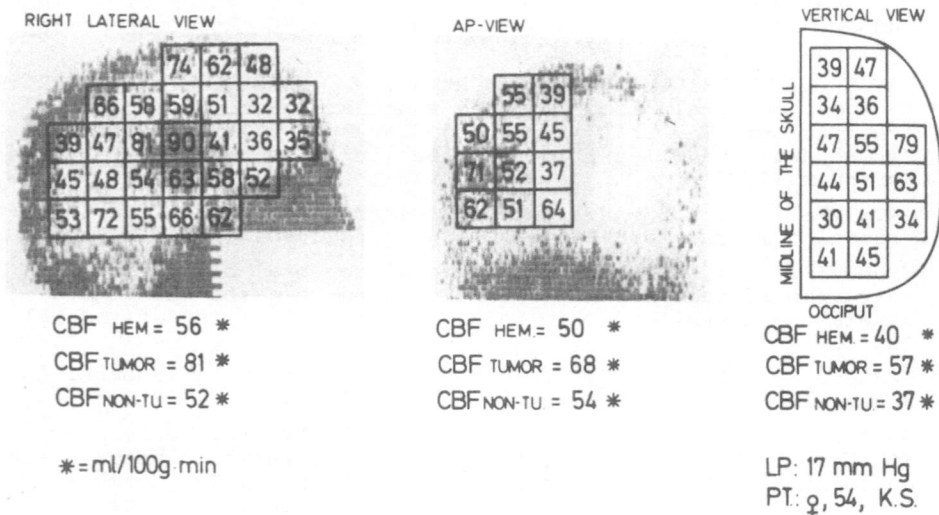

RIGHT LATERAL VIEW

CBF ᴴᴱᴹ = 56 *
CBF ᵀᵁᴹᴼᴿ = 81 *
CBF ɴᴏɴ-ᴛᵁ = 52 *

* = ml/100g·min

AP-VIEW

CBF ᴴᴱᴹ = 50 *
CBF ᵀᵁᴹᴼᴿ = 68 *
CBF ɴᴏɴ-ᴛᵁ = 54 *

VERTICAL VIEW

CBF ᴴᴱᴹ = 40 *
CBF ᵀᵁᴹᴼᴿ = 57 *
CBF ɴᴏɴ-ᴛᵁ = 37 *

LP: 17 mm Hg
PT: ♀, 54, K.S.

Fig. 1. rCBF in a case with a laterally superficially located neoplasm. Tumour-rCBF is highest when measured from lateral, but similar for $rCBF_{ap}$ and $rCBF_V$. Measuring $rCBF_V$ and $rCBF_{ap}$, there is more
tissue between tumour and brain surface, whereas in lateral aspect
there is nearly no brain tissue between tumour and the collimator

REGIONAL CEREBRAL BLOOD FLOW IN
INTRACRANIAL NEOPLASMS
(DEEP LESION)

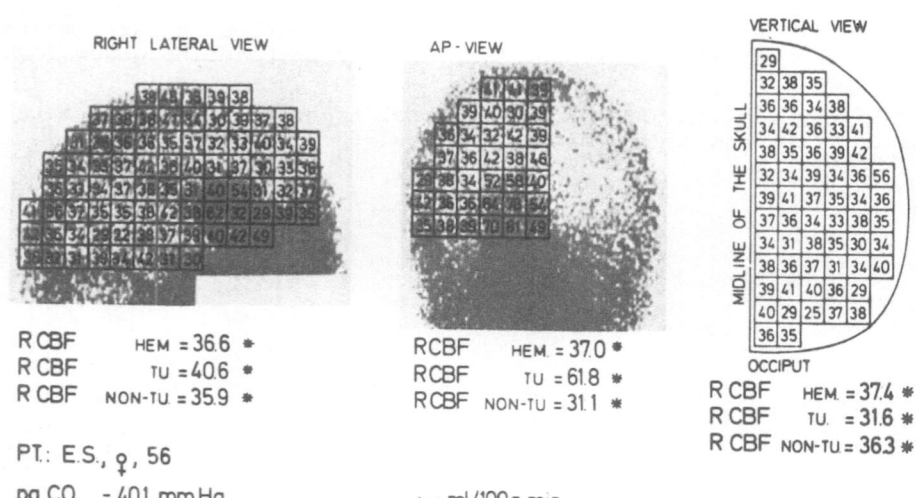

RIGHT LATERAL VIEW

R CBF ᴴᴱᴹ = 36.6 *
R CBF ᵀᵁ = 40.6 *
R CBF ɴᴏɴ-ᴛᵁ = 35.9 *

PT.: E.S., ♀, 56
pa CO_2 = 40.1 mmHg

AP-VIEW

RCBF ᴴᴱᴹ = 37.0 *
RCBF ᵀᵁ = 61.8 *
RCBF ɴᴏɴ-ᴛᵁ = 31.1 *

* = ml/100g min

VERTICAL VIEW

R CBF ᴴᴱᴹ = 37.4 *
R CBF ᵀᵁ = 31.6 *
R CBF ɴᴏɴ-ᴛᵁ = 36.3 *

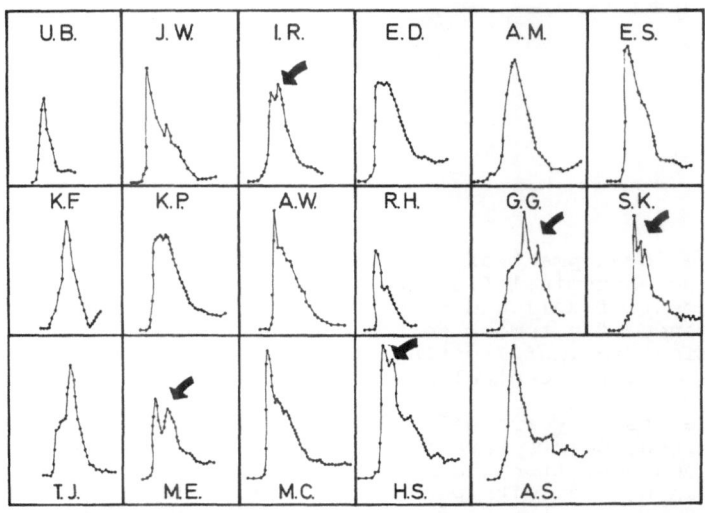

$^{99}Tc^m$ WASH-OUT-CURVES OVER TUMOR-AREAS
IN 17 PTS. WITH GLIOBLASTOMA MULTIFORME

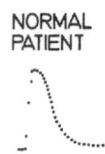

NORMAL
PATIENT

👆 = 2 PEAKS IN 1 CURVE

Fig. 2. rCBF from three sides in a patient with a deep tumour. The high flow is best detected from ap-aspect, worse from lateral aspect. Measuring $rCBF_V$ the tumour cannot be detected

◁

Fig. 3. Technetium 99m washout curves over tumour areas in 17 patients with intracerebral tumours. 8 patients showed peaks (steep in- and decrease of the washout curve) and 5 double peaks. We believe that peaks are due to arteriovenous shunts and double peaks due to several arteriovenous shunts, in which the tracer reaches the neoplasmatic tissue at different times. Time interval between two points is 0.2 seconds

419

Tumourdiagnosis by Cytology of Cerebrospinal Fluid

P. ENGELHARDT

Before the development of suitable methods, the finding of tumour cells in cerebrospinal fluid was a rare observation. Even after the establishment of cell and time saving techniques for cell separation, the adjacency of a tumour to the subarachnoid space as well as cell exofoliation remained limiting factors for cell differentiation in specimens of cerebrospinal fluid (1, 8, 10).

Within the last 4 years cell smears of 4,400 cerebrospinal fluids were examined. Smears were obtained by using millipore filters (M.F.) (3) or a sedimentation chamber (S.K. 7). Cells were differentiated after staining them with phenolic methylenblue-diamantfuchsin solution. Criteria for the differentiation of normal from tumour cells were chosen according to the data published by BISCHOFF (1), SPRIGGS (9) or JAEGER (2) respectively. Smears were examined using a Zeiss-Ultraphot III microscope and representative pictures were taken using Kodachrome II or Agfa-Ortho 25 film material.

The 52 tumours of the central nervous system examined comprised 13 primary and 39 secondary tumours (Table 1). While autochthonous brain tumours showed a less invasive growth according to observations made during open surgery or by different other methods (brain scan, arteriography), 24 out of 39 metastasis revealed a diffuse spreading, sometimes misleading to the diagnosis of a psychopathologic syndrome or a polyneuroradiculitis.

The establishment of the diagnosis of a secondary brain tumour out of the CSF was possible in 39 of 52 cases in contrast to 13 of 52 patients having a primary brain tumour. This was an unexpected finding, since over the past 12 years we have observed only 191 brain metastases (16,5%) out of a total of 1155 brain tumours (6). Our experience, e.g. the rare finding of an exact diagnosis of primary brain tumours by CSF cytology in contrast to brain metastases (4, 5, 10) may be explained by the following facts:

(1) Although primary brain tumours are frequently associated with a symptomatic meningitis, they rarely exfoliate tumour cells into the CSF.

(2) According to shape and size tumours cells in patients with primary brain tumours are hardly to differentiate from atypical cells seen in symptomatic meningitis, which are functionally equivalent to reticulum cells. Therefore the diagnosis of a primary brain tumour according to CSF cell-differentiation has to be established very carefully and critically and thus includes the danger of false negative diagnosis (Fig. 1).

(3) According to our experience a good differentiation is possible regarding medulloblastomas and more seldom ependymomas. The finding of

Table 1. Synopsis of primary and secondary brain tumours in 52 patients with tumour cell findings in CSF

Type of Tumour	Diffuse Growth	Circumscribed Growth	
Medulloblastoma		3	
Glioblastoma		4	
Tumour of 3rd ventricle		1	
Ependymoma		1	
Spinal meningioma		3	
Spinal neurinoma		1	
			13
Bronchial carcinoma	4	4	
Carcinoma of breast	5	4	
Melanoma	3	4	
Malignant lymphoma	5		
Ovarial carcinoma	2	1	
Hypernephroid carcinoma		1	
Carcinoma of rectum	1		
Carcinoma of pancreas	1		
Carcinoma of stomach	1	1	
Primary tumour unknown	2		
	24	28	52

a psammoma corpuscle may be taken as a hint for the presence of a meningeoma (Fig. 2).

In contrast secondary brain tumours are usually followed by quite distinct cytologic abnormalities in cerebrospinal fluid.

(1) Large polymorphe cells are easily differentiated from normal cells in most cases.

(2) The finding of pathologic cells is favoured by a high frequency of exfoliation which is typical for secondary brain tumours.

(3) In most cases similar to primary brain tumours the rounded atypical cells found in brain metastasis do not suffice to identify the tumour. Exceptions, however, are pigmented melanomas, sometimes adeno-carcinomas with a still preserved secretory and storage activity (Fig. 3). Furthermore immature lymphocyte like cells with a high degree of mitosis may give at least a hint of the existence of a lympho- or reticular cell sarcoma (Fig. 4).

Regarding the diagnostic value of CSF-cytology in primary brain tumours and circumscribed brain metastases, it does not comply with information given by various other diagnostic procedures such as brain scan or angiography. CSF-cytology, however, may be of great help in brain hemorrhage or midline tumours. In polytopic metastasis or diffuse carcinomatosis cytology often gives the only assurance of the neoplastic origin, while negative or positive contrast methods do not provide any definite result. Because of the simple method used for cytologic differentiation of CSF it should always be performed on patients suspected of having a brain tumour. Only those patients suffering from high intracranial pressure should be excluded.

Summary

Cell differentiation in the cerebrospinal fluid was performed on 52
Patients, 13 having a primary and 39 a secondary brain tumour. The
important criteria as well as the difficulties regarding the differentiation of CSF cells are discussed. Especially in meningeal carcinomatosis is CSF-cytology superior to other methods; however, the diagnosis of autochthonous brain tumours or isolated well circumscribed
metastasis only rarely occurs.

REFERENCES

1. BISCHOFF, A.: Der derzeitige Stand der Liquor-Cytodiagnostik.
   Schweiz. med. Wschr. 90, 479-487 (1960).

2. JAEGER, M.: Cerebrospinal fluid cytology in tumour-diagnosis.
   Inaugural-Dissertation, Zürich 1970.

3. KISTLER, G.S., BISCHOFF, A.: Zur exfoliativen Cytologie kleiner
   Flüssigkeitsmengen. Schweiz. med. Wschr. 92, 863-866 (1962).

4. MARSAN, C., KOURIE, M.: Renseignements fournis par l'étude cyto-
   logique du liquide céphalo-rachidien. Cab. Col. Med. Hôp. (Paris)
   5, 327-330 (1964).

5. McMENEWEY, W.H., CUMMINGS, J.N.: The value of the examination of
   the cerebrospinal fluid in the diagnosis of intra-cranial tumours.
   J. Clin. Path. 12, 400-411 (1959).

6. PATZOLD, U., HALLER, P.: Die Klinik zerebraler Metastasen. Münch.
   med. Wschr. 117, 301-306 (1975).

7. SAYK, J.: Ergebnisse neuer liquorcytologischer Untersuchungen mit
   dem Sedimentierkammerverfahren. Ärztl. Wschr. 9, 1042-1046 (1954).

8. SAYK, J.: Cytologie der Cerebrospinalflüssigkeit. Jena: Fischer
   1960.

9. SPRIGGS, A.I.: Malignant cells in cerebrospinal fluid. J. Clin.
   Path. 7, 122-130 (1954).

10. WIECZOREK, V.: Erfahrungen mit der Tumorzelldiagnostik im Liquor
    cerebrospinalis bei primären und metastatischen Hirngeschwülsten.
    Dtsch. Z. Nervenheilk. 186, 410-432 (1964).

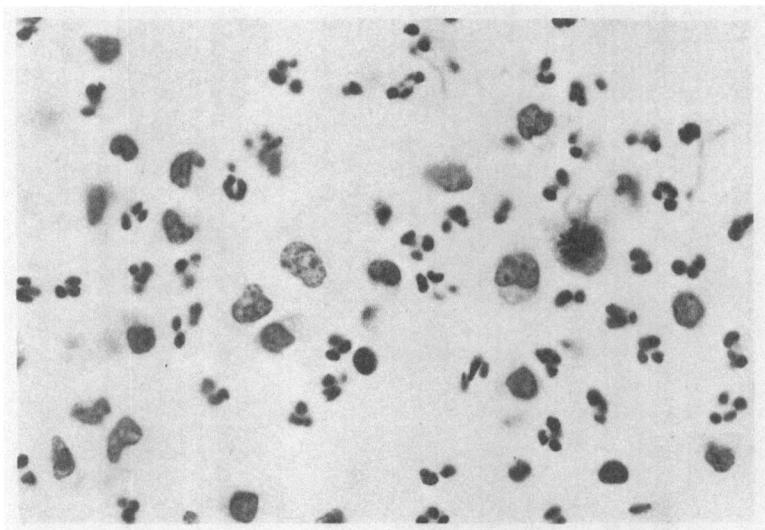

Fig. 1. Symptomatic meningitis accompanying glioblastoma of the frontal lobe, false negative finding (M.F. 250 x)

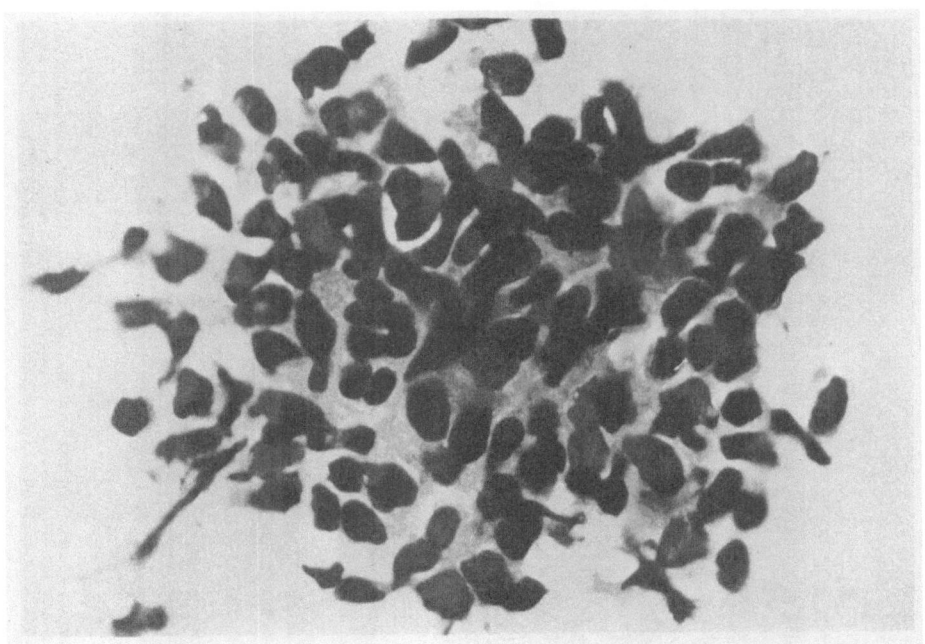

Fig. 2. Cytology of cerebrospinal fluid in medulloblastoma (M.F. 250 x)

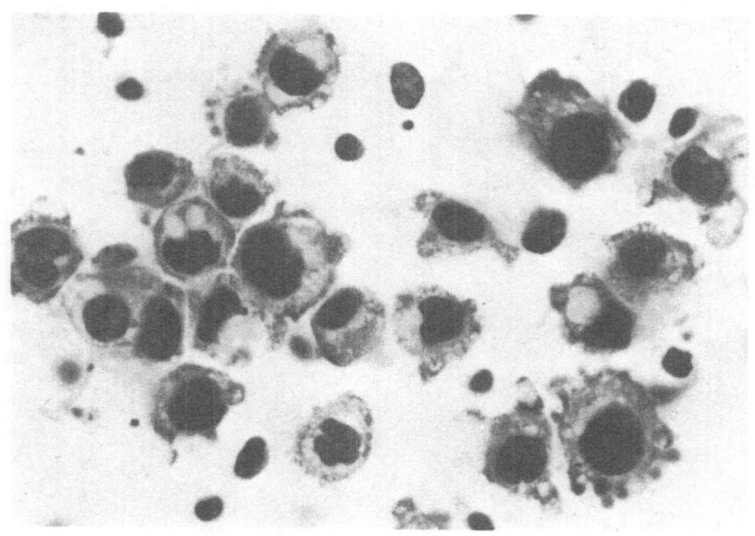

Fig. 3. Meningeosis carcinomatosa in a case with an unknown primary
tumour, presumably adeno-carcinoma (M.F. 250 x)

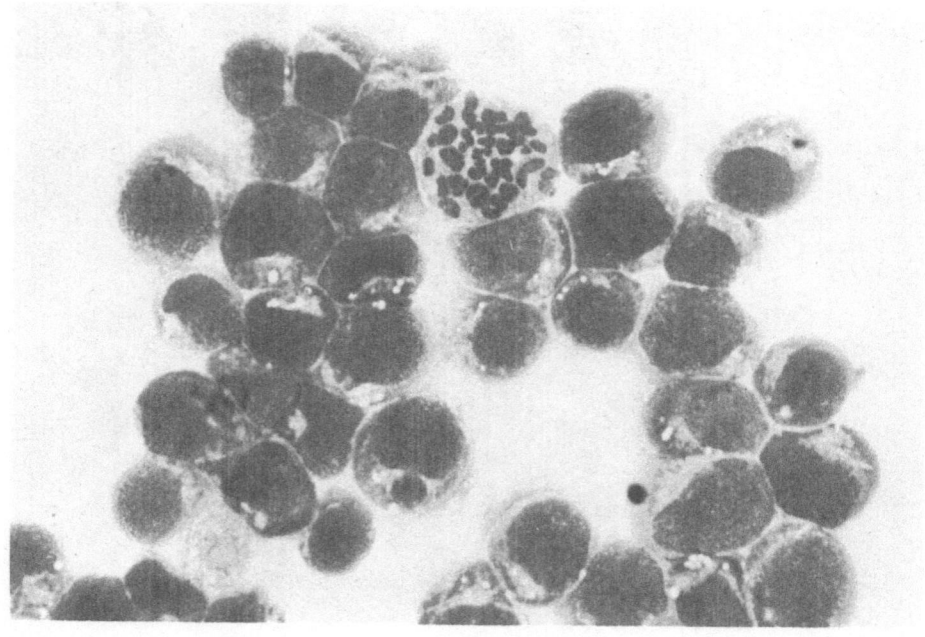

Fig. 4. Lymphosarkomatosis of Leptomeninges (S.K. 250 x)

Vascular Neoplasms of the Brainstem: A Place for Profound Hypothermia and Circulatory Arrest

R. H. Patterson, Jr. and R. A. R. Fraser

The reported surgical experience with hemangioblastoma adherent to the brainstem has not been satisfactory. Although some of these tumors may have a superficial attachment and can be removed safely, others are deeply imbedded in the brainstem, which makes extirpation risky because the surgical manipulations required to control hemorrhage may damage neural structures. Recently the use of deep hypothermia and circulatory arrest allowed us to remove safely a large hemangioblastoma imbedded in the brainstem even though this had not been possible at two previous operations using conventional techniques. This case and our experience with six other such tumors form the basis for this report.

Clinical Material

One patient, a 46 year old man, was not operated. He was in the hospital being treated for duodenal ulcer when he developed headache, dysphagia, and drowsiness. Air studies were done but not considered diagnostic. Death followed soon thereafter, and autopsy revealed a hemangioblastoma entirely within the middle of the brainstem.

The tumor in two of our patients could be removed without difficulty. Both were males aged 15 and 24 years respectively. In the former the tumor was attached to the brainstem at the obex. Postoperatively he hemorrhaged from a duodenal ulcer and was subjected to vagotomy and pyloroplasty. He also was dysphagic and aspirated oral feedings, but this proved self-correcting within two months. The 24 year old man had a tumor imbedded in the cerebellar peduncle in the left cerebello pontine angle, his fourth hemangioblastoma. This was removed without difficulty.

Three patients underwent partial removal of the hemangioblastoma. One was a 59 year old man who had had the tumor, which was in the right cerebellopontine angle, partially removed and radiated 24 years before. At reoperation, only about one half of the tumor could be removed. He had a stormy postoperative course, including gastrointestinal hemorrhage, and died one year later of recurrent tumor. A second patient was a 42 year old man with a hemangioblastoma attached to the obex. This was treated by partial removal and postoperative radiation. He remains well at three years. The last patient in this group was a 40 year old man also with an attachment of the tumor to the obex and also treated by partial removal and radiation therapy. He remains well at five years.

The seventh patient was a 42 year old woman who had two previous attempts at age 35 and 41 to excise a tumor located in the upper part of the fourth ventricle imbedded in the brainstem and superior cere-

bellar peduncle near the lower end of the iter. Radiation therapy had
been administered after the first operation, and persistant ventricular obstruction after the second prompted the placement of a ven-
triculoatrial shunt. Within a year symptoms recurred. Ataxia was
sufficient to make her bed ridden, and intellectual function was
dulled. A marked intention tremor involved particularly the left extremities. Besides a palsy of left cranial nerves III, V and VI, bilateral deafness was present as was a left Babinski reflex. An angiogram demonstrated the large, vascular neoplasm (Fig. 1).

At operation she was positioned on the left side with the head turned
even more toward a prone position. The old posterior fossa incision
was reopened while the heart and one femoral artery were exposed.
Although we favor deep hypothermia induced by the cannulation of peripheral vessels, this is difficult or impossible to accomplish for
posterior fossa surgery. After the top of the tumor was exposed by
dividing the transverse sinus and tentorium, the dura was sewed
firmly against the skull to prevent troublesome epidural bleeding.
The patient was heparinized, cannulas placed in the right atrium and
right femoral artery, and cardiopulmonary bypass begun. After 25 minutes cardiac action ceased, and the esophageal temperature had fallen
to 10°C. and the rectal temperature to 20°C. The head was tipped up,
and the blood allowed to drain into the extracorporeal circuit. The
tumor, now shrunken and avascular, was removed in 19 minutes using
bipolar electrocoagulation to coagulate any filmy connection that
might harbour an empty vessel. After the tumor was out, the table
was leveled and rewarming accomplished in 34 minutes. The heart required two electric shocks to convert ventricular fibrillation to a
normal sinus rhythm. Bleeding from the tumor bed and craniotomy
wound was minor and constituted no problem.

Her postoperative course was characterized by slow neurological improvement interrupted by a gastric resection for a bleeding duodenal
ulcer. Hearing quickly returned to normal, but after 7 months she
still has substantial dysarthria and requires some help to walk. Intellectual function appears normal.

Comment

Hemangioblastomas that involve the brainstem are not common. In
OLIVECRONA's series of 958 posterior fossa tumors; 70 (7%) were hemangioblastomas, and of these 5 (0.5%) involved the brainstem. Despite their rarity, these tumors assume importance because of the
morbidity that may follow attempts at removal. A review of the literature since 1950 has revealed 21 operated cases among which 11 postoperative deaths occurred, and of the patients that survived partial
removel, two died suddendly some years later (1-7). This kind of
experience prompted WALKER, JOHNSON, and BROWNE to comment that "the
therapy of vascular tumors of the fourth ventricle would seem to be
other than surgical".

Profound hypothermia has been used in the past for the repair of
difficult saccular aneurysms, but we are unaware of its being employed before in the surgery of a posterior fossa tumor. The principal technical difference arises from the need to place the patient
in a lateral or facedown position, which makes connections to the
pump-oxygenator by cannulation of the femoral vessels impractical
(8,9). Instead a thoracotomy appears necessary. Table 1 compares the
parameters of the perfusion in the present care with the last 19
aneurysms that we have operated under deep hypothermia in which all

patients were hooked up to the pump oxygenator through the femoral vessels without a thoracotomy. The time required to cool and rewarm the patients are comparable. The principal difference lies in the total amount of blood required, which is less if a thoracotomy is not performed.

Table 1. A comparison of the perfusion paramters in deep hypothermia for excision of brain tumor and saccular aneurysm.

	Hemangioblastoma	Aneurysm
N	1	19
Cooling Time	25 min	21 min
Arrest Time	19 min	18 min
Brain Temperature	-	14 C
Rewarming Time	34 min	28 min
Blood Used	2500 ml	1160 ml

Our experience in the past shows that these tumors can be operated with a low mortality provided the surgeon is willing to settle for partial removal if the attachment to the brainstem is extensive. With radiation therapy a remission measured in years may follow. However, when the tumor recurs, the prognosis is bleak, and excision under the avascular conditions of deep hypothermia and cardiac arrest merits consideration.

This remedy should be considered before the patient is devastated by irreversible neurological defects.

REFERENCES

1. ARCHER, C.R., ROBERSON, G.H., TAVERAS, J.M.: Posterior medullary hemangioblastoma. Radiology, 103, 323 (1972).

2. CHOU, S.N., ERICKSON, D.L., ORTIZ-SUAREZ, H.J.: Surgical treatment of vascular lesions in the brainstem. J. Neurosurg. 42, 23 (1975).

3. LIEBNER, E.J.: A case of Lindau's disease simulating anorexia nervosa. A roentgenologic report. Am. J. of Roentgen. 78, 283 (1957).

4. MYERS, J., SCOTT, M., SILVERSTEIN, A.: Cystic hemangioblastoma of the pons. J. Neurosurg. 18, 694 (1961).

5. OLIVECRONA, H.: The cerebellar angioreticulomas. J. Neurosurg. 9, 317 (1952).

6. STEIN, A.A., SCHILP, A.O., WHITFIELD, R.D.: The histogenesis of hemangioblastoma of the brain. A review of 21 cases. J. Neurosurg. 17, 751 (1960).

7. WALKER, A.E., JOHNSON, H.C., BROWNE, K.M.: Hemangiomas of the fourth ventricle. J. Neuropath. Exp. Neurol. 17, 103 (1952).

8. PATTERSON, R.H. Jr., RAY, B.S.: Profound hypothermia for intra-cranial surgery: Laboratory and clinical experiences with extra-corporeal circulation by peripherel cannulation. Ann. Surg. 156, 377 (1962).

9. PATTERSON, R.H. Jr., RAY, B.S.: Profound hypothermia for intracranial surgery using a disposable bubble oxygenator. J. Neurosurg.
   13, 184 (1965).

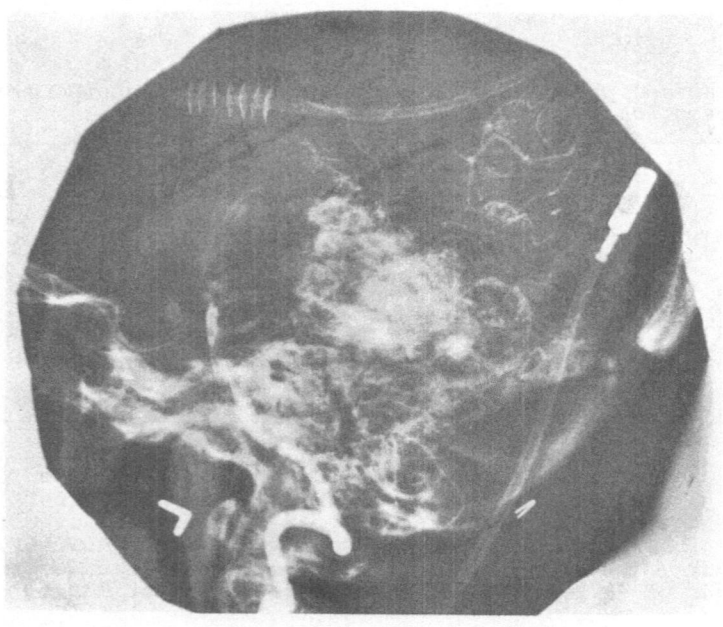

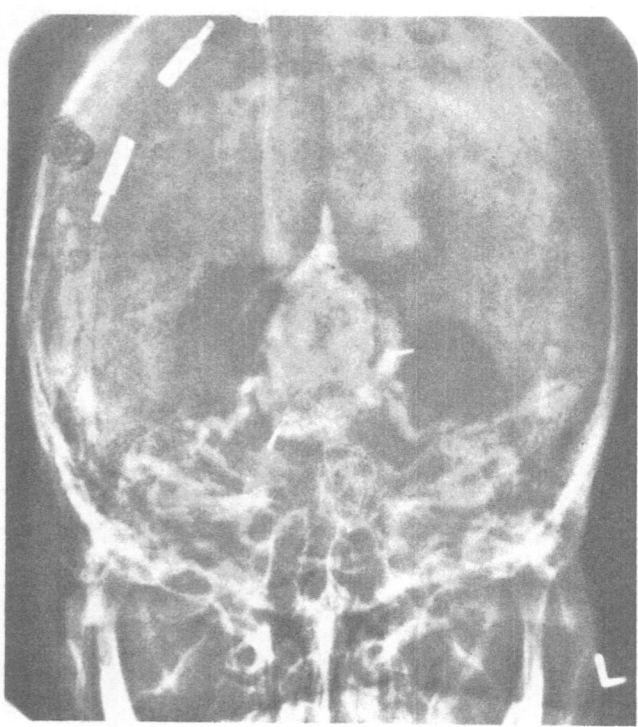

Fig. 1.
Upper: Lateral angio-
gram of the tumor in the
upper portion of the
fourth ventricle.
Lower: A-P projection of
the tumor

Coagulation Changes Following Intracranial Operations

A. WEIDNER, H. WIEGAND, and H. DIETZ

The disseminated intravascular coagulation (DIC) has received increasing attention during the past few years. Different publications
have appeared (2, 3) reporting that destruction of brain tissue may
lead to DIC. For this reason we have chosen to do research on the
influence of intracranial operations on hemostasis.

Tests were performed on 102 patients (35 female, 67 male); their ages
were 42 ± 17 years. The operations lasted 220 ± 80 minutes and were
performed under neuroleptic analgesia. The operative diagnoses were
as follows: 33 supratentorial tumors, 11 infratentorial tumors, 17
angiomas and aneurysmas and 3 abscesses. 38 patients were operated
on because of an acute head injury. The administration of colloids
(dextrane 6%, molecular weight 60000) was 600 ± 30 ml, the administration of blood 750 ± 850 ml during operation.

The following coagulation parameters were investigated: number of
thrombocytes, QUICK prothrombin time, partial thromboplastin time
(PTT), thrombin time, fibrinogen (method of CLAUSS), factors II and
V (1).

The tests were performed before and immediately after operation and
on the first postoperative day - about 20 hours after surgery. The
signigicance relies on the t-test for paired samples with two-sided
probability.

Results

Figs. 1 and 2 illustrate our results: a significant reduction in the
number of thrombocytes was observed immediately after surgery and
could still be noted on the first postoperative day. The QUICK prothrombin time is also significantly reduced immediately following
surgery and the PTT is reduced at the end of surgery but is elevated
again on the first postoperative day. The thrombin time continues to
be reduced postoperatively. Fig. 2 shows the different coagulation
patterns of the plasmatic factors. Reduction and re-elevation of
fibrinogen are significant whereas the activities of factors II and
V are almost unchanged.

We found a postoperative reduction in the number of thrombocytes and
of the fibrinogen level in 55 patients. 5 patients had to be given
medication because of manifest coagulopathia.

Discussion

The reduction in number of thrombocytes and of fibrinogen points to
an abnormally increased intravasal coagulation; the increased tendency

429

for coagulation reveals itself in the reduced PTT and thrombin time
(1). This disturbance occurs immediately following surgery and may
be due to the intraoperative release of tissue-thromboplastin which
brain tissue is very rich in (3). The increased tendency for coagulation persists on the first postoperative day; however, the re-elevation of PTT points toward spontaneous re-establishment of hemostatic
regulation. The global hemostasis tests PTT and above all thrombin
time do not indicate a marked reactive hyperfibrinolysis.

Fig. 3 shows a comparison of coagulation changes of our own intracranial operations with 71 extracranial operations of comparable
severeness, reviewed by VINAZZER (4). The comparison is based on data
from preoperative tests which are set at 100%. Intracranial operations
have shown a more marked consumption of thrombocytes and fibrinogen.

Reduction in the number of thrombocytes and of the level of fibrinogen, with factors II and V unchanged, are signs of a latent defibrination. Hemorrhagic diathesis, occurring as the potential of hemostasis,
is consumed by the elevated intravasal coagulation. Before this the
perfusion of the capillary system deteriorates through the intravasal
deposit of fibrinogen. Symptoms like oliguria and tachypnoea are
clinical signs of defibrination. The counterregulation of the organism
- the fibrinolysis - re-establishes capillary perfusion. Medication
of antifibrinolytica is therefore contraindicated.

Therapy consists of the interruption of the coagulation by heparin
induced by tissue-thromboplastin together with the substitution of
factors consumed by the increased coagulation.

Summary

(1) After intracranial operations there is an increased tendency of
intravascular coagulation.

(2) 55 out of 102 patients showed a latent defibrination which was
commonly normalized by the organism itself.

(3) Controls of coagulation tests are necessary in order to see
whether the disturbance is compensated for by the organism or whether
therapy is needed.

REFERENCES

1. BARTHELS, M., POLIWODA, H.: Gerinnungsanalyse. Stuttgart: Georg
   Thieme 1975 (in press).

2. GOODNIGHT, S.H., KENOYER, G., RAPAPORT, S.I., PATCH, M.J., LEE,
   J.A., KURZE, Th.: Defibrination after brain-tissue destruction.
   The New Engl. J. of Med. 290, 1043-1047 (1974).

3. PRESTON, F.E., MALIA, R.G., SWORN, M.J., TIMPERLEY, W.R., BLACK-
   BURN, E.K.: Disseminated intravascular coagulation as a consequence of cerebral damage. J. of Neurol. Neurosurg. Psychiat. 37,
   241-248 (1974).

4. VINAZZER, H.: Die postoperative Thrombosebereitschaft. Stuttgart:
   F.K. Schattauer 1969.

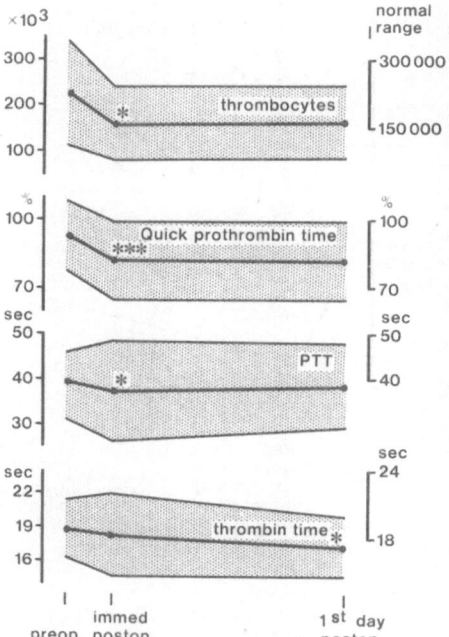

Fig. 1. Average levels and standard deviation of coagulation parameters before and after intracranial operation

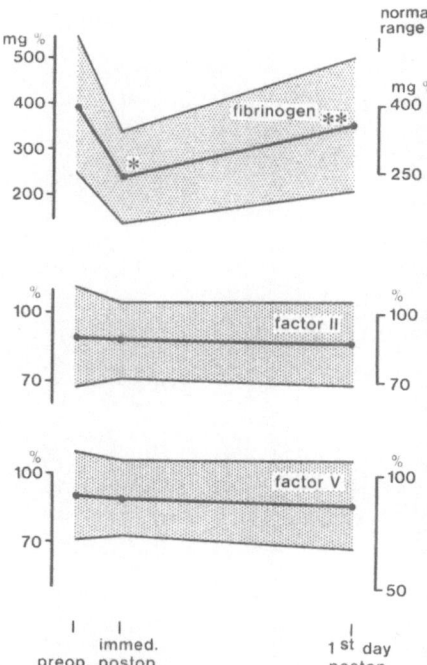

Fig. 2. Average levels and standard deviation of coagulation parameters before and after intracranial operation

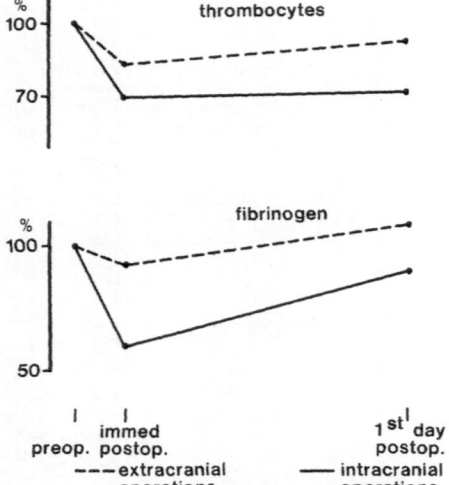

Fig. 3. Comparison of the number of
thrombocytes and of fibrinogen level
after our own intracranial operations
and extracranial operations of others
(4); initial dara set at 100%

Report on One Hundred Pituitary Adenomas

M. SAMII, K. SCHÜRMANN, and P. SCHMITZ

This paper reports on one hundred cases of pituitary adenomas, the follow-up period extending over 18 years. The suprasellar extension and the tendency of recurrence were particularly analyzed. According to the histological and clinical findings the pituitary adenomas were divided into four groups:

(1) chromophobe adenomas,
(2) acidophilic adenomas,
(3) mixed adenomas without clinical signs of acromegalia,
(4) mixed adenomas with clinical signs of acromegalia.

BAILEY and CUSHING (1928) already distinguished six different types of adenomas. They found that there is correlation between the clinical and the histological findings of mixed adenoma. Our simple division into four groups of adenomas doesn't require any quantitative histological studies in the case of mixed adenomas.

By means of air studies 5 different groups were distinguished with respect to suparasellar extension of the tumor. Fig. 1 shows an example of the first group with absolute intrasellar location of pituitary adenoma.

Fig. 2 is an example of the second group. The suprasellar portion of the tumor reaches the optic chiasm. An example of the third group (Fig. 3) shows the suprasellar extension to reach the floor of the third ventricle.

In the fourth group (Fig. 4) the floor of the third ventricle is elevated.

The last group (Fig. 5) includs tumors reaching the Foramen of Monro.

In 47 cases we were able to examine the adonemas by means of air studies.

Table 1 shows the different types of histological and clinical findings horizontally and the different groups of suparasellar extension vertically. Of 47 adenomas, 22 were chromophobic; 10 were mixed adenomas without acromegalia; 7 were mixed adenomas with acromegalia and 8 adenomas were acidophilic. Slightly more than one quarter of all chromophobic adenomas (6 out of 22) were located intrasellarly. More than half of the chromophobic adenomas reached the floor of the third ventricle.

There is equal distribution of the 10 mixed adenomas without acromegalia among the various tumors showing suprasellar extension. While only 2 out of 22 chromophobic adenomas (9%) elevated higher than to the floor of the third ventricle, exactly half of the mixed adenomas without acromegalia reached stages 4 and 5.

Mixed adenomas with acromegaly tend to have approximately the same distribution as mixed adenomas without acromegalia.

The majority of acidophilic adenomas (5 out of 8) is located intra-sellarly. Only 2 acidophilic tumors belong to the group reaching the floor of the third ventricle. Larger acidophilic tumors were not seen.

The correlation of visual disturbance with the individual suprasellar groups of pituitary adenomas was studied, and each eye was evaluated separately.

Table 1. Suprasellar extention of 47 air-studied cases of pituitary adenomas

Degree of suprasellar extension		Chromo-phobe adenomas	Mixed adenomas without acro-megalia	Mixed adenomas with acro-megalia	Acido-philic adenomas	Total
I	intrasellar or with slight dia-phragm elevation	6	1	2	5	14
II	suprasellar until optic chiasm or slight chiasm elevation	2	2	–	1	5
III	suprasellar until the floor of third ventricle	12	2	3	2	19
IV	suprasellar with elevation of the floor of third ventricle	2	2	1	–	5
V	suprasellar until Monroi foramina	–	3	1	–	4
Total		22	10	7	8	47

Table 2 shows the correlation between vision and the various supra-sellar groups. All cases belonging to the first and second group still have normal vision. In the third group approximately half of the eyes involved show high degree of visual impairment. In the last two groups the number of visual disturbance has increased. We have not. fortunately, encountered Blindness, fortunately, was not encountered any of our 47 cases of pituitary adenomas who had undergone air studies. It is noteworthy that, despite compression of the chiasm, half of all eyes in the third and fourth groups, maintained normal eyesight.

Table 3 shows the correlation between visual-field defects and the individual suprasellar groups of pituitary adenomas. A jump from one group of the table to the next higher one is accompanied by an in-crease of the visual-field defect. The unusual defect of lower nasal quadrantanopia has only been seen in one eye of group five.

While in the first and second groups visual-field defects occurred in
varying degrees, no visual disturbances below 5/7, however, were observed. Special clarification is necessary on three eyes in the first
group — two of which belonged to one patient. In both cases we an
intrasellar tumor was seen in air studies and later confirmed at
surgery. An explanation for visual loss in these cases may be seen in
an unusually basal location of the optic chiasm as a anatomical variation, or in an interrupted blood supply.

Table 2. Vision dependent on suprasellar extension total number of
eyes examined: 72

| Vision | Different groups: | | | | |
	I	II	III	IV	V
normal (till 5/7)	22	8	15	4	1
until 5/15	-	-	7	1	2
until 5/50	-	-	4	-	2
under 5/50	-	-	1	2	-
Finger count and hand movement	-	-	1	-	-
Lightshine	-	-	-	1	-
Blindness	-	-	-	-	-
Amblyopy	-	-	-	-	1
Total	22	8	28	8	6

Table 3. Visual field findings in individual groups of suprasellar
extension

| Visual field | Groups | | | | |
	I	II	III	IV	V
normal	19	2	4	1	-
upper temporal defect	3	2	5	-	-
partial temporal defect	-	2	2	2	4
total temporal defect	-	4	20	4	-
lower nasal defect	-	-	-	-	1
Total	22	10	31	7	5

Table 4 shows the results of follow-up of our patients according to
recurrence and survival rate in individual types of adenoma. The
number of cases decreased with the duration of our follow-up. For
example, 46 chromophobic adenomas and 13 mixed adenomas without
acromegalia were followed up for 3 years, while only 15 chromophobic
and 3 mixed adenomas without acromegalia could be follow-up over more
than 10 years. There is no remarkable difference between individual
types of adenomas according to their rates of survival. After 8 years
of follow-up observation, two-thirds of our patients were still alive.

Table 4. Survival rates and number of recurrences within 10 years of follow-up

Duration of follow-up in years	Type of tumor	Total number of cases	Number of sur- vivals	Survi- vals in %	Number of recur- rences
1	chro.a.	56	44	79	0
	mix.a.with acr.	10	8	80	0
	mix.a.without acr.	16	12	75	0
	acid.a.	10	8	80	0
2	chro.a.	49	35	71	1
	mix.a.with acr.	10	8	80	0
	mix.a.without acr.	16	12	75	2
	acid.a.	8	5	63	0
3	chro.a.	46	31	67	2
	mix.a.with acr.	7	6	86	0
	mix.a.without acr.	13	10	77	2
	acid.a.	7	5	71	0
5	chro.a.	33	24	73	2
	mix.a.with acr.	6	5	83	0
	mix.a.without acr.	10	5	50	3
	acid.a.	5	3	60	0
8	chro.a.	21	13	62	3
	mix.a.with acr.	3	2	67	0
	mix.a.without acr.	6	4	67	5
	acid.a.	3	2	67	0
10	chro.a.	15	8	53	2
	mix.a.with acr.	-	-	-	-
	mix.a.without acr.	3	3	100	3
	acid.a.	1	1	100	0

chro.a. = chromophobe adenoma; mix.a.with acr. = mixed adenoma with acromegalia; mix.a.without acr. = mixed adenoma without acromegalia; acid.a. = acidophilic adenoma

Table 5 compares the rates of survival as reported in literature with our own observations. The results are similar.

Table 6 shows the rate of recurrence of our pituitary adenoma in individual types. Those patients who died of a cause other than recurrence of pituitary adenoma, are not included. No recurrence was seen one year following operation. 2 years after operation the rate of recurrence is, 3% in the case of chromophobic adenomas, and 17% in the case of mixed adenoma without acromegalia. After 5 years, 8% of the patients with chromophobic adenoma had a recurrence, and 20% after 10 years. In the case of mixed adenomas without acromegalia the rate of 5 years 3 out of 7 show recurrence. After a 10 year follow-up recurrence had occurred in the only three cases left in this group. Acidophilic adenomas do not appear to show grow again.

Table 5. Survival rates of pituitary adenomas by different authors compared to our results

Author	Follow-up in years							
	1	2	3	4	5	6	8	10
YOUNGHUSBAND, HORRAX and Co-workers (1952)	81				72			
JACKSON (1958)					81			43
HEIMBACH (1959)	86		89		84			68
BAKAY (1950)								
chromophobe		81		75		79		76
acidophilic		76		64		57		54
together		80		73		75		73
Our results								
chromophobe	79	71	67		73		62	53
acidophilic	80	63	71		60		(67)	(100)
all types together	78	72	71		69		64	62

Table 6. Recurrence rates within 10 years of follow-up

Duration of follow-up in years	Type of tumor	Total number	Number of recurrences	Recurrence Quota in %
1	chro.a.	44	0	0
	mix.a.with acr.	8	0	0
	mix.a.without acr.	12	0	0
	acid.a.	8	0	0
2	chro.a.	35	1	3
	mix.a.with acr.	8	0	0
	mix.a.without acr.	12	2	17
	acid.a.	5	0	0
3	chro.a.	32	2	6
	mix.a.with acr.	6	0	0
	mix.a.without acr.	10	2	20
	acid.a.	5	0	0
5	chro.a.	25	2	8
	mix.a.with acr.	5	0	0
	mix.a.without acr.	7	3	43
	acid.a.	3	0	0
8	chro.a.	15	3	20
	mix.a.with acr.	2	0	0
	mix.a.without acr.	6	5	83
	acid.a.	2	0	0
10	chro.a.	10	2	20
	mix.a.with acr.	-	-	-
	mix.a.without acr.	3	3	100
	acid.a.	1	0	0

chro.a. = chromophobe adenoma; mix.a.with acr. = mixed adenoma with acromegalia; mix.a.without acr. = mixed adenoma without acromegalia; acid.a. = acidophilic adenoma

Table 7 again shows the recurrence tendency of chromophobic and mixed adenomas without acromegalia (in percentages) over 10 years of follow-up. The dotted column demonstrates the percentage of mixed adenoma recurring, and the striped column stands for chromophobic adenomas without acromegalia. There is a significant difference of recurrence between these two groups of pituitary tumors.

Table 7. Recurrence rate in percentages of chromophobe adenomas (striped columns) and mixed adenomas without acromegalia (dotted columns) within 10 years of follow-up

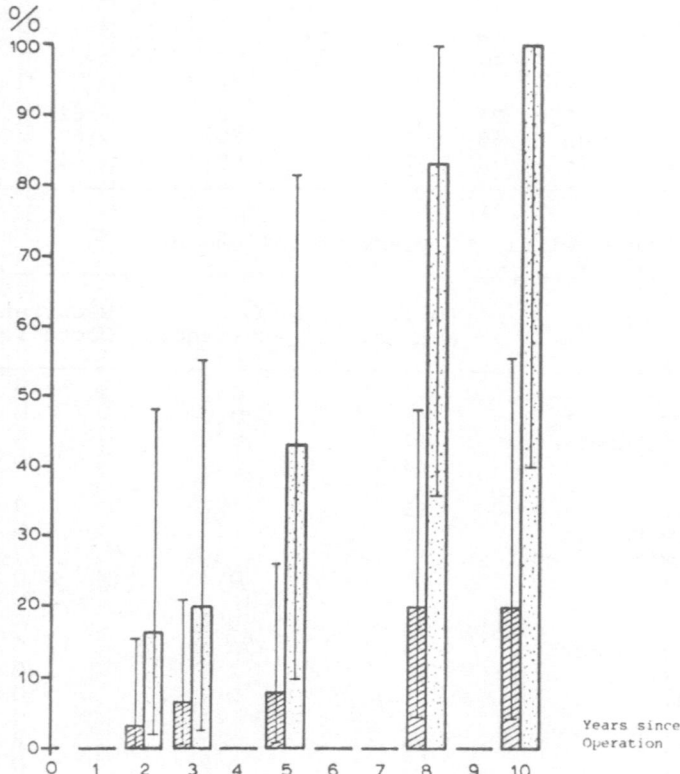

Summary

Air-studies have shown that most pituitary adenomas had outgrown the sella turcica and reached the floor of third ventricle, while only six out of 22 chromophobic adenomas were located intrasellarly. A large number of acidophilic adenomas didn't leave the intrasellar region (5 out of 8). The largest tumors confronted were, histologically, of the mixed-adenoma variety. Our comparative study showed, that mixed-adenomas without acromegalia had a greater recurrence tendency than the chromophobic adenomas. Acidophilic adenomas do not recur.

The pituitary adonomas did not show a wide margin of difference in their survival rates. 5 years after operation 69% of the patients were alive, while after 10 years 63% were still living.

REFERENCES

BAILEY, P., CUSHING, H.: The microscopical structure of adenomas in acrogemalic dyspituitarism (fugitive acromegaly). Am. J. Path. 4, 545-565 (1928).

BAKAY, L.: The results of 300 pituitary adenoma operations (Olivecrona's series). J. Neurosurg. 7, 240-255 (1950).

HEIMBACH, S.B.: Follow-up studies on 105 cases of verified chromophobe and acidophile pituitary adenomata after treatment by transfrontal operation and X-ray irradiation. Acta Neurochir. (Wien) 7, 101-155 (1959).

JACKSON, H.: Discussion on pituitary tumors. Proc. Roy. Soc. Med. 51, 907-916 (1958).

RUF, H., von WILD, K., NEUBAUER, M.: Follow-up studies on 33 craniopharyngiomas and 95 cases of chromophobe and acidophil pituitary adenomas after treatment by transfrontal operation. Excerpta Medica, International Congress Series No. 306, 152-161 (1972).

von WILD, K., RÖTTGER, P., KRÜCKE, W.: Recurrent adenoma of the adenohypophysis in connection with polyadenomatosis of endocrine glands, pheochromocytoma and alopecia totalis. Excerpta Medica, International Congres Series No. 306, 175-179 (1972).

YOUNGHUSBAND, O.Z., HORRAX, G., HURXTHAL, L.M., HARE, H.F., POPPEN, J.L.: Chromophobe pituitary tumors. I. Diagnosis. J. clin. Endocr. 12, 611-630 (1952).

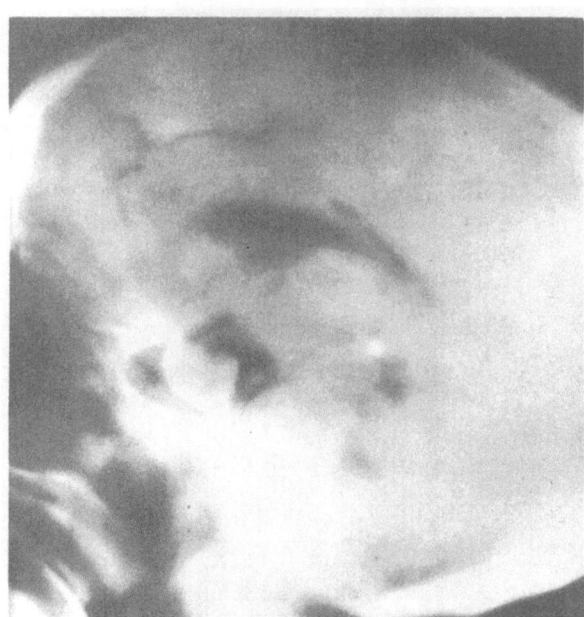

Fig. 1. Example of the first group with absolute intrasellar location (by air study) of pituitary adenomas

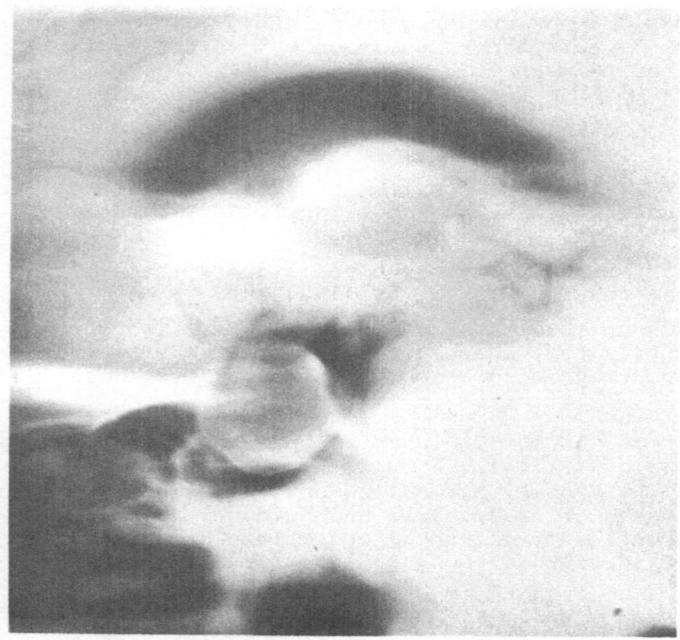

Fig. 2. Intrasellar adenoma with a slight suprasellar extension by air study. The suprasellar portion of the tumor reaches the optic chiasm (Group 2)

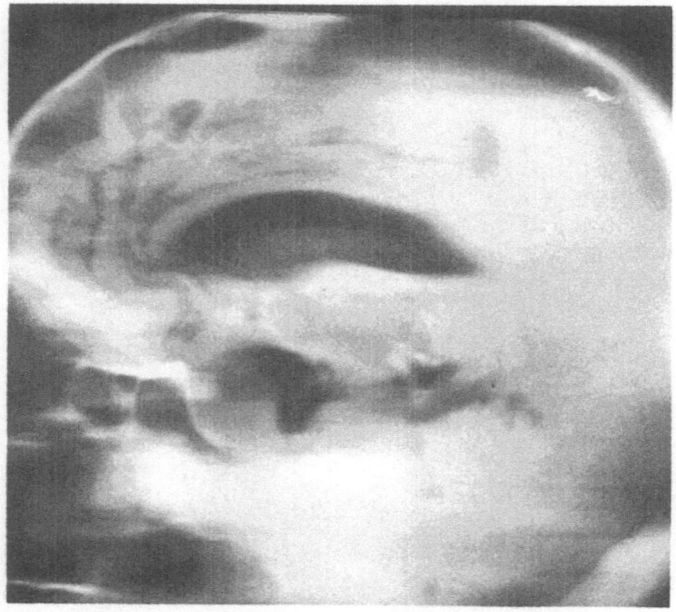

Fig. 3. Intra- and suprasellar pituitary adenoma by air study. The suprasellar extension reaches the floor of the third ventricle (Group 3)

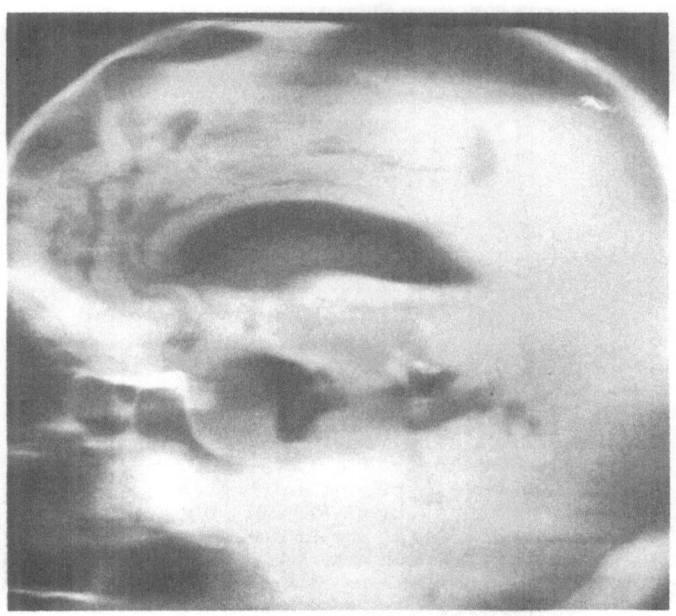

Fig. 4. Intra- and suprasellar pituitary adenoma by air study. The floor of the third ventricle is elevated (Group 4)

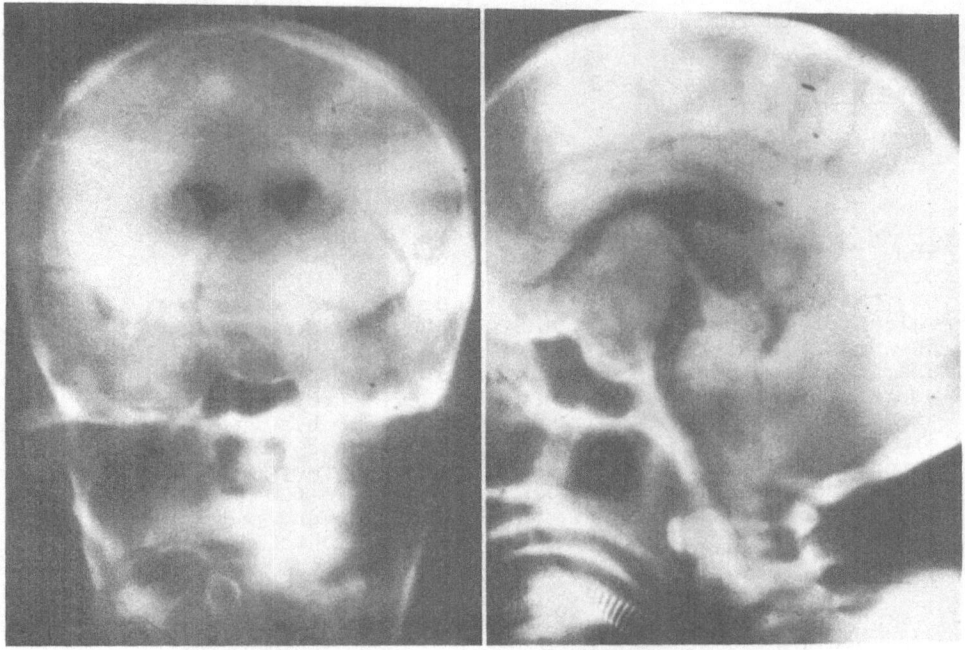

Fig. 5. Pituitary adenomas by air study with more suprasellar extension which nearly reach the Foramen Monroi (Group 5)

Gelastic Epilepsy in Tumors of the Hypothalamic Region

G. PENDL

Introduction

Laughter is a rare ictal phenomenon. One must differentiate uncontrollable laughter as a result of several other pathological causes
from those rare types of epileptic seizures, which were named
gelastic epilepsy by DALY and MULDER (3). The criteria used by GASCON
and LOMBROSO (7) and by REY-PIAS (19) for a true case of laughter as
an epileptic symptom may also be applied to two cases which were
encountered in the last two years at our Neurosurgery Service: They
include sterotype recurrence; absence of external precipitants; con-
comitance with other manifestations generally accepted as epileptic,
such as tonic or clonic movements, loss of consciousness, automa-
tisms; presence of interictal and, where it can be recorded, ictal
epileptiform discharges on EEG tracings; and absence of neurological
signs characteristic of conditions in which pathological laughter
may occur, i.e., bilateral cortico-bulbar lesions, multiple sclerosis,
amyotrophic lateral sclerosis, lacunar states, bilateral frontal lobe
disease, and various emotional states (2, 11).

Case Material[1]

Case 1, E.B.

E.B. is a 16-year-old boy. At the age of 10 weeks he had already had
fits of uncontrollable laughter of 30 to 60 seconds' duration. The
family history was non-contributory. His mother had hyperemesis in
the first trimester of pregnancy. Pre-eclampsia developed 2 weeks
prior to delivery, and X-ray studies were performed at that time. The
boy was delivered as the first of homozygote twins with a birth
weight of 2160 g and a lenght of 48 cm. In contrast to his brother,
he was reported to have been pale and extremely calm postpartum.
Statico-motor development was in full keeping with his age, but 3
weeks retarded in comparison to his twin brother. In the first years
of life, mental development was normal for his age, but mental abili-
ties were found to deteriorate later. At age 10 weeks episodes of
uncontrollable laughter were first noted. They were associated with
a distorsion of the facial muscles of 30 to 60 seconds' duration.
Mental cloudiness was, however, not proven and post-ictal abnormalities were absent. The episodes recurred 20 to 25 times a day, sometimes rousing the infant from his sleep. Since 1957, at age 3 years,

[1]*Acknowledgement.* I should like to acknowledge the assistance of Prof.
Dr. med. H. Doose, Neuropediatric Department, Pediatric Service,
University of Kiel Medical School, in supplying clinical details of
the two cases presented and critically reviewing the manuscript.

repeated therapeutic attempts had been made at other hospitals with
anticonvulsants. There was, however, no lasting improvement. In 1967,
at age 11 years, secondary sexual characteristics made their appearance. In comparison to his twin brother, the onset of puberty was
clearly precocious. At this time the boy was a head taller than his
homozygote brother. In 1972, at the age of 16, he was first admitted
to the Pediatric Service, University of Kiel Medical School, for
systematic anticonvulsant therapy. On admission, attacks were preceded by a short aura, which the boy was unable to describe accurately. This was followed by the occurrence of a set facial expression with occasional slight twitching of the mouth of a few seconds'
duration. Neurological findings were normal during the seizures,
electoencephalography showed pronounced diffusely abnormal tracings
with slowed rhythms. Steep paroxysmal patterns alternated with dys-
rhythmic groups and groups of 4/sec. waves notched by minor spikes
and peak-like potentials were also present. Left side accentuation
was noted in some sections of the EEG pattern. There was, however,
no clear-cut focality. In spring 1974 the patient was admitted to the
Neurosurgery Service, University of Kiel Medical School, for neuroradiological evaluation of a possible space-occupying process on the
floor of the third ventricle. This was suspected on the basis of his
laughing episodes and the precocious puberty, which the boy had
shown. On pneumoencephalography the midline tomogram revealed a tumour the size of a cherry, which was localized in the posterior portion of the hypothalamus and buldged into the basal cisterns. The
tumour apparently occupied a site in the area of the mamillary bodies.
While the aqueduct was normal, the third ventricle appeared to be
compressed from behind and the lateral ventricles showed some hydrocephalic distension (Fig. 1). Carotid angiogram and brain scan were
normal. Since the frequency of the attacks had increased in the last
few years inspite of 3 tablets MYLEPSIN and 4 1/2 tablets TEGRETAL
daily (the boy's mental and emotional make-up had progessively
changed and agressiveness had become more prominent) the hypothalamic
region was explored. Through a right subtemporal craniotomy the temporal lobe was lifted and the hypothalamic region exposed immediately
above the incisura tentorii. This revealed a whitish tumour with a
diameter of 3 cm. Under the surgical microscope hardly any vessels
were seen to course through the tumour tissue after careful incision.
To preserve the surrounding hypothalamic structures and the cranial
nerves embedded in the superficial tumour tissue the tumour capsule
was emptied but left in place. This produced a cavity of approximately 3 cm diameter (Fig. 2). The histological examination revealed
an almost acellular hamartoma with scant ganglionic cells. The postoperative course was satisfactory. The patient was soon mobilized
and only had two episodes of uncontrollable laughter of some seconds'
duration in the first two postoperative months. Electroencephalography 1 month after surgery showed an extremely flat pattern with generalized abnormalities and slow polymorphous basal activity. The boy
received TEGRETAL, 3 tablets daily. Two months postoperatively, while
free from laughing episodes, he again became increasingly aggressive
towards his environment, which was also noted in the last two years
prior to surgery. In addition, his short-term memory was apparently
deranged. During the postoperative follow-up period of 1 year, only
occasional attacks of uncontrollable laughter were noted. While the
patient's aggresive behaviour had prevented his social and vocational
integration prior to surgery, behavioral therapy (now) ensured his
social rehabilitation.

Case 2, F.W.

F.W. is a 9-year-old boy, who had psychomotor seizures from age 3 years. The family history was non-contributory. Delivery was spontaneous and uncomplicated after a normal pregnancy. The post-partum period was uneventful and development in early infancy normal. At age 3 years the parents noted attacks of uncontrollable laughter, which occurred with increasing frequency. They were associated with right upward rotation of the eyes, blinking and twiching of the right side of the face. During seizures the boy would occasionally utter peculiar sounds. He was unresponsive during the 20 seconds' duration of the attacks. Six months later the parents noted that the child appeared to anticipate the seizures. He would, for instance, say: "I feel I'll be laughing soon." At that time seizures assumed a different quality. They were initiated by a jerky movement of the head towards the right side and right upward rotation of the eyes. The boy would make fumbling and searching movements with his hands and become tense. Unresponsiveness would only last for some seconds, following which the boy would become drowsy. He would, however, not fall down and clonic spasms were absent. During this type of seizure, twichtching of the right side of the face was rare, and the boy would only occasionally break into peculiar laughter, utter strange sounds and swallow hard. This seizure pattern occurred once or twice a day in addition to his minor daily attacks. At irregular intervals the boy also had nocturnal seizures. These were again associated with jerky movements of the head towards the right, right upward rotation of the eyes, fumbling and searching movements of the hands, occasionally laughs, swallowing and blushing. Immediately after nocturnal seizures the child would continue to sleep. At this time the boy received anticonvulsants at another hospital (OSPOLOT MITE and ZENTROPIL). This medication reduced the frequency of seizures, but did not completely suppress them either during the day of night. For this reason he was again admitted to the hospital 3 months later. Antiepileptic medication had to be altered, since aggressiveness had been noted, and the boy had 1 or 2 episodes of slight drowsiness a day. These were of short duration and were not followed by sleep. On electroencephalography a right temporal focus was found to be present at that time. In the following 5 years, i.e., from 1968 to 1973, EEG's were recorded at regular intervals. The patient received an anticonvulsant therapy consisting of 3 tablets OSPOLOT MITE and 2 tablets of TEGRETAL. At intervals of about 2 days he would have short episodes of drowsiness; nocturnal seizures did not occur. At the end of 1973, at age 7 years, the patients condition deteriorated. Seizures occurred with increasing frequency, particularly at night. Repeated replacement of anticonvulsants did not produce any substantial improvement, and aggressive tendencies recurred particularly with MYLEPSIN medication. At that time the boy started doing poorly in school and to show signs of withdrawal from his environment. Seizures now occurred at least twice a day. In summer 1974, attacks progressively increased in frequency to about 25 episodes of drowsiness in 1 hour. Towards the end of 1974 he had about 10 seizures a day. These followed a definite pattern: He would have wide eyes, head and eyes would make jerky movements towards the right. There would also be strange laughter, sometimes blushing, and frequently a rubbing of the nose with his right index finger. Unresponsiveness would only last for a few seconds. In January 1975 the patient was admitted to the Pediatric Service, University of Kiel Medical School, for evaluation. Neurologic findings upon admission were negative. The electroencephalogram revealed abnormal theta and delta rhythms with increased amplitudes in the right frontal tracings and a monomorphous delta wave pattern. In addition, the right frontal tracing showed focally slowed activity with an increasing number of superimposed and interrupting spikes and polymorphous wave patterns with a rate of 2 to 3/sec. The latter were found to be generalized over short segments of the right hemispheral tracings. The right frontal pattern was suggestive of isolated peak potentials. Although the abnormal rhythms were indicative of a constitutional component to be involved in the psychomotor seizures, the patient was referred to the Neurosurgery Service to rule out any intracerebral processes. By lumbar pneumoencephalography the midline tomogram revealed a normal configuration of the ventricular system and an approximately rectangular tumour mass the size of a cherry, which was localized in the hypothalamic region and protruded into the basal cisterns (Fig. 3). Since the rate of the seizures dropped to 1 per day with TEGRETAL, 6 tablets daily, and MALIASIN, 4 tablets daily, surgical extirpation of the lesion has, for the time being, been refrained from.

Discussion

Laughter is the result of a complex interaction of facial and respiratory movements. It is controlled by the cortex, mediated by the posterior hypothalamus and executed at the level of the brain stem (13). The complexity of the phenomenon of laughter raises the question of the possible existence of a 'laughing center', which might be located in the hypothalamus, as proposed by MARTIN (16). Lesions in various regions other than this area of predilection may be responsible for triggering attacks of uncontrollable laughter, which need not necessarily be of epileptic origin (23).

The localization of lesions responsible for both triggered and epileptic involuntary laughter is probably widespread, but laughter as an epileptic symptom may be expected to be associated with lesions in the hypothalamic region, in the walls of the third ventricle, the temporal lobe and basal ganglia (6, 8, 24). This does not imply that the laughing phenomenon is triggered as a consequence of destruction of a certain area.

Our 2 cases of gelastic epilepsy with verified brain lesions in the hypothalamic region therefore document, as do similar cases reported in research literature (10), that a common circuit of an anatomical structure referred to as the 'limbic system' was activated by discharges originating in the hypothalamus, which itself forms part of this system.

Since the limbic system for control of emotion and behaviour is closely related with all the regions and structures mentioned above (14, 15, 21), the phenomenon of epileptic involuntary laughter should be regarded as the result of irritation within or near the limbic system (25).

Precocious puberty in patients with hypothalamic tumours who show ictal laughter, as our first case and some of those reported by other authors (1, 4, 5, 12, 18), must be regarded as a additional symptom aside from the epileptic disorder, as a result of an irridation of hypothalamic centers involved in controlling sexual function.

Since we have to regard these laughing seizures in tumours of the hypothalamus as symptomatic seizures (the lesion triggering the hypothalamic circuits of the limbic system), surgical removal of the lesion, which proved to be a hamartoma, was attempted in one of our cases in order to influence the seizure frequency (9). The result seems favourable, but in the second case the low seizure frequency thus far presents a good argument for not approaching this deep seated lesion surgically.

Tumours of the hypothalamus are rare and only very few cases of surgical approach are available for comparison, however, not in connection with gelastic epilepsy. ROBERSON and TILL (20) call lesions of this location clinically malignant and not accessible for surgical approach. In one of LIST's cases (12) with precocious puberty only a biopsy was taken from the anterior and posterior portion of the mass, which was thought to be a hamartoma. In another case he has discussed in research literature, death ensued after attempted removal of the lesion. MATSON (17) reports successful removal of hypothalamic tumours of various histological types either by subfrontal or subtemporal approach.

Radiotherapy on a lesion of the hypothalamus compatible with a hamartoma is not commendable, since they will not respond to it. ROBERSON and TILL (20) even doubt that hypothalamic gliomas are responsive to radiotherapy, but still it had a definite beneficial effect in 10 of their 20 reported cases of these gliomas verified by biopsy. STEIN et al. (22) in a report on 25 cases of tumours of the third ventricle recommend surgical exposure and histological confirmation of all tumours within the third ventricle, although they stress that the inferiorly situated third ventricular tumours are not amenable to surgical removal and respond poorly to radiotherapy.

Summary

Two cases of gelastic epilepsy in young male patients with tumours in the hypothalamic region are presented. The lesions were verified on pneumoencephalographic tomograms. In the first case of a 17 year old boy subtemporal surgery was performed and the tumour removed with subsequent improvement of seizures. In the second case of a 10 year old boy surgery was not attempted, since the seizure frequency has been ultimately rather low. A possible correlation of these special types of seizures with lesions within the structures of the limbic system is discussed.

REFERENCES

1. BIERICH, J.R., BLUNCK, W., SCHÖNBERG, D.: Frühreife bei cerebral-organischen Erkrankungen. Mschr. Kinderheilk. 115, 509-516 (1965).

2. CHEN, R., FORSTER, F.M.: Cursive epilepsy and gelastic epilepsy. Neurology, 23, 1019-1029 (1973).

3, DALY, D., MULDER, D.: Gelastic epilepsy. Neurology, 7, 189-192 (1957).

4. DOTT, N.M.: Surgical aspects of the hypothalamus. In: The hypothalamus, morpholocical, functional, clinical and surgical aspects (eds. W.E. CLARK, J. BEATTIE, G. LE GROS, G. RIDDOCH, N.M. DOTT), pp. 179. Edinburgh: OLIVER and BOYD 1938.

5. DRIGGS, M., SPATZ, H.: Pubertas praecox bei einer hyperplastischen Mißbildung des Tuber cinereum. Arch. path. Anat. 305, 567-592 (1939).

6. DRUCKMAN, R., CHAO, D.: Laughter in epilepsy. Neurology 7, 26-36 (1957).

7. GASCON, G.G., LOMBROSO, C.T.: Epileptic (gelastic) laughter. Epilepsia 12, 63-76 (1971).

8. GUMPERT, J., HANSOTIA, P., UPTON, P.: Gelastic epilepsy. J. Neurol. Neurosurg. Psychiat. 33, 479-483 (1970).

9. HEPPNER, F.: Eingriffe am limbischen System. Zbl. Neurochir. 17, 140-151 (1957).

10. IRONSIDE, R.: Disorders of laughter due to brain lesions. Brain 79, 589-609 (1956).

11. LEHTINEN, L., KIVALO, A.: Laughter epilepsy. Acta neurol. Scand. 41, 255-261 (1965).

12. LIST, C.F., DOWMAN, C.E., BAGCHI, B.K., BEBIN, J.: Posterior hypothalamic hamartomas and gangliogliomas causing precocious puberty. Neurology 8, 164-174 (1958).

13. LOISEAU, P., COHADON, F., COHANDON, S.: Gelastic epilepsy. A review and report of five cases. Epilepsia 12, 313-323 (1971).

14. MACLEAN, P.D.: The limbic system ('visceral brain') and emotional behaviour. Arch. Neurol. Psychiat. 73, 130-134 (1955).

15. MACLEAN, P.D.: The limbic galaxy. In: Limbisches System und Epilepsie (ed. F. HEPPNER), p. 52. Bern: HANS HUBER 1973.

16. MARTIN, J.P.: Fits of laugther (shame mirth) in organic brain disease. Brain 73, 453-464 (1950).

17. MATSON, D.D.: Neurosurgery of infancy and childhood. Springfield/Ill.: CHARLES C. THOMAS 1969.

18. MONEY, J., HOSTA, G.: Laughing seizures with sexual precocity. Report of two cases. John Hopkins Med. J. 120, 326-336 (1967).

19. REY-PIAS, J.M.: Gelastic epilepsy (laughing seizures). Schweizer Arch. Neurol. Neurochir. Psychiat. 111, 29-35 (1972).

20. ROBERSON, C., TILL, K.: Hypothalamic gliomas in children. J. Neurol. Neurosurg. Psychiat. 37, 1047-1052 (1974).

21. SMYTHIES, J.R.: Brain mechanisms and behaviour. Oxford: BLACKWELL 1970.

22. STEIN, B.M., FRASER, R.A.R., TENNER, M.S.: Tumours of the third ventricle in children. J. Neurol. Neurosurg. Psychiat. 35, 776-788 (1972).

23. STUTTE, H.: Zwangsaffekte und paroxysmale Lach- und Weinausbrüche als Epilepsie-Symptom. Nervenarzt 34, 290-295 (1963).

24. SWASH, M.: Released involuntary laughter after temporal lobe infarction. J. Neurol. Neurosurg. Psychiat. 35, 108-113 (1972).

25. WEIL, A., NOSIK, W.A., DEMMY, N.: Electroencephalographic correlation of laughing fits. Amer. J. med. Sciences 235, 301-308 (1958).

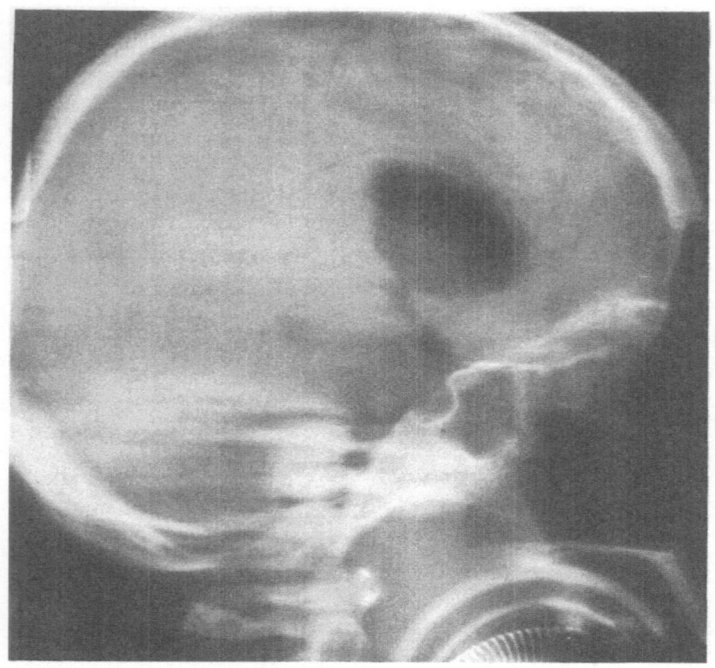

Fig. 1. Pneumoencephalography, midline tomogram, case 1: Clearly visualized tumour mass in the hypothalamic region and deformity of the posterior portion of the third ventricle

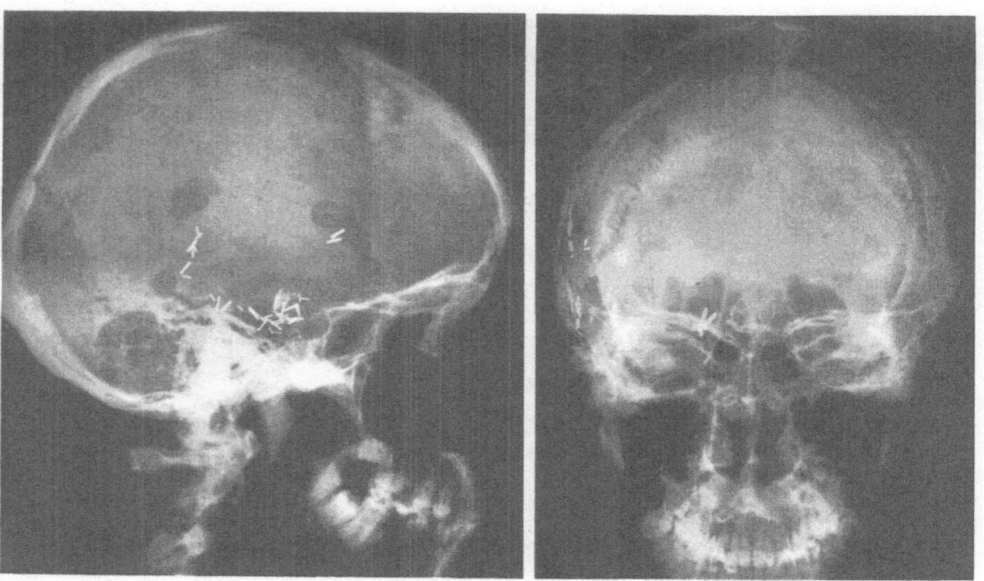

Fig. 2. Plain skull X-ray, postoperative, case 1: Tumour cavity in the hypothalamic region visualized with tantalum powder on a.-p. and lateral films

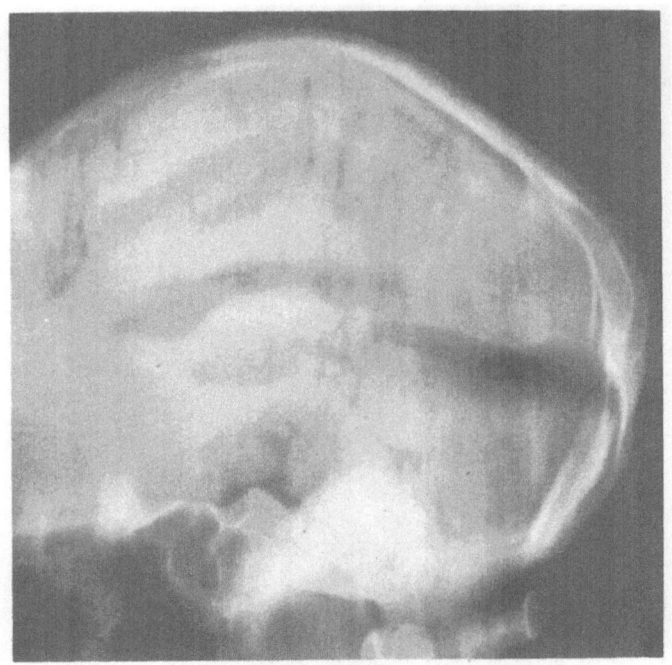

Fig. 3. Pneumoencephalography, midline tomogram, case 2: Somewhat tuberous, smoothly demarcated tumour mass in the hypothalamic region protruding into the prepontine basal cisterns

Subject Index

Abscess brain, post-traumatic 394
Achondroplastic dwarf 331
Acidophilic adenoma 433
Acidosis, hypercapnic 35
-, lactic 56, 82
-, respiratory 26, 82
-, tissue 34, 35
Acoustic neurinoma 365
Acromegalic rheumatism 269
Acromegaly 269, 271, 434
Action potentials 299
Activity, convulsion 34
Acupuncture 289
Acute disc rupture 357
Adenine nucleotides 56
Adenoma, acidophilic 433
-, chromophobe 433
-, pituitary 365, 433
Adrenalectomy 271
Alcohol destruction 301, 306
- injection 277, 289, 302, 320,
  321, 326
Alkali-reserve 20
Alkalosis, respiratory 44, 96
Alveolar hypoxia 14
Amplifier 314
Amputation stump 244
Anaerobic glycolysis 26, 87, 408
Anaesthesia 120
-, corneal 278, 280
- dolorosa 148, 229, 244, 249,
  280, 287, 293, 298 - 299, 302,
  306, 317, 325, 327
- methohexital 281
- neurolept 275, 303
Analgesia, differential 279
- dolorosa 280
- of the tongue 308
Analgetic drugs 268
Analysis, computer 320
Anastomosis microvascular 115
Anemic hypoxia 54
Aneurysm 366
- of the internal carotid 291
Angioendothelioma 382
Angiography, cerebral 116

-, selective 381
Anoxia 25
- ischemic 59
Anterior approach 179
- discectomy 357
- fusion 357
Anterolateral cordotomy
  161 - 166, 170
--, complications 165, 170 -173
--, indication 165
--, post-operative complaints
  165
--, results 170 - 173
- column 162, 165, 169
Apallic syndrome 3
Aphasia 279, 316
Aplastic anemia 287
Apnoea 332
Approach, endodural (DCS) 211
Approach to percutaneous
  cordotomy 185
---, anterior 179
---, lateral 179
---, posterior 179
Arachnoiditis 333
Areflexic tetraplegia 334, 336,
  337
Arnold-Chiari malformation 331
Arrest, circulatory 425
Arterial blood pressure 130
--- changes 130
--- fluctuations 130
- hypoxemia 42, 43
- occlusion 401
- partial pressure 130
- supply of dura 382
Arteriosclerosis 324
Artery, basilar 277
-, carotid 276
-, cerebral 401
-, external occipital 381
-, internal carotid 298, 401
-, -- aneurysm 291
-, middle meningeal 381
-, occipital 386
-, subclavian 331
-, vertebral 381

451

Other books of interest:

Advances in Neurosurgery

Vol. 1: **Brain Edema.** Pathophysiology and Therapy.
Cerebello Pontine Angle Tumors. Diagnosis and Surgery
Editors: K. Schürmann, M. Brock, H.-J. Reulen, D. Voth

Vol. 2: **Meningiomas.** Diagnostik and Therapeutic Problems. **Multiple Sclerosis.**
Misdiagnosis. **Forensic Problems in Neurosurgery.** Proceedings of the 25th
Annual Meeting of the „Deutsche Gesellschaft für Neurochirurgie" Bochum,
September 22-25, 1974. Editors: W. Klug, M. Brock, M. Klinger, C. Spoerri

K.J. ZÜLCH: **Atlas of Gross Neurosurgical Pathology**

T. NOMURA: **Atlas of Cerebral Angiography**

Radiological Exploration of the Ventricles and Subarachnoid Space
By G. Ruggiero et al.

Cerebral Blood Flow
Clinical and Experimental Results. International Symposium on the Clinical
Applications of Isotope Clearance Measurement of Cerebral Blood Flow,
Mainz, April 1969. Editors: M. Brock et al.

Cerebral Circulation and Metabolisms
Sixth International CBF Symposium, June 6-9, 1973
Editors: T.W. Langfitt et al.

Springer-Verlag Berlin Heidelberg New York

Cerebral Angiomas
Advances in Diagnosis and Therapy. Editors: H.W. Pia et al.

Gliomas
Current Concepts in Biology, Diagnosis and Therapy. Symposium on
"Cerebral Gliomas" held at the University of Chicago, May 18-19, 1974
(Recent Results in Cancer Research, Vol. 51)

**A. RAEDLER, J. SIEVERS: Influences of Experimental Brain Edema on the
Development of the Visual System**
(Advances in Anatomy, Embryology and Cell Biology, Vol. 51, Part 2)

Malignant Lymphomas of the Nervous System
International Symposium. Organized by the Österreichische Arbeitsgemein-
schaft für Neuropathologie and the Research Group of Neuropathology of the
World Federation of Neurology, Vienna, August 29-31, 1974
Editors: K. Jellinger, F. Seitelberger
(Acta Neuropathologica, Supplementum 6)

F. LÁHODA, A. ROSS, W. ISSEL: EMG Primer
A Guide to Practical Electromyography and Electroneurography
With a Preface by A. Schrader. English Version by J. Payan

Fundamentals of Neurophysiology
By R.F. Schmidt, J. Dudel, W. Jänig, M. Zimmermann
Editor: R.F. Schmidt (Springer Study Edition)

R. HEENE: Experimental Myopathies and Muscular Dystrophy
Studies in the Formal Pathogenesis of the Myopathy of 2,4-Dichlorophenoxy-
acetate.
(Schriftenreihe Neurologie / Neurology Series, Vol. 16)

Springer-Verlag Berlin Heidelberg New York